Blood Disorders in the Elderly

The developed world has an increasingly aging population, with approximately 10% of the population aged over 65 years. As the incidence and prevalence of blood disorders increases with age, these conditions are a heavy burden on healthcare systems.

Blood Disorders in the Elderly will provide hematologists, geriatricians, and all clinicians involved in the care of patients with blood disorders with clear clinical advice on the diagnosis and management of these conditions.

The introductory section reviews the epidemiology of aging and anemia, and provides a comprehensive approach to the management of cancer in the aging patient. This is followed by a full discussion of hematopoiesis and the changes it undergoes in aging. The remaining sections cover the diagnosis and management of all major disorders: anemia, malignancy, and hemostasis disorders, including hemophilia. A detailed chapter on antithrombotic therapies is also included.

Lodovico Balducci is the Division Chief of the Senior Adult Oncology Program at the H. Lee Moffitt Cancer Center and Research Institute, Tampa, Florida, and Professor of Oncology and Medicine.

William Ershler is Director of the Institute for Advanced Studies in Aging and Geriatric Medicine, Washington DC.

Giovanni de Gaetano is Director of the Research Laboratories at the Centre for High Technology Research and Education in Biomedical Sciences, Catholic University, Campobasso, Italy.

Blood Disorders in the Elderly

EDITED BY

Lodovico Balducci

H. Lee Moffitt Cancer Center and Research Institute, Florida

William Ershler

Institute for Advanced Studies in Aging and Geriatric
Medicine, Washington DC

Giovanni de Gaetano

Catholic University, Campobasso

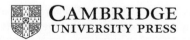

CAMBRIDGE
UNIVERSITY PRESS

CAMBRIDGE UNIVERSITY PRESS
Cambridge, New York, Melbourne, Madrid, Cape Town, Singapore, São Paulo, Delhi

CAMBRIDGE UNIVERSITY PRESS
The Edinburgh Building, Cambridge CB2 8RU, UK

Published in the United States of America by Cambridge University Press, New York

www.cambridge.org

For information on this title: www.cambridge.org/9780521875738

First published 2008

Printed in the United Kingdom at the University Press, Cambridge

A catalogue record for this publication is available from the British Library

ISBN 978-0-521-87573-8 hardback

Every effort has been made in preparing this book to provide accurate and up-to-date information
which is in accord with accepted standards and practice at the time of publication. Although case
histories are drawn from actual cases, every effort has been made to disguise the identities of the
individuals involved. Nevertheless, the authors, editors and publishers can make no warranties that
the information contained herein is totally free from error, not least because clinical standards are
constantly changing through research and regulation. The authors, editors and publishers therefore
disclaim all liability for direct or consequential damages resulting from the use of material contained
in this book. Readers are strongly advised to pay careful attention to information provided by the
manufacturer of any drugs or equipment that they plan to use.

Contents

List of contributors

Todd J. Alekshun, M.D.
Hematology & Oncology, H. Lee Moffitt Cancer
Center & Research Institute, 12902 Magnolia Drive,
Tampa, FL 33612, USA

Melissa Alsina, M.D.
Head of Multiple Myeloma, Malignant Hematology,
H. Lee Moffitt Cancer Center & Research Institute,
12902 Magnolia Drive, Tampa, FL 33612, USA

Andrew S. Artz, M.D., M.S.
Section of Hematology/Oncology, University of
Chicago, Chicago, IL 60616, USA

Lodovico Balducci, M.D.
Division of Geriatric Oncology, Senior Adult
Oncology Program, H. Lee Moffitt Cancer Center &
Research Institute, 12902 Magnolia Drive, Tampa,
FL 33612, USA

Oscar Ballester, M.D.
Feist–Weiller Cancer Center, Louisiana State
University, Shreveport, LA 71130, USA

Francesco Baudo, M.D.
Thrombosis and Hemostasis Unit, Department of
Hematology, Niguarda Hospital, Piazza Ospedale
Maggiore 3, 20162 Milano, Italy

Claudia Beghe, M.D.
James A. Haley Veterans Hospital, 13000 Bruce B
Downs Blvd, Tampa, FL 33612, USA

Salvador Bruno, M.D.
Cancer Therapy and Research Center, 7979
Wurzbach Road, San Antonio, TX 78229, USA

Marco Cattaneo, M.D.
Hematology and Thrombosis Unit, San Paolo
Hospital, University of Milan, Via di Rudinì 8,
20142 Milan, Italy

Oscar A. Cepeda, M.D.
Division of Geriatric Medicine, St. Louis University
School of Medicine, 1402 South Grand Blvd,
St. Louis, MO 63104, USA

Chiara Cerletti, M.D.
Laboratory of Cell Biology and Pharmacology
of Thrombosis, Research Laboratories, John
Paul II Center for High Technology Research
and Education in Biomedical Sciences, Catholic
University, 86100 Campobasso, Italy

Harvey Jay Cohen, M.D.
Center for the Study of Aging and Human
Development, Duke University Medical Center,
Durham, NC 27710, USA

Francesco de Cataldo, M.D.
Department of Hematology, Niguarda Hospital,
Piazza Ospedale Maggiore 3, 20162 Milano, Italy

Giovanni de Gaetano, M.D.
Research Laboratories, John Paul II Center for
High Technology Research and Education in
Biomedical Sciences, Catholic University, 86100
Campobasso, Italy

Yuping Deng, M.D.
The Glennan Center for Geriatrics and Gerontology,
Department of Internal Medicine, Eastern Virginia
Medical School, Norfolk, VA 23507, USA

Rita B. Effros, Ph.D.
Department of Pathology and Laboratory Medicine,
David Geffen School of Medicine, University of
California, Los Angeles, CA 90095, USA

William B. Ershler, M.D.
Clinical Research Branch, National Institute on
Aging, 3001 S. Hanover Street, Baltimore,
MD 21225, USA

Youssef Gamal, M.D.
1105 N Glassell Street, Orange, CA 92867, USA

Julie K. Gammack, M.D.
Division of Geriatric Medicine, St. Louis University
School of Medicine, 1402 South Grand Blvd,
St. Louis, MO 63104, USA

Tomas Ganz, Ph.D., M.D.
Departments of Medicine and Pathology, David
Geffen School of Medicine, University of California,
Los Angeles, CA 90095, USA

Giancarla Gerli, M.D.
Hematology and Thrombosis Unit, San Paolo
Hospital, University of Milan, Via di Rudinì 8,
20142 Milan, Italy

**Stefan Gravenstein, M.D., C.M.D.,
M.P.H., F.A.C.P.**
The Glennan Center for Geriatrics and Gerontology,
Department of Internal Medicine, Eastern Virginia
Medical School, Norfolk, VA 23507, USA

Jack M. Guralnik, Ph.D., M.D.
Laboratory of Epidemiology, Demography, and
Biometry, National Institute on Aging, National
Institute of Health, Gateway Building, Suite
3C-309, 7201 Wisconsin Avenue, Bethesda,
MD 20814, USA

Cheryl L. Hardy, Ph.D.
University of Mississippi School of Medicine,
2500 N. State Street, Jackson, MS 39216, USA

David N. Haylock, M.D.
Australian Stem Cell Centre, 3rd Floor Building
75 (STRIP), Monash University, Wellington Road,
Clayton, VIC 3800, Australia

Marc F. Hoylaerts, Ph.D.
Center for Molecular and Vascular Biology,
University of Leuven, Herestraat 49, B-3000 Leuven,
Belgium

Nicole Jacobi, M.D.
University Clinic Hamburg–Eppendorf,
Martinistrasse 52, 20246 Hamburg, Germany

Bindu Kanapuru, M.D.
Clinical Research Branch, National Institute on Aging,
3001 S. Hanover Street, Baltimore, MD 21225, USA

Samuel Kerr, M.D.
2102 Harrisburg Pike, Lancaster, PA 17604, USA

Jeffrey Lancet, M.D.
Department of Interdisciplinary Oncology,
University of South Florida College of Medicine;
and H. Lee Moffitt Cancer Center, 12902 Magnolia
Drive, Tampa, FL 33612, USA

France Laurencet, M.D.
25, rue Jacques-Grosselin, CH-1227 Carouge,
Switzerland

Thomas P. Loughran, M.D.
Penn State Cancer Institute, Penn State College of
Medicine, 500 University Drive, Hershey, PA 17033,
USA

Daniela Mari, M.D.
Department of Medical Sciences, University of
Milan; and IRCCS Ospedale Maggiore, Mangiagalli
and Regina Elena Foundation, Via Francesco Sforza
35, 20122 Milan, Italy

Fermina Mazzella, M.D.
Department of Pathology and Laboratory
Medicine, University of Connecticut Health Center,
Farmington, CT 06030, USA

Magda Melchert, M.D.
Department of Interdisciplinary Oncology,
University of South Florida College of Medicine;
and H. Lee Moffitt Cancer Center, 12902 Magnolia
Drive, Tampa, FL 33612, USA

John E. Morley, M.B., B.Ch.
Division of Geriatric Medicine, St. Louis University
School of Medicine, 1402 South Grand Blvd,
St. Louis, MO 63104, USA

Elizabeta Nemeth, Ph.D.
Department of Medicine, David Geffen School of
Medicine, University of California, Los Angeles, CA
90095, USA

Susan K. Nilsson, M.D.
Australian Stem Cell Centre, 3rd Floor Building
75 (STRIP), Monash University, Wellington Road,
Clayton, VIC 3800, Australia

Kushang V. Patel, Ph.D.
Laboratory of Epidemiology, Demography, and
Biometry, National Institute on Aging, National
Institutes of Health, Gateway Building,
Suite 3C-309, 7201 Wisconsin Avenue, Bethesda,
MD 20814, USA

Bruce A. Peterson, M.D.
Professor of Medicine, Division of Hematology,
Oncology and Transplantation, University of
Minnesota, Minneapolis, MN 55455, USA

Arati V. Rao, M.D.
Division of Medical Oncology and Division of
Geriatrics, Duke University Medical Center and
Durham Veterans Affairs Medical Center, Durham,
NC 27710, USA

Holger Schünemann, M.D., Ph.D.
Italian National Cancer Institute Regina Elena,
Via Elio Chianesi 53, 00144 Rome, Italy

Alexander S. D. Spiers, Ph.D., M.D.
Professor of Medicine, Department of
Haematology, John Radcliffe Hospital, Oxford, UK

Jerry L. Spivak, M.D.
Director, Johns Hopkins Center for the Chronic
Myeloproliferative Disorders, Traylor 924, 720
Rutland Avenue, Johns Hopkins University School
of Medicine, Baltimore, MD 21205, USA

Sally P. Stabler, M.D.
Department of Medicine/Division of Hematology,
University of Colorado Health Sciences Center,
Denver, Colorado 80262, USA

Laura Terranova, M.D.
Hematology and Thrombosis Unit, San Paolo
Hospital, University of Milan, Via di Rudinì 8,
20142 Milan, Italy

Gary Van Zant, Ph.D.
Division of Hematology/Oncology, University of
Kentucky, Markey Cancer Center, 800 Rose Street,
Lexington, KY 40536, USA

Jozef Vermylen M.D., Ph.D.
Center for Molecular and Vascular Biology,
University of Leuven, Herestraat 49, B-3000 Leuven,
Belgium

Jeffrey Yates, Ph.D.
Division of Hematology/Oncology, University of
Kentucky, Markey Cancer Center, 800 Rose Street,
Lexington, KY 40536, USA

Preface

The aging of the population is the most consequential epidemiologic event of our times. The whole societal organization, including medicine and public health, needs to accommodate the evolving demographic landscape, and to focus on the management of chronic diseases, disability, and functional dependence, as well as on the most effective utilization of limited resources.

The management of an aging society is based on the twofold hypothesis that death cannot be indefinitely postponed, but disease and functional decline may be delayed until the latest stages of life. "Compression of morbidity" is the main goal of geriatric medicine, and it involves rehabilitation and provision of a supportive environment where the elder is able to thrive, in addition to medical care and disease prevention. The achievement of this goal implies the ability to define aging, and to estimate the risk of aging-related events such as death, disease, and disability, as well as the reversibility of this risk.

Perhaps the most complete definition holds aging as "loss of entropy" and "loss of fractality." Loss of entropy implies a progressive decline in functional reserve of multiple organs and systems, and consequently reduced tolerance of stress, loss of fractality a progressive decline in the ability to coordinate different activities and to negotiate the environment. In the absence of precise measurements of entropy and fractality, aging is best assessed by its consequences, including progressive loss of function, emerging comorbidities, and the degree of chronic inflammation, reflected in the concentrations of inflammatory markers in the circulations. Chronology reflects very poorly the physiologic age of each individual, which can only be estimated on the basis of individual assessment.

In *Blood Disorders of the Elderly* we propose a novel look at aging. By identifying the influence of aging on the development of blood disorders, and the influence of these disorders on the progression of aging, we acknowledge the dynamic, and to some extent circular, aspect of aging. Recognizing that the incidence and prevalence of blood disorders increases with age, we explore the possibility that the study of the blood may reveal an individual's age, and that the correction of blood disorders may limit the risk of aging-related events, including death, disease, and disability.

We elected to study blood disorders in the aged, because blood disorders are our area of expertise. Luckily, hematopoiesis and hemostasis are also a common crossroads of diseases and environmental stresses. So, it is not far-fetched to expect that the different events that contribute to individual aging leave their fingerprints on that individual's blood. It is well known, for example, that aging is associated with a progressive reduction of marrow cellularity, a progressive increase in the prevalence of myeloid dysplasia, and increased concentration of coagulation markers, such as the D-dimer, in the circulation. It is also well known that the hemoglobin levels and levels of circulating coagulation markers are related to the risk of death, disability, and cognitive decline.

Given the rapid accumulation of new information related both to blood disorders and to aging, and given the dynamic nature of aging, this book is conceived as a new clinical paradigm for physicians involved in the management of older patients, as a springboard for scientists interested in the biology of aging and its clinical consequences, and as an operating system able to organize incoming knowledge for students of biological, clinical, and social sciences.

The reception of this book will represent the best measure of our success in pursuing our goals. Irrespective of our personal success, however, we hope to have inspired other clinicians and scientists to take a new and novel look at aging that will be translated into new publications, new research projects, and new approaches to clinical practice.

We wish to thank Cambridge University Press for supporting this project, our coauthors for their hard work, and especially Anita Klamo for the difficult task of coordinating the different contributions.

PART I

Epidemiology

PART

Epidemiology

Epidemiology of aging

Lodovico Balducci, William B. Ershler

Descriptive epidemiology

In the Western world the older population has undergone a progressive and accelerated expansion during the past 50 years, and the increment in the number of individuals 65 and older (Fig. 1.1) has been associated with a progressive prolongation of average life expectancy, which in the USA in 2000

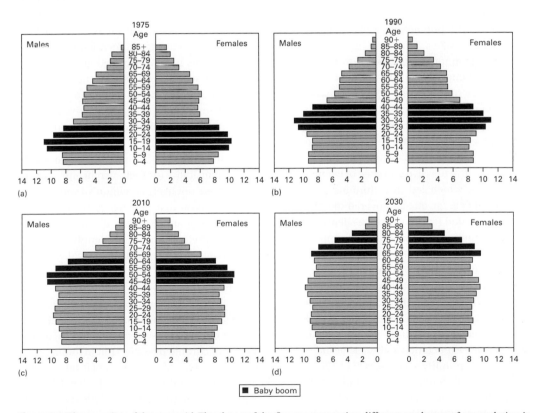

Figure 1.1 The squaring of the pyramid. The shape of the figure representing different age layers of a population is becoming closer and closer to a square, due to a reduction in the younger population and an increment in the older one. From Yancik & Ries, 2004 [1], with permission.

Blood Disorders in the Elderly, ed. Lodovico Balducci, William Ershler, Giovanni de Gaetano.
Published by Cambridge University Press. © Cambridge University Press 2008.

was 80 for women and 76 for men [1]. A progressive decline in birth rate has occurred, due to more effective birth control and family planning. At the same time, the mortality rate has also decreased, due to improved health and hygiene, the conquering of most infectious diseases, and the absence of worldwide conflicts and epidemics. Reduced natality and mortality rates have produced the so-called "squaring of the pyramid," which refers to the change in the shape of the figure describing the population subdivided in different age layers (Fig. 1.1). In 1975, this figure looked like a pyramid with a large base of young people, becoming narrower and narrower with increasing age. By the year 2030 the figure will become closer to a square, with a smaller basis of younger people and a larger representation of the older population [1]. In some countries, such as Italy and Japan, one may start seeing an "inversion of the pyramid," as the population over 65 already outnumbers that below 20 [2,3].

The aging of the population has been associated with social changes that may influence the care and the welfare of the elderly. Most noticeable are the increased mobility of the population, which makes lasting relationships more difficult and social support less predictable, the reduction in the number of young children available to take care of their aging parents, the massive entrance of women into the workforce, which led to a thinning pool of traditional home caregivers, and overall the dissolution of the extended family, which has deprived the elders both of their traditional source of support and of their traditional social roles [4].

The medical and social implications of the aging of the population are only partially understood. In part, this is due to the fact that the older population is very diverse in terms of health and function and it is difficult to predict on the basis of aging alone what is a person's life expectancy, ability to live independently, and susceptibility to diseases [5,6]. When the life expectancy of different cohorts of older individuals is subdivided into quartiles, one notices a marked discrepancy among the upper, intermediate, and lower quartiles (Fig. 1.2) [7]. Germane to this discussion, the upper life-expectancy quartile of

the 85+ cohort is longer than the lower quartile of the 70–75 cohort, underlying how aging refers to a highly diverse physiological event rather than to a chronologic one. Also, to some extent aging is a moving target: we cannot assume that the aging population today presents the same characteristics as that of only a few decades ago. To this point, the case of social security is paradigmatic. In the USA, the age at which a person can draw social security has increased from 65 to 67 as more and more individuals keep working beyond age 65, which represents a substantial change from the time when social security was instituted. One may conclude that the functional status of the elders has improved as their life expectancy has become more prolonged. The older population of today and that of the recent past may also differ on the basis of cultural changes, with important influences on medical care. While even in the recent past older individuals were likely to accept their physicians' recommendations without argument [8], this is rapidly changing. In part this is due to easier access to the media, and in particular to the Internet illustrating medical advances in a timely fashion and proposing alternative forms of medical treatment. In addition, we are witnessing the aging of the so-called generation of "pre-boomers" and "boomers," who are used to taking primary responsibility for their own health care, an attitude they are not likely to relinquish with aging.

The recognition that the aging population is rapidly increasing and is highly diverse raises the question of whether one may identify common aging trends – in physiological, functional, medical, and social terms – that may define this group of individuals.

There is general agreement that age is associated with a progressive decline in the functional reserve of multiple organs and systems [9], and increased prevalence of chronic diseases [10], including conditions that are typical of aging, albeit not unique, called "geriatric syndromes" [11] (Table 1.1). The consequences of these changes include reduced life expectancy and tolerance of stress, and increased risk of disease and functional dependence. Functional dependence implies that a person may not

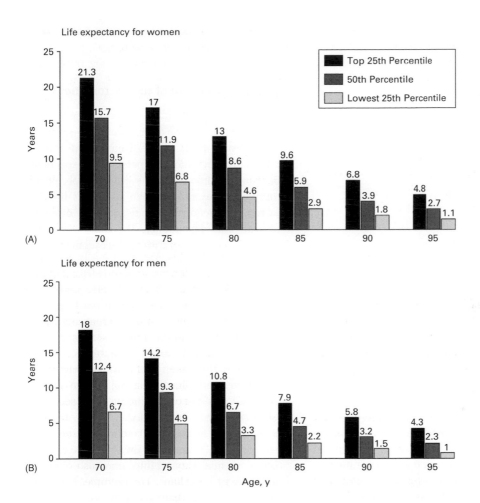

Figure 1.2 Life expectancy divided into quartiles: upper, middle, and lower quartiles for women (A) and men (B) at selected ages. From Walter & Covinsky, 2001 [7], with permission.

Table 1.1. Examples of geriatric syndromes.

Dementia

Severe depression

Delirium, caused by conditions that do not affect the central nervous system (medications, infections, pain, myocardial infarction, etc.)

Osteoporosis with spontaneous bone fractures

Falls

Dizziness

Failure to thrive

Neglect and abuse

be safe when living alone. Functional dependence is a broad term that encompasses different degrees of functional needs, such as the inability to carry on the activities necessary for independent living (instrumental activities of daily living, IADLs) [12] as well as basic activities of daily living (ADLs) [13] (Table 1.2). Clearly, loss of ADLs involves a higher degree of functional dependence than loss of IADLs, and may require a live-in caregiver or admission to a nursing home. Loss of IADLs may be compensated by a visiting caregiver or may be taken care of in an assisted living facility.

Table 1.2. Activities of daily living.

(A) Instrumental activities of daily living (IADLs)
    Use of transportation
    Shopping
    Taking medication
    Providing one's own meals
    Using the telephone
    Managing money
(B) Activities of daily living (ADLs)
    Transferring
    Bathing
    Going to the bathroom
    Grooming
    Dressing
    Eating

Functional dependence should be distinguished from disability, which also becomes more common with age [14], and which may or may not lead to functional dependence. Disability refers to the inability to perform a certain activity due to a particular functional loss. For example, loss of strength of the lower extremities (*loss of function*) may impede one's ability to climb stairs (*disability*). By itself this disability does not lead to functional dependence as long as an elevator or a wheelchair ramp allows the disabled person to transfer to the upper floors. In the absence of an elevator the disability becomes a *handicap* and leads to functional dependence (inability to transfer). Together with disease and functional decline, disability is a cause of functional dependence, but is not by itself functional dependence.

As an introduction to the themes of this book, we will examine medical and social implications of aging.

Medical implications of aging

The aging of the population has led to shifts in the paradigm of medical diagnosis and medical treatment. The most important medical implications of aging include increased prevalence of chronic conditions, increased mortality from acute conditions,

and change in the goals of treatment, from cure to avoidance of disease progression.

Increased prevalence of chronic conditions

The prevalence and the incidence of chronic diseases increase with age. Some of these conditions, including congestive heart failure, cancer, and chronic renal insufficiency, shorten a person's life expectancy [15]. Other conditions, such as arthritis or peripheral neuropathy, may not threaten a person's life, but may reduce functional capacity and cause disability and functional dependence. The consequences of increased prevalence of chronic diseases include:

- Changes in disease manifestations [16,17]. Some of these changes have been well described: these include delayed diagnosis due to *masking*, as is the case when bone pain due to metastatic cancer is mistakenly ascribed to worsening arthritis; or development of unusual symptoms, such as delirium in the presence of a urinary tract infection or myocardial ischemia that may be due to a *summation* of factors, including increased levels of circulating inflammatory cytokines, reduced number and function of cerebral neurons, and reduced oxygen supply to the brain due to coexistent anemia. Comorbidity may also alter the intensity of symptoms. For example, hypertension is associated with reduced and depression with enhanced perception of pain [18].
- Polypharmacy. The risk of drug complications and interactions increases progressively with the ongoing emergence of new drugs [19]. Older individuals are the most vulnerable to adverse events of polypharmacy, due to reduced functional reserve and coexistent diseases. One should not forget, however, that sometimes common drugs may also have positive effects. For example chronic use of non-steroidals has led to a reduction in cancer of the large bowel [20], while the use of statins may be associated with reduced risk of cancer of the large bowel, the breast, and the prostate [21].
- Estimate of life expectancy and disease prognosis. The presence of multiple comorbid conditions in

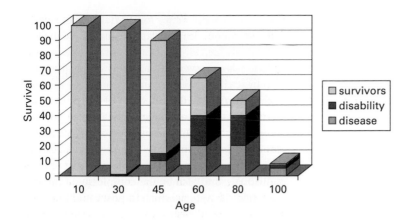

Figure 1.3 The percentage of people surviving at different ages, and the percentage affected by disease and disability. Compression of morbidity refers to bringing these curves closer together, to close the gap between death, disease, and functional impairment.

the same person may complicate the estimate of that person's prognosis and life expectancy. In the presence of conditions associated with rapid mortality, such as acute myeloid leukemia, metastatic cancer, or massive cerebrovascular accident, the influence of other conditions on life expectancy becomes negligible. More commonly, however, one has to account for the combined influence on life expectancy of conditions such as hypertension, well-controlled diabetes, arthritis, chronic lymphocytic leukemia, or low-grade lymphoma, none of which represent an immediate threat to a person's life. Furthermore, different forms of comorbidity may interact with each other. For example, it has become clear that in the presence of the so-called "metabolic syndrome" the risk of recurrence of colorectal cancer after surgery increases [22], and that cancer may enhance the risk of dementia [23].

Increased morbidity and mortality from acute conditions

It is not surprising that the stress represented by an acute illness might overwhelm the limited functional reserve of older individuals. Age is a risk factor for increased mortality following emergency surgery [24], increased risk of complications and hospitalization from elective surgery [24], increased risk for mortality and more prolonged hospitalization for infections [25,26], and increased risk of complications of cytotoxic chemotherapy, including myelodepression, mucositis, peripheral neuropathy, and cardiotoxicity [11].

Goals of medical treatment

While human life expectancy is in continuous expansion, human lifespan seemingly cannot be modified. Lifespan refers to the time one is allowed to live in the absence of disease and trauma, if death was due to the wearing out of one's functional reserve. This consideration, combined with the fact that the majority of chronic conditions affecting older individuals are incurable, may shift the goals of treatment in older individuals from cure toward preservation of function and quality of life. Notwithstanding acute and/or reversible conditions, such as pneumonia or localized cancer, the major goal of medical intervention in older individuals is compression of morbidity rather than elimination of diseases. Compression of morbidity (Fig. 1.3) refers to the delay of disability, functional dependence, and geriatric syndromes to the latest stage of life, and may be achieved with disease prevention, rehabilitation, and management of chronic diseases [27]. Reversal of anemia, even mild anemia, may play an important role in compression of morbidity, as anemia is an independent risk factor for functional decline [28].

Social implications of aging

The aging of the population involves a number of social implications that are only partly understood. Of particular concern is the dissolution of the traditional sources of support for the elderly at the very same time that the number of elderly is increasing. There is general agreement that the aging of the population will lead to a substantial cost in health care for at least three reasons:

- Increased incidence and prevalence of diseases.
- Increased cost of managing an individual's diseases. As already mentioned, infectious diseases may require a more prolonged hospitalization in older than in younger patients, and age is a risk factor for a wide array of treatment complications. Functional dependence, one of the most expensive aspects of aging, is also a common complication of prolonged hospitalization.
- Emergence of new and expensive treatments, beneficial in diseases such as cancer, hypertension, or diabetes that affect preferentially older individuals.

In addition, one should consider a basic economic difference between the management of younger and older individuals. The restoration of health to a younger patient may be considered an investment toward that person's gaining capacity. The restoration of health to an older individual is associated with little if any economic gain, and predisposes this individual to more diseases and more health-related expenses. Clearly, we are not proposing that older individuals should not receive the best medical care in the name of economic considerations. We are simply highlighting the need to minimize the cost of care by choosing the most effective care delivery. This may include adoption of a healthy lifestyle, interventions aimed at the prevention of disability and functional dependence, chemoprevention of and screening and early detection for common diseases, and avoidance of polypharmacy. For the purposes of this book it is important to underline how mild anemia, which is both a sign of underlying

disease and a risk factor for mortality and functional dependence, is largely under-diagnosed in older individuals [28,29]. Most causes of anemia in older individuals are reversible, and this simple intervention by itself may restore and preserve the function and the health of a large number of elderly people.

The delivery of cost-effective health care to older individuals is hampered by the scarcity of practitioners, especially primary care physicians, experienced in the assessment and management of these individuals, and also by the complexity of the current medical system, which imposes multiple visits to different specialists and may require older people to negotiate the hazards of urban traffic and the complex organization of large medical centers, not to mention the maze of rules governing Medicare and health insurance. Clearly, coordination of care and user-friendly healthcare delivery are the foundation of medical treatment of older individuals.

Conclusions

The world population is aging, and this process is particularly accelerated in the Western world. The aging of the population is associated with increased prevalence of disability, functional dependence, and chronic diseases, as well as increased risk of morbidity and mortality from acute conditions. While prevention of deaths and of chronic complications is always a goal of medical treatment, in older individuals compression of morbidity should be the focus of this treatment. Compression of morbidity may be achieved through a number of interventions, including the institution of a healthy lifestyle, the prevention of mobility and balance disorders, the chemoprevention and early detection of common diseases, and the avoidance of polypharmacy.

Coordination of care, and healthcare delivery in an elder-friendly environment, represent the major challenges to cost-effective care of the elderly.

The hematopoietic and blood coagulation systems represent a crossroads of multiple pathologic events involving different organs and systems. The study and the management of blood disorders in the elderly may thus have an important role in the preservation of the health and function of older individuals.

REFERENCES

1. Yancik R, Ries LAG. Cancer in older persons: magnitude of the problem and efforts to advance the aging/cancer research interface. In Balducci L, Lyman GH, Ershler WB, Extermann M, eds, *Comprehensive Geriatric Oncology*, 2nd edn (London: Taylor and Francis, 2004), 38–46.
2. Carpenter GI. Aging in the United Kingdom and Europe: a snapshot of the future? *J Am Geriatr Soc* 2005; **53**: S310–13.
3. Fukuda Y, Nakamura K, Takano T. Municipal socio-economic status and mortality in Japan: sex and age differences, and trends in 1973–1998. *Soc Sci Med* 2004; **59**: 2435–45.
4. Barberis M. America's elderly: policy implications. *Popul Bull* 1981; **35** (Suppl 4): 1–13.
5. Balducci L, Ershler WB. Cancer and ageing: a nexus at several levels. *Nat Rev Cancer* 2005; **5**: 655–62.
6. Balducci L, Aapro M. Epidemiology of cancer and aging. *Cancer Treat Res* 2005; **124**: 1–15.
7. Walter LC, Covinsky KE. Cancer screening in elderly patients: a framework for individual decision making. *JAMA* 2001; **285**: 2750–6.
8. Fox SA, Roetzheim RG. Barriers to cancer prevention in the older person. In Balducci L, Lyman GH, Ershler WB, Extermann M, eds, *Comprehensive Geriatric Oncology*, 2nd edn (London: Taylor and Francis, 2004), 376–86.
9. Duthie EH. Physiology of aging: relevance to symptom perception and treatment tolerance. In Balducci L, Lyman GH, Ershler WB, Extermann M, eds, *Comprehensive Geriatric Oncology*, 2nd edn (London: Taylor and Francis, 2004), 207–22.
10. Parmelee PA, Thuras PD, Katz IR, Lawton MP. Validation of the cumulative illness rating scale in a geriatric residential population. *J Am Geriatr Soc* 1995; **43**: 130–7.
11. Carreca I, Balducci L, Extermann M. Cancer in the older person. *Cancer Treat Rev* 2005; **31**: 380–402.
12. Lawton MP. Scales to measure competence in everyday activities. *Psychopharm Bull* 1988; **24**: 609–14, 789–91.
13. Katz S, Ford A, Moskowitz R, Jackson BA, Jaffe MW. Studies of illness in the aged: the index of ADL – a standardized measure of biological and psychosocial function. *JAMA* 1993; **185**: 914–19.
14. Wood PH. Appreciating the consequences of disease: the international classification of impairments, disabilities, and handicaps. *WHO Chron* 1980; **34**: 376–80.
15. Walter LC, Brand RJ, Counsell SR, *et al.* Development and validation of a prognostic index for 1-year mortality in older adults after hospitalization. *JAMA* 2001; **285**: 2987–94.
16. Fried LP, Stoner DJ, King DE, Lodder F. Diagnosis of illness presentation in the elderly. *J Am Geriatr Soc* 1991; **39**: 117–23.
17. Jarrett PG, Rockwood K, Carver D, *et al.* Illness presentation in elderly patients. *Arch Intern Med* 1995; **155**: 1060–4.
18. Balducci L. Management of cancer pain in geriatric patients. *J Support Oncol* 2003; **1**: 175–91.
19. Corcoran MB. Polypharmacy in the senior adult patient. In Balducci L, Lyman GH, Ershler WB, Extermann M, eds, *Comprehensive Geriatric Oncology*, 2nd edn (London: Taylor and Francis, 2004), 502–9.
20. Chan AT, Giovannucci EL, Meyerhardt JA, Schernhammer ES, Curhan GC, Fuchs CS. Long term use of aspirin and other non-steroidal anti-inflammatory drugs and risk of colon cancer. *JAMA* 2005; **294**: 914–25.
21. Poynter JN, Gruber SB, Higgins PDR, *et al.* Statins and the risk of colorectal cancer. *N Engl J Med* 2005; **352**: 2184–92.
22. Meyerhardt JA, Tepper JE, Niedwiecki D, *et al.* Impact of body mass index on outcomes and treatment-related toxicity in patients with stage II and III rectal cancer: findings from Intergroup Trial 0114. *J Clin Oncol* 2004; **22**: 648–57.
23. Heflin LH, Meyerowitz BE, Hall P, *et al.* Cancer as a risk factor for long term cognitive deficit and dementia. *J Natl Cancer Inst* 2005; **97**: 854–6.
24. Kemeny MM, Busch-Devereaux E, Merriam LT, O'Hea BJ. Cancer surgery in the elderly. *Hematol Oncol Clin North Am* 2000; **14**: 169–92.
25. Chrischilles E, Delgado DI, Stolshek BS, *et al.* Impact of age and colony stimulating factor use in hospital length of stay for febrile neutropenia in CHOP treated non-Hodgkin's lymphoma patients. *Cancer Control* 2002; **9**: 203–11.
26. Greene, J. N. Management of infectious complications in the aged cancer patient. In Balducci L, Lyman GH, Ershler WB, Extermann M, eds, *Comprehensive Geriatric*

Oncology, 2nd edn (London: Taylor and Francis, 2004), 803–12.

27. Doblhammer G, Kytir J. Compression or expansion of morbidity? Trends in healthy-life expectancy in the elderly Austrian population between 1978 and 1998. *Soc Sci Med* 2001; **52**: 385–91.

28. Chaves PH, Semba RD, Leng SX, *et al.* Impact of anemia and cardiovascular disease on frailty status of community-dwelling older women: the Women's Health and Aging Studies I and II. *J Gerontol A Biol Sci Med Sci* 2005; **60**: 729–35.

29. Guralnik JM, Eisenstaedt RS, Ferrucci L, Klein HG, Woodman RC. Prevalence of anemia in persons 65 years and older in the United States: evidence for a high rate of unexplained anemia. *Blood* 2004; **104**: 2263–8.

2

Epidemiology of anemia in older adults

Kushang V. Patel, Jack M. Guralnik

Introduction

The US Census Bureau enumerated 35.0 million adults aged 65 years and older in the 2000 decennial census [1]. Older adults comprised 12.4% of the total US population. By 2050, this segment is projected to grow to 86.7 million, and one out of every five persons will be elderly [2]. Further, the oldest old (those 85 years and older) will grow approximately 400% and represent the fastest-growing age group in the USA. However, the USA is not alone in experiencing population aging, and in fact it is now ranked the 38th oldest country [3]. While population aging is occurring in all regions of the world, rapid declines in fertility rates have generated faster growth rates in the proportion of older adults in developing countries than in developed ones. In view of global population aging and the multiple morbidities associated with aging, the prevention and treatment of conditions that impair functional capacity and quality of life is a major priority of geriatric medicine.

Anemia is a common hematologic condition among older adults, with prevalence estimates increasing as a function of age. Contrary to widely held beliefs that anemia is an innocuous condition of old age, recent evidence suggests that anemia does not reflect a normal aging process, but rather is a marker of underlying pathology and/or a cause of further physiological dysregulation. For instance, in a study of adults aged 85 and older, anemia as defined by the World Health Organization (WHO) was associated with a two fold 5-year mortality risk, independent of age, sex, and medical conditions [4].

Among older adults hospitalized for acute myocardial infarction, lower hematocrit on admission was associated with poorer 30-day survival, while transfusion in those with hematocrit less than 34% was associated with better 30-day survival [5]. In addition to the independent effects anemia has on cardiovascular outcomes [6,7], a number of studies have also shown that lower hemoglobin levels independently predict poor physical function in older adults (see Chapter 15). Given that anemia is not a benign condition in old age, greater attention to the diagnosis and management of anemia in the elderly population is needed. This chapter reviews the distribution and types of anemia among older adults.

Prevalence of anemia in older adults

A number of studies have estimated the prevalence of anemia using the WHO definition of hemoglobin concentration less than 12 g/dL in women and 13 g/dL in men. However, these estimates vary substantially because of biased source populations (e.g., clinic/referral populations) and restricted age ranges. Population-based studies of older adults have provided more stable and consistent prevalence estimates. For example, 15.2% of male and 12.6% of female participants (>70 years) in the Established Populations for Epidemiologic Studies of the Elderly were classified as anemic [8]. Similarly, the InCHIANTI study showed that 11.1% of men and 11.5% of women aged 65 years and older living in two communities in Tuscany, Italy, had anemia [9]. Most recently, Guralnik

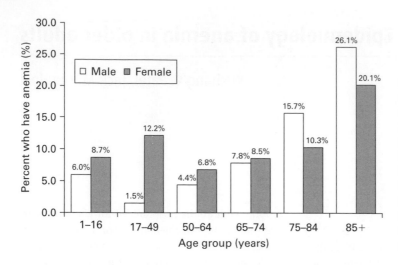

Figure 2.1 Percentage of persons anemic according to age and sex (NHANES III, Phases I and II, 1988–94). Originally published in *Blood*: Guralnik JM, Eisenstaedt RS, Ferrucci L, Klein HG, Woodman RC. Prevalence of anemia in persons 65 years and older in the United States: evidence for a high rate of unexplained anemia. *Blood* 2004; **104**: 2263–8 [10]. © The American Society of Hematology.

and colleagues analyzed data from the third National Health and Nutrition Examination Survey (NHANES III, 1988–94), which was not only designed to provide prevalence information for the non-institutionalized US population but also powered to investigate medical conditions in adults aged 65 years and older [10]. According to these data, the overall prevalence of anemia in elderly men and women was 11.0% and 10.2%, respectively. These estimates are similar to ones reported in other community-based samples of older adults [11,12]; however, they are substantially lower compared to prevalence estimates reported in institutionalized settings, which range between 30% and 48% [13–15].

The NHANES III data also indicated that anemia varied by age, sex, and racial/ethnic subgroups [10]. Figure 2.1 displays prevalence estimates stratified by age and sex. Men are least likely to experience anemia between ages 17 and 49, while for women prevalence is lowest after their reproductive years between 50 and 64. Prevalence increases with advancing age for both men and women after age 64. Whereas men and women have similar estimates at ages 65 to 74, prevalence doubles for men and increases by only 21% in women at ages 75–84. Highest prevalence of anemia occurs after age 84 for both sexes (26.1% for men and 20.1% in women). Consistent with other community-based studies, anemia occurs more frequently in men than in women aged 75 years and

older [8,11,12]. While the effect of age on anemia prevalence appears more dramatic in older men than in older women, the differential effect might result from the more conservative WHO definition applied to women.

The WHO criteria were primarily based on the distribution of hemoglobin in a study of apparently healthy adults (cutoffs were based on two standard deviations below the mean for each sex) [16,17]. Hemoglobin levels of 12–13 g/dL are considered normal in women but abnormal in men. If the same WHO definition for anemia in men were applied to women, then the prevalence of anemia in women aged 65 and older would increase to 32.5% [10]. Indeed, relative to men, the entire distribution of hemoglobin is shifted left towards lower values for women (Fig. 2.2) [10]. Considering that older women are well past menopause, researchers are questioning the application of the more conservative cutoff point in older women. For instance, the Women's Health and Aging Study I (WHAS I) has shown all-cause mortality rates are lowest among elderly women with hemoglobin levels approaching 14 g/dL [18]. Additionally, elderly men and women with hemoglobin values 0 to 1 g/dL above the WHO cutoffs were at increased risk of death compared to those 1 to 2 g/dL above the WHO cutoffs independent of potential confounders [19]. Similar findings have been observed for physical function outcomes. Although more replication

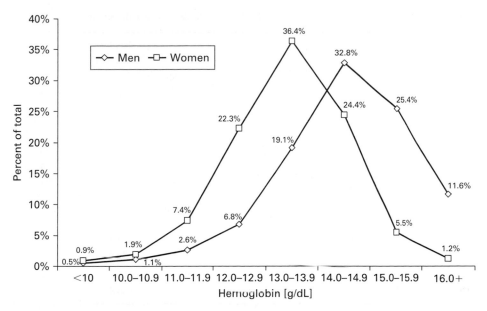

Figure 2.2 Distribution of hemoglobin in persons aged 65 and older by sex (NHANES III, Phases I and II, 1988–94). Originally published in *Blood*: Guralnik JM, Eisenstaedt RS, Ferrucci L, Klein HG, Woodman RC. Prevalence of anemia in persons 65 years and older in the United States: evidence for a high rate of unexplained anemia. *Blood* 2004; **104**: 2263–8 [10]. © The American Society of Hematology.

studies and further research are needed before revising the definition of anemia in older adults, these observations suggest that older adults with "low-normal" hemoglobin levels might benefit from treatments that increase their hemoglobin values.

In addition to the differential distributions by age and sex, prevalence of anemia in the elderly US population varies by race/ethnicity. According to NHANES III estimates (Table 2.1), older non-Hispanic Whites are least likely to have anemia compared to other racial/ethnic groups [10]. Older Mexican Americans, a rapidly growing segment of the US elderly population, had slightly higher prevalence of anemia (10.4%) than non-Hispanic Whites (9.0%). In contrast, older non-Hispanic Blacks were three times more likely to have anemia compared to non-Hispanic Whites. This differential has been previously reported, and is unexplained even after adjusting for multiple diseases, nutritional status, and health behavior [8,20–22]. Indeed, there is evidence that the distribution of hemoglobin values

Table 2.1. Percentage of persons age 65 and older who are anemic, by race/ethnicity and sex (NHANES III, Phases I and II, 1988–94).

Race/Ethnicity	Males (%)	Females (%)	Total (%)
Non-Hispanic White	9.2	8.7	9.0
Non-Hispanic Black	27.5	28.0	27.8
Mexican American	11.5	9.3	10.4
Other	20.4	7.5	14.0
Total	11.0	10.2	10.6

This research was originally published in *Blood*: Guralnik JM, Eisenstaedt RS, Ferrucci L, Klein HG, Woodman RC. Prevalence of anemia in persons 65 years and older in the United States: evidence for a high rate of unexplained anemia. *Blood* 2004; **104**: 2263–8 [10]. © The American Society of Hematology.

among Blacks is shifted toward lower values, even in young healthy Blacks, compared to Whites [23]. These observations have led some to consider race-specific criteria for defining anemia. However, further research is needed to determine whether

Table 2.2. Distribution of types of anemia in persons age 65 and older, USA (NHANES III, Phase II, 1991–4).

	Number in USA	Percent	Percent of all anemia
Nutrient deficiency-related anemia			
Iron deficiency only	466 715	48.3	16.6
Folate deficiency only	181 471	18.8	6.4
B_{12} deficiency only	165 701	17.2	5.9
Folate and B_{12} deficiencies	56 436	5.8	2.0
Iron with folate and/or B_{12} deficiencies	95 221	9.9	3.4
Total	965 544	100.0	34.3
Anemia without nutrient deficiencies			
Renal insufficiency only	229 686	12.4	8.2
Anemia of chronic disease, no renal insufficiency	554 281	30.0	19.7
Renal insufficiency and anemia of chronic disease	120 169	6.5	4.3
Unexplained anemia of aging	945 195	51.1	33.6
Total	1 849 331	100.0	65.7
Total, all anemia	**2 814 875**		**100.0**

This research was originally published in *Blood*: Guralnik JM, Eisenstaedt RS, Ferrucci L, Klein HG, Woodman RC. Prevalence of anemia in persons 65 years and older in the United States: evidence for a high rate of unexplained anemia. *Blood* 2004; **104**: 2263–8 [10]. © The American Society of Hematology.

the excess anemia experienced by the elderly non-Hispanic black population predicts excess morbidity and mortality.

Types of anemia

Anemia with nutrient deficiency

Identifying the cause of anemia is often difficult in older adults because of the high levels of comorbidity and polypharmacy in this population. Indeed, approximately two-thirds of older adults with anemia in NHANES III had two or more medical conditions [10]. Nonetheless, anemia can be broadly classified according to whether or not it is associated with nutrient deficiency. Among the 3 million older adults with anemia in the USA [10], 34% had anemia related to iron, folate, and/or vitamin B_{12} deficiency (Table 2.2). Deficiency in any of these nutrients can impair erythropoiesis [24]. Iron deficiency causes anemia by reducing the production of hemoglobinized erythrocytes (microcytic and

normocytic anemia), while deficiency in folate or vitamin B_{12} can impair deoxyribonucleic acid synthesis, reduce production of hematopoietic precursors, and cause erythroblast apoptosis (macrocytic and normocytic anemia) [24,25]. Given the low cost of therapy, identifying nutrient deficiency in elderly anemic patients provides opportunity to potentially remediate not only anemia but also other sequelae associated with nutrient deficiency [10].

Iron deficiency accounted for approximately a fifth of all anemia cases and over half of cases associated with nutrient deficiency in NHANES III (Table 2.2) [10]. Most cases of anemia associated with iron deficiency result from blood loss through gastrointestinal lesions [26,27], although some cases might arise from dietary behavior as well [28]. Diagnosing iron deficiency in older adults and distinguishing it from other causes of anemia is difficult [29]. Serum ferritin has, until recently, been considered the best laboratory test of iron storage, with values less than or equal to $12 \mu g/L$ indicating iron deficiency [30]; however, ferritin levels are known to increase with age and chronic medical conditions [31,32]. It is therefore not surprising that conventional diagnostic measures, such as ferritin, serum iron, and transferrin saturation levels, are reported to be insensitive in hospitalized adults above 80 years in age [33]. Thus, prevalence of iron-deficiency anemia based on these measures is likely underestimated in older adults [10].

An alternative measure of iron storage in older adults is serum transferrin receptor. The expression of transferrin receptor is regulated by the amount of iron reaching pro-erythroid cell surfaces [29]. When iron stores are low, transferrin receptors are overexpressed and appear in blood serum because of proteolysis [29]. The ratio of serum transferrin receptor level to log ferritin (hereafter referred to as the transferrin receptor–ferritin index) has a sensitivity of 88% and specificity of 93% (using cutoff value of 1.5) for detecting iron-deficiency anemia in older adults when compared to the more definitive and painful bone-marrow aspirate examination of normoblasts [33]. The transferrin receptor–ferritin index, therefore, outperforms routine laboratory tests in diagnosing iron-deficiency anemia in older adults [33]. A recent community-based study in Seoul, South Korea, reported that, compared to the "gold standard" transferrin receptor–ferritin index, a serum ferritin level less than or equal to $22\mu g/L$ had a sensitivity and specificity of 89% in classifying older adults with iron-deficiency anemia [34]. The new serum ferritin cutoff is lower than the previously recommended criterion of $45\mu g/L$ in older adults with anemia, but it is still higher than the $12\mu g/L$ cutoff used in younger adults [30,35]. Although this lower value is useful in settings where serum transferrin receptor assays are not readily available, it is unknown how the serum ferritin cutoff value of $22\mu g/L$ compares to bone aspirate examination and therefore using the transferrin receptor–ferritin index is preferable to establish iron deficiency in older adults with anemia.

Folate and vitamin B_{12} deficiencies are also fairly common among older adults, and are associated with at least 14% of all anemia cases (Table 2.2) [10]. Whereas folate deficiency results from inadequate dietary intake and absorption problems, vitamin B_{12} deficiency is primarily caused by problems with either releasing vitamin B_{12} from food, caused by decreased gastric acidity and decreased production of gastrin (i.e., the food-cobalamin malabsorption syndrome), or absorbing vitamin B_{12} through mucosal cells because of inadequate (or deficient) levels of intrinsic factor (i.e., pernicious anemia) [25,36]. Diagnosis of either deficiency cannot be made by serum concentrations alone, rather other metabolites must also be considered. Specifically, vitamin B_{12} deficiency is associated with higher levels of methylmalonic acid (MMA) and/or total homocysteine, while folate deficiency is only associated with higher homocysteine concentration and not MMA level [25,37]. Therefore, vitamin B_{12} deficiency is diagnosed when vitamin B_{12} concentration is low and MMA is high, and folate deficiency exists when folate is low, homocysteine is high, and MMA is normal [25]. Specific cutoff values for these parameters are not well established because currently there are no gold-standard tests for these vitamin deficiencies [36,38].

Anemia of chronic inflammation (chronic disease)

In addition to nutrient deficiency, anemia can also be caused by a number of chronic medical conditions that are characterized by inflammation and chronic immune activation, which has been aptly termed anemia of chronic inflammation (ACI) or anemia of chronic disease [39]. Conditions that are frequently associated with ACI include chronic infections (e.g., tuberculosis, human immunodeficiency virus), cancer (hematologic and solid tumors), autoimmune disorders (e.g., rheumatoid arthritis, inflammatory bowel disease), diabetes, and congestive heart failure [39–42]. Generally, the severity of anemia correlates positively with the severity of the underlying medical condition. For example, in a clinic sample of 820 Australian adults with diabetes, the overall prevalence of unrecognized anemia was 23%; however, anemia was two times more likely in microalbuminuric patients and ten times more likely in macroalbuminuric patients compared to diabetic patients with normal albumin levels and preserved renal function [40]. In addition to disease severity, anemia prevalence also varies by therapeutic intervention among cancer patients. Recent findings from the European Cancer Anemia Survey showed that the prevalence of anemia was 39% among 15367 cancer patients [41]. Of those who were not anemic at baseline, anemia incidence was 63% in those undergoing chemotherapy alone, 42% in those receiving a combination of chemotherapy and radiotherapy, and 20% in those treated with radiotherapy alone [41].

Among older adults, ACI is one of the most common forms of anemia, with an estimated prevalence of 19.7% (Table 2.2) [10]. This high prevalence of ACI likely reflects the low-grade pro-inflammatory state often experienced by older adults with multiple morbidities, and therefore identifying a putative disease underlying ACI in older adults is difficult [43]. Nonetheless, in addition to having higher prevalence of elevated levels of C-reactive protein and rheumatoid-factor positivity, older adults with ACI in the NHANES III were significantly more likely to have arthritis and diabetes compared to non-anemic older adults [10]. Also, the proportion of non-Hispanic Blacks among older adults with ACI was significantly higher than the proportion in the non-anemic older adult population (43.6% versus 15.1%) [10]. The biological and social–behavioral causes underlying this racial disparity remain unexplained.

Although several mechanisms contribute to the pathogenesis of ACI, each of them is immune driven [29,39]. Elevated levels of cytokines, such as interleukin 1, interleukin 6 (IL-6), and tumor necrosis factor α (TNF-α), and cells from the reticuloendothelial system impair iron delivery, proliferation of erythroid progenitor cells, and production of erythropoietin as well as reduce red cell survival [29,39]. The precise mechanisms linking pro-inflammatory cytokines to ACI is currently under active investigation; however, IL-6 has recently been shown to be a necessary and sufficient cytokine to induce expression of a small hepatic polypeptide called hepcidin [44]. Hepcidin is an iron regulatory hormone that induces (1)

degradation of the iron-exporting ferroportin in macrophages, and (2) decreased duodenal absorption of iron, which ultimately leads to inhibition of erythropoiesis [45,46]. The clinical utility of hepcidin as a potential marker for screening for ACI has not been investigated because of limited assay availability and development [29].

Anemia of chronic inflammation is normocytic and typically mild, with hemoglobin values ranging from 10 to 12 g/dL in older adults [10,39]. Distinguishing ACI from iron-deficiency anemia can be difficult in older adults because of potentially coexisting blood loss and the effects of medications. In both types of anemia, serum iron and transferrin saturation levels are reduced. To differentiate between ACI and iron-deficiency anemia, evaluation of ferritin levels as well as serum transferrin receptor levels is useful because ferritin levels are typically normal or increased in ACI while expression of the transferrin receptor is downregulated by pro-inflammatory cytokines. Therefore, a transferrin receptor–ferritin index value of less than 1 suggests ACI, while a value greater than 2 would indicate iron-deficiency anemia [39]. However, in the case where a patient has both ACI and iron-deficiency anemia, the transferrin receptor–ferritin index would also be high (>2) but accompanied with clinical or biochemical evidence of inflammation. It has also been suggested that the percentage of hypochromic red cells or reticulocyte hemoglobin content can also help identify patients with both types of anemia [47].

Anemia of chronic kidney disease

Chronic kidney disease (CKD) is another major medical condition that causes anemia by impairing the production of erythropoietin [48]. Approximately 8.2% of older adults with anemia have CKD, and an additional 4.3% have both CKD and ACI (Table 2.2) [8]. The relationship between age, kidney function, and anemia prevalence has been examined in the NHANES III [49]. The prevalence of anemia (defined as hemoglobin <12 g/dL) declined as a function of creatinine clearance in both older

(61–70 years) and younger (31–40 years) men and women. At every level of kidney function, the prevalence of anemia was higher in older than in younger men, while an opposite pattern was observed in women. After adjusting for age and race/ethnicity, the creatinine clearance threshold at which hemoglobin levels were significantly reduced was below 60 mL/minute in men and below 50 mL/minute in women [49]. Similar threshold effects have been observed in other studies, although different threshold values have been reported [50,51]. For example, in a population-based study of community-dwelling older adults living in Italy, a creatinine clearance threshold of below 30 mL/minute was associated with anemia, but milder levels of renal impairment (30–89 mL/minute) were not associated with anemia [51]. While further research is needed to better characterize the relationship between kidney function and anemia among older adults, recent results from the Prevalence of Anemia in Early Renal Insufficiency study suggest that there is no age variation in the prevalence of anemia among patients with CKD [48].

Unexplained anemia

Approximately one-third of anemia cases in community-dwelling older adults were unexplained (Table 2.2) [10]. This prevalence estimate might be upwardly biased because not every potential cause of anemia could be identified with the examination and laboratory test data available in NHANES III. For example, thalassemia minor, hereditary spherocytosis, or autoimmune hemolytic anemia are other causes of anemia that could not be evaluated in the NHANES III data, although these are fairly uncommon conditions. A condition that would perhaps account for the largest portion of unexplained anemia cases in NHANES III is myelodysplastic syndrome (MDS) [10]. While bone-marrow examination is needed to identify early MDS, more advanced cases of MDS are characterized by macrocytosis and are frequently accompanied by neutropenia or thrombocytopenia [10]. However, only 17.2% of unexplained anemia cases (5.8% of all anemia cases) in NHANES III were accompanied by leukopenia,

thrombocytopenia, or macrocytosis, which is a liberal definition of MDS that likely overestimates the number of MDS cases. Nonetheless, this suggests the proportion of unexplained anemia among older adults with anemia would still exceed 25% even if a more complete assessment for MDS were performed on the sample [10]. Similar estimates of unexplained anemia were reported in a Swedish study of hospitalized patients aged 70–81 in which the cause of anemia was not identified in 23–36% of anemic patients even after bone-marrow testing [52]. These findings indicate that unrecognized myelodysplastic syndrome accounts for only a small proportion of unexplained anemia cases in older adults [10,29]. More recently, the cause of anemia in elderly nursing-home residents was not identified in 45% of cases, although bone-marrow evaluation was not completed in this study and therefore bone-marrow failure and early myelodysplasia could not be ruled out [53].

Some researchers have speculated that production of erythropoietin in response to declining hemoglobin levels might be blunted in some older adults with unexplained anemia. For example, one study of older Japanese adults demonstrated the typical inverse relationship between erythropoietin and hemoglobin concentration in patients with iron-deficiency anemia; however, in patients with unexplained anemia, no relationship between erythropoietin and hemoglobin was observed [54]. In addition, a British study showed that older patients (≥70 years) with normocytic anemia and no iron deficiency had significantly lower levels of erythropoietin compared to younger patients (<70 years) with normocytic anemia and older patients with iron-deficiency anemia [55]. It has been suggested that impairment of renal endocrine function, not undetected nephron dysfunction or CKD, contributes to unexplained anemia because renal interstitial cells are responsible for erythropoietin production rather than renal glomeruli or tubules [51]. Alternatively, reduced erythropoietin production might reflect incipient renal insufficiency, which has been suggested to occur with diabetic nephropathy [56,57].

Summary

Anemia is a common condition among older adults that requires appropriate clinical intervention and should not be viewed as a normal part of aging. About one-third of anemia cases in older adults are related to nutrient deficiency that is amenable to safe and inexpensive therapy. Chronic kidney disease and other chronic conditions associated with inflammation account for another third of anemia cases, which can potentially be improved with erythropoietin therapy. The remaining cases of anemia do not have an identifiable cause. Considering the potential negative impact anemia can have on physical function and survival in older adults, it is important to recognize the underlying conditions that might contribute to anemia in order to guide diagnosis and management. Further research is needed to understand the pathogenesis and consequences of anemia in older adults, as well as to develop interventions and guidelines to improve treatment and management of this disorder.

REFERENCES

1. Hetzel L, Smith A. *The 65 Years and Older Population, 2000. Census 2000 Brief.* C2KBR/01-10 (Washington, DC: US Census Bureau, 2001).
2. US Census Bureau. U.S. Interim Projections by Age, Sex, Race, and Hispanic Origin. http://www.census.gov/ipc/www/usinterimproj. Accessed March 16, 2007.
3. Kinsella K, Phillips DR. Global aging: the challenge of success. *Popul Bull* 2005; **60**: 1–42.
4. Izaks GJ, Westendorp RGJ, Knook DL. The definition of anemia in older persons. *JAMA* 1999; **281**: 1714–17.
5. Wu WC, Rathore SS, Wang Y, Radford MJ, Krumholz HM. Blood transfusion in elderly patients with acute myocardial infarction. *N Engl J Med* 2001; **345**: 1230–6.
6. Esekowitz JA, McAlister FA, Armstrong PW. Anemia is common in heart failure and is associated with poor outcomes: insights from a cohort of 12,065 patients with new-onset heart failure. *Circulation* 2003; **107**: 223–5.
7. Sabatine MS, Morrow DA, Giugliano RP, *et al.* Association of hemoglobin levels with clinical outcomes in acute coronary syndromes. *Circulation* 2005; **111**: 2042–9.
8. Salive ME, Cornoni-Huntley J, Guralnik JM, *et al.* Anemia and hemoglobin levels in older persons: relationship with age, gender, and health status. *J Am Geriatr Soc* 1992; **40**: 489–96.
9. Penninx BW, Pahor M, Cesari M, *et al.* Anemia is associated with disability and decreased physical performance and muscle strength in the elderly. *J Am Geriatr Soc* 2004; **52**: 719–24.
10. Guralnik JM, Eisenstaedt RS, Ferrucci L, Klein HG, Woodman RC. Prevalence of anemia in persons 65 years and older in the United States: evidence for a high rate of unexplained anemia. *Blood* 2004; **104**: 2263–8.
11. Anía BJ, Suman VJ, Fairbanks VF, Melton LJ. Prevalence of anemia in medical practice: community versus referral patients. *Mayo Clin Proc* 1994; **69**: 730–5.
12. Inelmen EM, D'Alessio M, Gatto MR, *et al.* Descriptive analysis of the prevalence of anemia in a randomly selected sample of elderly people living at home: some results of an Italian multicentric study. *Aging Clin Exp Res* 1994; **6**: 81–9.
13. Kalchthaler T, Tan ME. Anemia in institutionalized elderly patients. *J Am Geriatr Soc* 1980; **28**: 108–13.
14. Chernetsky A, Sofer O, Rafael C, Ben-Israel J. Prevalence and etiology of anemia in an institutionalized geriatric population. *Harefuah* 2002; **141**: 591–4, 667.
15. Artz AS, Fergusson D, Drinka PJ, *et al.* Prevalence of anemia in skilled-nursing home residents. *Arch Gerontol Geriatr* 2004; **39**: 201–6.
16. World Health Organization. *Nutritional Anaemias: Report of a WHO Scientific Group* (Geneva: World Health Organization, 1968).
17. Wintrobe MM. Blood of normal men and women. *Bull Johns Hopkins Hosp* 1933; **53**: 118–30.
18. Chaves PH, Xue QL, Guralnik JM, Ferrucci L, Volpato S, Fried LP. What constitutes normal hemoglobin concentration in community-dwelling disabled older women? *J Am Geriatr Soc* 2004; **52**: 1811–16.
19. Penninx BW, Pahor M, Woodman RC, Guralnik JM. Anemia in old age is associated with increased mortality and hospitalization. *J Gerontol A Biol Sci Med Sci* 2006; **61**: 474–9.
20. Pan WH, Habicht JP. The non-iron-deficiency-related difference in hemoglobin concentration distribution between blacks and whites and between men and women. *Am J Epidemiol* 1991; **134**: 1410–16.
21. Johnson-Spear MA, Yip R. Hemoglobin difference between black and white women with comparable iron status: justification for race-specific anemia criteria. *Am J Clin Nutr* 1994; **60**: 117–21.

22. Jackson RT. Separate hemoglobin standards for blacks and whites: a critical review of the case for separate and unequal hemoglobin standards. *Med Hypotheses* 1990; **32**: 181–9.

23. Perry GS, Byers T, Yip R, Margen S. Iron nutrition does not account for the hemoglobin differences between blacks and whites. *J Nutr* 1992; **122**: 1417–24.

24. Koury MJ, Prem P. New insights into erythropoiesis: the roles of folate, vitamin B_{12}, and iron. *Annu Rev Nutr* 2004; **24**: 105–31.

25. Balducci L. Epidemiology of anemia in the elderly: information on diagnostic evaluation. *J Am Geriatr Soc* 2003; **51**: S2–S9.

26. Coban E, Timuragaoglu A, Meric M. Iron deficiency anemia in the elderly: prevalence and endoscopic evaluation of the gastrointestinal tract in outpatients. *Acta Haematol* 2003; **110**: 25–8.

27. Rockey DC, Cello JP. Evaluation of the gastrointestinal tract in patients with iron-deficiency anemia. *N Engl J Med* 1993; **329**: 1691–5.

28. Drewnowski A, Shultz JM. Impact of aging on eating behaviors, food choices, nutrition, and health status. *J Nutr Health Aging* 2001; **5**: 75–9.

29. Woodman R, Ferrucci L, Guralnik J. Anemia in older adults. *Curr Opin Hematol* 2005; **12**: 123–8.

30. Guyatt GH, Patterson C, Ali M, *et al.* Diagnosis of iron-deficiency anemia in the elderly. *Am J Med* 1990; **88**: 205–9.

31. Casale G, Bonora C, Migliavacca A, Zurita IE, de Nicola P. Serum ferritin and aging. *Age Ageing* 1981; **10**: 119–22.

32. Witte DL. Can serum ferritin be effectively interpreted in the presence of the acute-phase response? *Clin Chem* 1991; **37**: 484–5.

33. Rimon E, Levy S, Sapir A, *et al.* Diagnosis of iron deficiency anemia in the elderly by transferrin receptor–ferritin index. *Arch Intern Med* 2002; **162**: 445–9.

34. Choi CW, Cho WR, Park KH, *et al.* The cutoff value of serum ferritin for the diagnosis of iron deficiency in community-residing older persons. *Ann Hematol* 2005; **84**: 358–61.

35. Holyoake TL, Stott DJ, McKay PJ, *et al.* Use of plasma ferritin concentration to diagnose iron deficiency in elderly patients. *J Clin Pathol* 1993; **46**: 857–60.

36. Andrès E, Loukili NH, Noel E, *et al.* Vitamin B_{12} (cobalamin) deficiency in elderly patients. *CMAJ* 2004; **171**: 251–9.

37. Savage DG, Lindenbaum J, Stabler SP, *et al.* Sensitivity of serum MMA and total homocysteine determinations for diagnosing cobalamin and folate deficiencies. *Am J Med* 1994; **96**: 239–46.

38. Klee GG. Cobalamin and folate evaluation: measurement of methylmalonic acid and homocysteine vs vitamin B_{12} and folate. *Clin Chem* 2000; **46**: 1277–83.

39. Weiss G, Goodnough LT. Anemia of chronic disease. *N Engl J Med* 2005; **352**: 1011–23.

40. Thomas MC, MacIsaac RJ, Tsalamandris C, Power D, Jerums G. Unrecognized anemia in patients with diabetes: a cross-sectional survey. *Diabetes Care* 2003; **26**: 1164–9.

41. Birgegard G, Aapro MS, Bokemeyer C, *et al.* Cancer-related anemia: pathogenesis, prevalence and treatment. *Oncology* 2005; **68** (Suppl 1): 3–11.

42. Lindenfeld J. Prevalence of anemia and effects on mortality in patients with heart failure. *Am Heart J* 2005; **149**: 391–401.

43. Ferrucci L, Corsi A, Lauretani F, *et al.* The origins of age-related proinflammatory state. *Blood* 2005; **105**: 2294–9.

44. Nemeth E, Rivera S, Gabayan V, *et al.* IL-6 mediates hypoferremia of inflammation by inducing the synthesis of the iron regulatory hormone hepcidin. *J Clin Invest* 2004; **113**: 1271–6.

45. Laftah AH, Ramesh B, Simpson RJ, *et al.* Effect of hepcidin on intestinal iron absorption in mice. *Blood* 2004; **103**: 3940–4.

46. Rivera S, Nemeth E, Gabayan V, *et al.* Synthetic hepcidin causes rapid dose-dependent hypoferremia and is concentrated in ferroportin-containing organs. *Blood* 2005; **106**: 2196–9.

47. Brugnara C. Iron deficiency and erythropoiesis: new diagnostic approaches. *Clin Chem* 2003; **49**: 1573–8.

48. McClellan W, Aronoff SL, Bolton WK, *et al.* The prevalence of anemia in patients with chronic kidney disease. *Curr Med Res Opin* 2004; **20**: 1501–10.

49. Hsu CY, McCulloch CE, Curhan GC. Epidemiology of anemia associated with chronic renal insufficiency among adults in the United States: results from the Third National Health and Nutrition Examination Survey. *J Am Soc Nephrol* 2002; **13**: 504–10.

50. Cumming RG, Mitchell P, Craig JC, Knight JF. Renal impairment and anaemia in a population-based study of older people. *Intern Med J* 2004; **34**: 20–3.

51. Ferrucci L, Woodman RC, Penninx BW, *et al.* Unrecognized renal insufficiency and blunted EPO responses in the anemia of older persons: The InCHIANTI Study. *Blood* 2003; **102**: 512a.

52. Nilsson-Ehle H, Jagenburg R, Landahl S, Svanborg A, Westin J. Haematological abnormalities and reference intervals in the elderly. A cross-sectional comparative study of three urban Swedish population samples aged 70, 75 and 81 years. *Acta Med Scand* 1988; **224**: 595–604.

53. Artz AS, Fergusson D, Drinka PJ, *et al*. Mechanisms of unexplained anemia in the nursing home. *J Am Geriatr Soc* 2004; **52**: 423–7.

54. Kario K, Matsuo T, Kodama K, Nakao K, Asada R. Reduced erythropoietin secretion in senile anemia. *Am J Hematol* 1992; **41**: 252–7.

55. Carpenter MA, Kendall RG, O'Brien AE, *et al*. Reduced erythropoietin response to anaemia in elderly patients with normocytic anaemia. *Eur J Haematol* 1992; **49**: 119–21.

56. Inomata S, Itoh M, Imai H, Sato T. Serum levels of erythropoietin as a novel marker reflecting the severity of diabetic nephropathy. *Nephron* 1997; **75**: 426–30.

57. Bosman DR, Winkler AS, Marsden JT, Macdougall IC, Watkins PJ. Anemia with erythropoietin deficiency occurs early in diabetic nephropathy. *Diabetes Care* 2001; **24**: 495–9.

3

Cancer in the older person: a comprehensive approach

Oscar A. Cepeda, Julie K. Gammack, John E. Morley

Introduction

Cancer is a very common disease of the older adult; it is primarily a disease of the elderly, with a high index of mortality and disability [1]. The definition of "elderly" is somewhat arbitrary. The medical literature and epidemiologic data typically characterize the population as older than or younger than 65 years. Some studies, however, label patients as "older" when they are over 75 years and further categorize those patients over 85 years as the "oldest old" [2–4].

By the year 2030, one in five Americans will be older than 65 years [5]. The number of individuals over 75 will triple, and the number of those over 85 will double in the same period. Currently the average life expectancy for a 75-year-old individual is 11.3 years, and for an 85-year-old it is 6.3 years. As the size of the elderly population continues to increase, healthcare professionals can expect to see a steadily growing number of elderly patients with cancer [6,7].

Cancer deaths accounted for 23% of all deaths in the USA in 2002, second only to heart disease [8]. This major public health problem disproportionately affects older rather than younger persons. Increasing age is directly associated with increased rates of cancer, corresponding to an 11-fold greater incidence in persons over the age of 65 years. Around 60% of all cancers occur in this age group, where the mortality rate can be as high as 70% [7].

The incidence of cancer is higher in men than in women, and this difference is more evident after 64 years of age. There is a sharp incident rise after this age for both men and women, but it is higher for men (500 per 100 000 men ⩾65 years vs. 420 per 100 000 women). Lung cancer is the most common malignant entity in both men and women older than 60 years (30% of all cancer deaths in this group). The age group of 60–79 years have the second highest incidence of breast and colorectal cancer for women, and of colorectal and prostate cancer for men [8]. The incidence of some other malignant conditions such as brain tumors and skin cancer has increased in older persons for the last 30 years. Although the reasons for this increase are not totally clear, it is believed that age-related molecular alterations increase the likelihood of susceptibility to environmental carcinogens [9].

Elderly patients with cancer: how much does it cost?

Based on estimations from the National Institutes of Health, the annual direct medical cost of cancer treatment in the USA is around $60 billion. Healthcare costs vary depending on the therapeutic approach and type of malignancy. Within the Medicare system, for example, lung and colorectal cancer generate the highest costs ($17 500 per person per year) on average for the initial treatment, while the lowest cost is for breast cancer ($8913) [10].

Some tumors have a more benign profile in terms of economic impact, as is the case with prostate cancer, which has demonstrated an age-related decrease

Blood Disorders in the Elderly, ed. Lodovico Balducci, William Ershler, Giovanni de Gaetano.
Published by Cambridge University Press. © Cambridge University Press 2008.

in the costs of initial care. Cost reduction is due in part to a commonly used strategy of watchful waiting rather than active therapy in patients with a shorter life expectancy. The Group Health Cooperative study also showed that the costs of continuing care decreased with age for colon and breast cancer regardless of disease, stage, or age [10].

Chemotherapy-related side effects, such as neutropenia and myelosuppression, lead to febrile neutropenia, more frequent hospital admissions, longer lengths of stay, and thus higher direct costs [11,12]. Most of these complications can be treated with supportive care. The use of colony-stimulating factors after each chemotherapy cycle can reduce the length of the neutropenic period, resulting in lower hospitalization costs. On the other hand, outpatient care seems to be more cost-effective and comfortable for the patient, but it also has indirect costs that must be paid by patients or their families; these indirect costs include transportation to treatment sites, meals away from home, caregiver's time lost from work, and the intangible costs like emotional distress, pain, anger, and suffering [13,14].

Before starting any treatment

The aging process is a highly individualized and heterogeneous process, but these patients have common social, psychological, and physical characteristics that can influence how they should receive cancer treatment. Moreover, due to this individual process of aging, patients of the same chronologic age can differ greatly in physiologic age. Aging factors can have negative effects on the expected benefits of treatment and must be considered in the strategy of a patient's care [15,16].

No general agreement exists on the definition of frailty, which includes dependence in one or more activities of daily living (ADLs), three or more comorbid conditions, and one or more geriatric syndromes. It appears reasonable to thoroughly screen persons aged 85 and older for frailty, as the incidence of geriatric syndromes and functional dependence increases after this age. Frailty is a clear example of depleted functional reserve, and treatment with chemotherapy

may cross the thin line of equilibrium, resulting in severe side effects or even death [4,17]. Alzheimer disease and cognitive impairment are frequent findings in those older than 85 years. Depression, hearing impairment, and cognitive deficits can make complicated treatment regimens difficult to carry out effectively. Therapies that require active patient involvement and participation are even more difficult for patients with a superimposed reading or comprehension deficit [15].

Social issues, such as living far away from the treatment center, can be expensive and uncomfortable for patients who are not able to drive, and who need the help of friends or family to arrange transportation. In 2002, 19% of Americans lived in rural areas, but the figure was 24% for those aged 65 years and older. Between 1992 and 2002 the total rural population of the USA decreased by 4%, but among those over 50 it increased by 9% [18].

It is also very important to address the functional impairments and psychological sequelae associated with cancer treatment. Elderly patients require extra support whenever depression or anxiety becomes an obstacle during treatment. If the patient has a caregiver, it is necessary to evaluate the caregiver's competence and skills and also to assess the burden and stress that is generated while giving care and attention to the patient. Caregiver burden can be deleterious to both the caregiver and the patient [19].

Pharmacologic treatment of either the symptoms or the cancer should be carried out with extreme caution because of the higher likelihood of drug interactions and additive toxicity. This aspect is also important when selecting the appropriate chemotherapy regimen. Anthracyclines are considered toxic in older patients with some degree of cardiovascular disease and are contraindicated; newer agents of this class (e.g., epirubicin) are less toxic [16]. Successful treatment may also depend on nonmedical factors. For example, oral chemotherapeutic agents can be easily administered as an outpatient (at home), but non-compliance and erroneous dose administration are potential concerns [15].

It is of paramount importance always to look for orthostatic hypotension and postprandial hypotension, since these two syndromes are very common, and very easy to diagnose. Polypharmacy is often due to multiple hypertension medications, and can cause a sudden drop in the blood pressure, especially in the presence of other medications such as antipsychotics and narcotics. The importance of polypharmacy is reflected in a higher incidence of falls and hip fractures with orthostatic hypotension. The one-year mortality rate in elderly adults after hip fracture is 25%.

Comprehensive geriatric assessment

The history of the comprehensive geriatric assessment (CGA) dates back approximately 70 years. CGA was started in the United Kingdom by Dr. Marjory Warren at a hospital for chronic diseases where patients were elderly, neglected, and bedridden. Dr. Warren used a systematic approach to evaluate each patient and was therefore able to identify patients who might benefit from medical interventions and rehabilitation. The majority of these patients were then successfully discharged to their homes after receiving the comprehensive intervention. Warren soon demonstrated that the use of a strategy approach and multi-disciplinary intervention to assess elderly patients reduced placement in nursing homes. She became a leader in promoting the comprehensive assessment as a mainstay to evaluate elderly patients [20].

Over time, the practice of CGA has evolved to incorporate an extensive medical history, functional evaluation, social-work assessment, and other aspects of behavioral and social sciences. CGA is now employed routinely worldwide and has a key role in many venues of geriatric care, not only at the point of entry into nursing facilities [21].

Controlled clinical trials have showed that CGA is extremely useful in the recognition and management of a number of common geriatric problems, such as maintenance of independence and the prevention of institutionalization, delirium, and hospital readmission. It detects new and unsuspected problems in 76% of elderly persons living at home, and if it is done yearly, the incidence of new problems is reduced (Table 3.1) [22,23].

CGA is a multidimensional, interdisciplinary diagnostic process to determine the medical, psychological, and functional capabilities of a frail elderly person in order to develop a coordinated and integrated plan for treatment and long-term follow-up. While integrating standard medical diagnostic evaluation, CGA emphasizes quality of life, functional status, prognosis, and outcome that require a workup of more depth and breadth. The hallmarks of CGA are the employment of interdisciplinary teams and the use of any number of standardized instruments to evaluate aspects of patient functioning, impairments, and social supports (Table 3.2) [24,25].

Currently, the CGA is performed in a large number of institutional and community settings. CGA plays a very important role in services such as hospital geriatric units, primary care units (as a standard medical evaluation), and also in community-based services such as programs that provide comprehensive care for frail and disabled elderly patients. The short form of the CGA is known as the Multidimensional Geriatric Assessment. This abbreviated screening approach is performed by community health professionals to help decide when a referral is needed to geriatric specialty programs for a more comprehensive evaluation and management [20]. In patients with cancer, CGA was shown to improve emotional limitation, mental health, and bodily pain. Performing the CGA did not affect length of hospitalization or overall hospital costs [26]. This evaluation was easily administered in an abbreviated form in the outpatient setting and was effective in identifying cognitive and functional deficits in cancer patients [27].

The focus of a more extensive CGA is on the elderly who are frail (i.e., at risk of loss of homeostasis and incident disability), disabled, or both. Frailty is a clinically recognized syndrome that is common in older adults. Using recently developed criteria, the prevalence of marked frailty is less than 10% in community-dwelling adults 65 years and older, with high risk of mortality over 3 and 7 years. While the prevalence of disability appears to be declining somewhat, approximately one in five older Americans lives with some established disability. Given increases in the

Table 3.1. Practical screening questions and confirmatory tests.

Multidimensional screening	Screening method	Confirmatory test
Depression	Do you often feel sad or depressed?	GDS, positive if >5/15, workup for depression
Mental status	Name three objects and ask the patient to repeat them now and a few minutes later	MMSE, positive if <24, workup for dementia SLUMS
Comorbidity	Confirm the presence of serious chronic medical conditions from the ROS	Grade severity of each comorbid condition
Nutrition	Inquire about weight loss Weigh and measure the patient	Mini nutritional assessment (MNA)
ADLs	Inquire about ability to do basic activities (e.g., bathing, grooming, eating, continence, dressing)	Katz ADL scale
IADLs	Inquire about ability to do instrumental activities (e.g., cooking, handling finances, using the telephone, shopping, use of public transportation)	IADL scale
Social support	Ask about friends or relatives who would be able to help in case of an emergency	If none, try to arrange for a caregiver Assess independence of the caregiver if he/she is the same age as the patient
Polypharmacy	Review number, type, and indication of all medications	If more than three medications, look for compliance and interactions
Home environment	Ask about frequent tripping on objects and problems using stairs	Home safety evaluation

older population, particularly in the oldest old, the number of frail and disabled Americans has increased in the past decade and will continue to grow [28,29].

From its inception, geriatric medicine has recognized that frail and disabled older adults are at the highest risk for adverse outcomes and are also most likely to benefit from geriatric care. Subsequent health services and clinical research has sought to define the healthcare delivery modalities as well as specific interventions that would mitigate or even prevent frailty and its outcomes. The CGA has been central to this approach and has the objectives of improving diagnostic accuracy, optimizing medical treatment and health outcomes, improving function and quality of life, extending community tenure, reducing use of unnecessary formal services, and

instituting or improving long-term care management [30].

Once patients have been identified as appropriate for CGA screening, the usual model evokes a multidisciplinary approach to assessment. These teams are charged with improving the quality of care given to an older person, and the goal can be accomplished by delegating tasks to the most appropriate member of the team. Such team care requires a set of principles and coordination, or it can result in redundant and uncoordinated care. First among these principles is an understanding of the role of each member of the team and mutual respect among the different professions.

A thorough assessment of patients with cancer can help determine those who are candidates for

Table 3.2. Comprehensive geriatric assessment (CGA).

	Assessment	Additional evaluation
Geriatric syndromes	SLUMS scale Folstein mini mental Geriatric depression scale List of medical problems Delirium/confusion	Falls Osteoporosis Delirium Failure to thrive Abuse and neglect
Nutritional status	Mini nutritional assessment (MNA)	Regular weight monitoring
Comorbidity	Charlson comorbidity index Cumulative illness rating scale for geriatrics (CIRS-G)	Periodic update of problem list
Socioeconomic issues	Social work evaluation Complete documents for advance directives and legal decision makers	Living conditions Caregiver competence/burden Transportation Income
Functional status	ADLs IADLs Performance status Karnofsky scale	Routine review of functional deficits
Polypharmacy	Medication count and compliance review	Medication reduction Assessment Drug interactions Herbal and over-the-counter medicines
Mobility	Tinetti gait and balance "Get up and go" test	Safety evaluation
Blood pressure	Orthostatic hypotension Postprandial hypotension	Routine postural blood pressure Falls risk reduction
Pain	Faces scale	Routine pain inquiry

standard treatment to prolong life, as well as those in whom the potential benefits of such treatment are outweighed by its risks. The CGA can identify vulnerable patients that may still benefit from modified regimens, by substituting less-toxic agents; it also can point to non-medical factors that can be managed to make the treatment safer and more convenient. Frailty is a guide for simple pharmacologic palliation of symptoms or low-dose chemotherapy for tumor control.

Many forms of geriatric assessment exist, although some of them are too time-consuming to be applied to all geriatric patients, or even the frail and cognitive-impaired population. The National Comprehensive Cancer Network (NCCN) recommends that all patients older than 70 years be screened with some form of geriatric assessment. The consensus panel established that the evaluation must address at a minimum the following areas [16,31]:

- functional status
- comorbidity
- socioeconomic issues
- nutritional status
- polypharmacy
- geriatric syndromes

Table 3.3. Basic and instrumental activities of daily living (ADLs and IADLs).

ADLs			IADLs		
Activity	Independent	Needs assistance or unable to perform	Activity	Independent	Needs assistance or unable to perform
Dressing	......	......	Shopping	......	......
Bathing	......	......	Food preparation	......	......
Toileting	......	......	Telephone use	......	......
Transfer	......	......	Laundry	......	......
Feeding	......	......	Housekeeping	......	......
Continence	......	......	Medication	......	......
			Transportation	......	......
			Finances	......	......

- quality of life
- palliative care (advanced directives)
- pain
- elder abuse

Components of comprehensive geriatric assessment

Although the CGA has not been standardized and the detailed elements may vary, virtually all CGAs include screening for medical, psychological, social, functional, and environmental components.

A CGA can be effective only if there is a process for identifying elderly patients who may benefit from it. In most cases, they are elderly individuals who are frail and disabled or have multiple inter-acting comorbid conditions. As opposed to relatively healthy older people, including those whose health conditions are well managed with traditional medical approaches, those with serious chronic conditions benefit from disease management by a primary care provider with input from other subspecialists. Examples of at-risk older patients include those who appear to be on a rapid downward trajectory toward nursing-home placement, or a previously functional senior who is requiring increasing assistance to accomplish daily tasks [20].

Functional dependency

At the heart of CGA is a review of patient functioning, as reflected most commonly in terms of measures of ADLs. The ADLs are conveniently divided into the basic and instrumental (Table 3.3). The basic activities include the ability to bathe, dress, transfer from bed to chair, toilet and maintain continence, and eat without assistance [32,33]. In addition to the required daily activities, complex instrumental activities (IADLs) that one may do oneself include activities like handling finances, taking medications, performing domestic chores, using the telephone, shopping, and using public transportation [34].

In community-dwelling older patients, dependence in the basic ADLs is uncommon, and fewer than 10% of elderly people need assistance. Rates are much higher, however, among institutionalized and hospitalized patients and those older than 75 years [35]. One-third of community-residing people aged 85 years or older need assistance with one or more of the ADLs. Dependency in the performance of ADLs is most frequently a result of progressive disabilities related to specific health conditions, such as dementia, cancer, cardiovascular diseases, and musculoskeletal diseases. Once very old patients are disabled, they rarely recover independence, emphasizing the importance of preventing physical disability.

Despite the importance of functional assessment and the potential impact of interventions to prevent functional decline, functional disabilities are often overlooked and frequently go undertreated by physicians and nurses [36,37]. Early detection of risk factors for functional decline, when linked to specific interventions, may help reduce the incidence of functional disability and dependency for older patients.

In a frail patient, functional reserve is severely reduced, and tolerance to even a small stress is compromised. These individuals have at least one of the following: dependence in one or more ADLs, three or more relevant comorbidities, and one or more geriatric syndromes. Functional dependence is associated with shortened survival, and life expectancy is reduced by three years [38,39]. Dependence in instrumental activities like shopping, use of transportation and telephone, and handling finances can predict the development of clinical dementia in the following two years [40].

In many cases, particularly in ambulatory clinical settings, patients and/or caregivers are asked to report on these items by filling out questionnaires. In other settings, functioning may receive more extensive clinical evaluation by nurses or therapy providers. Given the importance of mobility in most functional activities, and the incidence of harmful consequences after falling, assessment of exercise practices, activity level, gait, and balance have become important functional assessments in most settings.

Dependence in one or more IADLs is associated with reduced tolerance to chemotherapy and a higher risk of developing complications from cytotoxic agents. However, if quality of life is the focus, frail individuals can still benefit from chemotherapy with drugs with a lower rate of complications, such as weekly taxanes, gemcitabine, or navelbine.

Cognitive impairment

Cognitive dysfunction is associated with a high risk of adverse outcomes after surgery and hospitalization. Unsuccessful rehabilitation from acute or chronic diseases can be attributed to the patient's inability to learn or retain new information. Dementia is the most common cause of cognitive impairment in elderly patients in outpatient setting and is associated with decreased survival. Cognition becomes progressively compromised with age, and by 85 almost 50% of the population demonstrates some degree of dementia [41]. Cognitive function can be assessed during medical interview by asking questions that probe the patient's short-term memory. Those with memory gaps or who provide minimal responses should be considered for further cognitive testing.

Screening for cognitive deficits can be achieved with instruments such as the Mini-Mental State Examination (MMSE), the Saint Louis University Mental Status Examination (SLUMS), which has demonstrated effective identification of patients with minimal cognitive impairment (Fig. 3.1), and the Clock Drawing Test, among others [42–44].

The MMSE is the most commonly used tool in quantifying the degree of cognitive impairment, although age and education influence performance. A score of less then 24 is consistent with cognitive dysfunction but not necessarily with dementia. The diagnosis of dementia requires documentation of a decline in intellectual functioning sufficient to interfere with personal or occupational functioning. Higher cut-points are used in educated and younger individuals. Once a patient is found to have cognitive dysfunction, further evaluation for the causes and possible treatments should be undertaken [45,46]. Dementia may be worsened by cytotoxic chemotherapy and associated with decreased tolerance to anti-neoplastic agents.

Delirium, defined as an acute change (<4 weeks) in mental status, is characterized by inattention, incoherent thinking, and altered level of consciousness (either hypoactive or agitated type of delirium). Delirium needs to be ruled out, since this entity carries a high mortality rate (25–30%) when it goes unrecognized in elderly patients (Table 3.4). The Confusion Assessment Method (CAM) is a very helpful tool to be used either in the office or at the bedside to identify patients with probable delirium (Table 3.5) [47].

VAMC
SLUMS Examination

Questions about this assessment tool? E-mail aging@slu.edu.

Name ——————————————————— Age ———————————————
Is patient alert? ——————————————— Level of education ———————————

/1 ❶ 1. What day of the week is it?

/1 ❶ 2. What is the year?

/1 ❶ 3. What state are we in?

Department of Veterans Affairs

4. Please remember these five objects. I will ask you what they are later.

　　　Apple　　　Pen　　　Tie　　　House　　　Car

5. You have $100 and you go to the store and buy a dozen apples for $3 and a tricycle for $20.
　　❶　How much did you spend?
/3 ❷　How much do you have left?

6. Please name as many animals as you can in one minute.
/3 　　❶ 0-4 animals　❶ 5-9 animals　❷10-14 animals　❸ 15+ animals

/5 7. What were the five objects I asked you to remember? 1 point for each one correct.

8. I am going to give you a series of numbers and I would like you to give them to me backwards.
　　For example, if I say 42, you would say 24.
/2 　　❶ 87　　　❶ 649　　　❶ 8537

9. This is a clock face. Please put in the hour markers and the time at
　　ten minutes to eleven o'clock.
　❷　Hour markers okay
/4 ❷　Time correct

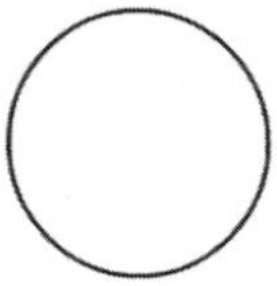

/2 ❶ 10. Please place an X in the triangle.

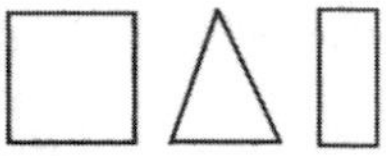

　　❶　Which of the above figures is largest?

11. I am going to tell you a story. Please listen carefully because afterwards, I'm going to ask you
　　some questions about it.
　　Jill was a very successful stockbroker. She made a lot of money on the stock market. She then met
　　Jack, a devastatingly handsome man. She married him and had three children. They lived in Chicago.
　　She then stopped work and stayed at home to bring up her children. When they were teenagers, she
　　went back to work. She and Jack lived happily ever after.
　❷ What was the female's name?　　　　❷ What work did she do?
/8 ❷ When did she go back to work?　　　❷ What state did she live in?

———— **TOTAL SCORE**

Department of Veterans Affairs

SAINT LOUIS UNIVERSITY

SCORING		
HIGH SCHOOL EDUCATION		**LESS THAN HIGH SCHOOL EDUCATION**
27-30	Normal	25-30
21-26	MNCD*	20-24
1-20	Dementia	1-19
* Mild Neurocognitive Disorder		

Figure 3.1 The Saint Louis University Mental Status (SLUMS) examination [43].

Table 3.4. Delirium mnemonic (Saint Louis University Delirium Mnemonics).

Drugs (polypharmacy)
Eyes and ears
Low O_2 state (MI, PE, Stroke)
Infection
Retention (feces, urine)
Ictal
Underhydration
Metabolic
Subdural

Table 3.5. Confusion Assessment Method (CAM) [47].

1 Acute onset and fluctuating
    Is there a change from the patient's baseline (usually
      <4 weeks)?
    Does abnormal behavior tend to come/go,
      increase/decrease in severity?
2 Inattention (or attention deficit)
    Could not complete days of the week backwards or
      numbers backwards, or patient easily distracted and
      cannot concentrate
3 Disorganized/incoherent thinking
    Rambling, irrelevant conversation
    Unclear/illogical flow of ideas
    Switching from subject to subject
4 Altered level of consciousness
    Is LOC something other than alert?
    Agitated/hyperalert, lethargic, stupor or coma

Diagnosis of delirium requires presence of 1 and 2, then either 3 or 4.

Depression

Depressive symptoms are common in the community-dwelling population, with some surveys suggesting that 10% of people over age 65 have depressive symptoms, and 1% have a major depressive disorder. Depression is associated with physical decline, in hospitalized and community-dwelling older adults, and also it has been associated with decreased survival. It is a frequent cause of weight loss and failure to thrive, and is considered a geriatric syndrome. Depression has also been associated with decreased survival in older individuals with cancer, and it reduces the motivation to receive treatment [22].

Screening for depression is very important given the common atypical presentations of this entity in the very old and the relation between depression and cognitive dysfunction, functional decline, and increased risk of suicide. Furthermore, depression can be easily treated with medications, psychotherapy, or even in the most severe cases electroconvulsive therapy (ECT). Screening for depression can be achieved using validated instruments, notably the short-form Geriatric Depression Scale (GDS) (Table 3.6) [48,49]. Patients with positive screens need further diagnostic evaluation and treatment, and this evaluation should include a complete workup for reversible causes of depression such as metabolic abnormalities, hypothyroidism, and hypogonadism.

Low testosterone levels (hypogonadism) in older men can mimic depression and also lead to sarcopenia and osteoporosis. A simple screening test is the Saint Louis University Androgen Deficiency in Aging Males (ADAM) questionnaire (Table 3.7) [50]. Chemotherapy has been shown to produce hypogonadism in cancer patients, secondary to testicular damage.

Falls and impaired mobility

Disorders of balance and gait increase with age and predispose elderly patients to falls. Accidental falls can be serious, and account for injuries including head trauma, hip fracture, and soft-tissue trauma. Chronic medical conditions, particularly musculoskeletal and neurologic disorders and polypharmacy, increase the risk of falls. Falls may lead to a fear of falling again, loss of mobility and decline in functional status.

It is important to recognize that frequent falls can be a symptom of delirium, and thus the patient needs to be evaluated for this condition. About 30% of community-residing elderly Americans fall each year, with rates as high as 50% among persons

Table 3.6. Patient assessment tool: Geriatric Depression Scale. Adapted from Yesavage *et al.* – [48], Sheikh & Yesavage 1986 [49].

Choose the best answer for how you felt this past week	Circle one	
* 1 Are you basically satisfied with your life?	yes	NO
2 Have you dropped many of your activities and interests?	YES	no
3 Do you feel that your life is empty?	YES	no
4 Do you often get bored?	YES	no
* 5 Are you in good spirits most of the time?	yes	NO
6 Are you afraid that something bad is going to happen to you?	YES	no
* 7 Do you feel happy most of the time?	yes	NO
8 Do you often feel helpless?	YES	no
9 Do you prefer to stay at home, rather than going out and doing new things?	YES	no
10 Do you feel you have more problems with memory than most?	YES	no
*11 Do you think it is wonderful to be alive now?	yes	NO
12 Do you feel pretty worthless the way you are now?	YES	no
*13 Do you feel full of energy?	yes	NO
14 Do you feel that your situation is hopeless?	YES	no
15 Do you think that most people are better off than you are?	YES	no

*Appropriate (non-depressed) answers = yes, all others = no.
Or count number of CAPITALIZED (depressed) answers.
Score = number of "depressed" answers.
Norms: 0–5, normal; 6–15, suggests depression.

Table 3.7. Androgen deficiency in the aging male (ADAM) scale for hypogonadism [50].

1 Do you have a decrease in libido?	yes/no
2 Do you have a lack of energy?	yes/no
3 Do you have a decrease in strength and/or endurance?	yes/no
4 Do you have a decreased enjoyment of life?	yes/no
5 Are you sad?	yes/no
6 Are you grumpy?	yes/no
7 Are your erections less strong?	yes/no
8 Have you noticed a recent deterioration in your ability to play sports?	yes/no
9 Are you falling asleep easily after dinner?	yes/no
10 Has there been any deterioration in your work performance?	yes/no

A positive score represents a *yes* to questions 1 or 7, or to any other three questions.

80 years and older [51]. Approximately 20% of elderly adults have some degree of difficulty walking and require the assistance of another person or assistive devices for independence. Almost 40% of patients older than 85 years need assistance with walking.

Screening and a detailed evaluation are therefore of high yield in identifying patients who should benefit from interventions [52,53], including tests of gait and mobility. A commonly used tool for evaluating ambulatory mobility is the Tinnetti gait and balance test (Fig. 3.2). Leg mobility and muscular strength can also be easily evaluated with the use of the "get up and go" test [54]. Upper-extremity mobility can be tested by asking the patient to raise arms straight up in the air, behind the neck, and behind the back [55]. A timed six-meter walk or the distance walked in six minutes can be used to provide objective information on physical performance. Balance platforms can provide further information on balance problems in older persons.

Orthostatic hypotension is common in older persons and can be a cause of falls. Orthostatic hypotension is a physical finding defined by the American Autonomic Society and the American Academy of Neurology as a systolic blood pressure decrease of at least 20 mm Hg or a diastolic blood pressure decrease of at least 10 mm Hg within three minutes of standing. The condition, which may be symptomatic or

Tinetti Assessment Tool: Balance

Patient: _____ Date: _____

Location: _____ Rater: _____

Initial Instructions: Subject is seated in a hard, armless chair. The following maneuvers are tested.

Task	Description of Balance	Score
1. Sitting balance:	Leans or slides in chair Steady, safe	= 0 = 1
2. Arises:	Unable without help Able, uses arms to help Able without using arms	= 0 = 1 = 2
3. Attempts to arise:	Unable without help Able, requires >1 attempt Able to arise, 1 attempt	= 0 = 1 = 2
4. Immediate standing balance	(first five seconds): Unsteady (swaggers, moves feet, trunk sway) Steady but uses walker or other support Steady without walker or other support	= 0 = 1 = 2
5. Standing balance	Unsteady Steady but wide stance (medial heels >4 in. apart) and uses cane or other support Narrow stance without support	= 0 = 1 = 2
6. Nudged	(subject at maximum position with feet as close together as possible, examiner pushes lightly on subject's sternum with palm of hand 3 times): Begins to fall Staggers, grabs, catches self Steady	 = 0 = 1 = 2
7. Eyes Closed	(at maximum position No. 6) Unsteady Steady	= 0 = 1
8. Turning 360 degrees	Discontinuous steps Continuous Unsteady (grabs, staggers) Steady	= 0 = 1 = 0 = 1
9. Sitting down	Unsafe (misjudges distance, falls into chair) Uses arms or not a smooth motion Safe, smooth motion	= 0 = 1 = 2

Balance Score: _____ /16

Source: The Journal of the American Geriatic Society by Carole Lewis Ph.D, PT

Tinetti Assessment Tool: Gait

Patient: _____ Date: _____

Location: _____ Rater: _____

Initial Instructions: Subject stands with examiner, walks down hallway or across room, first at "usual" pace, then back at "rapid, but safe" pace (using usual walking aids).

Task	Description of Gait	Score
10. Initiation of gait	(Immediately after told to "go") Any hesitancy or multiple attempts to start No hesitancy	= 0 = 1
11. Step length and height a. Right swing foot:	does not pass left stance foot with step passes left stance foot right foot does not clear floor completely with step right foot completely clears floor	= 0 = 1 = 0 = 1
b. Left swing foot:	does not pass right stance foot with step passes right stance foot left foot does not clear floor completely with step left foot completely clears floor	= 0 = 1 = 0 = 1
12. Step Symmetry	Right and left step length not equal (estimate) Right and left step appear equal	= 0 = 1
13. Step Continuity	Stopping or discontinuity between steps Steps appear continuous	= 0 = 1
14. Path	(estimated in relation to floor tiles, 12-inch diameter; observe excursion of 1 foot over about 10 ft. of the course.) Marked deviation Mild/moderate deviator or uses walking aid Straight without walking aid	 = 0 = 1 = 2
15. Trunk	Marked sway or uses walking aid No sway but flexion of knees or back or spreads arms out while walking No, sway, no flexion, no use of arms, and not use of walking aid	= 0 = 1 = 2
16. Walking Time	Heels apart Heels almost touching while walking	= 0 = 1

Gait Score: _____ /12

Balance + Gait Score: _____ /28

Source: The Journal of the American Geriatic Society by Carole Lewis Ph.D, PT

Figure 3.2 Tinetti assessment tool for balance and gait.

asymptomatic, is encountered commonly in the geriatric practice. In healthy persons, muscle contraction increases venous return of blood to the heart through one-way valves that prevent blood from pooling in dependent parts of the body. The autonomic nervous system responds to changes in position by constricting veins and arteries and increasing heart rate and cardiac contractility. When these mechanisms are faulty, or if the patient is hypovolemic, orthostatic hypotension may occur. In persons with orthostatic hypotension, gravitational opposition to venous return causes a decrease in blood pressure and threatens cerebral ischemia.

Several potential causes of orthostatic hypotension include medications; non-neurogenic causes such as impaired venous return, hypovolemia, and cardiac insufficiency; and neurogenic causes such as multisystem atrophy and diabetic neuropathy. Treatment generally is aimed at the underlying cause, and a variety of pharmacologic or non-pharmacologic treatments may relieve symptoms. Orthostatic hypotension has been observed in all age groups, but it occurs more frequently in the elderly, especially in persons who are sick and frail. It is associated with several diagnoses, conditions, and symptoms, including lightheadedness soon after standing, an increased rate of falls, and a history of myocardial infarction or transient ischemic attack; it also may be predictive of ischemic stroke.

Nutritional assessment

The prevalence of nutrient-specific malnutrition is higher in people over age 65. Older adults have a higher risk for undernutrition and weight loss than younger adults. Conditions associated with a higher prevalence of weight loss include severe chronic medical conditions, physical disability, difficulty chewing, social isolation, and limited income.

Based on the results of several surveys, it is known that the median energy intake for elderly adults is below the recommended levels, particularly among African-Americans and minorities. Weight loss is a marker of future malnutrition, depression, and dementia. Guidelines for the detection of

undernutrition in the elderly have been developed, and patients should be asked whether they have had a weight loss of 10% or more in the previous six months. If the answer is positive, then further screening and laboratory evaluation are warranted [56,57]. Anorexia, which is a common concomitant of cancer as well as aging, can be assessed by the Simplified Nutritional Questionnaire (SNAQ). The Mini Nutritional Assessment (MNA) is a validated approach to the nutritional status of the patient, and it requires no laboratory testing (Fig. 3.3) [58]. The use of albumin, pre-albumin, and retinol binding protein are limited as nutritional tools in cancer patients, as cytokine excess decreases values by displacing these proteins into the extravascular space.

The assessment of nutrition using the MNA is useful to recognize patients who are malnourished and at risk of developing malnutrition. Approximately 20% of persons older than 70 years have some degree of protein/energy malnutrition, and the prevalence is even higher when cancer is present at the same time. With timely intervention malnutrition may be prevented or reversed in older patients [58–60].

Malnutrition correlates with a greater risk for severe hematotoxic effects with chemotherapy. This is particularly true in the case of older patients, who already have decreased hematopoietic reserves.

Pain

Pain is now considered the fifth vital sign, and screening for pain is best done with a Likert-based rating scale. Faces depicting different levels of pain are generally better at eliciting the appropriate level of pain in older persons. Pain must be treated when identified, and a cause should be sought, since pain can be an isolated symptom of cancer. When this important symptom is not addressed properly it interferes deeply with the patient's quality of life, leading to disability, fear to mobilize, and depression.

Urinary incontinence

Urinary incontinence (UI) is defined as the involuntary loss of urine, of sufficient severity to be a health

Complete the screen by filling in the boxes with the appropriate numbers.
Add the numbers for the screen. If score is 11 or less, continue with the assessment to gain a Malnutrition Indicator Score.

Screening

A Has food intake declined over the past 3 months due to loss of appetite, digestive problems, chewing or swallowing difficulties?
  0 = severe loss of appetite
  1 = moderate loss of appetite
  2 = no loss of appetite ☐

B Weight loss during the last 3 months
  0 = weight loss greater than 3 kg (6.6 lbs)
  1 = does not know
  2 = weight loss between 1 and 3 kg (2.2 and 6.6 lbs)
  3 = no weight loss ☐

C Mobility
  0 = bed or chair bound
  1 = able to get out of bed/chair but does not go out
  2 = goes out ☐

D Has suffered psychological stress or acute disease in the past 3 months
  0 = yes   2 = no ☐

E Neuropsychological problems
  0 = severe dementia or depression
  1 = mild dementia
  2 = no psychological problems ☐

F Body Mass Index (BMI) (weight in kg)/(height in m)^2
  0 = BMI less than 19
  1 = BMI 19 to less than 21
  2 = BMI 21 to less than 23
  3 = BMI 23 or greater ☐

Screening score (subtotal max. 14 points) ☐ ☐
12 points or greater Normal – not at risk – no need to complete assessment
11 points or below Possible malnutrition – continue assessment

Assessment

G Lives independently (not in a nursing home or hospital)
  0 = no   1 = yes ☐

H Takes more than 3 prescription drugs per day
  0 = yes   1 = no ☐

I Pressure sores of skin ulcers
  0 = yes   1 = no ☐

Ref.: Guigoz Y, Vellas B and Garry PJ. 1994. Mini Nutritional Assessment: A practical assessment tool for grading the nutritional state of elderly patients. *Facts and Research in Gerontology*. Supplement #2:15-59.
Rubenstein LZ, Harker J, Guigoz Y and Vellas B. Comprehensive Geriatric Assessment (CGA) and the MNA: An Overview of CGA, Nutritional Assessment and Development of a Shortened Version of the MNA. In: "Mini Nutritional Assessment (MNA): Research and Practice in the Elderly". Vellas B. Garry PJ and Guigoz Y., editors. Nestlé Nutrition Workshop Series. Clinical & Performance Programme. vol. 1. Karger, Bale, in press.

J How many full meals does the patient eat daily?
  0 = 1 meal
  1 = 2 meals
  2 = 3 meals ☐

K Selected consumption markers for protein intake
  – At least one serving of dairy products
     (milk, cheese, yogurt) per day?   yes ☐ no ☐
  – Two or more servings of legumes
     or eggs per week?   yes ☐ no ☐
  – Meat, fish or poultry every day   yes ☐ no ☐
  0.0 = if 0 or 1 yes
  0.5 = if 2 yes
  1.0 = if 3 yes ☐.☐

L Consumes two or more servings of fruits or vegetables per day?
  0 = no   1 = yes ☐

M How much fluid (water, juice, coffee, tea, milk…) is consumed per day?
  0.0 = less than 3 cups
  0.5 = 3 to 5 cups
  1.0 = more than 5 cups ☐.☐

N Mode of feeding
  0 = unable to eat without assistance
  1 = self-fed with some difficulty
  2 = self-fed without any problem ☐

O Self view of nutritional status
  0 = views self as being malnourished
  1 = is uncertain of nutritional state
  2 = views self as having no nutritional problem ☐

P In comparison with other people of the same age, how does the patient consider his/her health status?
  0.0 = not as good
  0.5 = does not know
  1.0 = as good
  2.0 = better ☐.☐

Q Mid-arm circumference (MAC) in cm
  0.0 = MAC less than 21
  0.5 = MAC 21 to 22
  1.0 = MAC 22 or greater ☐.☐

R Calf circumference (CC) in cm
  0 = CC less than 31   1 = CC 31 or greater ☐

Assessment (max. 16 points) ☐ ☐.☐

Screening score ☐ ☐

Total Assessment (max. 30 points) ☐ ☐.☐

Malnutrition Indicator Score
17 to 23.5 points   at risk malnutrition ☐
Less than 17 points   malnourished ☐

Figure 3.3 The Mini Nutritional Assessment (MNA).

or social problem. It is a potentially disabling condition which is treatable and sometimes curable. The prevalence of UI increases in women over 65 years (10–15%) and in men and women older than 85 years (25%). Dementia and physical impairment are often associated with UI, and this explains the higher prevalence of this entity in nursing homes. Incontinence problems are often under-reported by patients and their families, and physicians frequently fail to ask about symptoms. Simple screening questions can be used when looking for incontinence: "Have you lost your urine on at least six separate days?" If the patient answers *yes* to this question, further evaluation is needed: infection must be excluded, and assessment for elevated post-void residual urine must be performed. A thorough assessment of UI symptoms includes a detailed voiding history, evaluation of current medications, pelvic and/or rectal examination, and assessment of bladder functioning. Much of this initial evaluation can take place in the primary care setting, although urogynecology referral may be necessary [61].

Visual and hearing impairment

Visual impairment increases sharply with advancing age. The prevalence of blindness increases from 1% in those 71–74 years old to 17% in those 90 years and older [62]. Age-related visual changes affect central visual acuity, peripheral vision, contrast sensitivity, and color vision. The most common cause of blindness is age-related macular degeneration. There are two preventable causes of blindness: cataracts and glaucoma. Whites are more susceptible to develop macular degeneration, whereas African-Americans more often have open-angle glaucoma. Visual impairment often goes unrecognized or undertreated, and is associated with functional dependency. The prevalence of bilateral blindness in nursing homes is around 17% and the prevalence of visual impairment is 19%, but these conditions are rarely listed as a medical diagnosis [63,64]. Ideally in an older person both field of vision and visual acuity should be assessed.

Hearing loss is present in about 24% of people 65–74 years old, and in 40% of those older than 75. Hearing loss is associated with significant emotional and social dysfunction even in patients with mild to moderate degrees of hearing loss. Only a few of older patients with hearing impairment use hearing aids, which suggests that better screening and assessment is needed. Intervention programs can help to improve the quality of life for this population [65,66].

Hearing loss is categorized as sensorineural, conductive, or both. Sensorineural hearing loss is caused by cochlear disease and is the most common cause of presbycusis. Conductive hearing loss results from impaired sound transmission to the inner ear. The most common causes for this condition are cerumen impaction and otosclerosis. A useful tool for office screening is an otoscope with built-in audiometer. Patients with abnormal audiometry testing require further evaluation. The whisper test is less precise than the audioscope, but can be completed quickly by an office assistant or during the physical examination. To check for hearing impairment, the examiner stands 30–35 cm (12–14 inches) behind the patient, covers one ear, and whispers three words in the uncovered ear. Inability to accurately repeat the words should prompt an examination to exclude cerumen impaction, before a referral to an audiologist.

Elder abuse

Elder abuse occurs in up to 5% of older persons. It is more common in the disabled, and it should be considered a possibility in any person with unexplained bruises, fractures, or poor-quality care. All medical professionals are required to report suspected abuse of adults age 65 or older. Abuse can be physical, mental, verbal, or sexual. Economic abuse also occurs commonly when older persons become vulnerable. Neglect by either a caregiver or by oneself is considered a form of abuse. Tools to assess caregiver strain and to screen for elder abuse allow medical professionals to identify stressors that can potentially lead to an abusive situation.

Quality of life

"Quality of life" (QOL) is a term commonly used by health professionals when trying to help patients and families make decisions concerning care near the end of life. Formal studies using QOL instruments are increasingly common in clinical trials, typically used as an outcome measurement before and after treatment. Implicit is the notion that if *quantity* of time left cannot be increased, then *quality* of life should be maximized.

But what does quality of life mean, and how should clinicians use this information in decision making? There are two key concepts about QOL: (1) it is multidimensional, and (2) it is most appropriately

Table 3.8. Karnofsky performance scale [68].

Condition	Percentage	Comments
(A) Able to carry on normal activity and to work	100	Normal, no complaints, no evidence of disease
No special care is needed	90	Able to carry on normal activity, minor signs or symptoms of disease
	80	Normal activity with effort, some signs or symptoms of disease
(B) Unable to work. Able to live at home, care for most personal needs. A varying degree of assistance is needed	70	Cares for self, unable to carry on normal activity or to do active work
	60	Requires occasional assistance, but is able to care for most of his/her needs
	50	Disease may be progressing rapidly: requires considerable assistance and frequent medical care
(C) Unable to care for self. Requires equivalent of institutional or hospital care	40	Disabled: requires special care and assistance
	30	Severely disabled: hospitalization is indicated although death not imminent
	20	Hospitalization necessary: very sick, active supportive treatment necessary
	10	Moribund: fatal processes progressing rapidly
	0	Dead

determined by the patient. Although family members, physicians, and other health professionals can make significant observations about QOL, studies consistently document important variances between patient- and surrogate-defined QOL. A quality-of-life assessment can be considered a review of systems of the patient's world.

Multidimensionality can be assessed by asking questions in the key domains of (1) physical, (2) functional, (3) emotional, (4) social, and (5) spiritual/existential. The sum of these questions can be a "snapshot" of the patient's world, and can give the clinician an idea of what is important to a patient, and what goals of care may be meaningful. For cancer patients, two of the most commonly used QOL scales are the FACT scale developed by Dr. D. Cella [67], which has been validated for a wide variety of tumors and gives an accurate sense of the QOL, and the Karnofsky scale (Table 3.8) [68], which is more focused on the functional status of the patient

and his or her ability to perform certain physical activities.

Conclusions

Potentially curative therapies should not be withheld from older patients because of their age alone. The routine use of the CGA provides valuable information about patient condition, functional status, and overall health risks. Based on the CGA, it is possible to recognize patients who are functional and independent, patients who are dependent in one or more IADLs with associated comorbid conditions, and patients who are very frail. When facing frail patients, symptom palliation and preservation of quality of life are the most important tasks for the healthcare team. The incidence and prevalence of changes associated with aging increases dramatically after the age of 70. It is reasonable practice for all patients aged 70 or older to have a complete geriatric evaluation, but it could also be indicated in persons younger than 70 years with decline in physical and cognitive performance.

Aging itself is a natural phenomenon, but the pace and severity of aging is a completely individualized process that is influenced by the environment and genetic background of each individual. Since frailty is poorly correlated with chronological age, functional ability is a better marker for initiating the multidisciplinary evaluation of older adults afflicted with a cancer diagnosis.

Understanding the quality of life of older persons represents an important step in allowing them to make rational treatment decisions. Overall the assessment of function in elderly patients with cancer is highly recommended, using assessment tools to improve the understanding of both the medical and the bio-psycho-social background of each patient.

REFERENCES

1. Balducci L. New paradigms for treating elderly patients with cancer: the comprehensive geriatric assessment and guidelines for supportive care. *J Support Oncol* 2003; **1** (4 Suppl 2): 30–7.

2. Ershler W. Cancer: a disease of the elderly. *J Support Oncol* 2003; **1** (4 Suppl 2): 5–10.

3. Yancik R, Ries LA. Aging and cancer in America: demographic and epidemiologic perspectives. *Hematol Oncol Clin North Am* 2000; **14**: 17–23.

4. Suzman RM, Willis DP. *The Oldest Old* (New York, NY: Oxford University Press, 1992).

5. Lichtman SM. Guidelines for the treatment of elderly cancer patients. *Cancer Control* 2003; **10**: 445–53.

6. Yancik R, Yates W. *Cancer in the Elderly: Approaches to Early Detection and Treatment* (New York, NY: Springer, 1989).

7. Edwards BK, Howe HL, Ries LA, *et al.* Annual report to the nation on the status of cancer, 1973–1999, featuring implications of age and aging on U.S. cancer burden. *Cancer* 2004; **94**: 2766–92.

8. Jemal A, Murray T, Samuels A, *et al.* Cancer statistics, 2003. *CA Cancer J Clin* 2003; **53**: 5–29.

9. Balducci L, Ballester OF. Non-Hodgkin's lymphoma in the elderly. *Cancer Control* 1996; **3** (5 Suppl 1): 5–14.

10. Riley GF, Potosky AL, Lubitz JD, Kessler LG. Medicare payments from diagnosis to death for elderly cancer patients by stage at diagnosis. *Med Care* 1995; **33**: 828–41.

11. Chrischilles E, Delgado DJ, Stolshek BS, *et al.* Impact of age and colony stimulating-factor use on hospital length of stay for febrile neutropenia in CHOP treated non-Hodgkin's lymphoma. *Cancer Control* 2002; **9**: 203–11.

12. Morrison VA, Picozzi V, Scott S. The impact of age on delivered dose intensity and hospitalizations for febrile neutropenia in patients with intermediate-grade non-Hodgkin's lymphoma receiving initial CHOP chemotherapy: a risk factor analysis. *Clin Lymphoma* 2001; **2**: 47–56.

13. Repetto L, Carreca I, Maraninchi D, *et al.* Use of growth factors in the elderly patient with cancer: a report from the Second International Society for Geriatric Oncology 2001 meeting. *Crit Rev Oncol Hematol* 2003; **45**: 123–8.

14. Spiegel D. Psychosocial aspects of breast cancer treatment. *Semin Oncol* 1997; **24**: S1.36–S1.47.

15. Monfardini S. Prescribing anti-cancer drugs in elderly patients with cancer. *Eur J Cancer* 2002; **38**: 2341–6.

16. Balducci L, Yates J. General guidelines for the management of older patients with cancer. *Oncology* 2000; **14**: 221–7.

17. Lichtman SM, Villani G. Chemotherapy in the elderly: pharmacologic considerations. *Cancer Control* 2000; **7**: 548–56.

18. American Association of Retired Persons (AARP). *Beyond 50.03: a Report to the Nation on Independent Living and Disability.* http://research.aarp.org/il/beyond_50_il.html. Accessed March 15, 2007.

19. Haley W. Family caregivers of elderly patients with cancer. understanding and minimizing the burden of care. *J Support Oncol* 2003; **1** (Suppl 2): 25–9.

20. Wieland D, Hirth V. Comprehensive geriatric assessment. *Cancer Control* 2003; **10**: 454–62.

21. Rubenstein LZ, Josephson KR, Wieland GD, English PA, Sayre JA, Kane RL. Effectiveness of a geriatric evaluation unit: a randomized clinical trial. *N Engl J Med* 1984; **311**: 1664–70.

22. Balducci L, Extermann M. Management of cancer in the older person: a practical approach. *Oncologist* 2000; **5**: 224–37.

23. Reuben DB, Frank JC, Hirsch SH, McGuigan KA, Maly RC. A randomized clinical trial of outpatient comprehensive geriatric assessment, coupled with an intervention, to increase adherence to recommendations. *J Am Geriatr Soc* 199; **47**: 269–76.

24. Kane RL, Kane RA. *Assessing Older Persons: Measures, Meaning and Practical Application* (New York, NY: Oxford University Press, 2000).

25. Gallo JJ, Fulmer T, Paveza GJ, Reichel W. *Handbook of Geriatric Assessment*, 3rd edn (Gaithersburg, MD: Aspen, 2000).

26. Extermann M, Aapro M, Bernabei R, *et al.* Use of comprehensive geriatric assessment in older cancer patients: recommendations from the Task Force on CGA of the International Society of Geriatric Oncology. *Crit Rev Oncol Hematol* 2005; **55**: 241–52.

27. Hurria A, Gupta S, Zauderer M, *et al.* Developing a cancer-specific geriatric assessment. *Cancer* 2005; **104**: 1998–2005.

28. Buchner DM, Wagner EH. Preventing frail health. *Clin Geriatr Med* 1992; **8**: 1–17.

29. Freedman VA, Martin LG, Schoeni RF. Recent trends in disability and functioning among older adults in the United States: a systematic review. *JAMA* 2002; **288**: 3137–46.

30. Rubenstein LZ. An overview of comprehensive geriatric assessment: rationale, history, program models, basic components. In Rubenstein LZ, Wieland D, Bernabei R, eds, *Geriatric Assessment Technology: the State of the Art* (New York, NY: Springer, 1995).

31. Lachs MS, Feinstein AR, Cooney LM, *et al.* A simple procedure for general screening for functional disability in elderly patients. *Ann Intern Med* 1990; **112**: 699–706.

32. Katz S, Ford A, Moskowitz R, Jackson BA, Jaffe MW. Studies of illness in the aged: the index of ADL – a standardized measure of biological and psychosocial function. *JAMA* 1993; **185**: 914–19.

33. Lawton MP, Brody EM. Assessment of older people: self-maintaining and instruments of daily living. *Gerontologist* 1969; **9**: 179–86.

34. Palmer R. Geriatric assessment. *Med Clin North Am* 1999; **83**: 1503–23.

35. Manton KG, Corder L, Stallard E. Chronic disability trends in elderly United States population: 1982–1994. *Proc Natl Acad Sci USA* 1997; **94**: 2593–8

36. Meldon SW, Emerman CL, Schubert DS. Recognition of depression in geriatric ED patients by emergency physicians. *Ann Emerg Med* 1997; **30**: 442–7.

37. Pinholt EM, Kroenke K, Hanley JF, Kussman MJ, Twyman PL, Carpenter JL. Functional assessment of the elderly: a comparison of standard instruments with clinical judgment. *Arch Intern Med* 1987; **147**: 484–8.

38. Reuben DB, Rubenstein LV, Hirsch SH, Hays RD. Value of functional status as predictor of mortality. *Am J Med* 1992; **93**: 663–9.

39. Siu AL, Morishita L, Blaustein J. Comprehensive geriatric assessment in a day hospital. *J Am Geriatr Soc* 1994; **42**: 1094–9.

40. Monfardini S, Ferrucci L, Fratino L, del Lungo I, Serraino D, Zagonel V. Validation of a multidimensional evaluation scale for use in elderly cancer patients. *Cancer* 1996; **77**: 395–401.

41. Hogan DB, Ebly EM, Fung TS. Disease, disability, and age in cognitively intact seniors: results from the Canadian Study of Health and Aging. *J Gerontol A Biol Sci Med Sci* 1999; **54**: M77–M82.

42. Folstein MF, Folstein SE, McHugh PR. Mini-mental state: a practical method of grading the cognitive state of patients for the clinician. *J Psychiatr Res* 1975; **12**: 189–98.

43. Tariq SH, Tumosa N, Chibnall JT, Perry MH, Morley JE. Comparison of the Saint Louis University mental status examination and the mini-mental state examination for detecting dementia and mild neurocognitive disorder: a pilot study. *Am J Geriatr Psychiatry* 2006; **14**: 900–10.

44. Sunderland T, Hill JL, Mellow AM, *et al.* Clock drawing in Alzheimer's disease: a novel measure of dementia severity. *J Am Geriatr Soc* 1989; **37**: 725–9.

45. Geldmacher DS, Whitehouse PJ. Evaluation of dementia. *N Engl J Med* 1999; **335**: 330–6.

46. Siu AL. Screening for dementia and investigating its causes. *Ann Intern Med* 1991; **115**: 122–32.

47. Inouye SK, van Dyck CH, Alessi CA, Balkin S, Siegal AP, Horwitz RI. Clarifying confusion: the confusion assessment method. A new method for detection of delirium. *Ann Intern Med* 1990; **113**: 941–8.

48. Yesavage JA, Brink TL, Rose TL, *et al.* Development and validation of a geriatric depression screening scale: a preliminary report. *J Psychiatr Res* 1982–3; **17**: 37–49.

49. Sheikh J, Yesavage JA. The Geriatric Depression Scale: recent evidence and development of a shorter version. *Clin Gerontol* 1986; **9**: 165–73.

50. Morley JE, Charlton E, Patrick P, *et al.* Validation of a screening questionnaire for androgen deficiency in aging males. *Metabolism* 2000; **49**: 1239–42.

51. Tinetti ME, Speechley M, Ginter SF. Risk factors for falls among elderly persons living in the community. *N Engl J Med* 1997; **319**: 1701–7.

52. Province MA, Hadley EC, Hornbrook MC, *et al.* The effects of exercise on falls in elderly patients. JAMA 1995; **272**: 1341–7.

53. Tinetti ME, Baker DI, McAvay G, *et al*. A multifactorial intervention to reduce the risk of falling among elderly people living in the community. *N Engl J Med* 1994; **331**: 821–7.

54. Mathias S, Nayak US, Isaacs B. Balance in elderly patients: the "get-up and go" test. *Arch Phys Med Rehabil* 1986; **67**: 387–9.

55. Foley K, Palmer RM. Office evaluation of the frail older: practical tips. *Home Med* 1996; **32**: 21.

56. Marwick C. NHANES III health data relevant for aging nation. *JAMA* 1997; **227**: 100–2.

57. Potter J, Langhorne P, Roberts M. Routine protein energy supplementation in adults: systematic review. *BMJ* 1998; **317**: 495–501.

58. Guigoz Y, Vellas B, Garry PJ. Mini nutritional assessment: a practical assessment tool for grading the nutritional state of elderly patients In *Facts, Research, Interventions in Geriatrics* (New York: Serdi, 1997), 15–60.

59. Balducci L, Wallace C, Khansur T, Vance RB, Thigpen JT, Hardy C. Nutrition, cancer and aging: an annotated review. *J Am Geriatr Soc* 1986; **34**: 127–36.

60. Aslani A, Smith RC, Allen BJ, Pavlakis N, Levi JA. The predictive value of body protein for chemotherapy-induced toxicity. *Cancer* 2000; **88**: 796–803.

61. Fantl JA, Newman DK, Colling J. *Urinary Incontinence in Adults: Acute and Chronic Management*. AHCPR publication No 96-0682 (Rockville, MD: US Department of Health and Human Services, 1996).

62. Salive ME, Guralnik J, Christen W, Glynn RJ, Colsher P, Ostfeld AM. Functional blindness and visual impairment in older adults from three communities. *Ophthalmology* 1992; **99**: 1840–7.

63. Sommer A, Tieslch JM, Katz J, *et al*. Racial differences in the cause-specific prevalence of blindness in east Baltimore. *N Engl J Med* 1991; **325**: 1412–17.

64 Tieslch JM, Sommer A, Witt K, Katz J, Royall RM. Blindness and visual impairment in an American urban population: the Baltimore Eye Survey. *Arch Ophthalmol* 1990; **108**: 286–90.

65. Macphee GJA, Crowther JA, McAlpine CH. A simple screening test for hearing impairment in elderly patients. *Age Ageing* 1988; **17**: 347–51.

66. Popelka MM, Cruickshanks KJ, Wiley TL, Tweed TS, Klein BE, Klein R. Low prevalence of hearing aid use among older adults with hearing loss. *J Am Geriatr Soc* 1998; **46**: 1075–8.

67. Cella DF, Tulsky DS, Gray G, *et al*. The Functional Assessment of Cancer Therapy scale: development and validation of the general measure. *J Clin Oncol* 1993; **11**: 570–9.

68. Karnofsky DA. Meaningful clinical classification of therapeutic responses to anticancer drugs. *Clin Pharm Ther* 1961; **2**: 709–12.

4

From fitness to frailty: toward a nosologic classification of the older aged person

Lodovico Balducci, Claudia Beghe

Introduction

In exploring the assessment of the older aged person, this chapter has two goals. The first is to estimate a person's life expectancy, tolerance of stress, medical, rehabilitative, and supportive needs in planning the management of hematologic conditions. The second is to relate hematologic findings to a physiologic rather than chronologic classification of age, reflecting the function and the health status of each individual. A special assessment is needed because aging occurs at different rates for different individuals, and, in the same individual, for different functions.

Various forms of geriatric assessment were developed by geriatricians with the goal to preserve or restore health and functional independence, that is the ability to survive alone. In the scope of these assessments, the older population was composed of two groups of individuals. The first group, which becomes larger with increasing age, includes people who are functionally dependent, for whom the goal of management is to restore function and to prevent further functional deterioration. These individuals may be affected by multiple medical conditions that contribute to their dependence. The second group, which becomes smaller with advancing age, includes people who are still independent. In this case, the assessment is aimed to identify those at risk of functional decline, disease, and death, and the goal of management is to try to prevent or delay these occurrences.

After an outline of the biology and physiology of aging we will review different forms of geriatric assessment and their clinical utilization, we will discuss the meaning of the common geriatric terms *frailty* and *disability*, and we will conclude by trying to integrate the different information in a nosologic classification of aging.

Biology and physiology of aging

Aging has been defined as a loss of entropy [1,2] and of fractality [3]. Loss of entropy implies that the energy available for daily activities diminishes progressively with aging, and the survival and the function of the elder hinge upon energy saving. Loss of fractality implies a progressive decline in the ability to deal with the surrounding world due to sensorial impairment, limited mobility, and waning social network. This construct of aging may be translated into measurable clinical data, including life expectancy, tolerance of stress, and ability of independent living.

Figure 4.1 illustrates the biology of aging and its ultimate clinical consequences, and suggests ways of assessing an individual's physiologic age. A progressive exhaustion of functional reserve of multiple organ systems occurs as a result of genetically determined programs (a very reasonable, albeit never conclusively proven, hypothesis), environmental impact, and disease. Both disease and reduced functional reserve conspire in reducing a person's life expectancy and tolerance of stress, and in increasing the risk of disease and functional dependence.

A number of systemic changes, such as increased concentration of cytotoxic cytokines in the circulation,

Blood Disorders in the Elderly, ed. Lodovico Balducci, William Ershler, Giovanni de Gaetano.
Published by Cambridge University Press. © Cambridge University Press 2008.

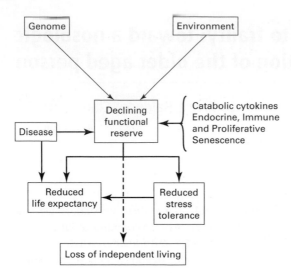

Figure 4.1 The biology of aging and its clinical consequences.

endocrine, immune, and proliferative senescence, effect and catalyze the decline in functional reserve and the susceptibility to stress and disease [4,5]. Inflammatory cytokines are responsible in part for sarcopenia [6–8], osteoporosis [9,10], and dysfunction of multiple organ systems [4,11–13], including the central nervous system [14–17] and the hematopoietic system [18,19]. Endocrine senescence involves decreased production of sexual hormones and chronic hypersecretion of adrenal corticosteroids [20] that together may lead to sarcopenia, osteoporosis, fatigue, and functional dependence. Immunosenescence involves progressive loss of cell-mediated immunity, which may predispose to infection by intracellular organisms, especially viruses [21], and to highly immunogenic tumors [21]. Proliferative senescence, best described in stromal cells, involves the loss of a cell's self-replicative capacity, associated with production of growth factors and lytic enzymes that may in the meantime destroy normal tissues and promote the growth of neoplastic ones [22].

Figure 4.1 suggests a number of ways of assessing a person's physiologic aging, including evaluation of function, of medical conditions, and of laboratory parameters. In the following discussion we will describe three forms of geriatric assessment – clinical, functional, and biochemical – and we will explore ways to integrate the geriatric assessment into a reproducible clinical classification of older individuals.

Clinical assessment of aging

Aging is multidimensional and involves decline in functional reserve as well as increased prevalence of chronic diseases, including a number of conditions, called "geriatric syndromes," that become more common with age. In addition, age involves emotional and social changes, such as increased prevalence of depression, waning economic resources, and social isolation, that may be associated with reduced access to care and poor nutritional and health habits. Not surprisingly, the most common and time-honored evaluation of the older aged person is a multidimensional assessment.

Comprehensive geriatric assessment (CGA)

Though the CGA has not been standardized, there is general agreement on its main components (Table 4.1) [23–31].

Function

Function is assessed as performance status (PS), activities of daily living (ADL), and instrumental activities of daily living (IADL). ADLs include transferring, bathing, dressing, eating, toileting, and continence; dependence in one or more of these activities, with the exception of incontinence, indicates that the person needs a home caregiver, and is associated with a two-year mortality rate of 27%. ADL dependence may prompt admission to an assisted living facility [32–35]. IADLs are necessary to maintain an independent life and include use of transportation, shopping, ability to take medications, provide for one's meals, use the telephone, and manage finances. Dependence in one or more

Table 4.1. Comprehensive geriatric assessment and clinical implications.

Functional status
  Activities of daily living (ADL) and instrumental
  activities of daily living (IADL)
	Dependence in one or more of these activities is associated with decreased life expectancy and with functional dependence

Comorbidity
  Number of comorbid conditions and comorbidity
  indices
	Comorbidity is associated with reduced life expectancy and with functional dependence. In addition, comorbidity may be associated with polypharmacy and may affect hematopoiesis and hemostasis

Emotional conditions Geriatric Depression Scale (GDS)	Depression has been associated with decreased life expectancy and function. It may reduce motivation for health care
Nutritional status Mini Nutritional Assessment (MNA)	Reversible condition. Possible relationship to survival. May affect hematopoiesis
Polypharmacy	Risk of drug interactions and hematopoietic suppression. Risk of drug-induced hemolytic anemia and bleeding

Geriatric syndromes
  Delirium, dementia, depression, falls, incontinence,
  spontaneous bone fractures, neglect and abuse,
  failure to thrive, vertigo
	Virtually all geriatric syndromes are associated with reduced life expectancy and with functional dependence

IADLs is associated with a 16% two-year mortality rate and indicates that the person cannot survive alone for a long period of time and needs the support of a caregiver, albeit not necessarily a home caregiver. In addition, dependence in one of more IADLs is harbinger of dementia in approximately 50% of cases [34, 35] and of complications from cytotoxic chemotherapy, especially neutropenic infections [36, 37]. Two studies found a poor correlation between functional dependence and PS, and recommended that both be evaluated [26, 27]. Though they are not part of the CGA, the advanced activities of daily living (AADL) are generating increasing interest. The AADLs are those that make life pleasurable and include leisure as well as professional and other working activities. Seemingly AADLs may represent an indirect measurement of the quality of life of the older person [38, 39].

Comorbidity

In the CGA, comorbidity refers mainly to chronic diseases. It is important to remember, however, that the mortality from acute conditions, especially infections and emergency surgery, increases with age [40,41]. Comorbidity is associated with decreased survival and function, and may affect hematopoiesis and hemostasis. For example, anemia of chronic inflammation and anemia of chronic renal insufficiency are among the most common forms of anemia in older individuals [42]. The assessment of comorbidity has not been standardized and is a subject of ongoing geriatric research. From a practical standpoint it is helpful to recognize that some comorbidities are independent risk factors of death. These include congestive heart failure and chronic renal insufficiency [43,44]. Of special interest to the readers of this book, anemia was also found to be an independent risk factor of mortality for individuals aged 65 and older [45–49], but it is not clear whether anemia itself is a cause of mortality or simply a marker of underlying diseases. After compiling a list of conditions associated with decreased survival in the general population, two approaches have been taken for the assessment of comorbidity. One approach is to sum the number of comorbid conditions [44]. The other utilizes comorbidity scales, accounting for the severity as well as the number of these conditions. The Charlson scale and the Cumulative Illness Rating Scale for Geriatrics (CIRS-G) have been used in the majority of studies [44]. The Charlson scale is suitable for epidemiologic studies, as it is simpler to use and may be scored based on data derived from medical and insurance records, whereas the CIRS-G appears more appropriate for individual assessment of comorbidity in clinical studies [41]. The CIRS-G is more cumbersome and time-consuming, but is more sensitive [44]. Another advantage of the CIRS-G is that its score may be translated into a Charlson score.

In addition to providing an estimate of physiologic aging, the assessment of comorbidity reveals conditions that may be reversed or arrested, at least in part, and whose management may delay aging. For the non-geriatrician this emphasis on comorbidity assessment may appear redundant, as it should be part of all good practice. The fact is, however, that disease manifestations in the elderly may often be neglected or misinterpreted by the patients themselves or by the healthcare provider, because they are attributed to a pre-existing condition or are wrongly considered normal manifestations of aging. For example, the diagnosis of bone cancer may be delayed as bone pain may be ascribed to pre-existing arthritis or to pain and ache typical of age. For this reason a careful medical history with special emphasis on new symptoms is recommended at each encounter with older patients. Atypical presentation of diseases is another reason why comorbidity may be under-diagnosed. Coronary ischemia in individuals over 70 may present as fatigue as commonly as it does with chest pain [50], and delirium is a harbinger of underlying organic disorders, such as infections, electrolyte imbalance, pain, and medication-related problems [51].

Geriatric syndromes

These conditions are typical of aging, if not specific, and include dementia, depression, delirium, incontinence, falls, spontaneous bone fractures, failure to thrive, neglect and abuse, and vertigo. They are associated with reduced life expectancy and almost always with some degree of functional dependence [34,35,51–57]. Effective management may reverse depression, falls, and osteoporosis, and may arrest the progression of other geriatric syndromes, including dementia. Screening older individuals for dementia, depression, osteoporosis, and risks of falling may be beneficial by allowing early diagnosis and timely management [51,58,59].

Failure to thrive, the inability to gain weight despite adequate food intake, is a sign of advanced aging and is seldom reversible. The cause is unknown in most cases and the mechanism may include overwhelming concentration of catabolic cytokines in the circulation leading to progressive sarcopenia [60]. Neglect and abuse is the least definable of the geriatric syndromes and is recognizable because patients are poorly kept and withdrawn. This is also a sign of advanced aging and of inadequate caregiving.

Geriatric syndromes are recognized as such when they interfere with a person's daily life. Dementia must be severe enough to disconnect an individual from daily activities; delirium must occur as a result of medications or organic diseases that do not commonly affect the central nervous system (e.g., urinary or upper respiratory infections); incontinence must cause a restriction of one's social life; depression must prevent pleasurable interactions and be associated with eating or sleeping disorders; falls must occur at least three times a month or the fear of falling must prevent regular activities, such as walking; vertigo must be continuous and so annoying as to cause a restriction in mobility.

Social resources

The adequacy of social resources is determined by individual needs. Those who are dependent in one or more ADLs do need a home caregiver, at least part of the time; those dependent in one or more IADLs do need a caregiver that is reachable and available on a short-time notice. Even for individuals who are fully independent and with negligible comorbidity it may be useful to identify a potential caregiver, as any acute disease or strenuous treatment, such as cancer chemotherapy, may precipitate functional dependence. Generally the caregiver or prospective caregiver is an older spouse with health problem of his/her own or an adult child, more often a daughter, who has to manage competing requests, from parents, from her/his family and from her/his profession. In addition to improving the quality of caregiving, appropriate planning may minimize the emotional stress [61,62].

Living conditions, access to transportation and to food, and income are interrelated and determine the quality of health even for individuals who are functionally independent. It is clear that a person in a wealthy retirement community, with close neighbors and shopping centers, and a choice of public transportations, has a better chance to survive an acute problem, causing momentary loss of function, than a person living in a run-down and unsafe neighborhood or one living alone in the countryside far from shops or public transportation.

Simple adjustments in home environment may go a long way in preventing common complications of aging. Good illumination, removal of carpets or obstacles, creation of a walking pathway where an individual can always find a support, prevent falls and allow the older person rapid access to the phone in case of emergency. In addition, changes in home environment, such as bathroom bars, may avoid the transformation of disability into handicap [63].

Nutrition

The prevalence of protein/calorie malnutrition increases with age [64]. Isolation, depression, economic restriction, reduced appreciation of hunger, may all contribute to insufficient food intake, while chronic diseases, inflammatory cytokines, and lack of exercise may impede the synthesis of new proteins [65]. The Mini Nutritional Assessment (MNA) is a simple nutritional screening test of worldwide use that identifies patients who are malnourished and those at risk of becoming malnourished, and allows the prevention and early reversal of malnutrition [66].

Polypharmacy

The prevalence of polypharmacy increases with age, and among cancer patients aged 70 and older was found as high as 41% [44,67]. Polypharmacy may include redundant prescriptions as well as dangerous drug interactions, and highlights a common problem of older individuals in developed countries: the absence of a primary care provider responsible for supervising the various medications. According to a recent study, more than 50% of individuals aged 70 and older in the USA, Canada, and Israel, while attending multiple specialty clinics, lacked a primary care physician [68].

Clinical application of the CGA

In general geriatric practice, the CGA has generated interventions able to preserve the health and independence of older individuals, resulting in a decline in admissions to hospital and to assisted living facilities. According to early studies, the CGA also improved the survival of older individuals [27–30].

In addition, the CGA may be used to estimate a person's life expectancy [69]. Walter and Covinsky integrated the results of the CGA with the US life tables. The life expectancy of each age cohort was subdivided into quartiles and the CGA determined to which quartile each individual belonged (Fig. 4.2). The same group of investigators established criteria to estimate the one-year mortality rate for older individuals discharged from the hospital (Table 4.2) [43] and the two-year mortality rate for home-dwelling older individuals based on function and comorbidity (Table 4.3) [70]. The benefits of the CGA extend beyond the realm of general geriatrics. In the management of cancer in older patients, the geriatric assessment has allowed the identification of a number of conditions including comorbidity, cognitive disorders, depression, and malnutrition that would have remained otherwise unrecognized [71–73], and it has identified risk factors for chemotherapy-related toxicity [37].

Of special interest to the readers of this book, the geriatric assessment may allow a nosologic classification of age based on physiologic rather than chronologic parameters. Hamerman has proposed a frame of reference for this classification (Table 4.4) [74].

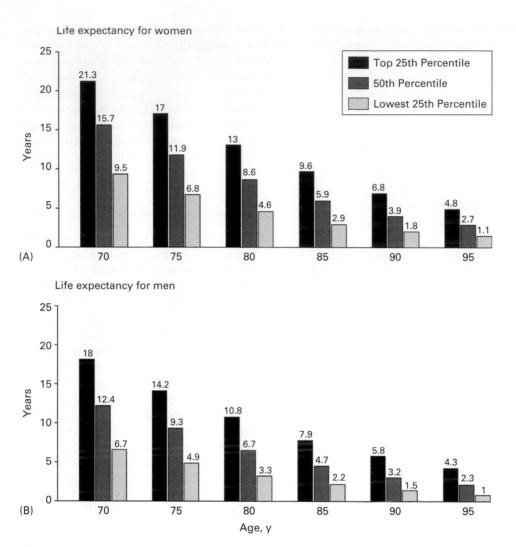

Figure 4.2 Estimate of life expectancy using the life tables: upper, middle, and lower quartiles for women (A) and men (B) at selected ages. From Walter & Covinsky, 2001 [69], with permission.

Limitation of the geriatric assessment

The CGA has allowed a formal, systematic, and largely reproducible exploration of aging and has demonstrated that aging is multidimensional, highly individualized, and poorly reflected in chronologic age. The clinical repercussions of the CGA include improved management of older individuals with preservation of function and quality of life and possibly improvement of comorbidity and of survival. The CGA may thus be considered the gold-standard geriatric evaluation and the reference for the development of new instruments. Several areas of geriatric assessment need improvement and fine-tuning, as suggested by its current limitations:

• Originally the CGA was designed to improve the management of patients with advanced

Table 4.2. Estimate of one-year mortality risk for individuals aged 70 and older discharged from hospital [43].

Scoring system

Risk factor	Odds ratio	*p*-value	Score
Male	1.4 (1.1–1.8)	<0.01	1
ADL			
1–4	2.1 (1.6–2.8)	<0.0001	2
all	5.7 (4.2–7.7)	<0.0001	5
Comorbidity			
CHF	2.0 (1.5–2.5)	<0.001	2
Early cancer	2.2 (1.2–3.2)	<0.001	3
Metastatic cancer	13.4 (6.2–39.0)	<0.001	8
Creatinine >3.0	1.7 (1.2–2.5)	<0.01	1
Serum albumin			
3.0–3.4	1.7 (1.2–2.3)	<0.001	1
<3.0	2.1 (1.4–3.0)	<0.001	2

One-year mortality risk

Score	Mortality risk
0–1	<10%
2–3	18%
4–6	31%
>6	62%

Table 4.3. Estimate of two-year mortality rate for home-dwelling individuals aged 70 and older [70].

Scoring system

Risk factor	*p*-value	Score
Male	<0.01	2
Age		
76–80	<0.05	1
>80	<0.01	2
Function		
Bathing	<0.01	1
Shopping	<0.0001	2
Walking more than 3 blocks	<0.001	2
Pulling or pushing	<0.05	1

Two-year mortality risk

Score	Mortality risk
0–2	3%
3–6	13%
>6	34%

Table 4.4. A nosologic classification of aging based on the geriatric functional continuum proposed by Hamerman [74].

Group	Characteristics
Primary	No functional dependence Negligible comorbidity
Intermediate	Dependence in one or more IADLs Stable comorbidity (for example stable angina, chronic renal insufficiency, etc.)
Secondary or frailty	One of the following criteria: • Dependence in one or more ADLs • Three or more comorbid conditions or one poorly controlled comorbid conditions • One or more geriatric syndrome
Tertiary	Near death

functional impairment and multiple comorbidities, such as those living in assisted living facilities and nursing homes, or attending outpatient geriatric clinics. As the majority of individuals over 65 enjoy good health and independence it is legitimate to ask two questions: Is a full CGA necessary and beneficial for these individuals? Is the CGA able to identify those healthy older individuals who are at risk of more rapid functional decline and for whom immediate management would be beneficial?

- The CGA has not been standardized, which makes it difficult to compare research and clinical data from different institutions and different practices. Its multidimensional nature makes standardization problematic. The two major variables include the number of different tools available for the assessment of each domain, and the person(s) performing the assessment. In many cases the CGA is based on patients' self-reports; in others it is performed by a nurse or a research assistant; and in others it involves different professionals (nurse, dietitian, social worker, pharmacist).
- The CGA may be redundant in the sense that it provides an excess of information. It is well

known that a correlation exists among the different parameters of the CGA (function and comorbidity, function and cognitive decline, function and depression, etc.) [35,75,76]. Ideally one would like to be able to compress the wealth of information into a small number of indexes predicting life expectancy and risk of functional decline, and identifying patients in need of special medical, nutritional, and social interventions.

- The CGA is complex, time-consuming, resource-intense and costly.

In the last ten years a number of short instruments have been developed to screen older individuals and identify those who may benefit from a CGA. Some of these instruments have also identified individuals at risk for functional decline, hospitalization, and death.

Shortened forms of assessment

There are several shortened forms of assessment that may be used to identify individuals in need of a full CGA. A review of all tests proposed to screen older individuals is beyond the scope of this chapter. We will provide three examples of tests that are widely used in clinical practice and in clinical studies.

In the "get up and go" test an individual is asked to get up from an armchair, walk 3 m (10 feet) forward and back, and sit down again. The performance requires less than a minute, and is scored from 0 (the best), to 3 (the worst). One point is assigned for using the arms in getting up, for taking more than 10 seconds to complete the exercise, and for unstable gait [77]. The higher the score, the higher is the risk of mortality and functional dependence. It appears reasonable to limit the full CGA to those individuals who score 1 or higher. This test, which has been validated in a prospective study, has the advantage of being very simple, but it may not be sensitive enough to identify healthy older individuals at risk for functional deterioration.

The Vulnerable Elders Survey (VES-13) is a 13-item questionnaire concerning age, self-reported health, selected ADL/IADL, and the performance

Table 4.5. The Vulnerable Elders Survey (VES-13) questionnaire for the definition of vulnerability [78].

Element of assessment	Score
Age	
75–84	1
≥85	3
Self-reported health	
Good or excellent	0
Fair or poor	1
ADL/IADL. Needs helps in	
Shopping	1
Money management	1
Light housework	1
Transferring	1
Bathing	1
Activities. Needs help in	
Stooping, crouching, or kneeling	1
Lifting or carrying 10 lb (4.5 kg)	1
Writing or handling small objects	1
Reaching or extending arm above shoulder	1
Walking 1/4 mile (0.4 km)	1
Heavy housework	1

of common activities (Table 4.5) [78]. In a group of 290 individuals aged 70 and over a score of 4 or higher indicated a fourfold increased risk of mortality or functional decline during the following five years. The main advantage of the VES-13 is that it is self-administered; the main disadvantage is the fact that it is age-weighted, that is chronologic age heavily influences the final score. Like the "get up and go" the VES-13 may not be sensitive enough to identify healthy individuals at risk for functional deterioration.

In the Cardiovascular Health Study (CHS), approximately 8500 home-dwelling individuals aged 65 and older have been followed yearly for 11 years. The primary goal of the CHS was to identify factors of risk for coronary artery disease and congestive heart failure in the elderly. At the same time data on mortality, hospitalization, and functional decline were collected. Of approximately 200 variables examined, five were independent factors of risk for mortality and functional decline (Table 4.6). Based

Table 4.6. Independent risk factors for mortality and functional decline in the Cardiovascular Health Study (CHS) [79].

Evaluation of frailty according to the CHS
1. Weight loss. Unintentional weight loss of ⩾10 lb (4.5 kg) in prior year, by direct measurement of weight
2. Grip strength <20% below standard for BMI, measured with Jamar Hydraulic Dynamometer (see below)
3. Walk time below a cutoff point for sex and height (see below)
4. Exhaustion, measured by two statements from the CES-D depression scale (see below)
5. Physical activity, measured on the short version of the Minnesota Leisure Time activity (see below). Men Kcal/week <383; women <270

Grip strength by body mass index (BMI) derived from height and body surface

BMI	Cutoff grip strength (kg)
Man	
⩽24	⩽29
24.1–26	⩽30
26.1–28	⩽30
>28	⩽32
Woman	
⩽23	⩽17
23.1–26	⩽17.3
26.1–29	⩽18
>29	⩽21

Walk time

Height (cm)	Cutoff point (seconds)
Man	
⩽173	⩾7
>173	⩾6
Woman	
⩽159	⩾7
>159	⩾6

Exhaustion: score 2 or 3 on two questions of the Center of Epidemiologic Studies Depression Scale (CES-D)
   a. I felt everything I did was an effort
   b. I could not get going
Score: 0 = never; 1 = 1–2 days a week; 2 = 3–4 days a week; 3 = most of the time

Physical activity. Patients are asked whether they engaged in any of the following activities in the past two weeks

High-intensity activities	Moderate or light-intensity activities
Swimming	Gardening
Hiking	Mowing
Anaerobics	Raking
Tennis	Golfing
Jogging	Bowling
Racquetball	Biking
Walked for exercise for	Dancing
at least 1 hour >4 miles/hour	
	Calisthenics
	Exercise cycle
	Walked for exercise for at least one hour at a strolling pace

Patients who did not engage in any of these activities over the past two weeks will be considered at low physical activity

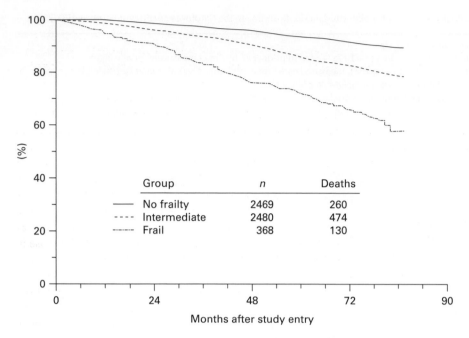

Figure 4.3 Survival of fit, pre-frail, and frail populations in the CHS study.

on the presence of these variables, three groups of individuals were identified: fit (those for whom all parameters were normal); pre-frail (those with one or two abnormal parameters), and frail (those who had three or more abnormal variables). Over 11 years, the three groups showed different risks of mortality (Fig. 4.3), of hospitalization, and of functional dependence [79]. As it has been validated in a large number of patients, for more than a decade, and is simple to perform, the CHS assessment appears almost ideal for screening apparently healthy older individuals for the risk of death and functional dependence. It has been proposed that the CHS classification be adopted as the official functional classification of older individuals. The CHS assessment is accurate in predicting which healthy older individuals are at risk of functional decline and therefore need an "in-depth" geriatric assessment. In its present form, however, it cannot be used for a nosologic classification of the whole older population. A large portion of older individuals, and more than 50% of the oldest old (that is, those 85 and over),

present some degree of functional dependence and of comorbidity that causes disability, shortens their life expectancy, and enhances their vulnerability to minimal stress. These individuals are not accounted for by the CHS assessment.

Practical applications of the geriatric assessment

From the discussion of geriatric assessment it is reasonable to conclude:

- Aging is multidimensional and its assessment should be multidimensional.
- A CGA is the most exhaustive form of evaluation of an older person.
- A CGA is clearly indicated in individuals presenting some degree of functional dependence or comorbidity, or one or more geriatric syndrome.
- For all other individuals, a CGA may be indicated if they are at increased risk of functional deterioration.

- Of the screening tests for risk of functional deterioration, the CHS assessment appears the best validated and probably the most practical; pre-frail and frail individuals should undergo a CGA.
- A nosologic classification of older individuals is still wanted. The CHS assessment offers the best-validated classification, but the frail subgroup encompasses a wide array of conditions and requires fine-tuning, based on functional dependence, comorbidity, nutrition, and other variables included in the CGA.

Other forms of geriatric assessment

In addition to the CGA, aging has been assessed with physical performance and laboratory tests.

Tests of physical performance

These tests evaluate the ability of a person to perform one or more simple physical activities. They may assess the actual performance of the activity or the individual's self-reports. The get-up-and-go tests, or the measurement of grip strength and walking speed in the CHS assessment, are examples of directly evaluated physical performances, while the VES-13 is an example of self-report [77,78]. Both approaches have proved reliable.

A list and description of all tests of physical performance is beyond the scope of this chapter. As a general rule these tests may be used to screen healthy individuals for risk of disability and functional dependence, and are not a substitute for geriatric assessment.

Laboratory assessment

Several studies have demonstrated that aging is associated with an increased concentration of inflammatory cytokines [5,16,60] and other markers of inflammation, such as the C-reactive protein and D-dimer, in the circulation. The concentration of these substances in the circulation is increased in most geriatric syndromes as well as in common diseases of aging, including dementia [16], osteoporosis [9,10], anemia [49], cardiovascular diseases [80], disability [7], and depression [81]. Interleukin 6 (IL-6) has probably been the best characterized of these substances.

A recent study in more than 1000 home-dwelling individuals aged 70 and older showed that the concentration of IL-6 and D-dimer in the circulation may be used to predict the risk of mortality and functional decline [5]. Those individuals in whom the concentration of both substances was below the upper quartile had a two-year risk of mortality or functional dependence less than 10%; for those in whom the concentration of either substance was in the upper quartile the risk was 20%; for those in whom the concentration of both substances was elevated the risk was approximately 40%. These results are very encouraging, and suggest that laboratory tests may become a routine part of the geriatric assessment in the near future. Any study involving older individuals should consider assessing IL-6 and D-dimer as part of the patient evaluation.

Frailty, real and elusive

Frail and *frailty* are recurrent terms in both geriatric and gerontology literature; for some, frail is almost synonymous with aged [79,82]. If asked to define a frail person, most of us would probably think of a curved older person, moving very slowly with the help of a walker and at risk of falling at any moment. The translation of this literary description into a clinical entity is lacking, however, and the clinical meaning of frailty remains elusive.

From the studies we have summarized one can see that the term *frailty* has been used by different authors in at least two different senses. In the classification proposed by Hamerman frailty means an almost complete exhaustion of functional reserve, that is a person unable to withstand even negligible stress [74]. In clinical terms this may be seen as a person dependent in one or more ADLs, with one or more geriatric syndromes and affected by severe life-limiting comorbidity [82]. In this construct, frailty is largely irreversible, and the main goal of management is to prevent further functional deterioration. For the investigators of the CHS, frailty means a predisposition to functional decline, that is the frail persons represent a subgroup of independent persons at increased risk of developing functional dependence. Seemingly, frailty may then be reversed by proper interventions including rehabilitation and treatment or prevention of diseases. This concept of frailty is predominant in the most recent literature [79].

Irrespective of the term being used, both conditions described as frailty are real and deserve to be recognized, but the reader of this book should be aware that a consensual definition of frailty is still wanted.

Functional dependence and disability

Prevention of functional dependence has been enounced as one of the goals of geriatrics, and functional dependence has been defined as inability to survive safely alone. Another common concept of geriatrics, linked to functional dependence but not to be confused with it, is disability.

Three terms related to disability have been well defined by the World Health Organization: functional impairment, disability, and handicap [83]. Functional impairment involves the deterioration of a specific function, such as walking or performing fine hand movements. Disability is the loss of a certain activity, such as climbing stairs, using the silverware, or driving, due to functional impairment. Clearly, not all forms of functional impairment are severe enough to cause disability. A disability becomes a handicap in the absence of environmental arrangements able to compensate for individual disability. For example, inability to walk or to climb stairs due to loss of the function of the lower extremities becomes a handicap in the absence of a wheelchair or an elevator, or a ramp allowing wheelchairs to climb to or descend from different levels of a building.

The prevalence of functional impairment, disability, and handicaps increases with age, and clearly these conditions may limit a person's ability for independent living. One of the goals of the tests of physical performance is to identify individuals at risk of disability and to prevent its development. Of special interest to the hematologist is the fact that anemia, even mild anemia, is associated with an increased risk of disability [48,49].

For the purpose of a classification of older individuals, however, it is important to distinguish functional dependence and disability and to realize that disability does not always cause functional dependence.

Toward a nosologic classification of aging

Though an official and consensual classification of aging is still wanted, the discussion related to the geriatric assessment allows us to distinguish some broad categories of older individuals. The outline proposed by Hamerman (Table 4.4) encompasses all different states of aging, but probably needs to be fine-tuned for clinical applications. In particular:

- The primary state should be subdivided according to the risk of functional deterioration. The CHS assessment [79], as well as the evaluation of circulating markers of inflammation, may allow this distinction.
- The intermediate state should include individuals with initial functional dependence (for example, IADL dependence) and disability who are amenable to rehabilitation, those with early geriatric syndromes (memory loss, depression, osteoporosis) that may be arrested with proper intervention, and those with a comorbidity that is function-impairing (for example, osteoarthritis), but not life-limiting.
- Whether we decide to call it frailty or not, the secondary state should include individuals who are dependent in one or more ADLs, those with more advanced geriatric syndromes, and those with life-limiting diseases (for example, congestive heart failure or some form of metastatic cancer).
- The third state should include individuals who have an average life expectancy of six months or less, for whatever reason.

The classification of aging in different states is undergoing continuous remodeling with the emergence of new data and the interpretation of existing data. Seemingly this process will never be concluded. Current information allows us to frame the hematology of aging in a context that is not purely chronologic and that takes into account function, comorbidity, the presence or absence of geriatric syndromes, as well as the social context of the older aged person.

REFERENCES

1. Lipsitz LA. Age-related changes in the "complexity" of the cardiovascular dynamics: a potential marker of vulnerability to disease. *Chaos* 1995; **5**: 102–9.
2. Marineo G, Marotta F. Biophysics of aging and therapeutic interventions by entropy-variation systems. *Biogerontology* 2005; **6**: 77–9.
3. Lipsitz LA. Physiological complexity, aging, and the path to frailty. *Sci Aging Knowl Environ* 2004; **16**: pe16.
4. Ferrucci L, Corsi A, Lauretani F, *et al.* The origins of age-related proinflammatory state. *Blood* 2005; **105**: 2294–9.
5. Cohen HJ, Harris T, Pieper CF. Coagulation and activation of inflammatory pathways in the development of functional decline and mortality in the elderly. *Am J Med* 2003; **114**: 180–7.
6. Payette H, Roubenoff R, Jacques PF, *et al.* Insulin-like growth factor 1 and interleukin 6 predict sarcopenia in very-old community-living men and women: the Framingham Heart Study. *J Am Geriatr Soc* 2003; **51**: 1237–43.
7. Ferrucci L, Penninx BW, Volpato S, *et al.* Change in muscle strength explains accelerated decline of physical function in older women with high interleukin-6 serum levels. *J Am Geriatr Soc* 2002; **50**: 1947–54.
8. Roubenoff R, Parise H, Payette HA, *et al.* Cytokines, insulin-like growth factor 1, sarcopenia, and mortality in very old community dwelling men and women: the Framingham Heart Study. *Am J Med* 2003; **115**: 429–35.
9. Abrahamsen B, Bonnevie-Nielsen V, Ebbesen EN, Gram J, Beck-Nielsen H. Cytokines and bone loss in a 5-year longitudinal study-hormone replacement therapy suppresses serum soluble interleukin 6 receptor and increases interleukin-1-receptor antagonist: the Danish Osteoporosis Prevention Study. *J Bone Miner Res* 2000; **15**: 1545–54.
10. Moffett SP, Zmuda JM, Cauley JA, *et al.* Association of the G-174C variant in interleukin-6 promoter region with bone loss and fracture risk in older women. *J Bone Miner Res* 2004; **19**: 1612–18.
11. Brunsgaard H, Pedersen BK. Age-related inflammatory cytokines and disease. *Immunol Allergy Clin North Am* 2003; **23**: 15–39.
12. Fernandez-Real JM, Vayreda M, Richart C, *et al.* Circulating interleukin 6 levels, blood pressure, and insulin sensitivity in apparently healthy men and women. *J Endocrinol Metab* 2001; **86**: 1154–9.
13. Pai JK, Pischon T, Ma J, *et al.* Inflammatory markers and risk of coronary heart disease in men and women. *N Engl J Med* 2004; **351**: 2599–610.
14. Alesci S, Martinez PE, Kelkar S, *et al.* Major depression is associated with significant diurnal elevations in plasma interleukin-6 levels, a shift of its circadian rhythm, and loss of physiological complexity in its secretion: clinical implications. *J Clin Endocrinol Metab* 2005; **90**: 2522–30.
15. Yaffe K, Lindquist K, Penninx BW, *et al.* Inflammatory markers and cognition in well-functioning African American and white elders. *Neurology* 2003; **61**: 76–8.
16. Wilson CJ, Cohen HJ, Pieper CF. Cross-linked fibrin degradation products (D-Dimer), plasma cytokines, and cognitive decline in community-dwelling elderly persons. *J Am Geriatr Soc* 2003; **51**: 1374–81.
17. Wilson CJ, Finch CE, Cohen HJ. Cytokines and cognition: the case for a head-to-toe inflammatory paradigm. *J Am Geriatr Soc* 2002; **50**: 2041–56.
18. Rothstein G. Disordered hematopoiesis and myelodysplasia in the elderly. *J Am Geriatr Soc* 2003; **51** (3 Suppl): S22–S26.
19. Balducci L, Hardy CL, Lyman GH. Hemopoiesis and aging. In Balducci L, Extermann M, eds, *Biological Basis of Geriatric Oncology* (New York, NY: Springer, 2005), 111–34.
20. Duthie EH. Physiology of aging: relevance to symptoms, perceptions, and treatment tolerance. In Balducci L, Lyman GH, Ershler WB, Extermann M, eds, *Comprehensive Geriatric Oncology*, 2nd edn (London: Taylor and Francis, 2004), 207–22.
21. Burns EA, Goodwin JS. Immunological changes of aging. In Balducci L, Lyman GH, Ershler WB, Extermann M, eds, *Comprehensive Geriatric Oncology*, 2nd edn (London: Taylor and Francis, 2004), 158–70.
22. Hornsby PJ. Replicative senescence and cancer. In Balducci L, Extermann M, eds, *Biological Basis of*

Geriatric Oncology (New York, NY: Springer, 2005), 53–74.

23. Balducci L, Cohen HJ, Engstrom P, *et al.* Senior adult oncology clinical practice guidelines in oncology. *J Natl Compr Canc Netw* 2005; **3**: 572–90.

24. Balducci L, Extermann M. Assessment of the older patient with cancer. In Balducci L, Lyman GH, Ershler WB, Extermann M, eds, *Comprehensive Geriatric Oncology*, 2nd edn (London: Taylor and Francis, 2004), 223–35.

25. Rao AV, Seo PH, Cohen HJ. Geriatric assessment and comorbidity. *Semin Oncol* 2004; **31**: 149–59.

26. Rockwood K, Mogilner A, Mitnitsky A. Changes with age in the distribution of a frailty index. *Mech Aging Dev* 2004; **125**: 517–19.

27. Cohen HJ, Feussner JR, Weinberger M, *et al.* A controlled trial of inpatient and outpatient geriatric evaluation and management. *N Engl J Med* 2002; **346**: 905–12.

28. Rubinstein LN. Comprehensive geriatric assessment: from miracle to reality. *J Gerontol A Biol Sci Med Sci* 2004; **59**: 473–7.

29. Kuo HK, Scandrett KG, Dave J, Mitchell SL. The influence of outpatient geriatric assessment on survival: a meta-analysis. *Arch Gerontol Geriatr* 2004; **39**: 245–54.

30. Caplan GA, Williams AJ, Day B, Abraham K. A randomized controlled trial of comprehensive geriatric assessment and multidisciplinary intervention after discharge of elderly patients from emergency department: the DEED II study. *J Am Geriatr Soc* 2004; **52**: 1417–23.

31. Balducci L. New paradigms for treating elderly patients with cancer: the comprehensive geriatric assessment and guidelines for supportive care. *J Support Oncol* 2003; **1** (4 Suppl 2): 30–7.

32. Reuben DB, Rubenstein LV, Hirsch SH, Hays RD. Value of functional status as predictor of mortality. *Am J Med* 1992; **93**: 663–9.

33. Inouye SK, Peduzzi PN, Robison JT, Hughes JS, Horwitz RI, Concato J. Importance of functional measures in predicting mortality among older hospitalized patients. *JAMA* 1998; **279**: 1187–93.

34. Ramos LR, Simoes EJ, Albert MS. Dependence in activities of daily living and cognitive impairment strongly predicted mortality in older urban residents in Brazil. *J Am Geriatr Soc* 2001; **49**: 1168–75.

35. Barberger-Gateau P, Fabrigoule C, Helmer C, Rouch I, Dartigues JF. Functional impairment in instrumental activities of daily living: an early clinical sign of dementia? *J Am Geriatr Soc* 1999; **47**: 456–62.

36. Zagonel V, Fratino L, Piselli P, *et al.* The comprehensive geriatric assessment predicts mortality among elderly cancer patients. *Proc Am Soc Clin Oncol* 2002; **21**: 365a, abs 1458.

37. Extermann M, Chen A, Cantor AB, *et al.* Predictors of tolerance to chemotherapy in older cancer patients: a prospective pilot study. *Eur J Cancer* 2002; **38**: 1466–73.

38. Katz P. Function, disability, and psychological well being. *Adv Psychosom Med* 2004; **25**: 41–62.

39. Avlund K, Vass M, Hendriksen C. Onset of mobility disability among community-dwelling old men and women: the role of tiredness in daily activities. *Age Ageing* 2003; **32**: 579–84.

40. Lloyd H, Ahmed I, Taylor S, Blake JR. Index for predicting mortality in elderly surgical patients. *Br J Surg* 2005; **92**: 487–92.

41. Arenal JJ, Bengoechea-Beeby M. Mortality associated with emergency abdominal surgery in the elderly. *Can J Surg* 2003; **46**: 111–16.

42. Weiss G, Goodnough LT. Anemia of chronic disease. *N Engl J Med* 2005; **352**: 1011–23.

43. Walter LC, Brand RJ, Counsell RS, *et al.* Development and validation of a prognostic index for 1 year mortality in older adults after hospitalization. *JAMA* 2001; **285**: 2987–93.

44. Extermann M. Biological basis of the association of cancer and aging comorbidity. In Balducci L, Extermann M, eds, *Biological Basis of Geriatric Oncology* (New York, NY: Springer, 2005), 173–88.

45. Izaks GJ, Westendorp RGJ, Knook DL. The definition of anemia in older persons. *JAMA* 1999; **281**: 1714–17.

46. Kikuchi M, Inagaki T, Shinagawa N. Five-year survival of older people with anemia: variation with hemoglobin concentration. *J Am Geriatr Soc* 2001; **49**: 1226–8.

47. Anía BJ, Suman VJ, Fairbanks VF, Rademacher DM, Melton JL. Incidence of anemia in older people: an epidemiologic study in a well defined population. *J Am Geriatr Soc* 1997; **45**: 825–31.

48. Chaves PH, Xue QL, Guralnik JM, Ferrucci L, Volpato S, Fried LP. What constitutes normal hemoglobin concentration in community-dwelling disabled older women? *J Am Geriatr Soc* 2004; **52**: 1811–16.

49. Woodman R, Ferrucci L, Guralnik J. Anemia in older adults. *Curr Opin Hematol* 2005; **12**: 123–8.

50. Tresch DD. Management of the older patient with acute myocardial infarction: difference in clinical presentations between older and younger patients. *J Am Geriatr Soc* 1998; **46**: 1157–62.

51. Weber JB, Coverdale JH, Kunik ME: Delirium: current trends in prevention and treatment. *Intern Med J* 2004 **34**: 115–21.

52. Stump TE, Callahan CM, Hendrie HC. Cognitive impairment and mortality in older primary care patients. *J Am Geriatr Soc* 2001; **49**: 934–40.

53. Blazer DG, Hybels CF. What symptoms of depression predict mortality in community-dwelling elderly? *J Am Geriatr Soc* 2004; **52**: 2052–6.

54. Tinetti ME, Williams CS. The effect of falls and fall injuries on functioning in community-dwelling older persons. *J Gerontol A Biol Sci Med Sci* 1998; **53**: M112–M119.

55. Kao AC, Nanada A, Williams CS, Tinetti ME. Validation of dizziness as a possible geriatric syndrome. *J Am Geriatr Soc* 2001; **49**: 72–5.

56. Verdery RB. Failure to thrive in old age: follow-up on a workshop. *J Gerontol A Biol Sci Med Sci* 1997; **52**: M333–M336.

57. Pavlik VN, Hyman DJ, Festa NA. Quantifying the problem of abuse and neglect in adults: analysis of a statewide data base. *J Am Geriatr Soc* 2001; **49**: 45–8.

58. Green AD, Colon-Emeric CS, Bastian L, Drake MT, Lyles KW. Does this woman have osteoporosis? *JAMA* 2004; **292**: 2890–900.

59. Fortinsky RH, Iannuzzi-Sucich M, Baker DI, *et al.* Fall-risk assessment and management in clinical practice. *J Am Geriatr Soc* 2004; **52**: 1522–6.

60. Hamerman D. Frailty, cancer cachexia and near death. In Balducci L, Lyman GH, Ershler WB, Extermann M, eds, *Comprehensive Geriatric Oncology*, 2nd edn (London: Taylor and Francis, 2004), 236–49.

61. Carreca I, Balducci L, Extermann M. Cancer in the older person. *Cancer Treat Rev* 2005; **31**: 380–402.

62. Haley WE, Burton AM, Lamonde LA. Family caregiving issues for older cancer patients. In Balducci L, Lyman GH, Ershler WB, Extermann M, eds, *Comprehensive Geriatric Oncology*, 2nd edn (London: Taylor and Francis, 2004), 843–52.

63. Baker DI, King MB, Fortinsky RH, *et al.* Dissemination of an evidence-based multicomponent fall risk-assessment and management strategy throughout a geographic area. *J Am Geriatr Soc* 2005; **53**: 675–80.

64. Fisher A. Of worms and women: sarcopenia and its role in disability and mortality. *J Am Geriatr Soc* 2004; **52**: 1185–90.

65. Goldspink G. Age-related muscle loss and progressive dysfunction in mechanosensitive growth factor signaling. *Ann NY Acad Sci* 2004; **1019**: 294–8.

66. Guigoz Y, Vellas B, Garry PJ. Mini nutritional assessment: a practical assessment tool for grading the nutritional state of elderly patients In *Facts, Research, Interventions in Geriatrics* (New York: Serdi, 1997), 15–60.

67. Corcoran MB. Polypharmacy in the senior adult patient. In Balducci L, Lyman GH, Ershler WB, Extermann M, eds, *Comprehensive Geriatric Oncology*, 2nd edn (London: Taylor and Francis, 2004), 502–9.

68. Clarfield AM, Bergman H, Kane R. Fragmentation of care for frail older people: an international problem. Experience from three countries: Israel, Canada, and the United States. *J Am Geriatr Soc* 2001; **49**: 1714–21.

69. Walter LC, Covinsky KE. Cancer screening in elderly patients: a framework for individual decision making. *JAMA* 2001; **285**: 2750–6.

70. Carey EC, Walter LC, Lindquist K, Covinsky KE. Development and validation of a functional morbidity index to predict mortality in community-dwelling elderly. *J Gen Intern Med* 2004; **19**: 1027–33.

71. Repetto L, Fratino L, Audisio RA, *et al.* Comprehensive geriatric assessment adds information to the Eastern Cooperative group Performance Status in Elderly cancer patients. An Italian Group for Geriatric Oncology Study. *J Clin Oncol* 2002; **20**: 494–502.

72. Ingram SS, Seo PH, Martell RE, *et al.* Comprehensive assessment of the elderly cancer patient: the feasibility of self-report methodology. *J Clin Oncol* 2002; **20**: 770–5.

73. Extermann M, Overcash J, Lyman GH, Parr J, Balducci L. Comorbidity and functional status are independent in older cancer patients. *J Clin Oncol* 1998; **16**: 1582–7.

74. Hamerman D. Toward an understanding of frailty. *Ann Intern Med* 1999; **130**: 945–50.

75. Lyness JM, King DA, Cox C, Yoediono Z, Caine ED. The importance of subsyndromal depression in older primary care patients. Prevalence and associated functional disability. *J Am Geriatr Soc* 1999; **47**: 647–52.

76. Kivela SL, Pahkala K. Depressive disorder as predictor of physical disability in old age. *J Am Geriatr Soc* 2001; **49**: 290–6.

77. Podsiadlo D, Richardson S. The timed "up & go": a test of basic functional mobility for frail elderly persons. *J Am Geriatr Soc* 1991; **39**: 142–8.

78. Saliba D, Elliott M, Rubenstein LZ, *et al.* The Vulnerable Elders Survey: a tool for identifying vulnerable older people in the community. *J Am Geriatr Soc* 2001; **49**: 1691–9.

79. Fried LP, Tangen CM, Walston J, *et al.* Frailty in older adults: evidence for a phenotype. *J Gerontol A Biol Sci Med Sci* 2001; **56**: M146–M156.

80. Ikeda U. Inflammation and coronary artery disease. *Curr Vasc Pharmacol* 2003; **1**: 65–70.

81. Illman J, Corringham R, Robinson D, *et al*. Are inflammatory cytokines the common link between cancer-associated cachexia and depression? *J Support Oncol* 2005; **3**: 37–50.

82. Balducci L, Stanta G. Cancer in the frail patient: a coming epidemic. *Hematol Oncol Clin North Am* 2000; **14**: 235–50.

83. Warshaw GA, Murphy JB. Rehabilitation and the aged. In Reichel W, ed, *Care of the Elderly: Clinical Aspects of Aging* (Baltimore, MD: Williams & Wilkins, 1995), 187–97.

PART II

Hematopoiesis

5

Stem cell exhaustion and aging

Jeffrey Yates, Gary Van Zant

Do hematopoietic stem cells show age-related loss of function?

The production of over 4×10^{15} erythrocytes, lymphocytes, and myeloid cells during the lifetime of an individual rests on the shoulders of the hematopoietic stem cell (HSC) [1]. While the demand placed upon the HSC may seem Sisyphean in its magnitude, it is hardly a futile endeavor. For instance, a single HSC can repopulate the entire hematopoietic system of a lethally irradiated mouse, and engraftment levels after secondary transplantation mirror those of the primary recipients [2,3]. While other transplantation protocols show that the numbers of primitive cells in the bone marrow (BM) of recipients remain depressed permanently, circulating blood cell numbers are not significantly different from non-transplanted mice [4]. This is a profound statement of the ability of these pluripotent stem cells to proliferate, differentiate, and perhaps most importantly, self-renew. Furthermore, BM cells can be serially transplanted up to five times before the marrow grafts fail to sustain hematopoiesis [5,6]. The transplantation process places extreme demand on the HSC population that is not encountered during normal aging, which leads to the suggestion that mouse BM cells have sufficient proliferative capacity to sustain hematopoiesis over multiple mouse lifespans [7,8]. Even more confounding is the finding by our laboratory and others that the absolute number of HSCs does not decrease but actually increases during the lifetime of the widely used C57BL/6 (B6) mouse strain [9–11]. Indeed, even human studies have shown that the ability of HSCs

to support hematopoiesis throughout life is reflected by the constancy of mature blood cell counts [12,13]. In light of this evidence it would seem pointless to suggest that HSCs become impaired as a result of the aging process. However, we now know that at the cellular level HSCs show aging-associated changes in processes integral for proper hematopoiesis. Here we present a brief yet comprehensive gathering of data that support the hypothesis that HSCs are significant targets of the aging process, which in turn result in the impairment and subsequent exhaustion of their functional capacity to maintain tissue homeostasis.

What do we mean by "exhaustion"? In the scope of this chapter, we refer to exhaustion as one of two outcomes: (1) the decreased hematopoietic capacity of HSCs, or (2) a decline in the number of HSCs to a threshold level that results in the impairment of steady-state and/or stress hematopoiesis. In this chapter we take a point-by-point approach to identify the parameters of stem cell function that may serve as substrates for the aging-associated decline of their function, while integrating putative mechanisms of aging, such as oxidative stress, DNA damage, and replicative senescence. Specifically, we will examine the processes of self-renewal, proliferation, and multi-lineage differentiation, a combination of characteristics that uniquely define a pluripotent stem cell. Furthermore, we will discuss aging-associated changes in stem cell mobilization and homing, processes that are required not only during BM transplantation but also during steady-state hematopoiesis. We will also explore how aging may lead to alterations in the integrity of the HSC genome

Blood Disorders in the Elderly, ed. Lodovico Balducci, William Ershler, Giovanni de Gaetano.
Published by Cambridge University Press. © Cambridge University Press 2008.

as well as the role that apoptosis plays in the regulation of the stem cell pool. Finally, we will summarize the recent developments in our lab relating to the genetic regulation of HSC aging.

Identification and study of the pluripotent HSC

The hematopoietic system is arguably the best-studied and most well-defined stem-cell-driven tissue in mammalian physiology. However, a consensus definition of the HSC, whether by functional assays or by cell surface phenotype, has been difficult to attain within the scientific community. This difficulty arises because most assays used to study HSCs rely on their clonogenic capacity, e.g., colony formation in spleen and methylcellulose or peripheral blood cell production after BM transplantation. In other words, the very cells being studied are lost due to the induction of proliferation and differentiation necessary for colony formation. Recent investigations have thus focused on applying these assays to BM subpopulations that are enriched and/or depleted for cell surface proteins. These cell surface antigens commonly consist of the c-kit receptor and stem cell antigen 1 (Sca-1) on a background that is devoid of lineage markers for differentiated cells, such as granulocytes, B cells, T cells, etc. (Lin-Sca1+ ckit+ or LSK). However, this paradigm of HSC identification has recently been challenged by the finding that cells expressing CD150 but not CD48 receptors of the signaling lymphocytic activation molecule family show remarkable purity for HSCs as defined by long-term repopulating ability [14]. Other approaches have targeted the ability of HSCs to efflux fluorescent dyes, such as Rhodamine 123 and Hoechst 33342 [15,16]. Indeed, it appears the most stringent definition of murine HSC activity may be found in the CD34-LSK fraction within the side population phenotype as assessed by Hoechst 33342 staining [17]. One caveat to studies using cell surface markers or vital dyes, however, is the fact that we do not yet know the full extent of how aging may affect the staining profiles of HSCs and their progeny. Evidence suggests that this may not be the case, with several studies showing unaltered staining profiles of the ckit, Sca-1, and lineage antigens in old mice [9,11,18].

Systemic versus cellular aging

What is aging? When does it begin? What are its targets? These are questions for which there are no easy answers. For instance, does aging begin at birth, at which point development has culminated in an independently functioning individual, or does it begin at puberty, when the individual has attained reproductive maturity, the putative endpoint of natural selection [19]? Furthermore, we can ask at what level the aging process occurs.

It has been proposed that there are two separate yet not necessarily mutually exclusive general levels of organismal aging – systemic and cell-autonomous. Systemic aging has been more formally proposed as the hormonal control of aging, where changes in humoral factors with age can cause system-wide changes in the homeostatic condition [20]. Support for this idea has gained traction from studies of mice expressing a mutant form of the *KLOTHO* gene product encoding a protein hormone that leads to phenotypic changes characteristic of accelerated aging [21]. Conversely, when the wild-type *KLOTHO* gene is overexpressed in mice it leads to a modest yet significant increase in both male and female lifespan [22].

The cell-autonomous theory on the other hand posits that individual cells are the targets of the aging process, via a time-dependent increase in homeostatic dysfunction. The potential mechanisms include increases in the production of reactive oxygen species, telomere shortening, and, not surprisingly, genomic instability. An implication of this theory is that long-lived cells in the organism, such as neurons, muscle, and importantly stem cells, would be the predominant substrates of aging, while those cells that undergo rapid and continuous turnover would be removed before they could exert an effect on tissue function. Here we take the view that aging targets the cell-intrinsic processes necessary for maintenance of tissue and thus organismal function. Specifically, we define aging as the detrimental and irreversible changes that occur during a cell's lifetime that lead to the inability of the resident tissue to maintain homeostasis both at steady-state levels and in response to stress. Importantly, this definition could also apply to the cellular changes that lead to carcinogenesis, a process bearing some of the common principles of aging. The fact that the incidence of most types of cancer escalates rapidly after the age of 65 and arises from accumulated genomic lesions is evidence that cancer is a manifestation of the aging process [23]. Thus, the changes in cellular biology that occur during oncogenesis should also be evident, in part, during successful aging.

Model systems of stem cell aging

The field of hematology has benefited immensely from the study of a wide variety of organisms. Studies of invertebrate systems such as *C. elegans* and *D. melanogaster* have yielded keen insight into stem cell biology and mechanisms of aging, but it has predominantly been the study of the mammalian hematopoietic system that has led to the current understanding of the physiology of hematopoiesis. The utilization of mouse genetics has only recently been fully realized as a tool, as it was this mammalian model that yielded the breakthrough discoveries of Till and McCulloch [24]. Most studies on the aging of HSCs have used the B6 strain due to its utility as a model for transplantation studies via the polymorphic CD45 locus. However, we now know that the B6 mouse strain is not necessarily representative of all other inbred mouse strains. We and others have shown that the HSCs of B6 mice differ markedly from other strains in proliferative kinetics, homing and engraftment properties, and pool size with age [25–27]. In addition, the B6 mouse strain is one of the longest-lived mouse strains, with a mean lifespan of 3 years, versus other mouse strains with mean lifespans of 1.5 to 2 years. Therefore, it is evident that the genetic background of a particular

mouse strain can have a profound effect on the biology of the HSC population as well as organismal longevity. Indeed, it is for this reason that it is difficult to compare findings from various laboratories where different mouse strains are used. Furthermore, caution must be exercised when attempting to extrapolate findings in homozygous laboratory mice to genetically heterogeneous humans.

The identification and study of human HSCs have lagged behind that of mouse and other mammalian HSCs primarily due to the difficulty in obtaining significant amounts of BM, particularly from very old donors. Furthermore, the field was hampered early on by the reliance on in-vitro clonogenic assays of putative HSC function in the absence of reliable in-vivo model systems such as those used by mouse researchers. A significant development in this regard has been the creation of severe combined immune deficient (SCID) mice that are able to support human HSC-derived hematopoiesis following BM transplant [28]. These mice have yielded key insights into the structure of the human hematopoietic hierarchy as well as the conservation of hematopoietic regulation between mouse and man. However, study of the long-term repopulating and self-renewal ability ascribed to HSCs, particularly as they relate to aging, is hampered by the large cell doses necessary for engraftment, the delayed time course of engraftment, and the relatively short repopulating period [28,29].

Regulation of aged HSC proliferation

A current model of HSC-directed hematopoiesis is based on the principle that one or at most a few HSCs of a highly quiescent population divide to produce highly proliferative progenitors with restricted developmental potential. These lineage-restricted transit-amplifying cells bear the proliferative load necessary for the production of the repertoire of cell types found in the peripheral blood. Thus, the ability of HSCs to carry out the demands of hematopoiesis hinges on their ability to proliferate in response to both intrinsic and extrinsic cues. The clonal selection theory of hematopoiesis [30] is supported by studies showing that when retrovirally marked HSCs were transplanted into a conditioned host, only a few clones contributed to mature blood cell production [31,32]. This observation was confirmed by Van Zant *et al.* [33], who, using the same retroviral marking strategy in B6-D2 chimeric mice, also showed the involvement of only a few clones in carrying out hematopoiesis. However, recent evidence suggests that the integration of these retroviral vectors into the DNA is not necessarily neutral in their effect on the fitness of the transformed cells. For example, the integration sites of clonally dominant HSCs often encode regulatory regions involved in the processes of HSC self-renewal and survival [34]. Furthermore, the transplantation studies that demonstrate oligoclonal hematopoiesis may not be representative of steady-state hematopoiesis in an unperturbed animal. Finally, when mice were continuously administered BrdU in their drinking water, the entire population of HSCs completed at least one round of replication within a two-month time period [35–37]. This finding implies that all HSCs in the BM contribute to steady-state hematopoiesis, thus arguing against an oligoclonal process.

The idea that the proliferative nature of HSCs may change during aging is consistent with the observation that the incidence of myeloproliferative disorders markedly increases with age in both mice and humans. One study showing that the frequency of HSCs in cycle old B6 mice was three times higher than in young animals seems to corroborate this finding. If true, this means that with an HSC frequency seven times higher in old mice, the increase in the absolute numbers of proliferating HSCs is quite profound [9]. Furthermore, studies using serial administration of hydroxyurea or irradiation of BM cells have shown no evidence for a decline in the capacity of HSCs to proliferate.

It should come as no surprise that most factors responsible for regulation of the cell cycle were discovered in the study of cancer, a disease of dysregulated cellular proliferation. A classic example is the retinoblastoma protein (pRb), which was first discovered as the affected gene product responsible for the development of retinal tumors during childhood. It has since been shown that members of the pRb family act to suppress entry into the active cell cycle and, upon their phosphorylation, allow for the assembly of the replicative machinery. Their phosphorylation is governed by the concerted actions of the cyclin-dependent kinases (cdks) and the cdk inhibitors (ckis). Chief among the ckis are $p16^{INK4a}$, $p21^{cip-1}$, and $p27^{kip-1}$. Their role in hematopoietic progenitor cell (HPC) proliferation was first shown by Mantel *et al.* [38], who demonstrated that p21 levels rise while those of p27 decrease after stimulation by the hematopoietic cytokines Steel factor and granulocyte colony-stimulating factor (G-CSF). Additionally, it has been shown that p27 has no effect on proliferation in the stem cell compartment, yet has a dramatic effect on the progenitor cell compartment [39]. It has also been shown that p21 plays a role in both stem cell proliferation and self-renewal [40]. Lewis *et al.* [41] demonstrated that mice null for the $p16^{INK4a}$ locus exhibit increased proliferation in the progenitor compartment. It was recently shown that transcriptional repressors, such as the Gfi-1 gene product, promote HSC quiescence and thus maintain the HSC in its pluripotent state [42,43]. While no studies have reported whether there are age-related alterations in the levels of these mitotic factors, it is tempting to hypothesize that these same molecular changes that contribute to tumorigenesis occur during "normal" aging as well.

Self-renewal of HSCs is altered during aging

In demonstration of the difficulty in parsing out changes in HSC proliferation and self-renewal, it has been shown that, while the self-renewal ability of murine HSCs undergoes progressive decline with serial transplantation [44], there are alterations in the frequency of cycling HSCs with age [9,10]. Moreover, many factors that play a role in the regulation of stem cell cycling also regulate self-renewal, particularly at the genomic level. Much excitement has been generated recently with the identification of the homeobox domain (Hox) family of transcription factors as potent regulators of stem cell function. The family member *HOXB4* can promote self-renewal as well as proliferation of HSCs while still allowing for effective differentiation. Other Hox family members implicated in HSC renewal, however, show pronounced effects on the differentiation pathways, often resulting in acute myeloid leukemia (AML). For example, the pro-leukemic *HOXB6* promotes HSC expansion and myeloid-directed differentiation at the expense of lympho- and erythropoiesis when overexpressed in mouse HSCs [45]. Similar results have also been shown with *HOXA9* and *HOXA10* [46,47].

Histone modification may play a role in the self-renewal of HSCs by modulating the transcriptional accessibility of the chromatin. Histones are targets of multiple classes of enzymes involved in acetylation, methylation, and phosphorylation whose function is to modify the DNA binding properties of the histones. In HSCs, members of the Polycomb gene family have been shown to play a key role in regulating self-renewal. The archetype of this group of chromatin modifiers is the *BMI-1* gene, whose function is to serve as a scaffold for the assembly of multimeric protein complexes consisting of histone methylases and deacetylases. In mice null for the *BMI-1* gene, the pool of HSCs shows accelerated exhaustion both in unperturbed and transplant settings [48]. The mel-18 gene product is another member of this group, and has been shown to result in the expansion of competitive repopulating units (CRUs) when overexpressed in mice [49].

The gold standard of proof for changes with age in the ability to self-renew comes from CRU studies of serially transplanted mice where the CRU frequency of young and old donors can be reliably measured in BM recipients. However, studies of B6 mice, where HSC numbers increase with age, have traditionally been the only available model to study competitive repopulation. Recently, Kamminga *et al.* [50] compared the renewal capacity of HSCs from B6 and D2 mice and showed that HSCs from D2 have a 1000-fold less capacity for expansion compared to B6 mice. It is tempting to speculate that changes in factors involved in self-renewal are altered during aging. In fact, a recent profiling of the transcriptional changes that occur in HSCs of B6 mice during aging found that 16 genes were upregulated with age that regulate hematopoiesis, including self-renewal [51].

Telomeres shorten with age

Telomeres have been postulated to serve as the mitotic clock underlying Hayflick's limit of replicative capacity [52]. Telomeres, the repetitive, noncoding DNA sequences at the ends of DNA strands, are the molecular solution to the end-replication problem of DNA synthesis. With each round of cell division, portions of these "dispensable" sequences are lost until a point is reached when they have contracted to a critically short length termed "crisis" [53]. This phenomenon commonly precedes cell death and/or senescence as well as oncogenic transformation. In renewing cell populations, it is believed that telomeres are resistant to replication-induced erosion through the activity of telomerase, the enzyme responsible for adding new sequences to the ends of telomeres. In fact, HSCs exhibit significant activity of this enzyme, thus potentially extending their proliferative capacity [54]. However, telomere shortening does indeed occur in the HSC compartment during aging and after HSC transplantation [55,56]. That telomeres also serve as docking regions for proteins regulating DNA integrity, such as TRF1, TRF2, and Ku, testifies to the impact of telomere shortening with age. Whether telomere shortening represents a molecular factor for the aging of HSCs or is merely correlative remains to be seen (for review see Greider [57] and Blackburn [58]). Furthermore, inbred mouse models may not be representative of telomere dynamics among mammals because inbred mice exhibit significantly longer telomeres than outbred mice [59] and thus they are not limiting in the proliferative potential of mouse HSCs during a typical lifespan [60]. However, because human telomeres are significantly shorter than mouse telomeres, telomere shortening may play a role in human HSC aging, especially after HSC transplantation.

Differentiation of stem cells

The ability of HSCs to provide adequate numbers of differentiated progeny is critical for the essential processes of oxygen transport, immune response, and blood coagulation. Indeed, in humans, aging is often accompanied by increased platelet activity, decreased immune responses, and changes in erythrocytes such as membrane deformability and oxygen carrying capacity. Whether these changes can be traced back to alterations in the HSCs is not yet clear. However, changes in the differentiation capacity of aged HSCs are supported by evidence that shows skewing of the ratios of the mature blood cell types. For instance, in older humans, as well as in mice, blood cell production is often skewed toward the myeloid lineage at the expense of both T- and B-cell production [11]. Furthermore, this phenomenon arises from a qualitative change in the HSC, as evidenced by an age-associated increase in phenotypic HSCs with increased myeloid potential. This finding was recently corroborated in experiments studying the homing of aged HSCs, where homed HSCs showed an aging-associated myeloid skewing with a concomitant deficiency in T-cell production in animals transplanted with old CRUs compared to young CRUs [9,61]. While a potential mechanism has yet to be defined, it is interesting that the cellular basis of acute myeloid leukemia is the production of myeloid progenitors arrested at the blast stage from a population of leukemic stem cells. It is feasible that the molecular changes during aging that cause myeloid skewing may also serve as one hit in the two-hit model of leukemogenesis [62].

Mobilization of stem cells

The frequency of stem cells in BM is determined not only by their proliferation and self-renewal but also by the balance of mobilization and homing. Here mobilization refers to the detachment of stem cells from their supporting stroma and subsequent entry into the systemic circulation. In clinical practice, this process has been manipulated using cytokines such as G-CSF in order to obtain sufficient numbers of cells for BM transplantation. However, it has become apparent that mobilization is a significant process during steady-state hematopoiesis as well. For instance, peripheral blood of mice contains low levels of BM progenitor cells. Furthermore, using parabiotic mice, these progenitor cells in the peripheral blood engraft non-conditioned BM of the partner mouse [63]. However, no studies have conclusively determined whether aging has an effect on either homeostatic or cytokine-induced HSC mobilization. Dose-response studies of G-CSF-induced mobilization of hematopoietic progenitors showed that 60% fewer CFU-GM-forming cells entered the circulation in old adults aged 70 to 80 years compared to young adults aged 20 to 30 years [64]. Furthermore, de la Rubia *et al.* [65] showed that the mobilization efficiency of CD34+ cells in response to G-CSF is two fold higher in patients younger than 18 versus those at older ages. In contrast, Boiret *et al.* [66] showed that the numbers of long-term culture-initiating cells in peripheral blood after G-CSF treatment do not differ between children and adults. Thus, more studies are needed to determine whether HSC mobilization is affected by the aging process, especially during steady-state hematopoiesis.

HSC homing during aging

The ability of transplanted BM cells to rescue hematopoiesis in lethally irradiated recipients requires that the injected cells migrate to the appropriate BM niche. This process of homing and ensuing engraftment is highly dependent on factors intrinsic to the HSCs and the BM microenvironment. Prior studies showing a decreased ability of aged cells to repopulate serially transplanted hosts compared to young cells have failed to adequately address the age-related changes in the ability of the cells to home to the proper microenvironment. While Morrison *et al.* [9] observed that old BM cells may not home as well to the BM as young cells, the study was not able to distinguish between the homing and actual engraftment of the HSCs.

We recently undertook to distinguish the individual roles that homing and engraftment played in the age-related changes in competitive repopulating ability of HSCs. Having shown that old progenitor cells homed to the BM one-third as well as young progenitor cells three hours after injection, we sought to determine whether more primitive BM cells from old animals also exhibited this characteristic deficiency in homing ability. By performing BM transplantation on myeloablated recipients and harvesting the BM 24 hours later, we could conceivably capture the primitive BM cells that had homed to the vacant marrow niche. We then injected these BM aspirates into secondary recipients in limiting doses to determine the CRU frequency of the homed cells. When the CRU seeding efficiency was compared between young and old donors transplanted into young hosts, we found that two fold more young HSCs had homed to the BM compared to old HSCs [61]. Additionally, the proliferative potential did not differ between young and old HSCs as assayed by clone size of individual CRUs.

DNA repair and genomic instability during aging

The fact that the HSC population must support hematopoiesis during the entire lifetime of the animal raises several interesting problems. First, these long-lived cells are under constant stress from both endogenous and exogenous genotoxins that can have profound effects on their DNA. Second, the proliferative nature of the HSCs and their immediate progeny makes them susceptible to DNA synthetic errors. Third, any unrepaired lesions that occur in the cells' DNA are necessarily passed on to their progeny. This last statement implies that upon self-renewal of cells containing DNA lesions, these lesions will be fixed in the genome of the HSC pool. To confront these potentially devastating processes, HSCs have been endowed with several defense mechanisms to ensure genomic stability (For review see Park & Gerson [67]). Murine HSCs preferentially express DNA repair genes compared to their mature

progeny [68,69]; however, human CD34+ cells have diverse responses to DNA damage with enhanced repair of UV-induced strand breaks, but impaired repair of nitrosourea-induced strand breaks [70,71].

Fanconi anemia is a rare autosomal recessive genetic disease that results in hematopoietic failure in children, and is composed of seven complementation groups. In mice, when the Fanconi anemia group C (*Fncc*) gene was knocked out, a significant decrease of 40–70% of primitive HSCs was found, with a corresponding increase in the sensitivity of these cells to the DNA-damaging agent mitomycin C at two months of age. This provides compelling evidence that DNA repair is an active process in HSCs and is critical for the maintenance of the HSC pool. A similar effect on the hematopoietic compartment has been observed in mice expressing a hypomorphic allele of the DSB repair gene *RAD50*, with complete BM failure occurring within four to eight weeks of birth [72].

While it is known that the ability of somatic cells to repair their DNA is altered during the aging process, evidence in HSCs is admittedly scant. Most studies that imply a role for decreasing DNA repair ability of HSCs rely on gene knockouts that result in progeroid, or premature-aging, phenotypes. For instance, mice null for the repair protein Ercc1 show progressive marrow failure resulting in a pancytopenia, while the mice exhibit several symptoms of premature aging [73]. However, no studies to date have demonstrated conclusively that diminished DNA repair capacity of HSCs with age results in their functional impairment, much less a decreased ability to repair DNA lesions with age.

Apoptosis

Surprisingly, there is a paucity of data on the role that apoptosis plays in the maintenance of HSC numbers. It is tempting to speculate that HSCs are subject to the same pro-apoptotic stimuli as other metabolically active cell types: reactive oxygen species, genomic damage, etc. Furthermore, apoptosis has been implicated as a gatekeeper mechanism of oncogenic transformation, a real consequence of the proliferative nature of stem cells [74]. To date the best evidence for the role of apoptosis in the regulation of the HSC pool comes from a study showing that overexpressing *Bcl-2* in mice resulted in a greater than two fold increase in primitive HSC numbers over wild-type mice. Furthermore, these transgenic HSCs manifested a competitive advantage over wild-type cells upon competitive repopulation [75]. In support of this observation, conditional deletion of the *Bcl-2* family member *Mcl-1* resulted in massive apoptosis of the BM with significant ablation of the HSC compartment [76]. Together, these studies suggest a critical role for the regulation of apoptosis in the size of the HSC pool. The role of apoptosis in the aging of HSCs has yet to be shown.

Genetic regulation of stem cell aging

Inbred mice have proved to be indispensable in the study of mammalian hematopoiesis, allowing for the definition of the hematopoietic hierarchy, molecular regulators of the various lineages, and theories of stem cell biology. However, only recently has it been recognized that inbred mouse strains exhibit pronounced heterogeneity in various parameters of HSC function. Indeed, our laboratory first became aware of this when we observed that the fraction of spleen colony-forming units (CFU-S) in cycle differed markedly among various inbred mouse strains. In particular we found a ten fold difference in the fraction of these proliferating hematopoietic progenitor cells between the B6 and D2 mouse strains, as assayed by a cell suicide technique [77].

This extreme difference in cycling cells between the two strains could be due to extrinsic factors regulating cellular proliferation or intrinsic factors that were present within the cells. To address this question, we constructed chimeric (allophenic) mice by combining pre-implantation embryos from B6 and D2 mice and injecting them into pseudo-pregnant female mice. In this way the extrinsic signals from the microenvironment would be common to the HSCs of both mouse strains, while the cell-autonomous differences would determine HSC function. We conducted blood cell chimerism studies for the duration of the individual allophenic lifetimes, which ranged from 1.5 to 3 years. In all animals tested, we found that both D2 and B6 HSCs contributed to hematopoiesis, as evidenced by the production of erythroid, lymphoid, and myeloid cell types during the first year of life. Interestingly, during the second year of life, the contribution of the D2 HSCs to hematopoiesis began to decline, until at two years, blood cell production was wholly B6 in origin [26]. It most likely is not a coincidence that this time point is also near the natural lifespan of the D2 mouse strain. In fact, as will be mentioned later, there is a striking correlation among various HSC parameters and organismal lifespan in the laboratory mouse.

With the observed differences in HSC cycling and hematopoiesis in chimeric mice, it is intriguing to invoke Hayflick's theory of the limited replicative capacity of proliferating somatic cells. In other words, did the D2 stem cell pool of chimeric mice reach its mitotic limit, thus allowing the slowly cycling B6 pool to take over blood cell production? To answer this, we transplanted BM of the allophenics in which D2 blood cell production had become undetectable into myeloablated recipients and found that initially D2 HSCs once again contributed to hematopoiesis. This, however, only lasted a few months, when once again blood cell production was solely of B6 origin. This interval of D2 blood cell production was even shorter in secondary transplants, thus showing the presence and reversible quiescence of the D2 HSC population [78]. Because some parameters of stem cell function were genetically regulated, we undertook genetic studies to identify molecular determinants of stem cell aging.

The genetic studies that we have undertaken are based on the premise that strain-specific differences in stem cell parameters are the result of unique combinations of genetic loci for which each mouse strain is homozygous. To parse out the individual genes that are responsible for these phenotypes, it is necessary to generate mice that have unique combinations of genetic loci derived from the parental strains, in order that quantitative changes in stem cell function can be correlated to specific chromosomal loci. In the context of our laboratory, we used the D2 and B6 mouse strains because of the strain-specific differences we have observed in HSC cycling and population dynamics with age. Furthermore, a recombinant inbred (RI) line of mice derived from these two strains was already in existence and being utilized for quantitative trait studies. The BXD RI mice consist of over 50 individual lines harboring unique homozygous combinations of B6 and D2 alleles. The high density of markers that have been mapped in these strains (over 2000) allows for the mapping of quantitative trait loci (QTL) with a resolution of one centimorgan (cM).

This approach clearly would not have been possible using previously described methods, due to the numbers of animals needed across the large number of BXD lines. Therefore, we applied a cell culture technique that relies on the survival, proliferation, and differentiation of HSCs in close association with a stromal cell monolayer. The cobblestone area-forming cell (CAFC) assay, as initially described by Dexter and Lajtha [79] and further developed by Cashman *et al.* [80] and Ploemacher *et al.* [81], is based on the observation that as HSC progeny transit the hematopoietic hierarchy, they expand in number and are increasingly in cycle. Limiting dilutions of BM cells are seeded onto FBMD-1 stromal cell monolayers in 96-well plates and assayed for the presence of CAFCs at one-week intervals starting on day 7. Indeed, the "primitiveness" of the stem cell is highly correlated to its quiescent state, such that cells that form cobblestones on day 35 are more primitive and less numerous than those that form cobblestones on day 28 and so on [81]. Furthermore, the cells that form CAFCs on day 35 are comparable to those able to initiate long-term cultures as well as engraft irradiated recipients long-term, and thus serve as a measure of stem cell activity in vitro [82].

We initially measured the frequency of day-7 CAFCs in cycle among eight inbred mouse strains and found that the percentage of the HPCs in S phase varied by more than ten fold from the highest to lowest cycling strains, as was seen previously using the CFU-S assay. Because we had previously observed that this trait seemed to correlate to lifespan in at least the D2 and B6 strains, we plotted the CAFC day-7 cycling data against the mean lifespan of the eight respective strains and found a striking inverse linear correlation of the two traits among all strains [10]. We had now supported our HSC cycling/lifespan hypothesis in three different experimental paradigms, and thus sought to identify the genetic regulators of these key traits. Our next step was to phenotype each of the BXD lines for the CAFC day-7 cycling trait to identify the responsible QTL. As a result, we identified two major loci on chromosomes 7 and 11 and two minor QTL on chromosomes 4 and 9 that accounted for at least part of the cycling phenotype. Using existing lifespan data of the existing BXD lines from Gelman *et al.* [83], we again showed a negative linear relationship between lifespan and HPC cycling. Importantly, on mapping the lifespan trait in the BXD lines, we found linkage to the same markers on chromosomes 7 and 11 responsible for CAFC day-7 cycling in addition to markers on chromosomes 2 and 4 [84]. Assuming a common gene underlies both loci, this would suggest but not necessarily prove causality between HSC/HPC cycling and lifespan.

The identification of QTL regulating stem cell function is just the first step in a long and potentially laborious path to identify the gene underlying the locus. A candidate-gene approach, whereby genes mapping to QTL-containing intervals are tested for their functional impact, is certainly a valid option in this context. However, the regions spanning the 95% confidence interval of the QTL are often megabases long and thus contain hundreds and perhaps thousands of genes. Instead, we approached the problem by selectively intercrossing and subsequently backcrossing B6 and D2 mice to move individual QTL from one strain onto the other strain's genetic background. These congenic mice allow us to determine whether the QTL truly contributes to the trait of interest if the phenotype follows the genotype. Thus, we would expect that when we move the B6 chromosome 7 locus controlling CAFC day-7 cycling onto a D2 background, the percentage of cycling day-7 CAFCs would more closely approximate that of the B6 strain and vice versa. Preliminary data have indeed borne out this expectation, while we do not yet know whether this locus affects organismal longevity.

A locus on chromosome 2 linked to aging of stem cells

It was mentioned previously that the B6 and D2 mouse strains markedly differ in various facets of HSC biology. For one, the B6 strain at young ages (<10 months) has two- to three fold fewer HSCs per femur than age-matched D2 mice. When the HSC pool was measured over the lifespan of these mice, the frequency of HSCs in B6 BM increased in a linear fashion along with that of D2 during the first year of life. However, after this point the HSC numbers dramatically fell in D2 mice while they continued to rise in the B6 mice. Thus, we surmised that the aging of the stem cells in these two strains differed according to their unique genetic background. QTL mapping revealed a locus on mouse chromosome 2 from 135 to150 Mbp that was linked to this particular trait. Intriguingly, we found that this locus overlapped a separately mapped locus involved in lifespan determination in these two strains. Congenic mice were then generated where we crossed the QTL-containing interval from the D2 strain onto a B6 background (B6.D2 Chr 2) to test the mapping data. Phenotyping of the congenic mice revealed a two-fold decrease in the HSC compartment of old mice compared to old B6 animals, thus confirming the role of the chromosome 2 locus in the aging-associated change in HSC numbers. Transplantation experiments where young BM from the congenic mice was competed against that of B6 revealed a significant decline in the contribution of B6.D2 HSCs to hematopoiesis one year after transplant. Furthermore, when BM from the primary recipients was injected into secondary recipients, a further drop in chimerism was observed in the B6.D2 compartment after only four months post-transplant. Given that the frequency of HSCs in BM was not different between the two strains at young age, it can be hypothesized that a decline in

the quality of the stem cells has already occurred and is only made manifest upon the transplantation process. To gain an understanding of what may be occurring mechanistically to cause this qualitative change in the stem cell compartment, we irradiated B6 and B6.D2 mice with either 0, 1, or 2 Gy of ionizing radiation, harvested their BM, and determined their competitive repopulating ability. As expected, at the 1 Gy dose, a significant effect was seen in the progenitor population, as evidenced by the reduced populating ability of BM from the B6.D2 mice at 8 and 12 but not 20 weeks post-transplant. However, at a dose of 2 Gy, virtually no B6.D2 contribution to peripheral blood cell counts was observed, and this was confirmed by analysis of BM chimerism. These data confirm that the functional capacity of HSCs from the congenic mice is compromised at an early age and that the defect may lie in the response to DNA damage. Whether this defect is the underlying cause of the decline in HSC numbers with age is yet to be determined.

Conclusion

It is now apparent that the HSC does not represent an immortal cell type, oblivious to the aging process while satisfying its tissue-specific demands at any cost. At the moment the only cell that comes near to fitting this description, in terms of both self-renewal capacity and developmental potency, is the embryonic stem cell [85]. Indeed, we have shown here that almost every parameter of HSC function is altered in some way during the aging process and may lead to functional exhaustion in a permissive genetic background. How this is relevant at the level of human HSC biology is not immediately clear. However, BM donation/transplantation is continuously being applied to older individuals. It is imperative that these BM grafts, when administered to young patients, must be able to support hematopoiesis for the remainder of that individual's life. There is little doubt that genetic alterations will have occurred within the repopulating population, and that this may predispose these cells to oncogenic transformation. However, long-term studies of transplant recipients of allografts are conspicuously absent. Will this patient show skewing of blood cell production? Will the incidence of leukemia, on a background of unknown mutational profile, rise? With the growing interest in stem-cell-based therapies, it is clear that these questions need to be addressed.

REFERENCES

1. Lansdorp PM. Stem cell biology for the transfusionist. *Vox Sang* 1998; **74**: 91–4.

2. Osawa M, Hanada K, Hamada H, Nakauchi H. Long-term lymphohematopoietic reconstitution by a single CD34-low/negative hematopoietic stem cell. *Science* 1996; **273**: 242–5.

3. Krause DS, Theise ND, Collector MI, *et al.* Multi-organ, multi-lineage engraftment by a single bone marrow-derived stem cell. *Cell* 2001; **105**: 369–77.

4. Iscove N, Nawa K. Hematopoietic stem cells expand during serial transplantation in vivo without apparent exhaustion. *Curr Biol* 1997; **7**: 805–8.

5. Siminovitch L, Till JE McCulloch EA. Decline in colony-forming ability of marrow cells subjected to serial transplantation into irradiated mice. *J Cell Comp Physiol* 1964; **64**: 23–31.

6. Ogden DA, Micklem HS. The fate of serially transplanted bone marrow cell populations from young and old donors. Transplantation 1976; **22**: 287–93.

7. Harrison DE, Astle CM, Delaittre JA. Loss of proliferative capacity in immunohemopoietic stem cells is caused by serial transplantation rather than aging. *J Exp Med* 1978; **147**: 1526–31.

8. Harrison D, Astle C. Loss of stem cell repopulating ability upon transplantation. Effects of donor age, cell number, and transplantation procedure. *J Exp Med* 1982; **156**: 1767–79.

9. Morrison SJ, Wandycz AM, Akashi K, Globerson A, Weissman IL. The aging of hematopoietic stem cells. *Nat Med* 1996; **2**: 1011–16.

10. de Haan G, Nijhof W, Van Zant G. Mouse strain-dependent changes in frequency and proliferation of hematopoietic stem cells during aging: correlation between lifespan and cycling activity. *Blood* 1997; **89**: 1543–50.

11. Sudo K, Ema H, Morita Y, Nakauchi H. Age-associated characteristics of murine hematopoietic stem cells. *J Exp Med* 2000; **192**: 1273–80.

12. Marley SB, Lewis JL, Davidson RJ, *et al.* Evidence for a continuous decline in haemopoietic cell function from birth: application to evaluating bone marrow failure in children. *Br J Haematol* 1999; **106**: 162–6.

13. Bagnara GP, Bonsi L, Strippoli P, *et al.* Hemopoiesis in healthy old people and centenarians: well-maintained responsiveness of CD34+ cells to hemopoietic growth factors and remodeling of cytokine network. *J Gerontol A Biol Sci Med Sci* 2000; **55**: B61–B70.

14. Kiel MJ, Yilmaz OH, Iwashita T, Yilmaz OH, Terhorst C, Morrison SJ. SLAM family receptors distinguish hematopoietic stem and progenitor cells and reveal endothelial niches for stem cells. *Cell* 2005; **121**: 1109–21.

15. Udomsakdi C, Eaves CJ, Sutherland HJ, Lansdorp PM. Separation of functionally distinct subpopulations of primitive human hematopoietic cells using rhodamine-123. *Exp Hematol* 1991; **19**: 338–42.

16. Goodell MA, Brose K, Paradis G, Conner AS, Mulligan RC. Isolation and functional properties of murine hematopoietic stem cells that are replicating in vivo. *J Exp Med* 1996; **183**: 1797–806.

17. Matsuzaki Y, Kinjo K, Mulligan RC, Okano H. Unexpectedly efficient homing capacity of purified murine hematopoietic stem cells. *Immunity* 2004; **20**: 87–93.

18. de Haan G, Szilvassy SJ, Meyerrose TE, Dontje B, Grimes B, Van Zant G. Distinct functional properties of highly purified hematopoietic stem cells from mouse strains differing in stem cell numbers. *Blood* 2000; **96**: 1374–9.

19. Schlessinger D, Ko MSH. Developmental genomics and its relation to aging. *Genomics* 1998; **52**: 113–18.

20. Wise PM, Krajnak KM, Kashon ML. Menopause: the aging of multiple pacemakers. *Science* 1996; **273**: 67–70.

21. Kuro-o M, Matsumura Y, Aizawa H, *et al.* Mutation of the mouse klotho gene leads to a syndrome resembling ageing. *Nature* 1997; **390**: 45–51.

22. Kurosu H, Yamamoto M, Clark JD, *et al.* Suppression of aging in mice by the hormone Klotho. *Science* 2005; **309**: 1829–33.

23. Edwards BK, Brown ML, Wingo PA, *et al.* Annual report to the nation on the status of cancer, 1975–2002, featuring population-based trends in cancer treatment. *J Natl Cancer Inst* 2005; **97**: 1407–27.

24. Till JE, McCulloch EA. Direct measurement of radiation sensitivity of normal mouse bone marrow cells. *Radiat Res* 1961; **14**: 213–22.

25. Harrison DE. Long-term erythropoietic repopulating ability of old, young, and fetal stem cells. *J Exp Med* 1983; **157**: 1496–504.

26. Van Zant G, Holland BP, Eldridge PW, Chen JJ. Genotype-restricted growth and aging patterns in hematopoietic stem cell populations of allophenic mice. *J Exp Med* 1990; **171**: 1547–65.

27. Chen J, Astle CM, Harrison DE. Development and aging of primitive hematopoietic stem cells in BALB/cBy mice. *Exp Hematol* 1999; **27**: 928–35.

28. Dick JE. Normal and leukemic human stem cells assayed in SCID mice. *Semin Immunol* 1996; **8**: 197–206.

29. Dick JE, Guenechea G, Gan OI, Dorrell C. In vivo dynamics of human stem cell repopulation in NOD/SCID mice. *Ann N Y Acad Sci* 2001; **938**: 184–90.

30. Kay HEM. How many cell-generations? *Lancet* 1965; **ii**: 418.

31. Dick JE, Magli MC, Huszar D, Phillips RA, Bernstein A. Introduction of a selectable gene into primitive stem cells capable of long-term reconstitution of the hemopoietic system of W/Wv mice. *Cell* 1985; **42**: 71–9.

32. Jordan CT, Lemischka IR. Clonal and systemic analysis of long-term hematopoiesis in the mouse. *Genes Dev* 1990; **4**: 220–2.

33. Van Zant G, Chen JJ, Scott-Micus K. Developmental potential of hematopoietic stem cells determined using retrovirally marked allophenic marrow. *Blood* 1991; **77**: 756–63.

34. Kustikova O, Fehse B, Modlich U, *et al.* Clonal dominance of hematopoietic stem cells triggered by retroviral gene marking. *Science* 2005; **308**: 1171–4.

35. Pietrzyk ME, Priestley GV, Wolf NS. Normal cycling patterns of hematopoietic stem cell subpopulations: an assay using long-term in vivo BrdU infusion. *Blood* 1985; **66**: 1460–2.

36. Bradford GB, Williams B, Rossi R, Bertoncello I. Quiescence, cycling, and turnover in the primitive hematopoietic stem cell compartment. *Exp Hematol* 1997; **25**: 445–53.

37. Cheshier SH, Morrison SJ, Liao X, Weissman IL. In vivo proliferation and cell cycle kinetics of long-term self-renewing hematopoietic stem cells. *Proc Natl Acad Sci USA* 1999; **96**: 3120–5.

38. Mantel C, Luo Z, Canfield J, Braun S, Deng C, Broxmeyer HE. Involvement of p21cip-1 and p27kip-1 in the molecular mechanisms of steel factor-induced proliferative synergy in vitro and of p21cip-1 in the maintenance of stem/progenitor cells in vivo. *Blood* 1996; **88**: 3710–19.

39. Cheng T, Rodrigues N, Dombkowski D, Stier S, Scadden DT. Stem cell repopulation efficiency but not pool size is governed by p27kip1. *Nat Med* 2002; **6**: 1235–40.

40. Cheng T, Rodrigues N, Shen H, *et al.* Hematopoietic stem cell quiescence maintained by p21(Cip1/waf1). *Science* 2000; **287**: 1804–8.

41. Lewis JL, Chinswangwatanakul W, Zheng B, *et al.* The influence of INK4 proteins on growth and self-renewal kinetics of hematopoietic progenitor cells. *Blood* 2001; **97**: 2604–10.

42. Hock H, Hamblen MJ, Rooke HM, *et al.* Gfi-1 restricts proliferation and preserves functional integrity of haematopoietic stem cells. *Nature* 2004; **431**: 1002–7.

43. Zeng H, Yucel R, Kosan C, Klein-Hitpass L, Moroy T. Transcription factor Gfi1 regulates self-renewal and engraftment of hematopoietic stem cells. *Embo J* 2004; **23**: 4116–25.

44. Albright J, Makinodan T. Decline in the growth potential of spleen-colonizing bone marrow stem cells of long-lived aging mice. *J Exp Med* 1976; **144**: 1204–13.

45. Fischbach NA, Rozenfeld S, Shen W, *et al.* HOXB6 overexpression in murine bone marrow immortalizes a myelomonocytic precursor in vitro and causes hematopoietic stem cell expansion and acute myeloid leukemia in vivo. *Blood* 2005; **105**: 1456–66.

46. Thorsteinsdottir U, Sauvageau G, Hough MR, *et al.* Overexpression of HOXA10 in murine hematopoietic cells perturbs both myeloid and lymphoid differentiation and leads to acute myeloid leukemia. *Mol Cell Biol* 1997; **17**: 495–505.

47. Thorsteinsdottir U, Mamo A, Kroon E, *et al.* Overexpression of the myeloid leukemia-associated Hoxa9 gene in bone marrow cells induces stem cell expansion. *Blood* 2002; **99**: 121–9.

48. Park IK, Qian D, Kiel M, *et al.* Bmi-1 is required for maintenance of adult self-renewing haematopoietic stem cells. *Nature* 2003; **423**: 302–5.

49. Kajiume T, Ninomiya Y, Ishihara H, Kanno R, Kanno M. Polycomb group gene mel-18 modulates the self-renewal activity and cell cycle status of hematopoietic stem cells. *Exp Hematol* 2004; **32**: 571–8.

50. Kamminga LM, van Os R, Ausema A, *et al.* Impaired hematopoietic stem cell functioning after serial transplantation and during normal aging. *Stem Cells* 2005; **23**: 82–92.

51. Rossi DJ, Bryder D, Zahn JM, *et al.* Cell intrinsic alterations underlie hematopoietic stem cell aging. *Proc Natl Acad Sci USA* 2005; **102**: 9194–9.

52. Hayflick L, Moorhead PS. The serial cultivation of human diploid cell strains. *J Exp Cell Res* 1961; **25**: 585–621.

53. Harley CB, Futcher AB, Greider CW. Telomeres shorten during ageing of human fibroblasts. *Nature* 1990; **345**: 458–60.

54. Morrison SJ, Prowse KR, Ho P, Weissman IL. Telomerase activity in hematopoietic cells is associated with self-renewal potential. *Immunity* 1996; **5**: 207–16.

55. Vaziri H, Dragowska W, Allsopp RC, Thomas TE, Harley CB, Lansdorp PM. Evidence for a mitotic clock in human hematopoietic stem cells: loss of telomeric DNA with age. *Proc Natl Acad Sci USA* 1994; **91**: 9857–60.

56. Allsopp RC, Cheshier S, Weissman IL. Telomere shortening accompanies increased cell cycle activity during serial transplantation of hematopoietic stem cells. *J Exp Med* 2001; **193**: 917–24.

57. Greider CW. Telomeres and senescence: the history, the experiment, the future. *Curr Biol* 1998; **8**: R178–R181.

58. Blackburn EH. Telomere states and cell fates. *Nature* 2000; **408**: 53–6.

59. Manning EL, Crossland J, Dewey MJ, Van Zant G. Influences of inbreeding and genetics on telomere length in mice. *Mamm Genome* 2002; **13**: 234–8.

60. Blasco MA, Lee HW, Hande MP, *et al.* Telomere shortening and tumor formation by mouse cells lacking telomerase RNA. *Cell* 1997; **91**: 25–34.

61. Liang Y, Van Zant G, Szilvassy SJ. Effects of aging on the homing and engraftment of murine hematopoietic stem and progenitor cells. *Blood* 2005; **106**: 1479–87.

62. Dash AB, Williams IR, Kutok JL, *et al.* A murine model of CML blast crisis induced by cooperation between BCR/ABL and NUP98/HOXA9. *Proc Natl Acad Sci USA* 2002; **99**: 7622–7.

63. Wright DE, Wagers AJ, Gulati AP, Johnson FL, Weissman IL. Physiological migration of hematopoietic stem and progenitor cells. *Science* 2001; **294**: 1933–6.

64. Chatta GS, Price TH, Allen RC, Dale DC. Effects of in vivo recombinant methionyl human granulocyte colony-stimulating factor on the neutrophil response and peripheral blood colony-forming cells in healthy young and elderly adult volunteers. *Blood* 1994; **84**: 2923–9.

65. de la Rubia J, Diaz MA, Verdeguer A, *et al.* Donor age-related differences in PBPC mobilization with rHuG-CSF. *Transfusion* 2001; **41**: 201–5.

66. Boiret N, Kanold J, Bons JM, *et al.* Granulocyte colony-stimulating factor-mobilized peripheral blood CD34+ cells from children contain the same levels of long-term culture-initiating cells producing the same numbers of colony-forming cells as those from adults, but display greater in vitro monocyte/macrophage potential. *Br J Haematol* 2001; **112**: 806–13.

67. Park Y, Gerson SL. DNA repair defects in stem cell function and aging. *Annu Rev Med* 2005; **56**: 495–508.

68. Ivanova NB, Dimos JT, Schaniel C, Hackney JA, Moore KA, Lemischka IR. A stem cell molecular signature. *Science* 2002; **298**: 601–4.

69. Ramalho-Santos M, Yoon S, Matsuzaki Y, Mulligan RC, Melton DA. "Stemness": transcriptional profiling of embryonic and adult stem cells. *Science* 2002; **298**: 597–600.

70. Myllyperkio MH, Vilpo JA. Increased DNA single-strand break joining activity in UV-irradiated CD34+ versus CD34− bone marrow cells. *Mutat Res* 1999; **425**: 169–76.

71. Buschfort-Papewalis C, Moritz T, Liedert B, Thomale J. Down-regulation of DNA repair in human CD34(+) progenitor cells corresponds to increased drug sensitivity and apoptotic response. *Blood* 2002; **100**: 845–53.

72. Bender CF, Sikes ML, Sullivan R, *et al.* Cancer predisposition and hematopoietic failure in Rad50(S/S) mice. *Genes Dev* 2002; **16**: 2237–51.

73. Prasher JM, Lalai AS, Heijmans-Antonissen C, *et al.* Reduced hematopoietic reserves in DNA interstrand crosslink repair-deficient Ercc1-/- mice. *Embo J* 2005; **24**: 861–71.

74. Kinzler K, Vogelstein B. Gatekeepers and caretakers. *Nature* 1997; **386**: 761–3.

75. Domen J, Cheshier SH, Weissman IL. The role of apoptosis in the regulation of hematopoietic stem cells: overexpression of BCL-2 increases both their number and repopulation potential. *J Exp Med* 2000; **191**: 253–63.

76. Opferman JT, Iwasaki H, Ong CC, *et al.* Obligate role of anti-apoptotic MCL-1 in the survival of hematopoietic stem cells. *Science* 2005; **307**: 1101–4.

77. Van Zant G, Eldridge PW, Behringer RR, Dewey MJ. Genetic control of hematopoietic kinetics revealed by analyses of allophenic mice and stem cell suicide. *Cell* 1983; **35**: 639–45.

78. Van Zant G, Scott-Micus K, Thompson BP, Fleischman RA, Perkins S. Stem cell quiescence/activation is reversible by serial transplantation and is independent of stromal cell genotype in mouse aggregation chimeras. *Exp Hematol* 1992; **20**: 470–5.

79. Dexter TM, Lajtha LG. Proliferation of haemopoietic stem cells in vitro. *Br J Haematol* 1974; **28**: 525–30.

80. Cashman J, Eaves AC, Eaves CJ. Regulated proliferation of primitive hematopoietic progenitor cells in long-term human marrow cultures. *Blood* 1985; **66**: 1002–5.

81. Ploemacher RE, van der Sluijs JP, van Beurden CA, Baert MR, Chan PL. Use of limiting-dilution type long-term marrow cultures in frequency analysis of marrow-repopulating and spleen colony-forming hematopoietic stem cells in the mouse. *Blood* 1991; **78**: 2527–33.

82. Breems DA, Blokland EA, Neben S, Ploemacher RE. Frequency analysis of human primitive hematopoietic stem cell subsets using a cobblestone are forming cell assay. *Leukemia* 1994; **8**: 1095–104.

83. Gelman R, Watson A, Bronson R, Yunis E. Murine chromosomal regions correlated with longevity. *Genetics* 1988; **118**: 693–704.

84. de Haan G, Van Zant G. Genetic analysis of hemopoietic cell cycling in mice suggests its involvement in organismal life span. *FASEB J* 1999; **13**: 707–13.

85. Donovan PJ, Gearhart J. The end of the beginning for pluripotent stem cells. *Nature* 2001; **414**: 92–7.

6

Hematopoietic microenvironment and age

David N. Haylock, Susan K. Nilsson

Introduction

Considerable evidence supports the concept that the localization of hematopoiesis to the bone marrow (BM) in adult mammals involves developmentally regulated interactions between primitive hematopoietic stem cells (HSCs) and the stromal cell-mediated hematopoietic microenvironment (HM) of the marrow. Moreover, it is well accepted that stromal cells and their extracellular biosynthetic products play a critical role in many aspects of hematopoiesis including the regulation, recruitment, and retention of hematopoietic stem and progenitor cells within preferred sites of the BM. Therefore, conceptually at least, there are two key cellular components for consideration when discussing the effects of aging on hematopoiesis: first the hematopoietic stem and progenitor cells themselves, and second those cells that comprise the hematopoietic microenvironment. In this chapter we review the current understanding of what constitutes the HM and how its components and functions change during aging and thereby impact specifically on primitive hematopoietic progenitor cells and hematopoiesis. In the final section, we highlight the unresolved questions concerning the effect of age on the HM and suggest a series of studies to further our understanding of this biology. Finally, we acknowledge the publications and contributions made by many investigators over the last four decades or more, and apologize to those whose work we may have inadvertently not referenced in this review.

HM and the HSC niche

Under steady-state conditions, HSCs have the unique ability to contribute indefinitely to the supply of mature blood elements, a property that is attributed, in part, to their ability to maintain blood cell production throughout life. The molecular mechanisms that regulate HSC quiescence are not completely defined, although it is well recognized that extrinsic cues provided by cells and extracellular matrix components of the stem cell microenvironment, or niche, are critical in stem cell regulation. In 1978, Schofield proposed the concept of an HSC niche as a distinct three-dimensional structure within a specific anatomical location in the BM [1]. He proposed that these fixed tissue spaces or niches were responsible for regulating stem cell fate and the size of the HSC pool. Since this initial proposal, it has been well accepted that the HSC niche comprises specific cell types together with their extracellular matrix proteins, which collectively would regulate HSC self-renewal, quiescence, and differentiation.

Functionally, the extrinsic control of hematopoiesis mediated by the HM is considered to operate at close range and to involve the same cellular and connective tissue elements that provide mechanical support for developing hematopoietic cells [2,3]. In this respect BM "stromal cells" are commonly attributed as the major cellular component of the supportive HM. The term "stromal" is ambiguous and includes a heterogeneous population of non-hematopoietic cells including fibroblasts, adipocytes, vascular smooth muscle cells, endothelium, and osteoblasts. Early evidence that stromal cells mediate hematopoiesis came from studies where severe damage or destruction of the BM stromal elements, induced by irradiation [4–6] or mechanical insult [7], resulted in permanent failure of the organ to support hematopoiesis. Experiments involving heterotopic transplantation also indicated that regeneration of stromal elements is required before onset of hematopoiesis [8–10]. The first attempts to define the morphology and function of marrow stromal cells came from Friedenstein when he showed that adherent "fibroblasts" cultured from murine BM, when implanted under the kidney capsule, could produce an environment that allowed hematopoiesis to develop [11]. These pioneering studies in the mouse were extended to the human setting [12–15] and collectively provided more direct evidence of marrow stromal cell precursors with the capacity to differentiate into mesenchymal cell types capable of supporting hematopoiesis. Additional in-vitro evidence for the ability of marrow stromal cells to support hematopoiesis came with development of long-term (3–6 weeks) murine BM culture systems demonstrating that active hematopoiesis was associated with the adherent fibroblast layer, where more primitive cells were located and divided [16,17]. The proliferation of primitive human hematopoietic progenitor cells, referred to as long-term culture (LTC)-initiating cells, on irradiated human marrow adherent cells provided further evidence of the importance of direct hematopoietic cell–stromal cell contact in regulation of primitive hematopoietic stem and progenitor cell regulation [18,19].

Although the niche model has remained unchallenged for almost 30 years the exact location of HSC niches and their regulation of HSC fate has only recently been addressed. Various studies [20–22] including our own [23–25] strongly suggest that the HSC niche is associated with bone and that HSCs actively migrate toward and reside within the endosteal region at the bone and BM interface. The importance of contact and interaction between HSCs and osteoblasts at the endosteal surface is also supported by studies reported by Zhang *et al.* [26], Calvi *et al.* [27], and Arai *et al.* [28]. Further evidence that osteoblasts directly regulate hematopoiesis is provided by studies

where conditional ablation of osteoblasts results in significant reduction of marrow hematopoiesis [29], although the factors responsible for this profound effect remain to be determined. In addition, in-vitro evidence indicates that osteoblastic cells can expand HSC numbers [30] and when co-transplanted with HSCs can improve engraftment [31].

Collectively, these findings suggest that osteoblasts are a key cell type within the HSC niche, and that molecules expressed by these cells may have previously unrecognized roles in regulating hematopoiesis. In this regard, osteoblasts within the endosteal region interact with and modulate HSC fate by stimulating and inhibiting HSC proliferation. The recent review by Taichman [32] describes in greater detail the central role of osteoblasts in hematopoiesis, and our own recent review [33] also highlights that osteopontin, the major protein synthesized by osteoblasts, has both a positive and a negative regulative influence on HSC regulation mediated by osteoblasts.

Furthermore, our studies of various molecules involved in the HSC niche have led us to expand the concept of the niche from that of having the sole role of regulating HSCs, to also include critical roles in the attraction, retention, and potentially release of the residing stem cells [33,34] (Fig. 6.1). The studies described above and the contributions made by many other investigators have significantly enhanced our understanding of the components of the HM. Change with aging in the number, anatomical location, and function of any one of the cell types comprising the niche or supportive HM can potentially impact on hematopoiesis. However, we propose that the effects of age on two cell types, osteoblasts and mesenchymal stem cells, will have the greatest impact on hematopoiesis, specifically HSCs and the size of the HSC pool. Before discussing these it is worthwhile to make some general comments on aging, HSCs, and senescence.

Definition of aging

Diminished proliferative, functional, and regenerative capacity is commonly accepted as the broad

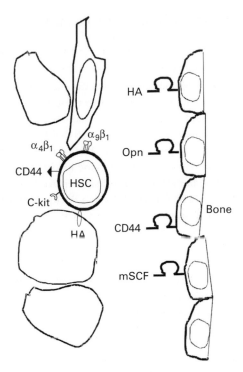

Figure 6.1 The hematopoietic stem cell niche: schematic of key interactions between niche molecules and their respective ligands on HSC.

system begins to "age" from that point in time when as an organ it has reached peak volume. According to this functional definition, aging in humans would commence soon after the teenage years, when body size and lean body weight is stabilized and the hematopoietic system is fully developed and able to meet the demands of the adult. Even though well-documented changes such as replacement of active "red" marrow areas with adipocyte-rich "yellow" marrow [40] and progressive atrophy of the thymus (reviewed by Aspinall *et al.* [41]) take place after this time, we contend that such changes represent normal physiological events rather than manifestations of aging, and as such these will not be discussed in the context of this review.

Hematopoietic stem cells and age

Of all cellular systems, aging in the hematopoietic system has been the most extensively studied [42]. Numbers of specific subsets of mature hematopoietic cells are known to be affected by age, including a reduction in B- and T-cell generation [43–45]. In aged mice, a decreased packed erythrocyte volume [46] and increased bleeding time [47] are commonly observed. In contrast, other hematopoietic subsets such as mycloid cells are unaffected by aging [48]. Potential age-related effects on the total number of HSCs within the BM remain unclear, with some studies suggesting maintenance or slight increases [49–53], while others suggest an age-related decrease in HSC numbers [54,55]. Much of this variability has been attributed to strain variations in intrinsic cell regulation [56,57]. Initially HSCs were thought to have unlimited self-renewal capacity, and hence to be exempt from aging. However, accumulating evidence over the past three decades compellingly argues that there is a significant impairment of function or aging of HSCs. Arguments both for and against the aging of stem cells in general are presented in two extensive reviews by Geiger and Van Zant [58], and Van Zant and Liang [59]. In summary, it would appear that HSCs are regulated in both a stage-specific and an age-specific manner [53].

definition of aging [35,36], and highlights the contribution of specific cells in cell replenishment and therefore their influence in lifespan. This definition also allows the separation of aging from other normal cellular processes such as senescence, which is defined as "*essentially the irreversible arrest of cell division*" [37,38], where there is question as to its importance for in-vivo aging [39]. However, the precise definition of cellular and/or organism aging remains unclear and is made more challenging when trying to distinguish between aging in vivo and prolonged passaging in vitro that may or may not represent "true" aging. For the purpose of this review we extend this definition to distinguish between normal physiological development and an age-related inability to maintain normal blood cell production. We propose that the hematopoietic

Studies analyzing an aging effect in HSC function, and specifically whether there is an effect on the ability of HSCs to reconstitute hematopoiesis post-transplant, have also produced varied results. Specific studies analyzing aging in HSCs suggest that HSCs isolated from both young and old mice are equally capable of reconstituting ablated recipients [60–62] but the proliferative potential of HSCs decreases with age [63]. Furthermore, while more recent studies suggest that HSCs from old or young mice are equally able to cure young W/W^v recipients, and that these cures are equally sustained through serial transplantation [64], other studies suggest that cells from old mice have a greater repopulating ability than those from young mice [65]. Botnick et al. [66] suggested that observed age-related changes in HSCs can be explained by stem cell heterogeneity, as well as the wide variety of assays and readouts of assays used to assess them. They proposed that during adult steady-state hematopoiesis, clones are selected on the basis of greatest divisional history, and thus an increase in average proliferative capacity occurs in the residual HSC population. However, the remaining population renewal capacity will remain unchanged as this is a measure of non-cycling highly primitive cells with maximal proliferative potential.

Recently, Liang et al., analyzing the effects of aging on the homing and engraftment of HSC, demonstrated that while the frequency of competitive repopulation units increased with age, the ability of these cells to home to the marrow decreased with age [67]. Furthermore, transplants involving aged HSCs and an aged HM resulted in a skewing of engraftment towards myelopoiesis. The authors suggest that this implies an age-related bias of intrinsic and extrinsic HSC regulation. Using a congenic mouse model to study the genetic regulation of HSC aging, Geiger et al. have defined a locus on murine chromosome 2 as controlling this process [35]. In addition, they provide evidence that links an HSC response to DNA double-strand breaks to cellular aging, hence suggesting that DNA integrity influences stem cell aging.

The hematopoietic microenvironment and age

Accumulating evidence suggests that age-related defects in hematopoiesis are primarily due to changes in the hematopoietic stroma rather than in HSC [68]. An age-related decrease in bone mass, the ultimate structural support of the HM, is well described [69–71]. The cellular mechanism for this is suggested to be an age-related increase in bone resorption and decrease in bone formation. The increase in bone resorption [72] corresponds with a decrease in levels of osteoprotegerin, which normally blocks the osteoclast-stimulatory effects of osteoprotegerin ligand, and therefore may increase the capacity of stromal cells to support osteoclastogenesis [73]. In parallel, the decrease in bone formation occurs in association with a decrease in the proliferative capacity of osteoprogenitor cells and consequently osteoblasts [74–78] and not a decrease in cellular function, with osteogenic potential of individual cells being maintained [79]. Correlating with a decrease in bone formation, an age-related decrease in the expression of bone-related genes such as osteocalcin and osteopontin has also been observed in older animals [80]. While an age-related quantitation of osteopontin synthesis and its direct effect on the HM and HSC has not been performed, it is highly likely that any changes in osteopontin synthesis will have significant effects. We have recently demonstrated that osteopontin plays a critical role in the attraction as well as the retention and regulation of HSCs within the microenvironmental HSC niche [25]. Specifically, osteopontin acts as a negative regulator of hematopoiesis by dampening the stimulatory influences of hematopoietic growth factors, and plays a critical role in regulating the size of the HSCs pool. It is therefore possible that with aging, osteopontin expression becomes deregulated at the endosteal region and domains with low or absent osteopontin are created. These osteopontin-depleted zones may promote increased rates of HSC proliferation and in time lead to an overall reduction in the HSC pool.

The level and function of other molecules within the HM with putative roles in HSC regulation may also change with age. For example, there is an age-related change in the expression and functional response of CXC chemokine receptors in human osteoblasts [81] including CXCR4, the known homing receptor for stromal cell-derived factor 1 (SDF-1) [82]. Whether the level of CXCR4 expression on hematopoietic cells, and specifically HSCs, alters as a function of age remains unknown. Even if CXCR4 expression by HSCs remains high their chemotactic response might be impaired thus adversely affecting the homing and reconstituting ability of transplanted aged HSCs. A more recent study suggests that the BM also contains a population of CXCR4+ highly motile non-hematopoietic tissue-committed stem cells (TCSCs), which are highly chemotactic to SDF-1 [83]. The numbers of these bone marrow TCSCs decrease significantly with age, and their direct involvement in diminished hematopoiesis remains to be determined.

Many studies suggest that one of the key HM cells, the mesenchymal stem cell (MSC), is both subject to aging and critical in the process of aging of hematopoiesis. Changes in the quantity, quality, and mobilization of MSCs with age have recently been extensively reviewed by Sethe et al. [36]. Early studies in rodents specifically analyzing age-related changes in the HM suggested that while much of the cellular content of the microenvironment may not alter with age, the stroma of older animals acquires an age-related defect [84] rendering it incapable of the normal control of hematopoietic cell proliferation [85]. As a consequence aged marrow has decreased proliferative capacity and is defective in its ability to form long-term BM cultures in vitro [86–88]. In vivo these changes result in a reorganization of the stromal microenvironment, as evidenced by an imbalance in the ratio of fibroblast colony-forming cells compared to granulocytic-macrophage precursors [89,90]. However, other studies provide evidence against an age-related decline in stromal proliferation and function. Matthews and Crouse demonstrated that long-term marrow cultures derived from old marrow had an increased ability

to support spleen colony-forming unit (CFU-S) production [86]. Furthermore, Schofield et al. [91] found that old marrow grew normally both in long-term BM cultures and in vivo when implanted as ectopic grafts in renal capsules.

A more recent study by Boggs et al. [92] showed a latent deficiency of the HM with age in vivo, revealed in W/W^v recipients by the stress of continuing demand on a limited number of donor HSCs. This resulted in older recipients being less capable of supporting donor wild-type erythropoiesis. The authors suggest that the BM microenvironments of aged mice lose their fine control of hematopoietic response following stress. The concept of an age-related deficiency in the HM during HSC engraftment was recently quantitated by Liang et al. [67], where they showed a greater than 50% reduction in the seeding efficiency of HSCs to an aged HM. The authors suggest that this deficiency reflects a decline in the marrow's ability to capture and/or retain engrafting stem cells. This possibility could be investigated by in situ cell tracking as developed by Nilsson et al. [23,93] to analyze the spatial distribution of transplanted HSCs within the HM (Fig. 6.2). It would be of particular interest to determine whether HSCs transplanted into old recipients show an altered spatial distribution and reduced preference for localization to the endosteum as compared to that observed in young recipients.

In addition, these deficiencies may also be attributed to alterations in the ability of stromal cells to produce cellular products such as extracellular matrix proteins and cytokines. For example, it is known that there is an age-related decrease in the solubility and denaturability of collagen [94], which has been suggested to make older tissues more vulnerable to damage when transplanted by inhibiting the removal of damaged tissue followed by tissue regeneration [95]. Even though there is evidence of an age-related increase in hyaluronan secretion by skin fibroblasts [96], significant age-related changes occur in the structure of aggrecan, link protein, and hyaluronan aggregates [97], with known effects on the stability of articular cartilage. The effects of these

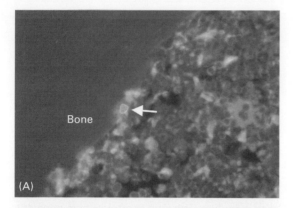

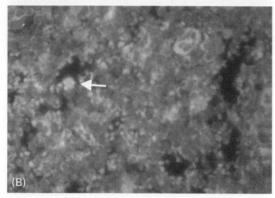

Figure 6.2 Analysis of spatial distribution following transplantation. CFSE-labeled cells (green) are designated as either endosteal (A) or central (B). *See color plate section.*

changes on the HM and in particular the HSC niche have not been analyzed. We have previously demonstrated that hyaluronan is critical in the attraction, retention, and regulation of HSCs in their microenvironmental niche [24], so any changes in the formation of the aggregate assembly necessary for the stability of hyaluronan is likely to have a direct effect on HSCs.

Stromal cells are the only cells in the marrow that produce interleukin 7 (IL-7) [98], which in combination with stromal contact is essential for B-cell production [99,100], but at least in vitro, aged stroma releases significantly decreased amounts of IL-7 [101]. However, not all stromal cells appear to be affected by age. For example, in-vitro studies

analyzing long-term BM cultures established with aged marrow show no change in the number of macrophages [102], nor in their ability to produce macrophage colony-stimulating factor (M-CSF) [101].

Other microenvironments capable of supporting hematopoiesis, such as the spleen, also show evidence of an age-related deficiency [103]. Harrison *et al.* [104] showed an impaired ability of spleens from older animals to reconstitute erythropoiesis when transplanted into Sl/Sl^d recipients. Hotta *et al.* [68] went on to demonstrate an age-related decline in splenic stromal ability to support CFU-S, which was confirmed by Wolf and Arora [105], who suggested that this loss of support was due to a decrease in proliferative capacity as fibroblasts do in vitro with passaging [106]. Recently a study by Liang *et al.* [67] showed an age-related decrease in the ability of hematopoietic progenitors to home to aged spleens, in the absence of a reduction in splenic size or cellularity, again suggestive of an altered and less receptive microenvironment.

Age-related changes in humans

The relevance to humans of many of the observed age-related changes in hematopoiesis in animals is unknown. In general there have been relatively few systematic studies assessing changes in human hematopoiesis with aging. In fact, we have not found any studies where a group of subjects has been prospectively monitored to document changes in hematopoiesis throughout life. Nevertheless, a number of studies have compared hematopoietic parameters and functions of specific hematopoietic cell types in groups of young and elderly humans [107–112]. One of the confounding factors in any study that assesses the effect of age on hematopoiesis is the interrelationship between changes as a result of age per se and those caused by dietary or environmental factors or presence of chronic disease. This is particularly relevant to hematopoiesis as any one of the latter, alone, can have profound effects on BM function. Anemia, the consequence of hematopoietic deregulation, is often observed in elderly humans [108,113]. While the cause of the anemia can usually not be identified, the fact that non-anemic elderly people also have reduced hematopoietic function strongly suggests that age contributes to the defect [108]. Aged subjects have reduced myelopoiesis [108], with previous studies identifying a defect in the aged host defense mechanisms, including an impaired ability to mount a neutrophil response to infection [114].

In animal models, it is much easier to assess the effect of age on the durability and functional capacity of the hematopoietic system. Damage can be sustained by physical or chemical means, and the rate of blood cell recovery can be used to assess hematopoietic potential, as a function of the age of the animal. Similar prospective studies cannot be performed in humans, and consequently alternative approaches have been used to assess the functional capacity of the human hematopoietic system with age.

The level of hematopoietic progenitor cells within the peripheral blood, or the ability to mobilize hematopoietic progenitors, can be considered as a surrogate measure of the capacity of the hematopoietic system. At least two studies have demonstrated that under steady-state conditions there is an inverse relationship between the number of peripheral-blood CD34+ cells or committed myeloid progenitors (CFU-GM) with age [115,116]. The first of these, by Egusa *et al.* [115], examined blood levels of CD34+ cells and CFU-GM in 50 normal volunteers with ages ranging between 20 and 90 years, whilst the second, by Bagnara *et al.* [116], measured these parameters in nine centenarians (median age 100.5 years), ten old people (median age 71 years) and ten young people (median age 35 years). In spite of a trend toward lower levels of circulating progenitors with age, the study conducted by Bagnara demonstrated that CD34+ cells from old people and centenarians exhibited equivalent responsiveness to cytokine stimulation (Fig. 6.3) and ability to form CFU-GM and erythroid colonies in vitro (Fig. 6.4). These data suggest that although individual progenitor cells from young and old people have similar proliferative potential the absolute number of progenitors within hematopoietic tissues available for

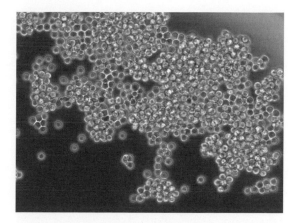

Figure 6.3 Example of CD34+ cells growing in serum-free culture in the presence of six stimulatory growth factors.

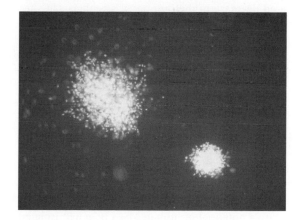

Figure 6.4 In-vitro colony-forming assay, used as a surrogate measure of hematopoietic potential. *See color plate section.*

mobilization and transplantation might reduce with age. This notion has been investigated, and data from multiple studies indicate that the in-vivo responsiveness to granulocyte colony-stimulating factor (G-CSF) and mobilization of CD34+ cells and CFU-GM declines with age [117–119], an outcome discordant with the equivalent proliferative response observed from CD34+ cells when stimulated by G-CSF under in-vitro assays. This disparity highlights the need to exercise caution in extrapolating results of in-vitro studies to the in-vivo setting, and also suggests that other factors apart from G-CSF responsiveness directly effect mobilization of hematopoietic progenitors with age.

Age-related changes to the HM, and specifically those related to osteogenesis, occur in mammals and directly contribute to the establishment and regulation of hematopoiesis [120,121]. Given the central role of osteoblasts within the HSC niche [26,122], and their demonstrated effect on HSC regulation, any change in their number is likely to directly regulate the HSC pool and HSC function. This notion has been proven experimentally using genetically modified mice [29], and by the administration of parathyroid hormone to mice to increase osteoblast numbers [27]. Humans lose bone mass with age and are consequently prone to osteoporosis. An associated decrease in the number of osteoblasts at sites of hematopoiesis is likely to diminish the HSC pool and in time lead to reduced levels of blood cells. However, studies conducted on human subjects have yielded conflicting results with regards to the incidence and function of mesenchymal cells with osteogenic potential isolated from BM [77,123–125]. The disparate results reported by these investigators reflect variations in colony assays, methods for assessing size and osteogenic potential of colonies, and, above all, differences in sites and techniques used for BM collection. Nevertheless, the decreased in-vitro lifespan and associated decrease in proliferative potential of human MSCs (Fig. 6.5) isolated from old as compared to younger donors suggests that a decrease in osteoblastic cell numbers, and not their function, leads to age-related decrease in bone formation and diminished hematopoiesis [78,126].

Apart from osteoblasts, other mesenchymal cells within the BM directly regulate HSCs and their progeny. Accordingly, studies to assess the incidence and functions of BM-derived MSCs and their specific differentiated progeny may provide some insight as to why hematopoiesis declines with age. Two recently published reviews of this subject tabulate and discuss the results of numerous studies conducted in humans and other mammals [36,127]. Notably these reviews discuss the question as to whether age-related changes in MSCs are due to intrinsic factors

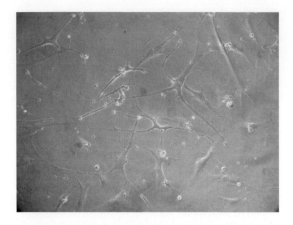

Figure 6.5 Human mesenchymal stem cells (MSCs) growing in culture.

or induced by their HM. Telomere length is considered to represent a biological clock and a key intrinsic regulator for cell lifespan. Aged human MSCs show a decline in both proliferation and differentiation potential, which is hypothesized to be a consequence of eroded telomeres [128,129]. However, there are conflicting reports on expression of telomerase in MSCs, although two recent studies suggest that a rare subset of MSCs might express high levels of the enzyme [130,131]. While the intrinsic properties of MSCs and other cells within the HM are clearly important with respect to age-related changes, most evidence supports the extrinsic theory [127].

Conclusions

There is now abundant evidence to show that the HM is critical in regulation of HSCs and for control of hematopoiesis in the adult mammal. However, age-related changes in the function and incidence of the cellular components of the HM have not been studied in great detail, particularly in humans. Although caution should be exercised in extrapolating findings from studies conducted in rodents to the human setting, valuable information about the roles of specific components of the HM during aging can be determined using a variety of murine models.

However, the field would be significantly advanced by well-designed long-term studies in non-human primates and humans to prospectively assess changes in the hematopoietic and non-hematopoietic compartments of the BM. Ideally, these studies should involve serial assessment of the hematopoietic system at defined time points of multiple individuals from neonate to old age. There are obvious inherent problems with this experimental strategy, including control of assay methodology over time, separating out the influences of other age-related changes secondary to disease or chronic illness, and also changes in environmental factors that will impact on human physiology. Not the least will be changes in diet and nutritional status, both of which are well recognized to impact on hematopoiesis. Another important objective for future studies is to further define and separate those age-related changes that are intrinsic to cells of the HM from those of the hematopoietic cells themselves. Finally, to date most investigations have been descriptive in nature and have paid limited attention to the molecular mechanisms that underpin changes in the function of defined cell populations within the supportive hematopoietic niche. It will be essential for the molecular basis of age-related changes to be defined before strategies and therapies can be developed to minimize or reverse the diminishing capacity of the hematopoietic system as we age.

REFERENCES

1. Schofield R. The relationship between the spleen colony-forming cell and the haemopoietic stem cell. *Blood Cells* 1978; **4**: 7–25.
2. Weiss L. The hematopoietic microenvironment of the bone marrow: an ultrastructural study of the stroma in rats. *Anat Rec* 1976; **186**: 161–84.
3. Lichtman MA. The ultrastructure of the hemopoietic environment of the marrow: a review. *Exp Hematol* 1981; **9**: 391–410.
4. Knospe WH, Blom J, Crosby WH. Regeneration of locally irradiated bone marrow: I. Dose dependent, long-term changes in the rat, with particular emphasis upon vascular and stromal reaction. *Blood* 1966; **28**: 398–415.
5. Maloney MA, Patt HM. Migration of cells from shielded to irradiated marrow. *Blood* 1972; **39**: 804–8.
6. Chamberlin W, Barone J, Kedo A, Fried W. Lack of recovery of murine hematopoietic stromal cells after irradiation-induced damage. *Blood* 1974; **44**: 385–92.
7. Tavassoli M, Ratzan RJ, Maniatis A, Crosby WH. Regeneration of hemopoietic stroma in anemic mice of S1-S1 d and W-W v genotypes. *J Reticuloendothel Soc* 1973; **13**: 518–26.
8. Perla D. The regeneration of autoplastic splenic transplants. *Am J Path* 1936; **12**: 665–75.
9. Tavassoli M, Crosby WH. Transplantation of marrow to extramedullary sites. *Science* 1968; **161**: 54–6.
10. Knospe WH, Husseini S, Trobaugh FE Jr. Hematopoiesis on cellulose ester membranes (CEM). II. Enrichment of the hematopoietic microenvironment by the addition of selected cellular elements. *Exp Hematol* 1978; **6**: 601–12.
11. Friedenstein AJ, Chailakhjan RK, Lalykina KS. The development of fibroblast colonies in monolayer cultures of guinea-pig bone marrow and spleen cells. *Cell Tissue Kinet* 1970; **3**: 393–403.
12. Castro-Malaspina H, Gay RE, Resnick G, et al. Characterization of human bone marrow fibroblast colony-forming cells (CFU-F) and their progeny. *Blood* 1980; **56**: 289–301.
13. Owen M. Marrow stromal stem cells. *J Cell Sci Suppl* 1988; **10**: 63–76.
14. Simmons PJ, Torok-Storb B. Identification of stromal cell precursors in human bone marrow by a novel monoclonal antibody, STRO-1. *Blood* 1991; **78**: 55–62.
15. Simmons PJ, Gronthos S, Zannettino A, Ohta S, Graves S. Isolation, characterization and functional activity of human marrow stromal progenitors in hemopoiesis. *Prog Clin Biol Res* 1994; **389**: 271–80.
16. Dexter TM, Lajtha LG. Proliferation of haemopoietic stem cells in vitro. *Br J Haematol* 1974; **28**: 525–30.
17. Dexter TM, Spooncer E, Toksoz D, Lajtha LG. The role of cells and their products in the regulation of in vitro stem cell proliferation and granulocyte development. *J Supramol Struct* 1980; **13**: 513–24.
18. Sutherland HJ, Eaves CJ, Eaves AC, Dragowska W, Lansdorp PM. Characterization and partial purification of human marrow cells capable of initiating long-term hematopoiesis in vitro. *Blood* 1989; **74**: 1563–70.
19. Sutherland HJ, Lansdorp PM, Henkelman DH, Eaves AC, Eaves CJ. Functional characterization of individual human hematopoietic stem cells cultured at limiting

dilution on supportive marrow stromal layers. *Proc Natl Acad Sci USA* 1990; **87**: 3584–8.

20. Lord BI, Testa NG, Hendry JH. The relative spatial distributions of CFU-S and CFU-C in the normal mouse femur. *Blood* 1975; **46**: 65–72.

21. Gong JK. Endosteal marrow: a rich source of hematopoietic stem cells. *Science* 1978; **199**: 1443–5.

22. Mason TM, Lord BI, Hendry JH. The development of spatial distributions of CFU-S and in-vitro CFC in femora of mice of different ages. *Br J Haematol* 1989; **73**: 455–61.

23. Nilsson SK, Johnston HM, Coverdale JA. Spatial localization of transplanted hemopoietic stem cells: inferences for the localization of stem cell niches. *Blood* 2001; **97**: 2293–9.

24. Nilsson SK, Haylock DN, Johnston HM, Occhiodoro T, Brown TJ, Simmons PJ. Hyaluronan is synthesized by primitive hemopoietic cells, participates in their lodgment at the endosteum following transplantation, and is involved in the regulation of their proliferation and differentiation in vitro. *Blood* 2003; **101**: 856–62.

25. Nilsson SK, Johnston HM, Whitty GA, *et al.* Osteopontin, a key component of the hematopoietic stem cell niche and regulator of primitive hematopoietic progenitor cells. *Blood* 2005; **106**: 1232–9.

26. Zhang J, Niu C, Ye L, *et al.* Identification of the haematopoietic stem cell niche and control of the niche size. *Nature* 2003; **425**: 836–41.

27. Calvi LM, Adams GB, Weibrecht KW, *et al.* Osteoblastic cells regulate the haematopoietic stem cell niche. *Nature* 2003; **425**: 841–6.

28. Arai F, Hirao A, Ohmura M, *et al.* Tie2/angiopoietin-1 signaling regulates hematopoietic stem cell quiescence in the bone marrow niche. *Cell* 2004; **118**: 149–61.

29. Visnjic D, Kalajzic Z, Rowe DW, Katavic V, Lorenzo J, Aguila HL. Hematopoiesis is severely altered in mice with an induced osteoblast deficiency. *Blood* 2004; **103**: 3258–64.

30. Taichman RS, Reilly MJ, Emerson SG. The hematopoietic microenvironment: osteoblasts and the hematopoietic microenvironment. *Hematol* 2000; **4**: 421–6.

31. El-Badri NS, Wang BY, Cherry, Good RA. Osteoblasts promote engraftment of allogeneic hematopoietic stem cells. *Exp Hematol* 1998; **26**: 110–16.

32. Taichman RS. Blood and bone: two tissues whose fates are intertwined to create the hematopoietic stem-cell niche. *Blood* 2005; **105**: 2631–9.

33. Haylock DN, Nilsson SK. Stem cell regulation by the hematopoietic stem cell niche. *Cell Cycle* 2005; **4**: 1353–5.

34. Nilsson SK, Simmons PJ. Transplantable stem cells: home to specific niches. *Curr Opin Hematol* 2004; **11**: 102–6.

35. Geiger H, Rennebeck G, Van Zant G. Regulation of hematopoietic stem cell aging in vivo by a distinct genetic element. *Proc Natl Acad Sci USA* 2005; **102**: 5102–7.

36. Sethe S, Scutt A, Stolzing A. Aging of mesenchymal stem cells. *Ageing Res Rev* 2006; **5**: 91–116.

37. Hayflick L, Moorhead PS. The serial cultivation of human diploid cell strains. *J Exp Cell Res* 1961; **25**: 585–621.

38. Campisi J. Cancer, aging and cellular senescence. *In Vivo* 2000; **14**: 183–8.

39. Hornsby PJ. Cellular senescence and tissue aging in vivo. *J Gerontol A Biol Sci Med Sci* 2002; **57**: B251–B256.

40. Rozman C, Feliu E, Berga L, Reverter JC, Climent C, Ferran MJ. Age-related variations of fat tissue fraction in normal human bone marrow depend both on size and number of adipocytes: a stereological study. *Exp Hematol* 1989; **17**: 34–7.

41. Aspinall R, Andrew D, Pido-Lopez J. Age-associated changes in thymopoiesis. *Springer Semin Immunopathol* 2002; **24**: 87–101.

42. Kay MM, Makinodan T. Immunobiology of aging: evaluation of current status. *Clin Immunol Immunopathol* 1976; **6**: 394–413.

43. Miller RA. The aging immune system: primer and prospectus. *Science* 1996; **273**: 70–4.

44. Kline GH, Hayden TA, Klinman NR. B cell maintenance in aged mice reflects both increased B cell longevity and decreased B cell generation. *J Immunol* 1999; **162**: 3342–9.

45. Labrie JE, Borghesi L, Gerstein RM. Bone marrow microenvironmental changes in aged mice compromise V(D)J recombinase activity and B cell generation. *Semin Immunol* 2005; **17**: 347–55.

46. Finch CE, Foster JR. Hematologic and serum electrolyte values of the C57BL-6J male mouse in maturity and senescence. *Lab Anim Sci* 1973; **23**: 339–49.

47. Harrison DE. Normal production of erythrocytes by mouse marrow continuous for 73 months. *Proc Natl Acad Sci USA* 1973; **70**: 3184–8.

48. Williams LH, Udupa KB, Lipshitz DA. Evaluation of the effect of age on hematopoiesis in the C57BL/6 mouse. *Exp Hematol* 1986; **14**: 827–32.

49. Chen MG. Age-related changes in hematopoietic stem cell populations of a long-lived hybrid mouse. *J Cell Physiol* 1971; **78**: 225–32.

50. Coggle JE, Gordon MY, Proukakis C, Bogg CE. Age-related changes in the bone marrow and spleen of SAS/4 mice. *Gerontologia* 1975; **21**: 1–9.

51. Morrison SJ, Wandycz AM, Akashi K, Globerson A, Weissman IL. The aging of hematopoietic stem cells. *Nat Med* 1996; **2**: 1011–16.

52. Sudo K, Ema H, Morita Y, Nakauchi H. Age-associated characteristics of murine hematopoietic stem cells. *J Exp Med* 2000; **192**: 1273–80.

53. Geiger H, True JM, Haan G, Van Zant G. Age- and stage-specific regulation patterns in the hematopoietic stem cell hierarchy. *Blood* 2001; **98**: 2966–72.

54. Harrison DE, Astle CM, Stone M. Numbers and functions of transplantable primitive immunohematopoietic stem cells. Effects of age. *J Immunol* 1989; **142**: 3833–40.

55. de Haan G, Van Zant G. Dynamic changes in mouse hematopoietic stem cell numbers during aging. *Blood* 1999; **93**: 3294–301.

56. Van Zant G, Holland BP, Eldridge PW, Chen JJ. Genotype-restricted growth and aging patterns in hematopoietic stem cell populations of allophenic mice. *J Exp Med* 1990; **171**: 1547–65.

57. Henckaerts E, Langer JC, Snoeck HW. Quantitative genetic variation in the hematopoietic stem cell and progenitor cell compartment and in lifespan are closely linked at multiple loci in BXD recombinant inbred mice. *Blood* 2004; **104**: 374–9.

58. Geiger H, Van Zant G. The aging of lympho-hematopoietic stem cells. *Nat Immunol* 2002; **3**: 329–33.

59. Van Zant G, Liang Y. The role of stem cells in aging. *Exp Hematol* 2003; **31**: 659–72.

60. Lajtha LG, Schofield R. Regulation of stem cell renewal and differentiation: possible significance in aging. *Adv Gerontol Res* 1971; **3**: 131–46.

61. Harrison DE. Normal function of transplanted marrow cell lines from aged mice. *J Gerontol* 1975; **30**: 279–85.

62. Ogden DA, Mickliem HS. The fate of serially transplanted bone marrow cell populations from young and old donors. *Transplantation* 1976; **22**: 287–93.

63. Albright JW, Makinodan T. Decline in the growth potential of spleen-colonizing bone marrow stem cells of long-lived aging mice. *J Exp Med* 1976; **144**: 1204–13.

64. Boggs DR, Boggs SS. Multipotent stem cells in vivo. In Golde DW, ed, *Methods in Hematology: Hematopoiesis* (New York: Churchill Livingstone, 1984).

65. Boggs DR, Boggs SS, Saxe DF, Gress LA, Canfield DR. Hematopoietic stem cells with high proliferative potential. Assay of their concentration in marrow by the frequency and duration of cure of W/Wv mice. *J Clin Invest* 1982; **70**: 242–53.

66. Botnick LE, Hannon EC, Obbagy J, Hellman S. The variation of hematopoietic stem cell self-renewal capacity as a function of age: further evidence for heterogenicity of the stem cell compartment. *Blood* 1982; **60**: 268–71.

67. Liang Y, Van Zant G, Szilvassy SJ. Effects of aging on the homing and engraftment of murine hematopoietic stem and progenitor cells. *Blood* 2005; **106**: 1479–87.

68. Hotta T, Hirabayashi N, Utsumi M, Murate T, Yamada H. Age-related changes in the function of hemopoietic stroma in mice. *Exp Hematol* 1980; **8**: 933–6.

69. Kragstrup J, Melsen F, Mosekilde L. Thickness of bone formed at remodeling sites in normal human iliac trabecular bone: variations with age and sex. *Metab Bone Dis Relat Res* 1983; **5**: 17–21.

70. Strates BS, Stock AJ, Connolly JF. Skeletal repair in the aged: a preliminary study in rabbits. *Am J Med Sci* 1988; **296**: 266–9.

71. Brockstedt H, Kassem M, Eriksen EF, Mosekilde L, Melsen F. Age- and sex-related changes in iliac cortical bone mass and remodeling. *Bone* 1993; **14**: 681–91.

72. Evanko SP, Angello JC, Wight TN. Formation of hyaluronan- and versican-rich pericellular matrix is required for proliferation and migration of vascular smooth muscle cells. *Arterioscler Thromb Vasc Biol* 1999, **19**. 1004–13.

73. Makhluf HA, Mueller SM, Mizuno S, Glowacki J. Age-related decline in osteoprotegerin expression by human bone marrow cells cultured in three-dimensional collagen sponges. *Biochem Biophys Res Commun* 2000; **268**: 669–72.

74. Termine JD. Cellular activity, matrix proteins, and aging bone. *Exp Gerontol* 1990; **25**: 217–21.

75. Nimni BS, Bernick S, Paule W, Nimni ME. Changes in the ratio of non-calcified collagen to calcified collagen in human vertebrae with advancing age. *Connect Tissue Res* 1993; **29**: 133–40.

76. Perkins SL, Gibbons R, Kling S, Kahn AJ. Age-related bone loss in mice is associated with an increased osteoclast progenitor pool. *Bone* 1994; **15**: 65–72.

77. Mueller SM, Glowacki J. Age-related decline in the osteogenic potential of human bone marrow cells cultured in three-dimensional collagen sponges. *J Cell Biochem* 2001; **82**: 583–90.

78. Stenderup K, Justesen J, Clausen C, Kassem M. Aging is associated with decreased maximal life span and accelerated senescence of bone marrow stromal cells. *Bone* 2003; **33**: 919–26.

79. Leskela HV, Risteli J, Niskanen S, Koivunen J, Ivaska KK, Lehenkari P. Osteoblast recruitment from stem cells does not decrease by age at late adulthood. *Biochem Biophys Res Commun* 2003; **311**: 1008–13.

80. Liang CT, Barnes J, Seedor JG, *et al.* Impaired bone activity in aged rats: alterations at the cellular and molecular levels. *Bone* 1992; **13**: 435–41.

81. Lisignoli G, Piacentini A, Toneguzzi S, *et al.* Age-associated changes in functional response to CXCR3 and CXCR5 chemokine receptors in human osteoblasts. *Biogerontology* 2003; **4**: 309–17.

82. Peled A, Petit I, Kollet O, *et al.* Dependence of human stem cell engraftment and repopulation of NOD/SCID mice on CXCR4. *Science* 1999; **283**: 845–8.

83. Kucia M, Ratajczak J, Ratajczak MZ. Bone marrow as a source of circulating CXCR4+ tissue-committed stem cells. *Biol Cell* 2005; **97**: 133–46.

84. Trentin JJ. Determination of bone marrow stem cell differentiation by stromal hemopoietic inductive microenvironments (HIM). *Am J Pathol* 1971; **65**: 621–8.

85. Chertkov JL, Gurevitch OA. Age-related changes in hemopoietic microenvironment. Enhanced growth of hemopoietic stroma and weakened genetic resistance of hemopoietic cells in old mice. *Exp Gerontol* 1981; **16**: 195–8.

86. Matthews KI, Crouse DA. An in vitro investigation of the hematopoietic microenvironment in young and aged mice. *Mech Ageing Dev* 1981; **17**: 289–303.

87. Mauch P, Botnick LE, Hannon EC, Obbagy J, Hellman S. Decline in bone marrow proliferative capacity as a function of age. *Blood* 1982; **60**: 245–52.

88. Lipschitz DA, Udupa KB. Effect of donor age on long-term culture of bone marrow in vitro. *Mech Ageing Dev* 1984; **24**: 119–27.

89. Sidorenko AV, Andrianova LF, Macsyuk TV, Butenko GM. Stromal hemopoietic microenvironment in aging. *Mech Ageing Dev* 1990; **54**: 131–42.

90. Gorskaya YF, Latzinik NV, Shuklina EU, Nesterenko VG. Age-related changes in population of stromal precursor cells in hematopoietic and lymphoid organs. *Russ J Immunol* 2000; **5**: 149–54.

91. Schofield R, Dexter TM, Lord BI, Testa NG. Comparison of haemopoiesis in young and old mice. *Mech Ageing Dev* 1986; **34**: 1–12.

92. Boggs SS, Patrene KD, Austin CA, Vecchini F, Tollerud DJ. Latent deficiency of the hematopoietic microenvironment of aged mice as revealed in W/Wv mice given +/+ cells. *Exp Hematol* 1991; **19**: 683–7.

93. Nilsson SK, Hulspas R, Weier HU, Quesenberry PJ. In situ detection of individual transplanted bone marrow cells using FISH on sections of paraffin-embedded whole murine femurs. *Histochem Cytochem* 1996; **44**: 1069–74.

94. Harrison DE, Archer JR, Sacher GA, Boyce FM. Tail collagen aging in mice of thirteen different genotypes and two species: relationship to biological age. *Exp Gerontol* 1978; **13**: 63–73.

95. Harrison DE, Astle CM, Delaittre J. Effects of transplantation and age on immunohemopoietic cell growth in the splenic microenvironment. *Exp Hematol* 1988; **16**: 213–16.

96. Vuillermoz B, Wegrowski Y, Contet-Audonneau JL, Danoux L, Pauly G, Maquart FX. Influence of aging on glycosaminoglycans and small leucine-rich proteoglycans production by skin fibroblasts. *Mol Cell Biochem* 2005; **277**: 63–72.

97. Dudhia J. Aggrecan, aging and assembly in articular cartilage. *Cell Mol Life Sci* 2005; **62**: 2241–56.

98. Funk PE, Stephan RP, Witte PL. Vascular cell adhesion molecule 1-positive reticular cells express interleukin-7 and stem cell factor in the bone marrow. *Blood* 1995; **86**: 2661–71.

99. Sudo T, Nishikawa S, Ohno N, Akiyama N, Tamakoshi M, Yoshida H. Expression and function of the interleukin 7 receptor in murine lymphocytes. *Proc Natl Acad Sci USA* 1993; **90**: 9125–9.

100. von Freeden-Jeffry U, Vieira P, Lucian LA, McNeil T, Burdach SE, Murray R. Lymphopenia in interleukin (IL)-7 gene-deleted mice identifies IL-7 as a nonredundant cytokine. *J Exp Med* 1995; **181**: 1519–26.

101. Stephan RP, Reilly CR, Witte PL. Impaired ability of bone marrow stromal cells to support B-lymphopoiesis with age. *Blood* 1998; **91**: 75–88.

102. Stephan RP, Lill-Elghanian DA, Witte PL. Development of B cells in aged mice: decline in the ability of pro-B cells to respond to IL-7 but not to other growth factors. *J Immunol* 1997; **158**: 1598–609.

103. Vacek A, Bartonickova A, Tkadlecek L. Age dependence of the number of the stem cells in haemopoietic tissues of rats. *Cell Tissue Kinet* 1976; **9**: 1–8.

104. Harrison DE, Astle CM, Delaittre JA. Loss of proliferative capacity in immunohemopoietic stem cells caused by serial transplantation rather than aging. *J Exp Med* 1978; **22**: 1526–31.

105. Wolf NS, Arora RK. Depletion of reserve in the hemopoietic system: I. Self-replication by stromal cells related to chronologic age. *Mech Ageing Dev* 1982; **20**: 127–40.

106. Hayflick L. The limited in vitro lifetime of human diploid cell strains. *Exp Cell Res* 1965; **37**: 614–36.

107. Giorno R, Clifford JH, Beverly S, Rossing RG. Hematology reference values. Analysis by different

statistical technics and variations with age and sex. *Am J Clin Pathol* 1980; **74**: 765–70.

108. Lipschitz DA, Udupa KB, Milton KY, Thompson CO. Effect of age on hematopoiesis in man. *Blood* 1984; **63**: 502–9.

109. Baldwin JG Jr. Hematopoietic function in the elderly. *Arch Intern Med* 1988; **148**: 2544–6.

110. Bao W, Dalferes ER Jr, Srinivasan SR, Webber LS, Berenson GS. Normative distribution of complete blood count from early childhood through adolescence: the Bogalusa Heart Study. *Prev Med* 1993; **22**: 825–37.

111. Marley SB, Lewis JL, Davidson RJ, *et al.* Evidence for a continuous decline in haemopoietic cell function from birth: application to evaluating bone marrow failure in children. *Br J Haematol* 1999; **106**: 162–6.

112. Cheng CK, Chan J, Cembrowski GS, van Assendelft OW. Complete blood count reference interval diagrams derived from NHANES III: stratification by age, sex, and race. *Lab Hematol* 2004; **10**: 42–53.

113. Marx JJ. Normal iron absorption and decreased red cell iron uptake in the aged. *Blood* 1979; **53**: 204–11.

114. Timaffy M. A comparative study of bone marrow function in young and old individuals. *Gerontol Clin (Basel)* 1962; **4**: 13–8.

115. Egusa Y, Fujiwara Y, Syaharuddin E, Sumiyoshi H, Isobe T, Yamakido M. Mobilization of peripheral blood stem cells in patients with advanced thoracic malignancies after irinotecan (CPT-11) administration. *Anticancer Res* 1998; **18**: 481–7.

116. Bagnara GP, Bonsi L, Strippoli P, *et al.* Hemopoiesis in healthy old people and centenarians: well-maintained responsiveness of CD34+ cells to hemopoietic growth factors and remodeling of cytokine network. *J Gerontol A Biol Sci Med Sci* 2000; **55**: B61–B70.

117. Chatta GS, Price TH, Allen RC, Dale DC. Effects of in vivo recombinant methionyl human granulocyte colony-stimulating factor on the neutrophil response and peripheral blood colony-forming cells in healthy young and elderly adult volunteers. *Blood* 1994; **84**: 2923–9.

118. Dreger P, Haferlach T, Eckstein V, *et al.* G-CSF-mobilized peripheral blood progenitor cells for allogeneic transplantation: safety, kinetics of mobilization, and composition of the graft. *Br J Haematol* 1994; **87**: 609–13.

119. de la Rubia J, Diaz MA, Verdeguer A, *et al.* Donor age-related differences in PBPC mobilization with rHuG-CSF. *Transfusion* 2001; **41**: 201–5.

120. Kuznetsov SA, Riminucci M, Ziran N, *et al.* The interplay of osteogenesis and hematopoiesis: expression of a constitutively active PTH/PTHrP receptor in osteogenic cells perturbs the establishment of hematopoiesis in bone and of skeletal stem cells in the bone marrow. *J Cell Biol* 2004; **167**: 1113–22.

121. Aguila HL, Rowe DW. Skeletal development, bone remodeling, and hematopoiesis. *Immunol Rev* 2005; **208**: 7–18.

122. Zhu J, Emerson SG. A new bone to pick: osteoblasts and the haematopoietic stem-cell niche. *Bioessays* 2004; **26**: 595–9.

123. Shigeno Y, Ashton BA. Human bone-cell proliferation in vitro decreases with human donor age. *J Bone Joint Surg Br* 1995; **77**: 139–42.

124. Oreffo RO, Bord S, Triffitt JT. Skeletal progenitor cells and ageing human populations. *Clin Sci (Lond)* 1998; **94**: 549–55.

125. Stenderup K, Justesen J, Eriksen EF, Rattan SI, Kassem M. Number and proliferative capacity of osteogenic stem cells are maintained during aging and in patients with osteoporosis. *J Bone Miner Res* 2001; **16**: 1120–9.

126. Muschler GF, Nitto H, Boehm CA, Easley KA. Age- and gender-related changes in the cellularity of human bone marrow and the prevalence of osteoblastic progenitors. *J Orthop Res* 2001; **19**: 117–25.

127. Fehrer C, Lepperdinger G. Mesenchymal stem cell aging. *Exp Gerontol* 2005; **40**: 926–30.

128. D'Ippolito G, Schiller PC, Ricordi C, Roos BA, Howard GA. Age-related osteogenic potential of mesenchymal stromal stem cells from human vertebral bone marrow. *J Bone Miner Res* 1999; **14**: 1115–22.

129. Sharpless NE, DePinho RA. Telomeres, stem cells, senescence, and cancer. *J Clin Invest* 2004; **113**: 160–8.

130. Zimmermann S, Voss M, Kaiser S, Kapp U, Waller CF, Martens UM. Lack of telomerase activity in human mesenchymal stem cells. *Leukemia* 2003; **17**: 1146–9.

131. Schieker M, Pautke C, Reitz K, *et al.* The use of four-colour immunofluorescence techniques to identify mesenchymal stem cells. *J Anat* 2004; **204**: 133–9.

7

Replicative senescence, aging, and cancer

Rita B. Effros

Introduction

One of the fundamental properties of mitotically competent human somatic cells is an innately programmed barrier to unlimited proliferation [1]. This process, known as replicative (or proliferative) senescence, may serve as one of many safeguards to maintain cellular integrity necessitated by the extended longevity of humans. Species such as rodents, which live for only a few years, can protect cells by such functions as DNA repair and antioxidant pathways. In humans, these conventional cellular defense strategies, which might otherwise fail over the many decades of human life, are bolstered by the mechanism of replicative senescence.

It is believed that a restriction in the number of cell divisions may serve as a protection against the potential for multiple mutations that are required for the development of a cancer cell from a cell that is normal [2]. The replicative senescence program is a strict characteristic of human, as opposed to mouse, cells, and in fact there is no documented case of a normal human cell undergoing spontaneous immortalization in cell culture. By contrast, mouse cells transform quite frequently in cell culture, becoming immortal cell lines [3]. Parallel observations have been made in vivo: mice show high rates of cancer within their three-year lifespan, whereas most human cancers occur after age 50. Thus, the process of replicative senescence may constitute a protective function against cancer in humans. Nevertheless, for some cell types, the replicative senescence program can lead to deleterious consequences, particularly

by old age. This chapter will provide an overview of the process of replicative senescence in one specific type of white blood cell, the T lymphocyte. Extensive research in this area has led to the notion that replicative senescence, particularly in the so-called CD8, or cytotoxic, T cells (CTL), not only hampers immune function itself, but may contribute to several of the pathologies of aging [4].

Proliferation is essential for immune function

During the complex transition from hematopoietic stem cells to mature lymphocytes, T cells generate their antigen receptors by a unique process of random joining of DNA segments from several different gene families. The outcome of this developmental program is that each lymphocyte expresses a unique receptor. When a particular lymphocyte becomes activated as a result of encounter with the appropriate antigen, it undergoes clonal expansion, and the identical receptor is expressed on all the resulting daughter cells [5].

The generation of antigen receptors by this stochastic process leads to an extremely large repertoire of antigen specificities, thereby enabling the immune system to have broad coverage over multiple and varied types of pathogens. However, precisely because of the huge spectrum of antigen specificities, the number of T cells that can respond to any single pathogen is extremely small, leading to the requirement for massive cell division and

Blood Disorders in the Elderly, ed. Lodovico Balducci, William Ershler, Giovanni de Gaetano.
Published by Cambridge University Press. © Cambridge University Press 2008.

clonal expansion of the few cells whose receptors recognize the invading pathogen. Once the antigen-specific T cells clear the pathogen, most of the expanded cell population dies by apoptosis, leaving only a few memory cells to handle possible future encounters with the same antigen.

Under normal circumstances, the proliferative limit of T cells would not be expected to interfere with immune responses. For example, an average proliferative lifespan of 35 population doublings (PDs), which would result in over 10^{10} cells, is more than sufficient to cover the response to at least two or three rounds of antigenic stimulation, even taking into account the fact that each wave of T-cell expansion is followed by the elimination of excess cells. However, in situations where antigen-specific T cells are chronically stimulated or encounter the same antigen multiple times over many decades, the proliferative limit may actually be reached by certain T cells, particularly by old age [6].

Replicative senescence in T cells

Much of the information on the process of senescence in human lymphocytes has emerged from experiments performed in cell culture using T cells derived from healthy donors. The basic protocol involves stimulation with antigen and the growth factor, interleukin 2 (IL-2), and allowing the responding cells to expand in culture for 3–4 weeks, at which time they become quiescent. This procedure of antigen-induced proliferation is repeated over many months, until the culture shows no further cell division in response to stimulation with antigen and/or IL-2 [7].

It should be emphasized that the specific stimulus used to induce proliferation is not relevant to the process of replicative senescence. Both CD4 and CD8 T cells have been shown to reach this end stage in cell culture, whether stimulated with alloantigen, viral antigens, mitogens, or activatory antibodies [4,8,9]. In other words, the driving force to the end stage of replicative senescence is the process of repeated cell division.

Cultures of senescent T cells show a variety of characteristics in addition to their cell-cycle arrest in G1. As with other cell types that have been studied longitudinally in cell culture, T cells undergo progressive telomere shortening [10–12]. Telomeres are the repeated DNA sequences at the ends of all linear chromosomes. Due to the mechanism of DNA replication, the extreme ends of the telomeres cannot be replicated during cell division, resulting in their gradual attrition. It is believed that telomeres (alone, or in concert with certain telomere-binding proteins) are the clock that registers the number of divisions a cell has undergone, and that when a critical telomere length is reached, a DNA damage signal occurs and the cell cycle is permanently arrested [13,14].

T cells that undergo extensive cell division in cell culture reach a mean telomere length of 5–7 kilobases (kb) at senescence, a substantial change from their original 10–11 kb size [15]. This observation was initially somewhat surprising, since T cells differ from most other somatic cells in that they can upregulate the telomere-extending enzyme, telomerase, in concert with activation [11,16]. Indeed, primary stimulation of T cells with either antigen or mitogen leads to levels of telomerase activity that are as high as those seen in tumor cells. Upregulation of telomerase activity has also been documented in antigen-specific T cells responding to an acute infection in vivo. During the first two weeks of infection with Epstein–Barr virus (EBV), the responding CD8 T cells show high telomerase activity and telomere length maintenance. However, one year after infection, when telomerase is longer active, antigen-specific CD8 T cells from the same individual have undergone telomere shortening, suggesting that telomerase upregulation may not be a permanent feature of T-cell activation [17].

In order to analyze telomerase dynamics during repeated rounds of antigen-induced T-cell activation, CD4 and CD8 T cells isolated from the same individual were followed longitudinally in cell culture. The initial stimulation with antigen resulted in equivalent levels of telomerase activity in both subsets. However, by the third and all subsequent stimulations, CD8 T cells were unable to upregulate telomerase activity. This early and permanent loss of telomerase upregulation is specific for CD8 T cells; CD4 T cells from the same individual are able to upregulate telomerase to high levels even after seven rounds of stimulation [18].

CD8 T cells that reach the end stage of replicative senescence are metabolically active and viable, and in fact under proper cell culture conditions can survive for long periods in their non-proliferative state. Moreover, senescent CD8 T cells are resistant to a variety of apoptotic stimuli that cause rapid cell death in early passage cultures from the same donor [19]. This inability to initiate programmed cell death is similar to other cell types that reach senescence in culture [20]. Another important cellular defense process that is altered in senescent T cells is the response to stress, specifically, the upregulation of heat shock protein 70 (hsp70), the major mammalian stress protein. This hsp family of cellular proteins protects cells during a wide spectrum of cellular stressors, including mild heat shock, viral infection, and temporary oxidative stress. Senescent T cells show a significantly blunted upregulation of hsp70 in response to a mild, short heat stress compared to their progenitors [21]. Finally, as cells age in culture, they show increased microsatellite instability, an indicator of reduced DNA mismatch repair capacity, which is capable of rectifying errors in DNA replication [22]. Thus, as T cells progress to the end stage of replicative senescence in cell culture, they are altered in a variety of processes reflecting cellular integrity and defense.

Elderly persons have high proportions of senescent T cells

One of the most significant outcomes that emerged from analysis of the process of T-cell replicative senescence under the controlled conditions of cell culture was the identification of a novel biomarker of senescence. This change in cell-surface antigen expression was detected by sequential flow cytometric analyses of a panel of T-cell-specific cell-surface molecules. In general, the expression level of a variety of markers reflecting subsets, memory status, adhesion, and degree of activation was unchanged as T cells progressed along the path to senescence. The sole exception was the key T-cell-specific signal transduction molecule, CD28, which was totally absent on cells in senescent cultures, despite its expression on >99% of the T cells used to initiate the cultures [23].

The complete loss of CD28 expression in senescent T-cell cultures facilitated the analysis of blood samples to determine whether cells with a similar phenotype accumulate in vivo. These studies clearly showed that the proportion of T cells that lack CD28 expression increases with age, and that the majority of such cells are within the CD8 subset, the type of T cell responsible for controlling viral infection. In fact, it has been shown that in some elderly persons, more than 50% of the peripheral CD8 T-cell pool consists of cells that are CD28-negative (CD28–) [24].

Comparison of individuals within different age groups has shown that the proportion of CD8 T cells with characteristics of senescence accumulates gradually over the entire lifespan, starting with <1% CD28– T cells present at birth [25]. Although aging is closely correlated with increased proportions of senescent CD8 T cells [26], it should be emphasized that it is not aging or chronological time per se that is critical, but rather chronic stimulation associated with extensive cell division. Indeed, younger individuals (including infants) infected with HIV show similarly high proportions of CD8 T cells that lack CD28 expression [27–32]. Moreover, increased proportions of CD28– T cells have been documented in a variety of other clinical situations, such as ankylosing spondylitis [33], multiple sclerosis [34], coronary artery disease [35], and certain forms of cancer [36,37].

In order to further investigate the potential similarities between CD28– T cells isolated from peripheral blood samples and cells that reach senescence in cell culture, several types of experiments were performed. First, telomere lengths were measured in subpopulations of lymphocytes that were purified by flow cytometry sorting procedures. Studies by several groups have shown that the telomere lengths of purified CD8+CD28– T cells are significantly shorter than CD8 T cells that express CD28 [27,38].

In addition, assays to evaluate proliferative capacity have shown that CD8+CD28– T cells show minimal proliferative activity, further confirming their similarity to senescent cultures [25,27]. Finally, one study on virus-specific CD8 T cells documented that the CD28– population tested immediately ex vivo was resistant to superantigen-induced apoptosis, again reminiscent of senescent cultures [39].

What is the driving force responsible for the accumulation of senescent CD8 T cells with age? It is believed that one of the major factors is chronic viral infection [40]. Viruses that establish latency require ongoing immune control to maintain the latent state, implying chronic exposure of the relevant virus-specific CD8 T cells to an antigenic stimulus. This notion is supported by the re-emergence of latent infections in immunodeficient individuals. For example, organ-transplant recipients who receive immunosuppressive drugs have an increased incidence of EBV-associated lymphomas. Similarly, persons infected with HIV often develop shingles, which involves reactivation of latent varicella zoster virus (VZV) infection. In the elderly, another latent infection, cytomegalovirus (CMV), seems to contribute to the generation of senescent CD8 T cells. Indeed, CMV seropositivity is correlated with high proportions of CD28– T cells and early mortality [41]. Based on these findings, one of the possible strategies that has been proposed to retard the generation of senescent CD8 T cells during aging might be the development of a vaccine to prevent primary CMV infection [40].

What are the in-vivo consequences of senescent CD8 T cells?

Data from longitudinal analysis of virus-specific CD8 T cells in long-term culture suggest that replicative senescence is associated with reduced ability to perform antigen-specific cytotoxicity and diminished production of the antiviral cytokine interferon gamma (IFN-γ) [42]. CD8 T cells with similar functional decrements accumulate progressively over time in persons chronically infected with

HIV [43]. Indeed, reduced potency of the virus-specific cytotoxic response and diminished proliferative potential are key components of the immune exhaustion that is the signature of HIV disease [44]. Conversely, one of the main immunological characteristics of long-term survivors infected with HIV is the presence of a population of virus-specific CD8 T cells with robust lytic function and high proliferative activity [45–47]. Thus, from both cell culture studies and clinical observations of chronic infections, it seems clear that one of the most immediate effects of replicative senescence in virus-specific CD8 T cells is loss of effective control over the infection.

A second aspect of the accumulation of CD28– T-cell populations in vivo relates to the observation that they are generally part of CD8 oligoclonal expansions [48–54]. Since the total number of T cells does not change (or may possibly even decrease) with age, the large expansions of certain T-cell clones would be predicted to narrow the overall repertoire of available specificities. Indeed, one study did in fact show that elderly persons with high proportions of CD8-T-cell clonal expansions have a more restricted repertoire [55]. In combination with the diminished export of naive T cells by the aging thymus, the restricted repertoire further limits the range of antigens to which many elderly persons can respond.

In addition to narrowing the available repertoire, it is possible that the high proportions of senescent T cells might lead to specific overall effects on health. Interest in the mechanism by which senescent CD8 T cells exert their effects has been bolstered by several studies showing correlations with a variety of deleterious outcomes. For example, longitudinal studies performed over several decades in Sweden have suggested that early mortality is correlated with an "immune risk phenotype" [56]. This cluster of parameters includes high proportions of CD8+CD28– T cells, and poor T-cell proliferation. In another study, the telomere length of lymphocytes derived from a group of 60-year-olds was evaluated in terms of subsequent mortality. Interestingly, those individuals whose telomere length fell in the lowest quartile at age 60 had a 7–8 times greater risk of dying from infectious causes compared to those individuals with the longest telomeres [57].

It should be emphasized that such correlative studies do not in any way suggest that it is telomere shortening per se that is the cause of mortality. Rather, it is more likely that the reduced telomere length is a biomarker of other physiological changes [58]. For example, in the case of shorter telomeres being associated with increased death from infectious causes, one possible mechanism that might be operating is that the T cells were working overtime (and eventually failing) to control a particular infection, and in the process undergoing extensive cell division and concomitant telomere shortening. Studies on HIV-infected persons are consistent with this notion, since over many years the chronic activation and proliferation of CD8 T cells does eventually lead to high proportions of CD8 T cells that lack CD28 expression and have shortened telomeres. An alternative possibility to explain the short-telomere/infection association relates to the observation that telomere length is a heritable trait [59–61], and may be linked to other genetic factors that are the true cause of the increased death risk from infections.

Given that infections are a major cause of morbidity and mortality in the elderly, vaccination is an important prophylactic strategy. Influenza, in particular, has been shown to be the fourth leading cause of death in elderly persons, so that this age group is a priority target population for influenza vaccination. Thus, it is highly relevant that two studies have shown a significant correlation between poor response to influenza vaccination and high proportions of senescent CD8 T cells. The underlying mechanism for this association has not been identified, but in other contexts, CD8 T cells that lack CD28 expression have been shown to have suppressor cell functions, leading to downregulation of antigen presentation as well as other T-cell activities [62]. CD8+CD28− T cells also accumulate and mediate liver damage in hepatitis C infection [63]. Suppressor functions have also been attributed to CD8 T cells that are CD57-positive, a phenotype associated with loss of CD28 expression. These putatively senescent CD8 T cells exert suppressive influences on effector functions of HIV-specific CTL [64].

Another interesting correlation that has emerged from clinical studies is the association between high proportions of senescent CD8 T cells and osteoporotic fractures in a group of elderly women [65]. Although this was a small-scale study, increasing evidence suggests that chronic immune activation is, in fact, associated with bone loss [66]. Moreover, the profile of cytokines produced by senescent T cells (e.g., increased IL-6 and reduced IFN-γ) would be predicted to favor maturation and activation of osteoclasts, the bone-resorbing cells. Further research in the relatively new field of osteoimmunology will undoubtedly uncover new and important mechanisms that link the immune system of the elderly with some of the well-documented age-related skeletal changes.

Senescent T cells and cancer

One of the fundamental questions spanning the fields of both cancer biology and immunology is whether immune surveillance plays a role in tumor initiation and progression. Although for cancers in general this issue has not been resolved, there is accumulating evidence suggesting that in certain virally related cancers, exhaustion of immune control over the virus may play a role in tumor initiation [67]. Immune deficiency is, in fact, closely correlated with several types of tumors that have viral etiologies. For example, in immunosuppressed individuals, virtually all lymphomas are EBV in origin, presumably resulting from the ultimate failure of T cells to effectively control EBV infection [68,69]. Another latent herpesvirus-associated tumor, Kaposi's sarcoma, is increased in HIV-infected persons, and cervical cancer, which also increases during immune suppression, is associated with certain strains of human papillomavirus.

Viruses that are able to establish latency develop a complex relationship with the host's immune system. Evasion of immune recognition as well as specific physiological effects on the T cells themselves are probably involved [70]. It is clear that the initial primary infection with these viruses does elicit an immune response. During the acute phase of infectious mononucleosis (EBV infection), for example, high levels of telomerase activity and activation markers can be detected on the antigen-specific CD8 T cells. Nevertheless, one year after infection, when presumably the virus has become latent, these same T cells show evidence of having experienced chronic antigenic stimulation, as indicated by telomere shortening of the tetramer-binding CD8 T cells [17]. These data suggest that, at least in the case of EBV, latency is associated with prolonged antigen-specific proliferation in vivo. Since EBV is involved not only in lymphomas, but also in invasive breast cancer and in some tumors of the prostate and of the liver [68], it is possible that immune exhaustion caused by replicative senescence of virus-specific CD8 T cells plays a role in the development of a broad spectrum of tumor types.

Persons with virally associated tumors do, in fact, have increased proportions of CD8 T cells with characteristics reminiscent of T cells that reach replicative senescence in cell culture, suggesting an association between loss of control over the virus and transformation of the latently infected cells [4]. Indeed, it has been shown that antigen-specific CD8 T cells in several chronic viral infections, such as HIV, CMV, and EBV, eventually lose their antiviral cytolytic function once the infection becomes chronic [71]. Interesting, in patients with certain EBV-associated nasopharyngeal tumors, such fundamental CD8-T-cell protective functions as secretion of IFN-γ and perforin expression by CD8 T cells are also impaired [72]. Moreover, in many of these cancer patients, reduced EBV-specific CTL precursor frequency has also been documented and, importantly, the deficit correlated with plasma viral burden [73]. Since the limiting dilution assay used to detect precursor frequency is critically dependent on proliferation, the above observation is consistent with a role for proliferative exhaustion. In addition, EBV-associated lymphomas are correlated with high tumor necrosis factor α levels, reminiscent of senescent T-cell cultures [74]. In sum, there is increasing evidence lending support to

the hypothesis that chronic exposure to antigens of latent viruses (e.g., EBV, HPV) may facilitate tumor progression and metastasis by driving the relevant antigen-specific T cells to senescence.

The potential to generate senescent antigen-reactive T cells may not be restricted to situations involving latent infections. Certain non-viral tumor-associated antigens may also be a source of chronic immune stimulation. For example, prostate-specific antigen (PSA), the blood levels of which increase in persons with prostate cancer, is also present in normal prostate tissue, and is thus an antigen to which T cells have had prolonged exposure [75]. CD8 T cells from patients with prostate cancer do, in fact, show reactivity to PSA peptides immediately ex vivo [76], consistent with the notion that they were previously primed in vivo to this antigen. Similarly, melanoma-specific antigens, which cause chronic activation of T cells, have been suggested to play a role in the loss of CD28 expression in some melanoma patients [77]. Thus, like antigens of viruses that establish latency, tumor-associated antigens also have the potential to cause chronic T-cell activation, possibly driving some antigen-specific cells to senescence.

As noted above, loss of CD28 expression is the signature change of CD8 T-cell senescence in cell culture. It is thus relevant to note that altered expression of CD28, and by implication replicative senescence, has also been associated with the clinical outcome of certain non-viral cancers. In advanced renal carcinoma, for example, the proportion of CD8 T cells that are CD57+ (a marker present on a majority of CD28– T cells) has predictive value with respect to patient survival [78]. Further, in patients with head and neck tumors, it has been shown that tumor resection is associated with a reduction in the CD8+CD28– T-cell subset, which had undergone expansion during the period of tumor growth [37]. Thus, replicative senescence of CD8 T cells, already implicated in defective immunity to chronic viral infections [44], may also play a role in the failed immune surveillance that may facilitate the development or metastasis of certain types of cancer.

In addition to possibly facilitating the development of some tumors, the process of CD8-T-cell replicative senescence also has an impact on adoptive immunotherapy for cancer, since sustained control over the tumor requires extensive T-cell proliferation and maintenance of functional integrity. The impediment of replicative senescence has, in fact, been documented in the case of EBV, where in-vitro expansion of EBV-specific CD8 T cells for the purpose of cancer immunotherapy is associated with loss of cytolytic function [79, 80]. This change is consistent with observations from cell culture studies on replicative senescence [81]. Thus, prevention or retardation of the process of replicative senescence will lead to improvement in immunotherapy directed at cancer, one of the major diseases of old age.

Solutions to the problem of T-cell replicative senescence

Given the spectrum of deleterious effects associated with senescent T cells, investigators are actively pursuing strategies to reverse, prevent or retard the process of replicative senescence. Based on the central role of telomere shortening in signaling the cell-cycle arrest, one of the major approaches has been manipulation of the enzyme telomerase, either by genetic or by pharmacologic methods. Gene transduction with the catalytic component of human telomerase (hTERT) has been extensively analyzed in human fibroblasts, epithelial cells, and keratinocytes. These studies have documented that the transduced cells show unlimited proliferation, telomere length stabilization, normalization of function, and, importantly, no evidence of altered growth or tumorogenesis in immunodeficient (SCID) mice.

In CD8 T cells, gene transduction with hTERT is able to reverse some, but not all, of the components of the replicative senescence program. CD8 T cells that are specific for tumors and for HIV have both been shown to acquire unlimited proliferative capacity following transduction with hTERT. Nevertheless, the ultimate loss of CD28 expression is not prevented by this strategy [81,82]. The importance of retaining CD28 expression has been documented in several studies of cancer immunotherapy and anti-tumor

vaccines, in which incorporation of the CD28 ligand, B7, enhanced treatment efficacy [34,83–85]. Genetic modulation of telomerase activity also fails to prevent the ultimate collapse of antigen-specific cytolytic function in virus-specific cultures [86]. Ongoing research is addressing whether combinations of hTERT and CD28 gene therapies will result in more comprehensive correction of the features of CD8-T-cell replicative senescence.

Because of the complexity and impractical aspects of gene-therapy approaches, efforts are also directed at identifying pharmacologic agents that might accomplish the same goals. It has been known for some time that cells of the immune system contain estrogen receptors; the original radioactive estrogen binding studies suggested that CD8 T cells, in particular, bind estrogen with high affinity [87]. Although little is known about the spectrum of T-cell genes that are modulated by estrogen, an estrogen-responsive element has been documented in the promoter region of IFN-γ [88], a cytokine that is often monitored in evaluating immune responses to viruses and cancer [89]. Interestingly, IFN-γ has also been recently shown to upregulate the enzyme telomerase in T cells [90].

Estrogen can also directly modulate telomerase activity; there is an estrogen-responsive element in the promoter of the *hTERT* gene in a variety of reproductive tissues [91]. Estrogen also affects calcium mobilization in T cells. Thus, evidence from a variety of systems suggests that estrogen has the potential to modulate several T-cell functions that are altered in senescent cells, and may therefore constitute a novel type of non-genetic strategy to modulate senescence. Clearly, application of these hormone-based approaches to cancer immunotherapy or to modulation of antiviral immunity will require identifying designer estrogens that specifically affect T cells, but not estrogen-sensitive tumor cells. Finally, research on non-hormonal modulators of T-cell telomerase activity may provide additional approaches to modulating replicative senescence, thereby expanding the efficacy of cancer immunotherapy and effective control over viral infections in the elderly [92].

ACKNOWLEDGEMENTS

The research described in this chapter has been supported in part by the NIH and the UCLA Center on Aging. Dr. Effros holds the Thomas and Elizabeth Plott Endowed Chair in Gerontology.

REFERENCES

1. Hayflick L, Moorhead PS. The serial cultivation of human diploid cell strains. *Exp Cell Res* 1961; **25**: 585–621.

2. Effros RB, Dagarag M, Spaulding CC, Man J. The role of CD8+ T-cell replicative senescence in human aging. *Immunol Rev* 2005; **205**: 147–57.

3. Akbar AN, Soares MV, Plunkett FJ, Salmon M. Differential regulation of CD8+ T cell senescence in mice and men. *Mech Ageing Dev* 2000; **121**: 69–76.

4. Effros RB, Cai Z, Linton PJ. CD8 T cells and aging. *Crit Rev Immunol* 2003; **23**: 45–64.

5. Janeway CA, Travers P, Walpert MSM. *The Immune System in Health and Disease*, 5th edn (New York, NY: Garland, 2001).

6. Effros RB, Pawelec G. Replicative senescence of T lymphocytes: does the Hayflick limit lead to immune exhaustion? *Immunol Today* 1997; **18**: 450–4.

7. Perillo NL, Walford RL, Newman MA, Effros RB. Human T lymphocytes possess a limited in vitro lifespan. *Exp Gerontol* 1989; **24**: 177–87.

8. Pawelec G, Rehbein A, Haehnel K, Meri A, Adibzadeh M. Human T cell clones in long-term culture as a model of immunosenescence. *Immunol Rev* 1997; **160**: 31–42.

9. Levine BL, Cotte J, Small CC, *et al.* Large-scale production of CD4+ T cells from HIV-1-infected donors after CD3/CD28 costimulation. *J Hematother* 1998; **7**: 437–48.

10. Harley C, Futcher AB, Greider C. Telomeres shorten during ageing of human fibroblasts. *Nature* 1990; **345**: 458–60.

11. Bodnar AG, Kim NW, Effros RB, Chiu CP. Mechanism of telomerase induction during T cell activation. *Exp Cell Res* 1996; **228**: 58–64.

12. Weng NP, Levine BL, June CH, Hodes RJ. Human naive and memory T lymphocytes differ in telomeric length and replicative potential. *Proc Natl Acad Sci USA* 1995; **92**: 11091–4.

13. Smogorzewska A, de Lange T. Regulation of telomerase by telomeric proteins. *Annu Rev Biochem* 2004; **73**: 177–208.

14. Blackburn EH. Telomeres and telomerase: their mechanisms of action and the effects of altering their functions. *FEBS Lett* 2005; **579**: 859–62.

15. Vaziri H, Schachter F, Uchida I, *et al.* Loss of telomeric DNA during aging of normal and trisomy 21 human lymphocytes. *Am J Hum Genet* 1993; **52**: 661–7.

16. Weng NP, Palmer LD, Levine BL, Lane HC, June CH, Hodes RJ. Tales of tails: regulation of telomere length and telomerase activity during lymphocyte development, differentiation, activation, and aging. *Immunol Rev* 1997; **160**: 43–54.

17. Maini MK, Soares MV, Zilch CF, Akbar AN, Beverley PC. Virus-induced CD8+ T cell clonal expansion is associated with telomerase up-regulation and telomere length preservation: a mechanism for rescue from replicative senescence. *J Immunol* 1999; **162**: 4521–6.

18. Valenzuela HF, Effros RB. Loss of telomerase inducibility in memory T cells with repeated antigenic stimulation. *FASEB J* 2000; **14**: A991.

19. Spaulding CS, Guo W, Effros RB. Resistance to apoptosis in human CD8+ T cells that reach replicative senescence after multiple rounds of antigen-specific proliferation. *Exp Gerontol* 1999; **34**: 633–44.

20. Wang E, Lee MJ, Pandey S. Control of fibroblast senescence and activation of programmed cell death. *J Cell Biochem* 1994; **54**: 432–9.

21. Effros RB, Zhu X, Walford RL. Stress response of senescent T lymphocytes: reduced hsp70 is independent of the proliferative block. *J Gerontol* 1994; **49**: B65–B70.

22. Krichevsky S, Pawelec G, Gural A, *et al.* Age related microsatellite instability in T cells from healthy individuals. *Exp Gerontol* 2004; **39**: 507–15.

23. Effros RB, Boucher N, Porter V, *et al.* Decline in CD28+ T cells in centenarians and in long-term T cell cultures: a possible cause for both in vivo and in vitro immunosenescence. *Exp Gerontol* 1994; **29**: 601–9.

24. Boucher N, Defeu-Duchesne T, Vicaut E, Farge D, Effros RB, Schachter F. CD28 expression in T cell aging and human longevity. *Exp Gerontol* 1998; **33**: 267–82.

25. Azuma M, Phillips JH, Lanier LL. CD28– T lymphocytes: antigenic and functional properties. *J Immunol* 1993; **150**: 1147–59.

26. Nilsson BO, Ernerudh J, Johansson B, *et al.* Morbidity does not influence the T-cell immune risk phenotype in the elderly: findings in the Swedish NONA Immune Study using sample selection protocols. *Mech Ageing Dev* 2003; **124**: 469–76.

27. Effros RB, Allsopp R, Chiu CP, *et al.* Shortened telomeres in the expanded CD28–CD8+ subset in HIV disease

implicate replicative senescence in HIV pathogenesis. *AIDS/Fast Track* 1996; **10**: F17–F22.

28. Borthwick NJ, Bofill M, Gombert WM. Lymphocyte activation in HIV-1 infection II: functional defects of CD28– T cells. *AIDS* 1994; **8**: 431–41.

29. Jennings C, Rich K, Siegel JN, Landay A. A phenotypic study of CD8+ lymphocyte subsets in infants using three-color flow cytometry. *Clin Immunol Immunopath* 1994; **71**: 8–13.

30. Brinchmann JE, Dobloug JH, Heger BH, Haaheim LL, Sannes M, Egeland T. Expression of costimulatory molecule CD28 on T cells in human immunodeficiency virus type 1 infection: functional and clinical correlations. *J Infect Dis* 1994; **169**: 730–8.

31. Pantaleo G, Koenig S, Baseler M, Lane HC, Fauci AS. Defective clonogenic potential of CD8+ T lymphocytes in patients with AIDS: expansion in vivo of a nonclonogenic CD3+CD8+DR+CD25– T cell population. *J Immunol* 1990; **144**: 1696–704.

32. Lewis DE, Tang DSN, Adu-Oppong A, Schober W, Rodgers JR. Anergy and apoptosis in CD8+ T cells from HIV-infected persons. *J Immunol* 1994; **153**: 412–20.

33. Schirmer M, Goldberger C, Wurzner R, *et al.* Circulating cytotoxic CD8(+) CD28(–) T cells in ankylosing spondylitis. *Arthritis Res* 2002; **4**: 71–6.

34. Foss FM. Immunologic mechanisms of antitumor activity. *Semin Oncol* 2002; **29** (3 Suppl 7): 5–11.

35. Jonasson L, Tompa A, Wikby A. Expansion of peripheral CD8+ T cells in patients with coronary artery disease: relation to cytomegalovirus infection. *J Intern Med* 2003; **254**: 472–8.

36. Pilch H, Hoehn H, Schmidt M, *et al.* CD8+CD45RA+CD27–CD28-T-cell subset in PBL of cervical cancer patients representing CD8+T-cells being able to recognize cervical cancer associated antigens provided by HPV 16 E7. *Zentralbl Gynakol* 2002; **124**: 406–12.

37. Tsukishiro T, Donnenberg AD, Whiteside TL. Rapid turnover of the CD8(+)CD28(–) T-cell subset of effector cells in the circulation of patients with head and neck cancer. *Cancer Immunol Immunother* 2003; **52**: 599–607.

38. Monteiro J, Batliwalla F, Ostrer H, Gregersen PK. Shortened telomeres in clonally expanded CD28–CD8+ T cells imply a replicative history that is distinct from their CD28+CD8+ counterparts. *J Immunol* 1996; **156**: 3587–90.

39. Posnett DN, Edinger JW, Manavalan JS, Irwin C, Marodon G. Differentiation of human CD8 T cells: implications for in vivo persistence of CD8+ CD28– cytotoxic effector clones. *Int Immunol* 1999; **11**: 229–41.

40. Pawelec G, Akbar A, Caruso C, Effros RB, Grubeck-Loebenstein B, Wikby A. Is immunosenescence infectious? *Trends Immunol* 2004; **25**: 406–10.

41. Wikby A, Johansson B, Olsson J, Lofgren S, Nilsson BO, Ferguson F. Expansions of peripheral blood CD8 T-lymphocyte subpopulations and an association with cytomegalovirus seropositivity in the elderly: the Swedish NONA immune study. *Exp Gerontol* 2002; **37**: 445–53.

42. Dagarag MD, Evazyan T, Rao N, Effros RB. Genetic manipulation of telomerase in HIV-specific CD8+ T cells: enhanced anti-viral functions accompany the increased proliferative potential and telomere length stabilization. *J Immunol* 2004; **173**: 6303–11.

43. Lieberman J, Shankar P, Manjunath N, Andersson J. Dressed to kill? A review of why antiviral CD8 T lymphocytes fail to prevent progressive immunodeficiency in HIV-1 infection. *Blood* 2001; **98**: 1667–77.

44. Appay V, Rowland-Jones S. Premature ageing of the immune system: the cause of AIDS? *Trends Immunol* 2002; **23**: 580–5.

45. Migueles SA, Laborico AC, Shupert WL, *et al.* HIV-specific CD8(+) T cell proliferation is coupled to perforin expression and is maintained in nonprogressors. *Nat Immunol* 2002; **3**: 1061–8.

46. Riviaere Y, McChesney MB, Porrot F, *et al.* Gag-specific cytotoxic responses to HIV type 1 are associated with a decreased risk of progression to AIDS-related complex or AIDS. *AIDS Res Hum Retroviruses* 1995; **11**: 903–7.

47. Rinaldo CJ, Beltz LA, Huang XL, Gupta P, Fan Z, Torpey DJ. Anti-HIV type 1 cytotoxic T lymphocyte effector activity and disease progression in the first 8 years of HIV type 1 infection of homosexual men. *AIDS Res Hum Retroviruses* 1995; **11**: 481–9.

48. Posnett DN, Sinha R, Kabak S, Russo C. Clonal populations of T cells in normal elderly humans: the T cell equivalent to "benign monoclonal gammopathy". *J Exp Med* 1994; **179**: 609–18.

49. Morley JK, Batliwalla FM, Hingorani R, Gregersen PK. Oligoclonal CD8+ T cells are preferentially expanded in the CD57+ subset. *J Immunol* 1995; **154**: 6182–90.

50. Weekes MP, Wills MR, Mynard K, Hicks R, Sissons JG, Carmichael AJ. Large clonal expansions of human virus-specific memory cytotoxic T lymphocytes within the CD57+ CD28– CD8+ T-cell population. *Immunology* 1999; **98**: 443–9.

51. Manfras BJ, Weidenbach H, Beckh KH, *et al.* Oligoclonal CD8+ T-cell expansion in patients with chronic hepatitis C is associated with liver pathology and poor

response to interferon-alpha therapy. *J Clin Immunol* 2004; **24**: 258–71.

52. Scheuring UJ, Sabzevari H, Theofilopoulos AN. Proliferative arrest and cell cycle regulation in CD8(+)CD28(–) versus CD8(+)CD28(+) T cells. *Hum Immunol* 2002; **63**: 1000–9.

53. McFarland EJ, Harding PA, Striebich CC, MaWhinney S, Kuritzkes DR, Kotzin BL. Clonal CD8+ T cell expansions in peripheral blood from human immunodeficiency virus type 1-infected children. *J Infect Dis* 2002; **186**: 477–85.

54. Khan N, Shariff N, Cobbold M, *et al.* Cytomegalovirus seropositivity drives the CD8 T cell repertoire toward greater clonality in healthy elderly individuals. *J Immunol* 2002; **169**: 1984–92.

55. Ouyang Q, Wagner WM, Wikby A, *et al.* Large numbers of dysfunctional CD8+ T lymphocytes bearing receptors for a single dominant CMV epitope in the very old. *J Clin Immunol* 2003; **23**: 247–57.

56. Ferguson FG, Wikby A, Maxson P, Olsson J, Johansson B. Immune parameters in a longitudinal study of a very old population of Swedish people: a comparison between survivors and nonsurvivors. *J Gerontol A Biol Sci Med Sci* 1995; **50**: B378–B382.

57. Cawthon RM, Smith KR, O'Brien E, Sivatchenko A, Kerber RA. Association between telomere length in blood and mortality in people aged 60 years or older. *Lancet* 2003; **361**: 393–5.

58. Aviv A. Telomeres and human aging: facts and fibs. *Sci Aging Knowledge Environ* 2004; **2004** (51): pe43.

59. Aviv A, Shay J, Christensen K, Wright W. The longevity gender gap: are telomeres the explanation? *Sci Aging Knowledge Environ* 2005; **2005** (23): pe16.

60. Unryn BM, Cook LS, Riabowol KT. Paternal age is positively linked to telomere length of children. *Aging Cell* 2005; **4**: 97–101.

61. Slagboom PE, Droog S, Boomsma DI. Genetic determination of telomere size in humans: a twin study of three age groups. *Am J Hum Genet* 1994; **55**: 876–82.

62. Suciu-Foca N, Manavalan JS, Scotto L, *et al.* Molecular characterization of allospecific T suppressor and tolerogenic dendritic cells: review. *Int Immunopharmacol* 2005; **5**: 7–11.

63. Kurokohchi K, Masaki T, Arima K, *et al.* CD28-negative CD8-positive cytotoxic T lymphocytes mediate hepatocellular damage in hepatitis C virus infection. *J Clin Immunol* 2003; **23**: 518–27.

64. Sadat-Sowti B, Parrot A, Quint L, Mayaud C, Debre P, Autran B. Alveolar CD8+CD57+ lymphocytes in human

immunodeficiency virus infection produce an inhibitor of cytotoxic functions. *Am J Respir Crit Care Med* 1994; **149**: 972–80.

65. Pietschmann P, Grisar J, Thien R, *et al.* Immune phenotype and intracellular cytokine production of peripheral blood mononuclear cells from postmenopausal patients with osteoporotic fractures. *Exp Gerontol* 2001; **36**: 1749–59.

66. Arron JR, Choi Y. Bone versus immune system. *Nature* 2000; **408**: 535–6.

67. Lanier LL. A renaissance for the tumor immunosurveillance hypothesis. *Nat Med* 2001; **7**: 1178–80.

68. Israel BF, Kenney SC. Virally targeted therapies for EBV-associated malignancies. *Oncogene* 2003; **22**: 5122–30.

69. Pardoll D. T cells and tumours. *Nature* 2001; **411**: 1010–12.

70. Petersen JL, Morris CR, Solheim JC. Virus evasion of MHC class I molecule presentation. *J Immunol* 2003; **171**: 4473–8.

71. Zhang D, Shankar P, Xu Z, *et al.* Most antiviral CD8 T cells during chronic viral infection do not express high levels of perforin and are not directly cytotoxic. *Blood* 2003; **101**: 226–35.

72. Zanussi S, Vaccher E, Caffau C, *et al.* Interferon-gamma secretion and perforin expression are impaired in CD8+ T lymphocytes from patients with undifferentiated carcinoma of nasopharyngeal type. *Cancer Immunol Immunother* 2003; **52**: 28–32.

73. Chua D, Huang J, Zheng B, *et al.* Adoptive transfer of autologous Epstein–Barr virus-specific cytotoxic T cells for nasopharyngeal carcinoma. *Int J Cancer* 2001; **94**: 73–80.

74. Mori A, Takao S, Pradutkanchana J, Kietthubthew S, Mitarnun W, Ishida T. High tumor necrosis factor-alpha levels in the patients with Epstein–Barr virus-associated peripheral T-cell proliferative disease/lymphoma. *Leuk Res* 2003; **27**: 493–8.

75. Kennedy-Smith AG, McKenzie JL, Owen MC, Davidson PJ, Vuckovic S, Hart DN. Prostate specific antigen inhibits immune responses in vitro: a potential role in prostate cancer. *J Urol* 2002; **168**: 741–7.

76. Chakraborty NG, Stevens RL, Mehrotra S, *et al.* Recognition of PSA-derived peptide antigens by T cells from prostate cancer patients without any prior stimulation. *Cancer Immunol Immunother* 2003; **52**: 497–505.

77. Hakansson A, Hakansson L, Gustafsson B, *et al.* Biochemotherapy of metastatic malignant melanoma: on down-regulation of CD28. *Cancer Immunol Immunother* 2002; **51**: 499–504.

78. Characiejus D, Pasukoniene V, Kazlauskaite N, *et al.* Predictive value of CD8highCD57+ lymphocyte subset in interferon therapy of patients with renal cell carcinoma. *Anticancer Res* 2002; **22**: 3679–83.

79. Carlens S, Liu D, Ringden O, *et al.* Cytolytic T cell reactivity to Epstein–Barr virus is lost during in vitro T cell expansion. *J Hematother Stem Cell Res* 2002; **11**: 669–74.

80. Straathof KC, Bollard CM, Rooney CM, Heslop HE. Immunotherapy for Epstein–Barr virus-associated cancers in children. *Oncologist* 2003; **8**: 83–98.

81. Dagarag MD, Ng H, Lubong R, Effros RB, Yang OO. Differential impairment of lytic and cytokine functions in senescent HIV-1-specific cytotoxic T lymphocytes. *J Virol* 2003; **77**: 3077–83.

82. Hooijberg E, Ruizendaal JJ, Snijders PJ, Kueter EW, Walboomers JM, Spits H. Immortalization of human CD8+ T cell clones by ectopic expression of telomerase reverse transcriptase. *J Immunol* 2000; **165**: 4239–45.

83. Mitchell MS. Cancer vaccines, a critical review: part I. *Curr Opin Investig Drugs* 2002; **3**: 140–9.

84. Gitlitz BJ, Belldegrun AS, Figlin RA. Vaccine and gene therapy of renal cell carcinoma. *Semin Urol Oncol* 2001; **19**: 141–7.

85. Townsend SE, Allison JP. Tumor rejection after direct costimulation of CD28+ T cells by B7-transfected melanoma cells. *Science* 1993; **259**: 368–70.

86. Dagarag MD, Effros RB. Ectopic telomerase expression prevents functional and phenotypic alterations associated with replicative senescence in virus-specific CD8 T cells. *Clin Immunol* (FOCIS meeting abstract book). 2003.

87. Cutolo M, Sulli A, Seriolo B, Accardo S, Masi AT. Estrogens, the immune response, and autoimmunity. *Clin Exp Rheumatol* 1995; **13**: 217–26.

88. Fox HS, Bond BL, Parslow TG. Estrogen regulates the IFN-gamma promoter. *J Immunol* 1991; **146**: 4362–7.

89. Pittet MJ, Zippelius A, Speiser DE, *et al.* Ex vivo IFN-gamma secretion by circulating CD8 T lymphocytes: implications of a novel approach for T cell monitoring in infectious and malignant diseases. *J Immunol* 2001; **166**: 7634–40.

90. Xu D, Erickson S, Szeps M, *et al.* Interferon alpha down-regulates telomerase reverse transcriptase and telomerase activity in human malignant and nonmalignant hematopoietic cells. *Blood* 2000; **96**: 4313–18.

91. Kyo S, Takakura M, Kanaya T, *et al.* Estrogen activates telomerase. *Cancer Res* 1999; **59**: 5917–21.

92. Fauce S, Jamieson BD, Chin A, *et al.* Telomerase activators increase HIV-specific CD8+ T cell function: a novel approach to prevent or delay immune exhaustion and progression to AIDS. In *Cold Spring Harbor Symposium on Telomeres and Telomerase 2005*, 197.

8

Qualitative changes of hematopoiesis

France Laurencet

Introduction

This chapter explores the association of aging and qualitative abnormalities of hematopoiesis. While incidence and prevalence of benign and malignant hematologic conditions increase with age, it is not clear whether quantitative or qualitative abnormalities of hematopoiesis underlie these changes. A definition of the mechanisms by which older individuals are more vulnerable to hematologic diseases is necessary for their prevention and treatment.

A common example of a hematologic abnormality in the elderly is unexplained anemia [1–8]. Controversy lingers over whether hematopoietic exhaustion, erythropoietic abnormalities due to genomic damage, increased vulnerability to environmental stress, or a combination of these factors may lead to anemia. Likewise, changes in lymphocytic phenotype, a decline in immune function (immunosenescence), and reduced chemotaxis and bactericidal capacity of neutrophils have been reported in older individuals [9–15]. Despite these changes, hematopoiesis appears adequate to maintain the homeostasis of the peripheral blood elements both in healthy elderly persons and in aging experimental animals, in the absence of hematopoietic stress [11–19].

Aging may be considered a condition of enhanced vulnerability to stress due to loss in functional reserve of multiple organ systems and simultaneous decline in personal and social resources [20–23]. Both environmental and genomic changes may conspire to restrict the functional reserve of the aged. Of the environmental changes the best defined is a condition of

progressive inflammation, associated with increased concentration of pro-inflammatory cytokines in the circulation, that may hamper immune response, alter the ratio of various subpopulations of B and T cells in the circulation, promote apoptosis of hematopoietic progenitors, and reduce their responsiveness to growth factors [9,24,25]. At the same time, genomic alteration of these progenitors may prevent their differentiation and also reduce their responsiveness to growth factors [23,26].

Environmental and genomic alterations appear to converge in the pathogenesis of myelodysplastic syndromes (MDS), a group of common hematologic malignancies after age 60, characterized by clonal hematopoiesis and dysmorphic changes in the bone marrow (Fig. 8.1) and peripheral blood (Fig. 8.2), due to increased proliferation, increased apoptosis, and reduced maturation (Fig. 8.3) [27]. In the following discussion we will explore the mechanisms of MDS as the best-established manifestation of qualitatively deficient hematopoiesis in the elderly.

Incidence of qualitative hematopoietic abnormalities

Most industrialized countries have experienced an increase in the elderly population due to more prolonged life expectancy and reduced birth rates [28]. In 2000, more than 20% of the people were older than 60 years, and this percentage is projected to increase in the foreseeable future [29,30]. Accumulation of oxidative damage to various organs and tissues is

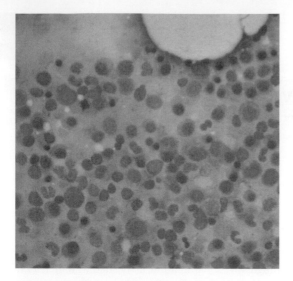

Figure 8.1 Aspirate smear showing hyperplastic and dysplastic features. *See color plate section.*

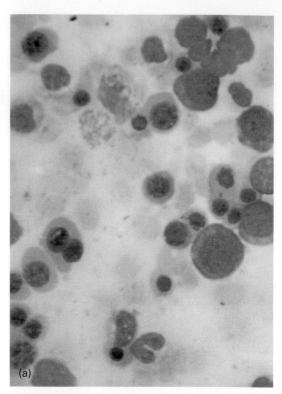

(a)

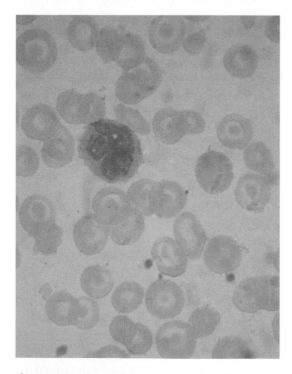

Figure 8.2 Blood smear from a patient with myelodysplastic syndrome, showing an abnormal monocyte. *See color plate section.*

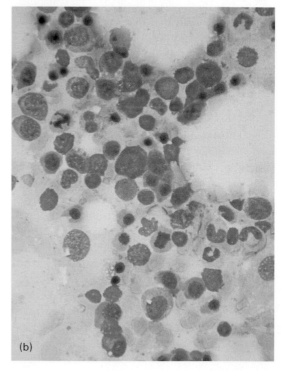

(b)

Figure 8.3 (a and b) Aspirate smear: myelodysplastic dyserythropoiesis and mitosis. *See color plate section.*

Table 8.1. Risk factors for MDS.

Age	
Environmental factors	
Drugs	INH, anti-tuberculosis drugs, chloramphenicol, Cycloserine, penicillamine, immunosuppressors
Toxins, drinking water	Ethanol, zinc, arsenic, cadmium, chloroform, halomethanes
Nutritional (malnutrition)	Copper and pyridoxine deficiency; phenols and hydroquinone
Occupational	Asbestos, paint products, benzene and organic solvents, ammonia, diesel fuel, or other petrochemicals
Chronic exposure	Pesticides, tobacco, agricultural chemicals, free radicals
Infections	Viruses
Genetic factors	Inherited mutations, karyotypic abnormalities, gene mutations, chromosomal instabilities, gender
Immunological factors	Lymphocytes and cytokines dysregulation
Others	Depression, obesity and endocrine status

partly responsible for age-related molecular changes [31,32]. In the hematopoietic system this damage may be manifested in minor dysplastic changes frequently observed in the bone marrow (BM) of elderly patients, the significance of which is still not understood. In particular it is not clear whether these changes signal the development of MDS or are benign and self-limiting [33–35]. The incidence of hematopoietic neoplasia [36–40] increases with age, but the incidence of MDS is difficult to define precisely, because of the heterogeneity of the disease. The more benign subtypes might be under-diagnosed and under-reported [39–41]. MDSs are rarely seen before the age of 50, and the median age is about 70 years [42,43]. The overall disease incidence is about 3–4 per 100 000, but this may rise to 20–30 per 100 000 in the over-70s and up to 89 per 100 000 in the over-80s [44,45].

In Germany the incidence of MDS appears to have increased in recent decades, though this finding is controversial [46–49]. In a French analysis of 100 patients in a geriatric hospital with a median age of 86 years, the prevalence of macrocytosis was 21% [50,51]. Some of these cases may certainly be ascribed to B_{12} and folate deficiency, or to drugs interfering with nuclear metabolisms. It is not farfetched to assume that at least in part these cases of macrocytosis represent early MDS or another form of qualitative hematopoietic defect.

In conclusion, the incidence and prevalence of MDS, one example of a qualitative defect of hematopoiesis,

increases with age. This finding suggests that the general prevalence of qualitative defects of hematopoiesis also increases with age. What is not yet clear is whether all forms of qualitative defects, and particularly macrocytosis, may end up as MDS.

Risk factors

The association of age and hematopoietic neoplasias may be accounted for by both constitutional and environmental factors [36,37,52]. The occurrence of qualitative abnormalities of hematopoiesis may represent a likely step toward neoplasia [27,39,40]. Risk factors for MDS are shown in Table 8.1.

Genetic factors

Many karyotypic abnormalities, inherited mutations, polymorphism of several genes, and chromosomal instabilities are associated with disturbance of normal hematopoiesis. Both gender and ethnic origin are important risk factors [53,54]. Of special interest in understanding the mechanism of hematopoietic abnormalities are the reports of familial MDS [55–61]. Inherited abnormalities as well as chromosomal instability may provide the initial genetic hit that predisposes to other hematopoietic abnormalities, including neoplasia [62,63]. Aging itself is associated with a number of genetic changes that may represent the initial steps predisposing to phenotypic abnormalities. The complex interaction of genetic and environmental factors is well illustrated by sideroblastic anemia, which is a heterogeneous group of disorders characterized by impaired heme synthesis and iron accumulation in the mitochondria [64]. The hereditary forms are primarily X-linked via a gene mutation or secondary to the deletion in the mitochondrial genome [65]. But there is also an acquired phenotype, induced by drugs, alcohol abuse, toxins, and deficiency in pyridoxine [65]. Interestingly, after removal of the toxic agents, morphological changes usually resolve, underlying the role of environmental factors in this setting.

Environmental factors

In older age, the role of constitutional factors is much less important than the role of acquired factors, related to infections, environment, immunosupression, and treatment. A pilot case–control study reviewed the association between environmental and occupational exposures and found a significant increase in MDS in subjects who had worked with ammonia, diesel fuel, or other petrochemicals [66]. Chronic exposure to tobacco, benzene, paints, petroleum products, and agricultural chemicals plays a major role in the alteration of hematopoiesis [38,41,67–69]. Phenols and hydroquinone produced by the gastrointestinal flora may also alter hematopoiesis [31,70]. Free radicals may damage various components of an organism and in particular DNA and mitochondria [71]. Elevated levels of tumor necrosis factor α (TNF-α) and other catabolic cytokines in the circulation of older individuals may induce DNA oxidative damage, hampering normal hematopoiesis [72].

Immunologic factors

Immunosenescence, characterized by involution of the thymus and diminished concentration and function of T cells, is associated with perturbations of the hematopoietic microenvironment and neoplasia [40,73,74]. This possibility is supported by the finding that patients with aplastic anemia (AA) treated with antithymocyte globulin have increased risk of subsequent MDS or acute myeloid leukemia (AML) [75]. It is also possible, however, that patients who recover from AA have pre-existing clonal abnormalities of hematopoietic progenitors [76–78].

Other factors

Hematopoietic abnormalities have also been associated with marital status, depression, pregnancies, modified endocrines status, and obesity [38,40,79–81].

History

A brief historical review may help to introduce the mechanisms of qualitative abnormalities and MDS. The major steps included the recognition of multipotential hematopoietic progenitors, the definition of ineffective erythropoiesis [82–86], and the discovery of clonality in hematopoietic malignancies [87–89]. In 1984, Lipschitz and colleagues showed an overall reduction in hematopoiesis in the anemic elderly [90]. This study demonstrated that the anemic elderly had reduced levels of committed macrophage/granulocyte progenitor cells (CFU-C) and erythroid and myeloid precursors, and that erythroid progenitors (CFU-E) were less responsive to erythropoietin (EPO). It was then established in the mouse model that basal hematopoiesis was not altered in aging, but that the reserve capacity was compromised when mice were submitted to stress [10,11,91]. During the last two decades there has been much progress in understanding the role of the immune system, pro-inflammatory cytokines [13], gene interactions [92], point mutations, and transcription factors [93,94]. These discoveries have enabled researchers to identify potential alterations in the hematopoietic steps associated with aging, and to define the mechanisms of dysplasia.

Dysplasia and hematologic characteristics

Dysplasia is characterized by qualitative defects in cells maturation and function. Dysplastic changes are often seen in the peripheral blood and are not specific [95,96]. A small number of dysplastic erythroid, granulocytic, or megakaryocytic cells can be seen in marrow specimens from normal individuals (Fig. 8.4a) [97]. Dysplastic features may be induced by viruses (HIV, parvovirus B19) [98,99], medications [100], nutritional deficiencies, alcohol, drugs, toxins, cancers [101], and chronic renal and liver diseases. All these conditions may be found in the older population, and should be investigated prior to diagnosing MDS [68,96,102–104]. This diagnosis should be confirmed by cytogenetics and immunophenotype [105–109].

Qualitative analysis of bone marrow of 54 healthy volunteers aged 60 years or more showed dysplastic changes in megakaryocytes in up to 89% of the cases, consisting of giant megakaryocytes, hypo- or non-lobulated megakaryocytes, macronormoblasts, and rarely reduced granulations in the myeloid lineage [33]. In addition, asynchrony in cellular development, abnormal mitosis, and nests of erythoblasts at the same stage of maturation may be observed. It is not clear whether these changes are always harbingers of MDS. In the peripheral blood dyserythropoiesis is manifested by anisocytosis, poikilocytosis, macrocytes, acanthocytes, and basophilic stippling [110], which also become more common with age. These abnormalities are particularly evident in MDS. Bone marrow often shows erythroid hyperplasia and dyserythropoietic abnormalities including nuclear budding, karryohexis, multinuclearity, and nuclear bridging (Fig. 8.3b) [95,111–113]. In sideroblastic anemias, the BM contains ring sideroblasts formed by the accumulation of iron within perinuclear mitochondria encircling the nucleus [67,112–116]. Dysgranulopoiesis may be prominent. Neutrophils show hypogranulations, dysgranulations, nucleus hyposegmentations (i.e., pseudo-Pelger–Huet anomalies) and sometimes nuclear hypersegmentation (Figs. 8.4b, 8.5). Secondary granules are often absent in myelocytes and more mature cells, and myeloperoxidase and alkaline phosphatase activities may be diminished, suggesting a diminished chemotaxis, phagocytosis, and bactericidal capacity [117–119]. Besides, some myeloid precursors stain with both specific

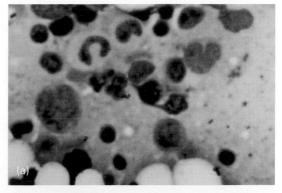

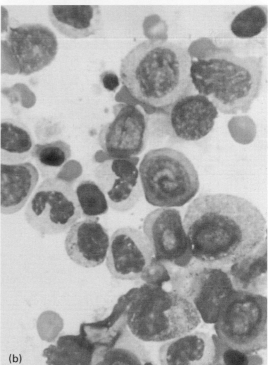

Figure 8.4 Dysgranulopoiesis. Aspirate smears from (a) a 48-year-old man with granule deficiency; (b) a 79-year-old man with bicytopenia and maturation defect in the granulopoiesis. *See color plate section.*

and non-specific esterases, suggesting infidelity between granulocytic and monocytic lineages in MDS [120]. Dysmegakaryopoiesis is manifested as thrombocytopenia resulting from maturation defect

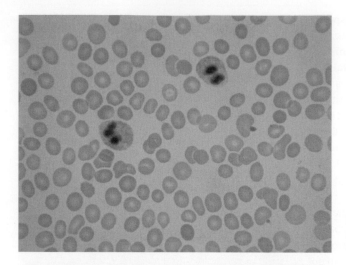

Figure 8.5 Blood smear from a patient with refractory cytopenia, showing two neutrophils with bilobed nuclei. *See color plate section.*

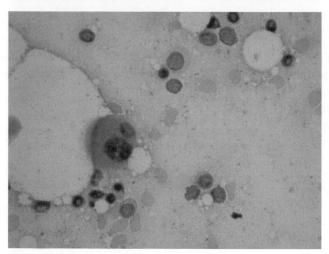

Figure 8.6 Dysplastic megakaryocyte: aspirate smear from a 77-year-old female with bicytopenia and thrombocytosis (5q– syndrome). *See color plate section.*

[121–123]. Secondary thrombocytosis may be associated with a particular cytogenetic alteration, the 5q-minus syndrome, or with sideroblastic anemia (Fig. 8.6) [124–125].

Qualitative changes in the healthy elderly

MDS is a frequent clonal disease with qualitative changes in the elderly, and some of the changes of MDS, such as macrocytosis, may be found in older individuals even without MDS [50,51,126,127]. It is

reasonable to ask then whether aging of the hematopoietic stem cells (HSCs) may be revealed by these changes, and what mechanisms lead to HSC aging. By age 70 and more, the hematopoietic cellularity of the iliac crest is diminished to about 30% in comparison to young subjects [128–130]. Williams *et al.* demonstrated in the mouse model that there were no age-related changes in basal hematopoiesis but that the marrow's reserve capacity was compromised in stress [10]. There is no conclusive evidence that the number of pluripotent HSCs declines with age, while the lifespan of peripheral blood elements does not appear shortened [131,132]. The self-renewal capacity of the HSCs appears well maintained in serial transfer experiments even at the end of an animal's lifespan [133–135], though clones of stem cells with reduced self-renewal capacity may appear. In this section we will explore the hematopoietic changes of aging, both described and potential.

The stem cell

While it is not established that the number of HSCs declines with age, qualitative changes appear likely and may affect their self-renewal potential [136]. Replication, stress, and aging may favor accumulation of mutations responsible for disordered hematopoiesis, MDS, or leukemia. Sharp *et al.* noted that BM cells from old mice manifest a more pronounced self-renewal and differentiation capacity than those of young animals [129]. De Haan *et al.* demonstrated that the HSC pool in unmanipulated mice continuously expands during the animal's lifetime, so that old mice have substantially more HSCs than young ones [137]. Harrison *et al.* suggested an accumulation of pluripotent progenitors with reduced self-replicative ability with age [91]. Different strains of mice have different lifespans and age at different rates [17,135,138–140], and it is not established which model, if any, most accurately reflects human aging [139–141]. The most primitive HSCs are mostly quiescent, residing in the G0 phase, and are then protected from depletion and exhaustion. In cases of increased demand, previously quiescent HSCs respond by entering proliferation and differentiation, which are regulated by extrinsic factors such as Flt3-ligand, Steel factor, and interleukin 11 (IL-11). These factors may be altered with aging [8,142]. With age, an increased proportion of HSCs may enter proliferation and become more susceptible to mutagenic environmental factors [8,16,140–145].

In-vitro cultures of hematopoietic tissues from healthy centenarians yield the same number of HSCs as cultures from younger individuals [21]. This system is unable to reflect the influence of hematopoietic stress, however. In these conditions, loss of sensitivity to growth factors and of self-renewal capacity may lead to delays and incomplete hematopoietic recovery [18, 21, 131,137,140,146–149]. There is evidence that the human HSC becomes more refractory to growth and differentiation factors and becomes incapable of producing lymphoid cells [135,150]. In addition to intrinsic abnormalities of the HSC, increased concentrations of cytokines, and abnormalities in growth factors and transcription factors, may underline these changes [139,142,151]. Since the cytokine network changes with age, the balance between the different cell lines might be disrupted (Fig. 8.7). Until now, the molecular mechanisms that regulate these age-related changes remain largely unknown [152]. An additional phenomenon that characterizes hematopoiesis in the elderly is clonal hematopoiesis. In older women this has been repeatedly demonstrated, utilizing as markers of clonality the enzymes encoded by genes in the X chromosomes [153–155].

The role of telomeres

Telomeres are the noncoding DNA sequences found at the ends of the chromosomes. Telomeres shorten as a function of age [156,157]. As a result, it is thought that critical genes at the ends of the chromosomes become either deleted or repressed, leading to senescence or death. Under normal physiologic conditions in vivo, even in old animals, the capacity of HSCs to replicate is not exhausted [158,159]. When telomere length and telomerase activity were measured in whole blood from individuals aged from 1 to 96 years, rapid telomere shortening was demonstrated in the first year of life, followed by a gradual slow decline [156]. This study suggests that the proliferative potential of HSCs is limited and decreases gradually with age [160], but that the hematopoietic reserves are adequate even at advanced age. Telomere length might represent the different injuries a person has suffered during his or her lifespan, and telomere shortening would be one of several factors that contribute to the onset of senescence in human cells [161]. Recent studies have provided important insights regarding the manner in which different stresses and stimuli activate the signaling pathways leading to senescence. Growing cells

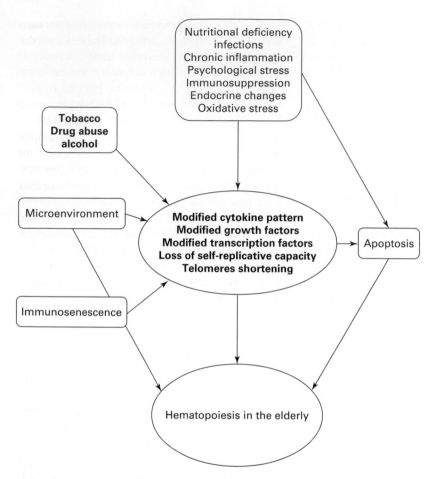

Figure 8.7 Effect of age on the natural history and pathogenesis of hematopoiesis.

might suffer from a combination of different physiologic stresses acting simultaneously. HSC transplantation studies have shown that telomeres in peripheral leukocytes from recipients were shorter than those from the donors, confirming that an increased replicative activity was associated with telomere shortening. Accelerated telomere shortening has also been demonstrated after exposure of HSCs to oxidative stress [162–165]. The signaling pathways activated by these stresses involve tumor-suppressor proteins – p53 and Rb – whose combined levels

of activity determine whether cells enter senescence [166]. Even emotional stress has been associated with accelerated telomere erosion in peripheral mononuclear cells from healthy women [167]. The importance of gender was revealed by a recent report demonstrating that women have longer telomeres than men, which implies a lower rate of telomere attrition [153]. Telomeric senescence itself seems unlikely to be solely responsible for HSC depletion, since mean telomere length, even in the ninth decade of life, remains well maintained [153,160,162,168,169].

The role of apoptosis

Apoptosis is programmed cell death leading to the elimination of cells that have exhausted their function [170]. Apoptosis is regulated by a complex network of cytokines, genes, enzymes, and membrane receptors. As myeloid precursors differentiate, they develop receptors for apoptogenic factors resulting in ligand-induced apoptosis and death [171]. p53, Bcl-2/Bax, caspases, granzyme, and Fas are some of the regulators of apoptosis [170]. Dysregulated cytokine production, including IL-1β, TNF-α, and interferon gamma (IFN-γ) may have a pro-apoptotic effect. A correlation between IL-1β production by marrow cells and the degree of apoptosis has been described [172]. Declining bone-marrow cellularity with aging might be ascribed partly to the increased apoptosis, modified cytokines, and alterations of the microenvironment [23,146].

Nutritional deficiencies may also lead to apoptosis. For example, human proerythroblasts undergo apoptosis in vitro in case of folate deficiency [172–174].

Growth and transcription factors

The production of growth factors is roughly maintained although modified in basal conditions in the aged mouse, but the sensitivity of HSC to growth factors is diminished [175]. After stimulation of stromal cultures, the production of GM-CSF and IL-3 decreases and that of stem cell factor increased in aging marrow [18]. Sex, parity, menopausal status, and lipid profile influence cytokine production [81,176]. Pro-inflammatory cytokines, whose level increases with age in the circulation, seem to inhibit erythropoiesis [177]. Altered response to growth factors in vivo is suggested by increased susceptibility to infection and more prolonged time to recovery from an infection in the aged [25]. Transcription factors have emerged as important in the differentiation process in hematopoiesis. It has been demonstrated that, depending on which of the members of the GATA family was lacking, precursors were not able to expand normally, or to differentiate in more mature cells. Other transcription factors such as NF-κB, KF-E2, PU.1, and C/EBP play a role in the differentiation process [151,177–180].

Microenvironment, stroma, and dendritic cells

Stromal cells are important sources of various growth and inhibitory factors. Senescent stromal cells might be unable to maintain a self-renewal capacity. TGF-β activity, which inhibits proliferation, declines [181]. Dendritic cells (DC) are the most powerful antigen-presenting cells able to activate T cells and partially regulate the adaptive and innate immune system. Age does not seem to affect the function of DC in healthy older individuals [130], but it is compromised in the frail elderly [182]. Another cause of altered stroma is cancer, whose prevalence increases with age [101].

B cells and T cells

Numerous deficiencies in the immune response in elderly mice and humans have been documented [8], and are discussed in other chapters. Immunosenescence corresponds to a state of dysregulated immune function that contributes to infections, cancer, and autoimmunity [183,184]. Well-defined changes include reduced proliferation of T cells, which may be restored by appropriate stimuli [185–187]; alteration in T-cell subsets such as reduction in concentration of CD4 cells and increased concentration of NK cells in centenarians [188,189], restricted ability to secrete new immunoglobulins, decreased production of IL-2 [23], and increased production of IFN especially after age 100 [188]. Studies in individuals aged 65 and older, including centenarians, suggest that the preservation of NK-cell function correlates with good health and autonomy [189,190].

Macrophages

The number of blood monocytes in elderly and young subjects appears to be very similar. However, there is a significant decrease in macrophage precursors as well as macrophages in the marrow of the elderly [146]. Macrophages have been implicated in unresponsiveness of aged mice to vaccine [191]. The increased incidence of infections suggests a possible defect in epithelial cells and in macrophage function. Macrophage changes include diminished production of reactive oxygen and nitrogen intermediates, essential for intracellular killing of micro-organisms and tumor lysis. Besides, macrophages secrete a wide range of cytokines, chemokines, growth factors, and enzymes in response to pathogens. Their dysregulation may contribute to the altered response.

Neutrophils

One of the most important cell components of the immune response is the neutrophil [192]. During differentiation, myeloblasts give rise to promyelocytes and acquire the primary azurophil granules containing the myeloperoxidase, and then evolve to myelocytes with the appearance of secondary granules [193]. Baseline neutrophil count in young and old persons is the same [174,194], but the phagocytic function of neutrophils (PMNs) is reduced in the aged [11,14,15,146,195]. To combat bacterial and fungal infections, functional specific receptors for cytokines such as GM-CSF, IL-8, and formyl-methionyl-leucyl-phenylalanine (FMLP) are needed. Fulop and colleagues demonstrated a significant age-related decrease in chemotaxis towards FMLP and a decrease in free radical production stimulated by FLMP [183]. Other functions that change with age include superoxide anion production, enzyme release, and apoptosis [15,183,188,194–196]. A decline in neutrophil antioxidant shield leads to increased cell oxidative load, which may increase the rate of apoptosis and cell loss [197]. This problem may be aggravated by a protein-free diet in aging mice [198]. Aged neutrophils showed a diminished capacity to respond to pro-inflammatory mediators, such as G-CSF and GM-CSF [174,183]. The expression of CD95, which correlates with the concentration of Fas, does not change with aging, indicating that older neutrophils are not more susceptible to apoptosis through the Fas pathway [188,199–201].

Qualitative defects in hematopoiesis: myelodysplasia

Ineffective hematopoiesis results from a complex interaction between hematopoietic progenitors and the microenvironment (Fig. 8.8). Myelodysplastic progenitors display deficient growth of multipotent and primitive progenitors, retarded maturation capacity, and impaired responsiveness to growth factors resulting in premature apoptotic death of progenitors and of their maturing progeny [16]. Furthermore, cells released in the peripheral blood have both functional and morphological abnormalities [170–202]. A number of factors already described may be responsible for the genomic damage to the HSCs [31,203]. With time, additional mutations can occur, driving to a clone that gives origin to acute leukemia [204,205]. Common genomic changes include hypermethylation [206], and increased concentration of genes that encode Ras, p53, PDGF, and CSF-1 receptors [103,207].

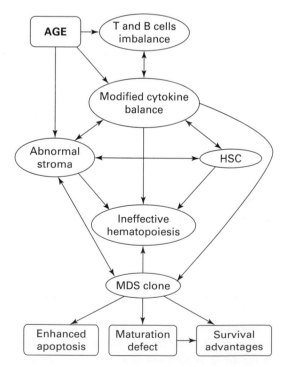

Figure 8.8 Interactions in the pathogenesis of MDS in the elderly.

Both plasma and bone marrow of patients with MDS produce increased amounts of inflammatory cytokines such as TNF-α and IL-1β. These cytokines promote apoptosis of primitive and committed hematopoietic progenitors [95], and increased concentration of vascular endothelial growth factor (VEGF).

Clonality and cytogenetic abnormalities

MDSs are clonal disorders [208]. The selective clonal advantage appears to derive from genetic mutations by which dysplastic cells become independent from normal growth constraints. The natural disease course is primarily determined by the type of progenitors that are clonally mutated and by the nature of clonal mutations [209–211]. The best-identified elements involved in MDS are CD34+ cells [212]. Some studies suggest that a mycloid-lymphoid HSC might be the cell from which the disease initiates [209,213], but lymphoid elements do not appear to be involved in MDS [214–217]. This discrepancy may be explained in several ways. One is that MDSs originate on a myeloid-only progenitor, the other that lymphocytes in the circulation have originated before the emergence of MDS [218]. Also, it is possible that circulating lymphocytes originate from persisting normal progenitors, while those derived from the mutated HSCs undergo earlier apoptosis [216]. In a recent study, the percentage of clonal granulocytes and CD14+ cells increased by four times between patients with early MDS and those with refractory cytopenia with multilineage dysplasia (RCMD). This may reflect the multistep pathogenesis of MDS cells [219]. So an age-related acquired or inherent genetic instability within the myelodysplastic clone may predispose to additional mutations and progression [209,220–224]. Clonal cytogenetic abnormalities are detectable in 20–60% of MDS and in up to 80% of patients with secondary or treatment-induced MDS [225,226]. The most frequent abnormalities are partial or complete loss of a chromosome (del(5q), -7, del(20q), and $-Y$) [227–231]. Spontaneous chromosomal instability and interstrand crosslink damage may contribute to the functional decline of the hematopoietic system associated with aging [232,233]. There is also evidence that DNA repair defects may be involved in the progression of MDS.

The 5q-minus syndrome consists of refractory anemia (RA), thrombocytosis, and abnormal megakaryocyte morphology with a relatively good prognosis [234–237]. The deleted region of chromosome 5 contains the genes for several hematopoietic growth factors and is of particular interest regarding the maturation defect in MDS. IL-3, IL-4, IL-5, IL-9, GM-CSF, the M-CSF receptor, and interferon regulatory factor 1 (IRF1) involved in signal transduction, are located in this region [238]. Although the pathogenic mechanism underlying this deletion is still not understood, this acquired mutation is present in multipotent progenitor cells giving rise to both erythroid and granulocytic lineages [208,212,214,236,237,239].

Loss of heterozygosity is noted on chromosomes 1 and 18, suggesting that these chromosomes may contain tumor suppressor genes. The del(7q) abnormality includes 7q22, containing genes involved in DNA repair [240]. The 17p syndrome is associated with dysgranulopoiesis and frequent loss of p53 [241]. Finally, when detailed microsatellite allelotypes are examined in MDS patients, a high percentage of loss of heterozygosity is identified on chromosomes 5q, 7q, 17p, or 20q. Progression to AML, however, may be influenced by epigenetic events. For example, silencing methylation of the proto-oncogene p15^{INK4b}, which is detected in more than 70% of patients experiencing AML evolution, may allow leukemic cells to escape inhibitory signals [242,243]. DNA aneuploidy and the presence of mutations affecting Ras or p53 may also influence the outcome [244–246]. In conclusion, cytogenetic and molecular studies support the stepwise accumulation of genomic damage in the hematopoietic progenitor compartment as the origin of the phenotypic presentation and natural course of MDS.

Apoptosis in MDS

Since the first demonstration, published in 1992, numerous studies have confirmed the high percentage of apoptotic cells in MDS [247–252]. Increased production of cytokines by the stroma, autoreactive T cells, and altered interaction between hematopoietic progenitors and extracellular matrix may promote apoptosis [209]. Typical Pelger–Huet-type cells appear to be apoptotic granulocytes [202,249]. But is apoptosis related to the molecular pathogenesis of MDS, or is it merely a logical consequence of progressive damage to genes essential for cell proliferation and survival? Apoptosis can also be considered as a rescue or suicide mechanism to avoid the acquisition of further genomic damage. The apoptotic rate is higher in RA, RA with ringed sideroblasts (RARS), and RA with excess blasts (RAEB), with a progressive decline when the disease acquires a more leukemic phenotype [209]. The level of apoptosis-related oncoproteins c-Myc (enhancer) and Bcl-2 (inhibitor) expressed within CD34+/− marrow cells of MDS patients reveals an imbalance between cell death (e.g., c-Myc) and cell survival (e.g., Bcl-2) that may contribute to the ineffective hematopoiesis in this disorder [250–254]. Defects in cytokine receptors or receptor-mediated intracellular signaling pathways have also been mentioned. There is also evidence that MDS marrow stroma cells may be abnormally sensitive to apoptosis [255]. The role of dysregulated cytokines such as IL-1β, TNF-α, TNF-related apoptosis-inducing ligand (TRAIL), TGF-β and IFN-γ is postulated as a pro-apototic event, and a correlation between IL-1β production and the degree of apoptosis has been reported [172,252]. Altered expression of CD95/FasL appears also to be of relevance in the dysregulation of hematopoiesis in MDS since Fas expression and TNF-α are higher in RA than in other MDS and diminish during leukemic transformation [256,257]. Rigolin *et al.* demonstrated that, in MDS, non-clonal progenitors are more prone to respond to rHuEpo and G-CSF [258]. Thus, growth-promoting cytokines such as EPO, IL-3, IL-6, and TPO, which are usually increased in MDS patients, may try to counterbalance the pro-apototic stimuli.

The role of the immune system

One mechanism underlying the marrow failure in MDS is immunologic attack on the HSCs, which may also be found in aplastic anemia and paroxysmal nocturnal hemoglobinuria (PNH). T lymphocytes may inhibit hematopoiesis in MDS [212]. Decrease of natural killer cells is routinely seen in MDS, but CD8

are slightly increased [73,259,260]. Immunoglobulin production may be decreased or modified, and monoclonal gammopathy is found in more than 10% of cases [261–263], predominantly in chronic myelomonocytic leukemia (CMML).

Angiogenic factors

Angiogenic factors play a crucial role in proliferation, survival, and mobility of the cells, and in the progression of MDS [264]. The in-vitro generation of microvessels is increased in RA, RARS, and RAEB in comparison with controls. The occurrence of large islands, formed by clusters of endothelial cells, unable to generate microcapillaries is also reported [265]. Angiogenic receptors are expressed on subsets of primary hematopoietic cells as well as leukemic cells. This suggests that chronic dysregulation of angiogenic factors may alter the microenvironment, dislocating marrow HSCs, modifying proliferation and differentiation in varying degrees, contributing to the qualitative defect of hematologic disorders [266–268]. Furthermore, secretion of cytokines and growth factors modulates angiogenesis in the marrow, leading to pathological increase of new vessels and sustenance of the clonal population [265,269].

The role of the microenvironment

Whether the microenvironment is normal in MDS has been a subject of debate [270]. An increased apoptotic rate in MDS stromal-cell culture [212] suggests dysregulation of the stroma. Mesenchymal SCs (MSCs) are key components of the hematopoietic microenvironment. In terms of morphology, as well as in the expression of certain cell markers, no differences have been found between MSCs from MDS patients and those derived from normal marrow. But in some MDS patients, MSCs and hematopoietic cells showed cytogenetic abnormalities suggesting that MSCs may also undergo clonal transformation [271]. The microenvironment regulates progenitor growth and survival by contact and via soluble factors. Misplaced megakaryocytes release pro-fibrotic factors, including platelet-derived growth factors and TGF-β, that modify the production of cytokines by the stroma [272]. Monocytes from MDS patients showed low potential to differentiate into dendritic cells, and exhibited a reduced endocytic capacity [273] and diminished response to TNF-α.

The role of *RB, TP53* and *RAS*

TP53 and *RB* are involved in the regulation of cell-cycle progression, and their inactivation leads to prolonged cellular lifespan. *RB* gene inactivation is a very rare event in MDS. *TP53* mutation, frequently found in the elderly, occurs in less than 10% of MDS [274], and it is more frequently associated with progression or transformation, as it is for *RAS* abnormality [241,275,276]. *TP53* mutations are significantly associated with 5q deletion, and in these situations confer a worse prognosis [244,277–281]. *RAS* mutation is the molecular abnormality most often found in MDS, followed by *p15* gene hypermethylation and *FLT3* duplications [229,282]. None of these abnormalities is specific for MDS. Besides, tumor-suppressor genes, growth-regulatory genes, and adhesion molecules are often silenced in hematopoietic malignancies by DNA hypermethylation [283]. They have been implicated in the lack of differentiation [284]. Hypermethylation of *p15* is almost constant in MDS, particularly in progression [285], and has been associated with deletion or loss of chromosome 7q. It might contribute to defective megakaryopoiesis in MDS [277,286]. Hypermethylation of the death-associated protein kinase (DAP-kinase) has been associated with myelodysplastic changes in the BM [287]. Agents preventing DNA methylation are associated with improved hematopoiesis, demonstrating indirectly the role of transcription factors in MDS [284,288–290].

Oxidative damage and mitochondrial mutations

Increased genomic damage can also be related to a reduction in the capacity to metabolize genotoxins and oxidants, facilitating the development of MDS [209]. Malfunction of the mitochondrial respiratory chain attributable to mutations of mitochondrial DNA to which aged individuals are more vulnerable has also

been described, and leads to intramitochondrial accumulation of ferric iron (Fe^{3+}) that can not be used for the last step on heme synthesis, contributing to ringed sideroblasts. Several mechanisms are apparently involved in this abnormal mitochondrial iron deposition: defects in enzymes or cofactors of the heme synthetic pathway, defects in the transport or processing of iron before it is incorporated into heme, altered mitochondria. Defective reduction of Fe^{3+} to ferrous iron (Fe^{2+}), which is necessary before incorporation into heme, with abnormal accumulation of Fe^{3+}, may damage mitochondria via free-radical formation [291,292].

Telomeres

The disruption of telomeric structure or its erosion may stimulate cell-cycle arrest or aberrant chromosomal end joinings [293]. Activation of telomerase may induce cell survival. To permit immortalization, a second event is necessary such as mutation of *TP53* or *RB*. Thus, it might well be that telomeres have two different roles, one in the early stage of cell transformation, during which telomere attrition limits cell proliferation and suppresses malignant transformation by limiting cell life, and a later stage during which too many suppressions have led to genomic instability that drives chromosome joining and leukemic transformation. This correlates with the fact that most MDSs show weak telomere fluorescence, corresponding to short telomeres [123], and shortened telomeres and high telomerase activity almost always correlate with disease severity in MDS [294–297].

A model

Leukemia is composed of cells with proliferative and survival advantages, and also diminished or poor differentiation, as compared to normal [298]. They are associated with chromosomal translocations, which juxtapose two unrelated genes, and their products, which lead to aberrant expression or function of a fusion protein. Studies in AML indicate that most translocations involve transcription factors or components of the transcriptional activation complex [298]. Activation of certain transcription factors leads to differentiation blockade. Then a second mutation related to a tyrosine kinase activation leads to limitless growth and survival, corresponding to leukemia. This second event may be age-related, and may also account for qualitative changes in hematopoiesis.

Conclusions

Aging is associated with a number of qualitative changes in hematopoiesis, including decreased self-replicative ability of HSCs, reduced responsiveness of these elements to growth factor, reduced activity of neutrophils, monocytes, dendritic cells, and some lymphocyte subsets. Anemia and macrocytosis are other common manifestations of these qualitative changes.

The qualitative changes of hematopoiesis may be related to alteration of the genome from environmental substances and oxidative stress, disruption of the hematopoietic microenvironment, and increased concentration of catabolic cytokines.

It is not clear whether all qualitative abnormalities do indeed preannounce MDS. Nonetheless, MDS represents a useful model to interpret the development and progression of hematopoietic changes. Under age-related conditions a number of genomic alterations occur. These alterations may lead to apoptosis or to malignancy. Telomeres may play a central role in this process, in that progressive shortening of telomeres may lead to cell death, and later, as a consequence of genetic instability, may lead to chromosome joining and immortalization. This model may explain the development and progression of MDS, as well as the reason why certain abnormalities do not progress to MDS, and it may be used as a framework of reference in the interpretation of other hematopoietic changes of aging.

REFERENCES

1. Thomas JH. Anaemia in the elderly. *Br Med J* 1973; **4**: 288–90.
2. Nilsson-Ehle H, Jagenburg R, Landahl S, Svanborg A. Blood haemoglobin declines in the elderly: implications for reference intervals from age 70 to 88. *Eur J Haematol* 2000; **65**: 297–305.
3. Cohen HJ. Anemia in the elderly: clinical impact and practical diagnosis. *J Am Geriatr Soc* 2003; **51** (3): S1.
4. Balducci L. Epidemiology of anemia in the elderly: information on diagnosis evaluation. *J Am Geriatr Soc* 2003; **51** (3): S2–S9.
5. Izaks GJ, Westendorp RG, Knook DL. The definition of anemia in older persons. *JAMA* 1999; **281**: 1714–17.
6. Wieczorowska-Tobis K, Niemir Z, Mossakowska M, Klich-Raczka A, Zyczkowska J. Anemia in centenarians. *J Am Geriatr Soc* 2002; **50**: 1311–13.
7. Ehlers WB. Biological interactions of ageing and anemia: a focus on cytokine. *J Am Geriatr Soc* 2003; **51** (3): S18–S21.
8. Fuller J. Hematopoietic stem cells and aging. *Sci Aging Knowledge Environ* 2002; **2002** (25): pe11–14.
9. Rossi MI, Yokota T, Medina Kl, Garrett KP, Comp PC, Schipul AH Jr, Kincade PW. B lymphopoiesis is active throughout human life, but there are developmental age-related changes. *Blood* 2003; **101**: 576–84.
10. Williams LH, Udupa KB. Lipschitz D. Evaluation of the effect of age on hematopoiesis in the C57BL/6 mouse. *Exp Hematol* 1986; **14**: 827–32.
11. Berkahn L, Keating A. Current clinical practice: hematopoiesis in the elderly. *Hematology* 2004; **9**: 159–63.
12. Boogaerts MA, Nelissen V, Roelant C, Goossens W. Blood neutrophil function in primary myelodysplastic syndromes. *Br J Haematol* 1983; **55**: 217–27.
13. Effros R. Ageing and the immune system. *Novartis Found Symp* 2001; **235**: 130–9.
14. Quaglino D, Ginaldi L, Furia N, De Martinis, M. The effect of age on hemopoiesis. *Aging Clin Exp Res* 1996; **8**: 1–12.
15. Fulop T, Foris G, Worum I, Paragh G, Leovey A. Age related variations of some polymorphonuclear leukocyte functions. *Mech Ageing Dev* 1985; **29**: 1–8.
16. Rothstein G. Disordered hematopoiesis and myelodysplasia in the elderly. *J Am Geriatr Soc* 2003; **51** (3): S22–S26.
17. Globerson A. Mini-review: hematopoietic stem cells and aging. *Exp Gerontol* 1999; **34**: 137–46.
18. Bagnara GP, Strippoli P, Bonifazi F, *et al.* Hemopoiesis in healthy old people and centenarians: well-maintained responsiveness of CD34+ cells to hemopoietic growth factors and remodelling of cytokine network. *J Gerontol A Biol Sci Med Sci* 2000; **55** (2): B61–B66.
19. Harrison, DE. Long-term erythropoietic repopulating ability of old, young and fetal stem cells. *J Exp Med* 1983; **157**: 1496–504.

20. Lipschitz D. Medical and functional consequences of anemia in the elderly. *J Am Geriatr Soc* 2003; **51** (3): S10–S13.

21. Balducci L, Hardy CL, Lyman GH. Hematopoietic growth factors in the older cancer patient. *Curr Opin Hematol* 2001; **8**: 170–87.

22. Seidman SN. Testosterone deficiency and mood in aging men: pathogenic and therapeutic interactions. *World J Biol Psychiatry* 2003; **4**: 14–20.

23. Baraldi-Junkins CA, Beck AC, Rothstein G. Hematopoiesis and cytokines: relevance to cancer and ageing. *Hematol Oncol Clin North Am* 2000; **14**: 45–61.

24. Krabbe KS, Pedersen M, Bruunsgaard H. Inflammatory mediators in the elderly. *Exp Gerontol* 2004; **39**: 687–99.

25. Bruunsgaard H, Pedersen M, Pedersen BK. Aging and proinflammatory cytokines. *Curr Opin Hematol* 2001; **8**: 131–6.

26. Gilliland DG, Dunbar CE. Myelodysplastic syndromes. In Handin RI, Lux SE, Stossel TP, eds, *Blood: Principles and Practice of Hematology*, 2nd edn (Philadelphia, PA: Lippincott Williams & Wilkins, 2003), 334–77.

27. Edelman AS, Fahri DC. Myelodysplastic syndromes. In Farhi DC, Chiling Chai C, Edelman AS, Parveen T, Thi Vo TL. *Pathology of Bone Marrow and Blood Cells* (Philadelphia, PA: Lippincott Williams & Wilkins, 2004), 241–64.

28. United Nations. *World Population Prospects. Volume II: Sex and Age* (New York, NY: United Nations, 1998).

29. Larkin M, Butler R. Championing a healthy view of ageing. *Lancet* 2001; **357**: 48–9.

30. Buckley BM. Healthy ageing: ageing safety. *Eur Heart J* 2001; **3** (Suppl N): N6–N10.

31. Golden TR, Hinerfeld DA, Melov S. Oxidative stress and aging: beyond correlation. *Aging Cell* 2002; **1**: 117–23.

32. Bell RB, Van Zant G. Stem cells, aging, and cancer: inevitabilities and outcomes. *Oncogene* 2004; **23**: 7290–6.

33. Girodon F, Favre B, Carli PM, *et al.* Minor dysplastic changes are frequently observed in the bone marrow aspirate in elderly patients without haematological disease. *Clin Lab Haematol* 2001; **23**: 297–300.

34. Malaguarnera M, Di Fazio I, Vinci E, *et al.* Haematologic pattern in healthy subjects. *Panminerva Med* 1999; **41**: 227–31.

35. Fernandez-Ferrero S, Ramos F. Dyshaemopoietic bone marrow features in healthy subjects are related to age. *Leuk Res* 2001; **25**: 187–9.

36. Nagura E, Minami S, Nagara K, *et al.* Acute myeloid leukemia in the elderly: 159 Nagoya case studies. Nagoya Cooperative Study Group for Elderly Leukemia. *Nagoya J Med Sci* 1999; **62**: 135–44.

37. Rossi G, Pelizzari AM, Bellotti D, Tonelli M, Barlati S. Cytogenetic analogy between myelodysplastic syndrome and acute myeloid leukemia of elderly patients. *Leukemia* 2000; **14**: 636–41.

38. Farhi DC, Chiling Chai C, Edelman AS, Parveen T, Thi Vo TL. Risk factors for hematopoietic neoplasia. In Farhi DC, Chiling Chai C, Edelman AS, Parveen T, Thi Vo TL. *Pathology of Bone Marrow and Blood Cells* (Philadelphia, PA: Lippincott Williams & Wilkins, 2004), 189–200.

39. Pautas E, Gaillard M, Chambon-Pautas C, Siguret V, Andreux JP, Gaussem P. Les syndromes myélodysplasiques: diagnostics et prise en charge des patients de plus de 70 ans. *La Presse Médiale* 1999; **28**: 1771–8.

40. Linton PJ, Dorshkind K. Age-related changes in lymphocyte development and function. *Nat Immunol* 2004; **5**: 133–9.

41. Steensma DP, Tefferi A. The myelodysplastic syndromes: a perspective and review highlighting current controversies. *Leuk Res* 2003; **27**: 95–120.

42. Bowen D, Culligan D, Jowitt S, *et al.* Guidelines for the diagnosis and the therapy of adult myelodysplastic syndromes. *Br J Hematol* 2003; **120**: 187–200.

43. Jaffé ES, Harris NL, Stein H, Vardiman JW. *WHO Classification of Tumours: Pathology and Genetics of Tumours of Haematopoietic and Lymphoid Tissues* (Lyon: IARC Press, 2001), 45–73.

44. Saba HI. Myelodysplastic syndromes in the elderly. *Cancer Control* 2001; **8**: 79–102.

45. Hamblin TJ, Oscier DG. The myelodysplastic syndrome: a practical guide. *Hematol Oncol* 1987; **5**: 19–34.

46. Aul C, Gattermann N, Schneider W. Age-related incidence and other epidemiological aspects of myelodysplastic syndromes. *Br J Haematol* 1992; **82**: 358–67.

47. Germing U, Strupp C, Kundgen A, *et al.* No increase in age-specific incidence of myelodysplastic syndromes. *Haematologica* 2004; **89**: 905–10.

48. Williamson PJ, Kruger AR, Reynolds PJ, Hamblin TJ, Oscier DG. Establishing the incidence of myelodysplastic syndromes. *Br J Haematol* 1994; **87**: 743–5.

49. Radlund A, Thiede T, Hansen S, Carison M, Engquist L. Incidence of myelodysplastic syndromes in a Swedish population. *Eur J Haematol* 1995; **54**: 153–6.

50. Anttila P, Ihalainen J, Salo A, Heiskanen M, Juvonen E, Palotie A. Idiopathic macrocytic anaemia in the aged: molecular and cytogenetic findings. *Br J Haematol* 1995; **90**: 797–803.

51. Dewulf G, Gouin I, Pautas E, *et al.* Syndromes myélo-dysplasiques diagnostiqués dans un hôpital géri-atrique: profil cytologique de 100 patients. *Ann Biol Clin* 2004; **62**: 197–202.

52. Lichtman MA, Rowe JM. The relationship of patient age to the pathobiology of the clonal myeloid diseases. *Semin Oncol* 2004; **31**: 185–97.

53. Gilbert HS. Familial myeloproliferative disease. *Bailleres Clin Haematol* 1998; **11**: 849–58.

54. Brubaker LH, Wasserman LR, Goldberg JD, *et al.* Increased prevalence of polycythemia vera in parents of patients on polycythemia vera study group proto-cols. *Am J Hematol* 1984; **16**: 367–73.

55. Mandla SG, Goobie S, Kumar RT, *et al.* Genetic analy-sis of familial myelodysplastic syndrome: absence of linkage to chromosomes 5q31 and 7q22. *Cancer Genet Cytogenet* 1998; **105**: 113–18.

56. Paul B, Reid MM, Davison EV, Abela M, Hamilton PJ. Familial myelodysplasia: progressive disease associ-ated with emergence of monosomy 7. *Br J Haematol* 1987; **65**: 321–3.

57. Li FP, Marchetto DJ, Vawter GF. Acute leukemia and preleukemia in eight males in a family: an X-linked dis-order? *Am J Hematol* 1979; **6**: 61–9.

58. Palmer CG, Heerema NA, Greist A, Tricot G, Hoffman R. Cytogenetic findings in siblings with a myelodysplastic syndrome. *Cancer Genet Cytogenet* 1987; **27**: 241–9.

59. Shannon KM, Turhan AG, Chang SS, *et al.* Familial bone marrow monosomy 7: evidence that the predisposing locus is not on the long arm of chromosome 7. *J Clin Invest* 1989; **84**: 984–7.

60. Marsden K, Challis D, Kimber R. Familial myelodys-plastic syndromes with onset late in life. *Am J Hematol* 1995; **49**: 153–6.

61. Mintzer D, Bagg A. Clinical syndromes of transforma-tion in clonal hematologic disorders. *Am J Med* 2001; **111**: 480–8.

62. Kumar T, Mandla SG, Greer WL. Familial myelodys-plastic syndromes with early age of onset. *Am J Hematol* 2000; **64**: 53–8.

63. Horwitz M, Goode EL, Jarvick GP. Anticipation in famil-ial leukemia. *Am J Hum Genet* 1996; **10**: 669–74.

64. Koc S, Harris JW. Sideroblastic anemias: variations on imprecision in diagnostic criteria, proposal for an extended classification of sideroblastic anemias. *Am J Hematol* 1998; **57**: 1–6.

65. Alcindor T, Bridges KR. Sideroblastic anemias. *Br J Haematol* 2002; **116**: 733–43.

66. Farrow A, Jacobs A, West RR. Myelodysplasia, chemical exposure, and other environmental factors. *Leukemia* 1989; **3**: 33–5.

67. Van Den Berghe H, Louwagie A, Broeckaert-Van Orshoven A, David G, Verwilghen R. Chromosome analysis in two unusual malignant blood disorders presumably induced by benzene. *Blood* 1979; **53**: 558–66.

68. Nisse C, Haguenoer LM, Grandbastein B, *et al.* Occupational and environmental risk factors of the myelodysplastic syndromes in the north of France. *Br J Haematol* 2001; **112**: 927–35.

69. Chang G, Orav EJ, McNamara T, Tong MY, Antin JH. Depression, cigarette smoking and hematopoietic stem cell transplantation outcome. *Cancer* 2004; **101**: 782–9.

70. McDonald TA, Holland NT, Skibola C, Duramas P, Smith MT. Hypothesis: phenol and hydroquinone derived mainly from diet and gastrointestinal flora activity are causal factors in leukemia. *Leukemia* 2001; **15**: 10–20.

71. Maugeri D, Santangelo A, Bonanno MR, *et al.* Oxidative stress and aging: studies on an East-Sicilian, ultraocta-genarian population living in institutes or at home. *Arch Gerontol Geriatr Suppl* 2004; **9**: 271–7.

72. Peddie CM, Wolf CR, McLellan LI, Collins AR, Bowen DT. Oxidative DNA damage in CD34+ myelo-dysplastic cells is associated with intracellular redox changes and elevated plasma tumor necrosis factor-alpha concentration. *Br J Haematol* 1997; **99**: 625–31.

73. Copplestone JA, Mufti GJ, Hamblin TJ, Oscier DG. Immunological abnormalities in myelodysplastic syn-dromes. *Br J Haematol* 1986; **63**: 149–59.

74. Greenberg BR, Miller C, Cardiff RD, MacKenzie MR, Walling P. Concurrent development of preleukaemic, lymphoproliferative and plasma cell disorders. *Br J Haematol* 1983; **53**: 125–33.

75. Socie G, Rosenfeld S, Frickhofen N, Gluckman E, Tichelli A. Late clonal diseases of treated aplastic ane-mia. *Semin Hematol* 2000; **37**: 91–101.

76. Young NS. The problem of clonality in aplastic ane-mia: Dr Dameshek's riddle, restated. *Blood* 1992; **79**: 1385–92.

77. Alter BP, Greene MH, Velazquez I, Rosenberg PS. Cancer in Fanconi anemia. *Blood* 2003; **101**: 2072.

78. Maciejewski JP, Risitano A. Hematopoietic stem cells in aplastic anemia. *Arch Med Res* 2003; **34**: 520–7.

79. Estey E, Thall P, Kantarjian H, Pierce S, Kornblau S, Keating M. Association between increased body mass

index and a diagnosis of acute promyelocytic leukaemia in patients with acute myeloid leukemia. *Leukemia*
1997; **11**: 1661–4.

80. Kiecolt-Glaser JK, Fisher LD, Ogrocki P, Stout JC, Speicher
CE, Glaser R. Marital quality, marital disruption, and
immune function. *Psychosom Med* 1987; **49**: 13–34.

81. Barrat FS, Lesourd BM, Louise AS, *et al.* Pregnancies
modulate B lymphopoiesis and myelopoiesis during
murine ageing. *Immunology* 1999; **98**: 604–11.

82. Rhoads CP, Barker WH. Refractory anemia. *JAMA* 1938;
110: 794.

83. Hamilton-Paterson JL. Pre-leukaemic anaemia. *Acta
Haematol* 1949; **2**: 309–16.

84. Vilter RW, Jarrold T, Will JJ, Mueller JF, Friedman BI,
Hawkins VR. Refractory anemia with hyperplastic
bone marrow. *Blood* 1960; **15**: 1–29.

85. Block M, Jacobson LO, Bethard WF. Preleukemic acute
human leukemia. *JAMA* 1953; **152**: 1018–28.

86. Dameshek W. Sideroblastic anemia: is this a malignancy? *Br J Haematol* 1965; **2**: 52–8.

87. Metcalf D. Cellular hematopoiesis in the twentieth
century. *Semin Hematol* 1999; **36** (Suppl 7): 5–12.

88. Till JE, Price GB, Mak TW, McCulloch EA. Regulation of
blood cell differentiation. *Fed Proc* 1975; **34**: 2279–84.

89. McCulloch EA, Buick RN, Till JE. Normal and leukemic
hemopoiesis compared. *Cancer* 1978; **42** (2 Suppl):
845–53.

90. Lipschitz DA, Udupa KB, Milton KY, Thompson CO.
Effect of age on hemopoiesis in man. *Blood* 1984; **63**:
502–9.

91. Harrison DE, Astle CM, Stone M. Numbers and functions of transplantable primitive immunohematopoietic stem cells: effects of age. *J Immunol* 1989; **142**:
3833–40.

92. Gabrilove JL. Cancer therapy: new strategies and treatment modalities for optimizing patient outcomes.
Semin Hematol 2001; **38** (3 Suppl 7): 1–7.

93. Speck NA. Core binding factor and its role in normal
hematopoietic development. *Curr Opin Hematol* 2001;
8:192–6.

94. Gilliland DG. Hematologic malignancies. *Curr Opin
Hematol* 2001; **8**: 189–91.

95. List AF. New approaches to the treatment of myelodysplasia. *Oncologist* 2002; **7** (Suppl 1): 39–49.

96. List AF, Vardiman J, Issa JP, DeWitte TM. Myelodysplastic syndromes. *Hematology* 2004; ASH Educational
Program book 2004: 297–317.

97. Bain BJ. The bone marrow aspirate of healthy subjects.
Br J Haematol 1996; **94**: 206–9.

98. Spivak JL, Selonick SE, Quinn TC. Acquired immune
deficiency syndrome and pancytopenia. *JAMA* 1983;
250: 3084–7.

99. Schneider DR, Picker LJ. Myelodysplasia in the
acquired immune deficiency syndrome. *Am J Clin
Pathol* 1985; **84**:144–52.

100. Breccia M, Gentile G, Martino P, *et al.* Acute myeloid
leukemia secondary to a myelodysplastic syndrome
with t(3;3) (q21;q26) in an HIV patient treated with
chemotherapy and highly active antiretroviral therapy. *Acta Haematol* 2004; **111**:160–2.

101. Castello A, Coci A, Magrini U. Paraneoplastic marrow
alterations in patients with cancer. *Haematologica*
1992; **77**: 392–7.

102. Hasselbalch HC, Juhl BR, Hansen PB. The myelodysplastic syndrome I. Pathogenesis, clinical symptoms,
diagnosis and differential diagnosis. *Ugeskr Laeger*
2002; **164**: 476–9.

103. Lawrence LW. Refractory anemia and the myelodysplastic syndromes. *Clin Lab Sci* 2004; **17**: 178–86.

104. Greenberg P, Cox C, LeBeau MM, *et al.* International
scoring system for evaluating prognosis in myelodysplastic syndromes. *Blood* 1997; **89**: 2079–88.

105. Goasguen JE, Bennett JM. Classification and morphologic features of the myelodysplastic syndromes.
Semin Oncol 1992; **19**: 4–13.

106. Mangi MH, Mufti GJ. Primary myelodysplastic syndromes: diagnostic and prognostic significance of
immunohistochemical assessment of bone marrow
biopsies. *Blood* 1992; **79**: 198–205.

107. Kass L, Elias JM. Cytochemistry and immunocyto-
chemistry in bone marrow examination: contempo-
rary techniques for the diagnosis of acute leukemia
and myelodysplastic syndromes. *Hematol Oncol Clin
North Am* 1988; **2**: 537–55.

108. Hokland P, Kerndrup G, Griffin JD, Ellegaard J. Analysis
of leukocyte differentiation antigens in blood and
bone marrow from preleukemia (refractory anemia)
patients using monoclonal antibodies. *Blood* 1986;
67: 898–902.

109. Stetler-Stevenson M, Arthur DC, Jabbou N, *et al.*
Diagnostic utility of flow cytometric immunophenotyping in myelodysplastic syndrome. *Blood* 2001; **98**:
979–87.

110. Doll DC, List AF, Dayhoff DA, Loy TS, Ringenberg QS,
Yarbro JW. Acanthocytosis associated with myelodysplasia. *J Clin Oncol* 1989; **7**: 1569–72.

111. Bethlenfalvay NC, Phaure TAJ, Phyliky RL, Bowman RP.
Nuclear bridging of erythroblasts in acquired

dyserythropoiesis: an early and transient preleukemic marker. *Am J Hematol* 1986; **21**: 315–22.

112. Vallespi T, Imbert M, Meducci C, Preudhomme C, Fenaux P. Recent advances in myelodysplastics syndromes: diagnosis, classification, and cytogenetics of myelodysplastic syndromes. *Haematologica* 1998; **83**: 258–75.

113. Head DR, Kopecky K, Bennett JM, *et al.* Pathogenetic implications of internuclear bridging in myelodysplastic syndrome: an Eastern Cooperative Oncology Group/Southwest Oncology Group Cooperative Study. *Cancer* 1989; **64**: 2199–202.

114. Matthes TW, Meyer G, Samii K, Beris P. Increased apoptosis in acquired sideroblastic anaemia. *Br J Haematol* 2000; **111**: 843–52.

115. Acin P, Florensa L, Andreu LL, Woessner S. Cytoplasmic abnormalities of erythroblasts as a marker for ringed sideroblasts in myelodysplastic syndromes. *Eur J Haematol* 1995; **54**: 276–8.

116. Hast R. Sideroblasts in myelodysplasia: their nature and clinical significance. *Scand J Haematol* 1986; **45**: 53–5.

117. Aractingi S, Bachmeyer C, Dombret H, Vignon-Pennamen D, Degos L, Dubertret L. Simultaneous occurrence of two rare cutaneous markers of poor prognosis in myelodysplastic syndrome: erythema elevatum diutinum and specific lesions. *Br J Dermatol* 1994; **131**: 112–17.

118. Roos D, Kuijpers TW, Mascart-Lemone F, *et al.* A novel syndrome of severe neutrophil dysfunction: unresponsiveness confined to chemotaxin-induced functions. *Blood* 1993; **81**: 2735–43.

119. Cech P, Markert M, Perrin LH. Partial myeloperoxidase deficiency in preleukemia. *Blut* 1983; **47**: 21–30.

120. Scott CS, Cahill A, Bynoe AG, Hough D, Roberts BE. Esterase cytochemistry in primary myelodysplastic syndromes and megaloblastic anaemias: demonstration of abnormal staining patterns associated with dysmyelopoiesis. *Br J Haematol* 1983; **55**: 411–18.

121. List AF, Doll DC. The myelodysplastic syndromes. In Lee GR, Foerster J, Lukens J, Paraskevas F, Greer JP, Rodgers GM, eds, *Wintrobe's Clinical Hematology*, 10th edn (Philadelphia, PA: Lippincott Williams & Wilkins, 2003) Chapter 89.

122. Najean Y, Lecomt T. Chronic pure thrombocytopenia in elderly patients: an aspect of the myelodysplastic syndrome. *Cancer* 1989; **64**: 2506–10.

123. Sashida G, Takaku TI, Shoji N, *et al.* Clinico-hematologic features of myelodysplastic syndrome presenting as isolated thrombocytopenia: an entity with a relatively favorable prognosis. *Leuk Lymphoma* 2003; **44**: 653–8.

124. Zeidman A, Sokolover N, Fradin Z, Cohen A, Redlich O, Mittelman M. Platelet function and its clinical significance in the myelodysplastic syndromes. *Hematol J* 2004; **5**: 234–8.

125. Brummitt DR, Barker HF, Pujol-Moix N. A new platelet parameter, the mean platelet component, can demonstrate abnormal platelet function and structure in myelodysplasia. *Clin Lab Haematol* 2003; **25**: 59–62.

126. Savage DG, Ogundipe A, Allen RH, Stabler SP, Lindenbaum J. Etiology and diagnostic evaluation of macrocytosis. *Am J Med Sci* 2000; **319**: 343–52.

127. Mahmoud MY, Lugon M, Anderson CC. Unexplained macrocytosis in elderly patients. *Age Ageing* 1996; **25**: 310–12.

128. Gilleece MH, Dexter TM. The biological ageing in bone marrow. *Rev Clin Gerontol* 1993; **3**: 317–25.

129. Sharp A, Zipori D, Toledo J, Tal S, Resnitzky P, Globerson A. Age-related changes in hemopoietic capacity of bone marrow. *Mech Ageing Dev* 1989; **48**: 91–9.

130. Pinto A, De Filippi R, Frigeri F, Corazzelli G, Normanno N. Aging and the hemopoietic system. *Crit Rev Oncol Hematol* 2003; **48**: S3–S12.

131. Van Zant G. Commentary on hemopoiesis in healthy old people and centenarians: well-maintained responsiveness of CD34+ cells to hemopoietic growth factors and remodelling of cytokine network. *J Gerontol A Biol Sci Med Sci* 2000; **55**: B67–B70.

132. Balducci L, Hardy CL, Lyman GH. Hemopoietic reserve in the older cancer patient: clinical and economic considerations. *Cancer Control* 2000; **7**: 539–47.

133. Botnick L, Hannon E, Obbagy J. The variation of hematopoietic stem cell self-renewal capacity as a function of age: further evidence for heterogeneity of the stem cell compartment. *Blood* 1982; **60**: 268–71.

134. Morrison SJ, Wandycz AM, Akashi K, Globerson A, Weissman IL. The aging of hematopoietic stem cells. *Nat Med* 1996; **2**: 1011–16.

135. Sudo K, Ema H, Morita Y, Nakauchi H. Age-associated characteristics of murine hematopoietic stem cells. *J Exp Med* 2000; **192**: 1273–80.

136. Van Zant G, Liang Y. The role of stem cells in aging. *Exp Hematol* 2003; **31**: 659–72.

137. de Haan G, Van Zant G. Intrinsic and extrinsic control of hemopoietic stem cell numbers: mapping of a stem cell gene. *J Exp Med* 1997; **186**: 529–36.

138. Van Zant G, de Haan G, Rich IN. Alternatives to stem cell renewal from a developmental viewpoint. *Exp Hematol* 1997; **25**: 187–92.

139. Geiger H, True JM, de Haan G, Van Zant G. Age- and stage-specific regulation patterns in the hematopoietic stem cell hierarchy *Blood* 2001; **98**: 2966–72.

140. De Benedictis G, Carotenuto L, Carrieri G, *et al.* Gene/ longevity association studies at four autosomal loci (REN, THO, PARP, SOD2). *Eur J Hum Genet* 1998; **6**: 534–41.

141. de Haan G, Szilvassy J, Meyerrose TE, Dontje B, Grimes B, Van Zant G. Distinct functional properties of highly purified hematopoietic stem cells from mouse strains differing in stem cell numbers. *Blood* 2000; **96**: 1374–89.

142. Krosl JK, Faubert A, Sauvageau G. Molecular basis for stem-cell self-renewal. *Hematol J* 2004; **5**: S118–S121.

143. Botnick LE, Hannon EC, Hellman S. Nature of the hematopoietic stem cells in vitro. *Blood Cells* 1979; **5**: 195–206.

144. de Haan G, Nijhof W, Van Zant G. Mouse strain-dependent changes in frequency and proliferation of hematopoietic stem cells during aging: correlation between lifespan and cycling activity. *Blood* 1997; **89**: 1543–50.

145. Hofmann WK, de Vos S, Komor M, Hoelzer D, Wachsman W, Koeffler HP. Characterization of gene expression of CD34+ cells from normal and myelodysplastic bone marrow. *Blood* 2002; **100**: 3553–60.

146. Ogawa T, Kitagawa M, Hirokawa K. Age-related changes of human bone marrow: a histometric estimation of proliferative cells, apoptotic cells, T cells, B cells and macrophages. *Mech Ageing Dev* 2000; **117**: 57–68.

147. Chatta GS, Andrews RG, Rodger E, Schrag M, Hammond WP, Dale DC. Hematopoietic progenitors and aging: alterations in granulocytic precursors and responsiveness to recombinant human G-CSF, GM-CSF, and IL-3. *J Gerontol* 1993; **48**: 207–12.

148. Kim SJ, Letterio SJ. Transforming growth factor-beta signaling in normal and malignant hematopoiesis. *Leukemia* 2003; **17**: 1731–7.

149. Morley A, Blake J. An animal model of chronic aplastic marrow failure. I. Late marrow failure after busulfan. *Blood* 1974; **44**: 49–56.

150. Cheshier SH, Morrison SJ, Liao X, Weissman IL. In vivo proliferation and cell cycle kinetics of long-term self-renewing hematopoietic stem cells. *Proc Natl Acad Sci USA* 1999; **96**: 3120–5.

151. Tenen DG, Hromas R, Licht JD, Zhang DE. Transcription factors, normal myeloid development, and leukemia. *Blood* 1997; **90**: 489–519.

152. Liang Y, Van Zant G. Genetic control of stem-cell properties and stem cells in aging. *Curr Opin Hematol* 2003; **10**: 195–202.

153. Christensen K, Kristiansen M, Hagen-Larsen H, *et al.* X-linked genetic factors regulate hematopoietic stem cell kinetics in females. *Blood* 2000; **95**: 2449–51.

154. Champion KM, Gilbert JG, Asimakopoulos FA, Hinshelwood S, Green AR. Clonal haemopoiesis in normal elderly women: implications for the myeloproliferative disorders and myelodysplastic syndromes. *Br J Haematol* 1997; **97**: 920–6.

155. Gale RE, Fielding AK, Harrison CN, Linch DC. Acquired skewing of X-chromosome inactivation patterns in myeloid cells of the elderly suggests stochastic clonal loss with age. *Br J Haematol* 1997; **98**: 512–19.

156. Robertson JD, Gale RE, Wynn RF, *et al.* Dynamics of telomere shortening in neutrophils and T lymphocytes during ageing and the relationship to skewed X chromosome inactivation patterns. *Br J Haematol* 2000; **109**: 272–9.

157. Aviv A. Telomeres and human aging: facts and fibs. *Sci Aging Knowledge Environ* 2004; **2004** (51): pe43.

158. Effros RB, Globerson A. Hematopoietic cells and replicative senescence. *Exp Gerontol* 2002; **37**: 191–6.

159. Proctor CJ, Kirkwood TB. Modelling cellular senescence as a result of telomere state. *Aging Cell* 2003; **2**: 151–7.

160. Vaziri H, Dragowska W, Allsopp RC, Thomas TE, Harley CB, Lansdorp PM. Evidence for a mitotic clock in human hematopoietic stem cells: loss of telomeric DNA with age. *Proc Natl Acad Sci USA* 1994; **91**: 9857–60.

161. Artandi SE, Attardi LD. Pathways connecting telomeres and p53 in senescence, apoptosis, and cancer. *Biochem Biophys Res Commun* 2005; **331**: 881–90.

162. Wynn RF, Cross MA, Testa NG. Telomeres and haemopoiesis. *Br J Haematol* 1998; **103**: 591–3.

163. Engelhardt M, Wasch R, Guo Y. Telomeres and telomerase in normal and leukemic hematopoietic cells. *Leuk Res* 2004; **28**: 1001–4.

164. Serra V, Grune T, Sitte N, Saretzki G, von Zglinicki T. Telomere length as a marker of oxidative stress in primary human fibroblast cultures. *Ann N Y Acad Sci* 2000; **908**: 327–30.

165. Fern L, Pallis M, Carter I, Seedhouse C, Russell N, Byrne J. Clonal haemopoiesis may occur after conventional chemotherapy and is associated with accelerated telomere shortening and defects in the NQo1 pathway: possible mechanisms leading to an increased risk of t-AML/MDS. *Br J Haematol* 2004; **126**: 63–71.

166. Ben-Porath I, Weinberg RA. The signals and pathways activating cellular senescence. *Int J Biochem Cell Biol* 2005; **37**: 961–76.

167. Epel ES, Blackburn EH, Lin J, *et al.* Accelerated telomere shortening in response to life stress. *Proc Natl Acad Sci USA* 2004; **101**: 17312–15

168. Chiu CP, Dragowska W, Kim NW, *et al.* Differential expression of telomerase activity in hematopoietic progenitors from adult human bone marrow. *Stem Cells* 1996; **14**: 239–48.

169. Zaucha JM, Yu C, Mathioudakis G, Seidel K, *et al.* Hematopoietic responses to stress conditions in young dogs compared with elderly dogs. *Blood* 2001; **98**: 322–7.

170. Israels LG, Israels ED. Apoptosis. *Stem Cells* 1999; **17**: 306–13.

171. Westwood NB, Mufti BJ. Apoptosis in the myelodysplastic syndromes. *Curr Hematol Rep* 2003; **2**: 186–92.

172. Mundle SD, Venugopal P, Cartlidge JD, *et al.* Indication of an involvement of interleukin-1 beta converting enzyme-like protease in intramedullary apoptotic cell death in the bone marrow of patients with myelodysplastic syndromes. *Blood* 1996; **88**: 2640–7

173. Koury MJ, Horne DW, Brown ZA, *et al.* Apoptosis of late-stage erythroblasts in megaloblastic anemia: association with DNA damage and macrocyte production. *Blood* 1997; **89**: 4617–23.

174. Horne MK. Nutritional deficiencies. In Rodgers GP, Young NS, eds, *Bethesda Handbook of Clinical Hematology* (Philadelphia, PA: Lippincott Williams & Wilkins, 2005), Chapter 2, 11–20.

175. Chatta GS, Price TH, Allen RC, Dale DC. Effects of in vivo recombinant methionyl human granulocyte colony-stimulating factor on the neutrophil response and peripheral blood colony-forming cells in healthy young and elderly adult volunteers. *Blood* 1994; **84**: 2923–9.

176. Barrat F, Lesourd B, Boulouis HJ, *et al.* Sex and parity modulate cytokine production during murine ageing. *Clin Exp Immunol* 1997; **109**: 562–8.

177. Fagiolo U, Cossarizza A, Scala E, *et al.* Increased cytokine production in mononuclear cells of healthy elderly people. *Eur J Immunol* 1993; **23**: 2375–8.

178. Shivdasani RA. The role of transcription factor NF-E2 in megakaryocyte maturation and platelet production. *Stem Cells* 1996; **14** (Suppl 1): 112–15.

179. Liu WF, Yu SS, Li YZ. NF-kappaB tumorigenesis and drug development. *Sheng Wu Gong Cheng Xue Bao* 2005; **21**: 12–18.

180. Tsai FY, Orkin SH. Transcription factor GATA-2 is required for proliferation/survival of early hematopoietic cells and mast cell formation, but not for erythroid and myeloid terminal differentiation. *Blood* 1997; **89**: 3636–43.

181. Tsuboi I, Morimoto K, Hirabayashi Y, *et al.* Senescent B lymphopoiesis is balanced in suppressive homeostasis: decrease in interleukin-7 and transforming growth factor-beta levels in stromal cells of senescence-accelerated mice. *Exp Biol Med* 2004; **229**: 494–502.

182. Uyemura K, Castle SC, Makinodan T. The frail elderly: role of dendritic cells in the susceptibility of infection. *Mech Ageing Dev* 2002; **123**: 955–62.

183. Fulop T, Larpi A, Douzieh N, *et al.* Signal transduction and functional changes in neutrophils with aging. *Aging Cell* 2004; **3**: 217–26.

184. DeVeale B, Brummel T, Seroude L. Immunity and aging: the enemy within? *Aging Cell* 2004; **3**: 195–208.

185. Sansoni P, Fagnoni F, Vescovini R, *et al.* T lymphocyte proliferative capability to defined stimuli and costimulatory CD28 pathway is not impaired in healthy centenarians. *Mech Ageing Dev* 1997; **96**: 127–36.

186. Paganelli R, Scala E, Rosso R, *et al.* A shift to Th0 cytokine production by CD4+ cells in human longevity: studies on two healthy centenarians. *Eur J Immunol* 1996; **26**: 2030–4.

187. Cossarizza A, Ortolani C, Paganelli R, *et al.* CD45 isoforms expression on CD4+ and CD8+ T cells throughout life, from newborns to centenarians: implications for T cell memory. *Mech Ageing Dev* 1996; **86**: 173–95.

188. Miyaji C, Watanabe H, Toma H, *et al.* Functional alteration of granulocytes, NK cells, and natural killer T cells in centenarians. *Hum Immunol* 2000; **61**: 908–16.

189. Mocchegiani E, Malavolta M. NK and NKT functions in immunosenescence. *Aging Cell* 2004; **3**: 177–84.

190. Mariani E, Ravaglia G, Meneghetti A, *et al.* Natural immunity and bone and muscle remodelling hormones in the elderly. *Mech Ageing Dev* 1998; **102**: 279–92.

191. Garg M, Luo W, Kaplan AM, Bondada S. Cellular basis of decreased immune responses to pneumococcal vaccines in aged mice. *Infect Immun* 1996; **64**: 4456–62.

192. Plowden J, Renshaw-Hoelscher M, Engleman C, Katz J, Sanbhara S. Innate immunity in aging: impact on macrophage function. *Aging Cell* 2004; **3**: 161–7.

193. Garwicz D, Lennartsson A, Jacobsen SE, Guiberg U, Lindmark A. Biosynthetic profiles of neutrophil serine proteases in a human bone marrow differentiation model. *Haematologica* 2005; **90**: 38–44.

194. Lipschitz KB, Udupa SR, Indelicato SR, Das M. Effect of age on second messenger generation in neutrophils. *Blood* 1991; **78**: 1347–54.

195. Mege JL, Capo C, Michel B, Gastaut JL, Bongrand P. Phagocytic cell function in aged subjects. *Neurobiol Aging* 1988; **9**: 217–20.

196. Gombart AF, Kwok SH, Anderson KL, Yamaguchi Y, Torbett BE, Koeffler HP. Regulation of neutrophil and eosinophil secondary granule gene expression by transcription factors C/EBP epsilon and PU.1. *Blood* 2003; **101**: 3265–73.

197. Tortorella C, Piazzolla G, Spaccavento F, Jirillo E, Antonaci S. Age-related effects of oxidative metabolism and cyclic AMP signaling on neutrophil apoptosis. *Mech Ageing Dev* 1999; **110**: 195–205.

198. Lekstrom-Himes JA, Gallin JI. Immunodeficiency diseases caused by defects in phagocytes. *N Engl J Med* 2000; **343**: 1703–14.

199. Tortorella C, Piazzolla G, Spaccavento F, Antonaci S. Effects of granulocyte-macrophage colony-stimulating factor and cyclic AMP interaction on human neutrophil apoptosis. *Mediators Inflamm* 1998; **7**: 391–6.

200. Gombart AF, Koeffler HP. Neutrophil specific granule deficiency and mutations in the gene encoding transcription factor C/EBP(epsilon). *Curr Opin Hematol* 2002; **9**: 36–42.

201. Larbi A, Douziech N, Fortin C, Linteau A, Dupuis G, Fulop T. The role of the MAPK pathway alterations in GM-CSF modulated human neutrophil apoptosis with aging. *Immun Ageing* 2005; **2**: 6.

202. Shetty V, Hussaini S, Broady-Robinson L, *et al.* Intramedullary apoptosis of hematopoietic cells in myelodysplastic syndrome patients can be massive: apoptotic cells recovered from high-density fraction of bone marrow aspirates. *Blood* 2000; **96**: 1388–92.

203. Merry BJ. Oxidative stress and mitochondrial function with aging: the effects of calorie restriction. *Aging Cell* 2004; **3**: 7–12.

204. Janssen JW, Buschle M, Layton M, *et al.* Clonal analysis of myelodysplastic syndromes: evidence of multipotent stem cell origin. *Blood* 1989; **73**: 248–54.

205. Raskind WH, Tirumali N, Jacobson R, Singer J, Fialkow PJ. Evidence for a multistep pathogenesis of a myelodysplastic syndrome. *Blood* 1984; **63**: 1318–23.

206. Ihalainen J, Pakkala S, Savolainen ER, Jansson SE, Palotie A. Hypermethylation of the calcitonin gene in the myelodysplastic syndromes. *Leukemia* 1993; **7**: 263–7.

207. Tabin CJ, Bradley SM, Bargmann CI, *et al.* Mechanism of activation of a human oncogene. *Nature* 1982; **300**: 143–9.

208. Oscier D. Myelodysplastic syndromes. *Ballieres Clin Haematol* 1987; **1**: 389–426.

209. Delforge M. Understanding the pathogeneis of myelodysplastic syndromes. *Hematol J* 2003; **4**: 303–9.

210. Hanahan D, Weinberg RA. The hallmarks of cancer. *Cell* 2000; **100**. 57 70.

211. Li X, Bryant CE, Deeg HJ. Simultaneous demonstration of clonal chromosome abnormalities and apoptosis in individual marrow cells in myelodysplastic syndrome. *Int J Hematol* 2004; **80**: 140–5.

212. Liesveld JL, Jordan CT, Phillips GL. The haematopoietic stem cell in myelodysplasia. *Stem Cells* 2004; **33**: 590–9.

213. White N, Nacheva E, Asimakopoulos F, Bloxham D, Paul B, Green A. Deletion of chromosome 20q in myelodysplasia can occur in a multipotent precursor of both myeloid cells and B cells. *Blood* 1994; **83**: 2809–16.

214. Lewis S, Oscier D, Boultwood J, *et al.* Hematological features of patients with myelodysplastic syndromes associated with a chromosome 5q deletion. *Am J Hematol* 1995; **49**: 194–200.

215. Abrahamson G, Boultwood J, Madden J, *et al.* Clonality of cell populations in refractory anaemia using combined approach of gene loss and X-linked restriction fragment length polymorphism-methylation analyses. *Br J Haematol* 1991; **79**: 550–5.

216. Delforge M, Demuynck H, Verhoef G, *et al.* Patients with high-risk myelodysplastic syndrome can have polyclonal or clonal haemopoiesis in complete haematological remission. *Br J Haematol* 1998; **102**: 486–94.

217. Lawrence HJ, Broudy VC, Magenis RE, *et al.* Cytogenetic evidence for involvement of B lymphocytes in acquired sideroblastic anemia. *Blood* 1987; **70**: 1003–5.

218. Amin HM, Jilani I, Estey EH, *et al.* Increased apoptosis in bone marrow B lymphocytes but not T lymphocytes in myelodysplastic syndrome. *Blood* 2003; **102**: 1866–8.

219. Cermak J, Belickova M, Krejcova H, *et al.* The presence of clonal cell subpopulations in peripheral blood

and bone marrow of patients with refractory cytopenia with multilineage dysplasia but not in patients with refractory anemia may reflect a multistep pathogenesis of myelodysplasia. *Leuk Res* 2005; **29**: 371–9.

220. Mecucci C. Molecular features of primary MDS with cytogenetic changes. *Leuk Res* 1998; **22**: 293–302.

221. Nilsson-Ehle H, Swolin B, Westin J. Bone marrow progenitor cell growth and karyotype changes in healthy 88-year-old subjects. *Eur J Haematol* 1995; **55**: 14–18.

222. Yunis JJ, Lobell M, Arnesen MA, *et al.* Refined chromosome study helps define prognostic subgroups in most patients with primary myelodysplastic syndrome and acute myelogenous leukaemia. *Br J Haematol* 1988; **68**: 189–94.

223. Knapp RH, Dewald GW, Pierre RV. Cytogenetic studies in 174 consecutive patients with preleukemic or myelodysplastic syndromes. *Mayo Clin Proc* 1985; **60**: 507–16.

224. Tricot G, Boogaerts MA, De Wolf-Peeters C, Van den Berghe H, Verwilghen RL. The myelodysplastic syndromes: different evolution patterns based on sequential morphological and cytogenetic investigations. *Br J Haematol* 1985; **59**: 659–70.

225. Dansey R, Myelodysplasia. *Curr Opin Oncol* 2000; **12**: 13–21.

226. Saba HI. Myelodysplastic syndromes in the elderly: the role of growth factors in management. Cancer. *Leuk Res* 1996; **20**: 203–19.

227. Lopez-Holgado N, Arroyo JL, Pata C, *et al.* Analysis of hematopoietic progenitor cells in patients with myelodysplastic syndromes according to their cytogenetic abnormalities. *Leuk Res* 2004; **28**: 1181–7.

228. Pierre R, Catovsky D, Mufti G, *et al.* Clinical cytogenetic correlations in myelodysplasia (preleukemia). *Cancer Genet Cytogenet* 1989; **40**: 149–61.

229. Side LE, Curtiss NP, Teel K, *et al.* RAS, FLT3, and TP53 mutations in therapy-related myeloid malignancies with abnormalities of chromosomes 5 and 7. *Genes Chromosomes Cancer* 2004; **39**: 217–23.

230. United Kingdom Cytogenetics Group. Loss of the Y chromosome from normal and neoplastic bone marrows. *Genes Chromosome Cancer* 1992; **5**: 83–8.

231. Wiktor A, Rybicki BA, Piao ZS, *et al.* Clinical significance of Y chromosome loss in hematologic disease. *Genes Chromosomes Cancer* 2000; **27**: 11–16.

232. Prasher JM, Lalai AS, Heijmans-Antonissen C, *et al.* Reduced hematopoietic reserves in DNA interstrand crosslink repair-deficient Ercc1-/- mice. *EMBO J* 2005; **24**: 861–71.

233. Ueda M, Ota J, Yamashita Y, *et al.* DNA microarray analysis of stage progression mechanism in myelodysplastic syndrome. *Br J Haematol* 2003; **123**: 288–96.

234. Van den Berghe H, Cassiman JJ, David G, Fryns JP. Distinct haematological disorder with deletion of long arm of No. 5 chromosome. *Nature* 1974; **251**: 437–8.

235. Van den Berghe H, Vermaelen K, Mecucci C, Barbieri D, Tricot G: The 5q- anomaly. *Cancer Genet Cytogenet* 1985; **17**: 189–255.

236. Sokal G, Michaux JL, Van Den Berghe H, *et al.* A new hematologic syndrome with a distinct karyotype: the 5q- chromosome. *Blood* 1975; **46**: 519–33.

237. Boultwood J, Fidler C, Strickson AJ, *et al.* Narrowing and genomic annotation of the commonly deleted region of the 5q- syndrome. *Blood* 2002; **99**: 4638–41.

238. Stephenson J, Mufti GJ, Yoshida Y. Myelodysplastic syndromes: from morphology to molecular biology. Part II. The molecular genetics of myelodysplasia. *Int J Hematol* 1993; **57**: 99–112.

239. Giagounidis AA, Germing U, Wainscoat JS, Boultwood J, Aul C. The 5q- syndrome. *Hematology* 2004; **9**: 271–7.

240. Le Beau MM, Espinosa R, Davis EM, Eisenbart JD, Larson RA, Green ED. Cytogenetic and molecular delineation of a region of chromosome 7 commonly deleted in malignant myeloid diseases. *Blood* 1996; **88**: 1930–5.

241. Lai JL, Preudhomme C, Zandecki M, *et al.* Myelodysplastic syndromes and acute myeloid leukemia with 17p deletion. An entity characterized by specific dysgranulopoiesis and a high incidence of P53 mutations. *Leukemia* 1995; **9**: 370–81.

242. Christiansen DH, Andersen MK, Pedersen-Bjergaard J. Methylation of p15(INK4B) is common, is associated with deletion of genes on chromosome 7q and predicts a poor prognosis in therapy-related myelodysplasia and acute myeloid leukemia. *Leukemia* 2003; **17**: 1813–19.

243. Quesnel B, Guillerm G, Vereecque R, *et al.* Methylation of the p15(INK4b) gene in myelodysplastic syndromes is frequent and acquired during disease progression. *Blood* 1998; **91**: 2985–90.

244. Horiike S, Kita-Sasai Y, Nakao M, Taniwaki M. Configuration of the TP53 gene as an independent prognostic parameter of myelodysplastic syndrome. *Leuk Lymphoma* 2003; **44**: 915–22.

245. Kita-Sasai Y, Horiike S, Misawa S, *et al.* International prognostic scoring system and TP53 mutations are inde-

pendent prognostic indicators for patients with myelodysplastic syndrome *Br J Haematol* 2001; **115**: 309–12.

246. Fenaux P. Chromosome and molecular abnormalities in myelodysplastic syndromes. *Int J Hematol* 2001; **73**: 429–37.

247. Hatfill SJ, Fester ED, Steytler JG. Apoptotic megakaryocyte dysplasia in the myelodysplastic syndromes. *Hematol Pathol* 1992; **6**: 87–93.

248. Yoshida Y. Hypothesis: apoptosis may be the mechanism responsible for the premature intramedullary cell death in the myelodysplastic syndrome. *Leukemia* 1993; **7**: 144–6.

249. Raza A, Mundle S, Iftikhar A, *et al.* Simultaneous assessment of cell kinetics and programmed cell death in bone marrow biopsies of myelodysplastics reveals extensive apoptosis as the probable basis for ineffective hematopoiesis. *Am J Hematol* 1995; **48**: 143–54.

250. Rajapaksa R, Ginzton N, Rott LS, Greenberg PL. Altered oncoprotein expression and apoptosis in myelodysplastic syndrome marrow cells. *Blood* 1996; **88**: 4275–87.

251. Parker JE, Mufti GJ, Rasool F, Mijovic A, Devereux S, Pagliuca A. The role of apoptosis, proliferation, and the Bcl-2 related proteins in the myelodysplastic syndromes and acute myeloid leukaemia secondary to MDS. *Blood* 2000; **96**: 3932–8.

252. Zang DY, Goodwin RG, Loken MR, Bryant E, Deeg HJ. Expression of tumor necrosis factor-related apoptosis-inducing ligand, Apo2L and its receptor in myelodysplastic syndrome. Effects on in vitro hemopoiesis. *Blood* 2001; **98**: 3058–65.

253. Yoshida Y. The aplasia-myelodysplasia enigma: a re-emerging question. *Int J Hematol* 1999; **70**: 65–7.

254. Shimazaki K, Ohshima K, Suzumiya J, Kawasaki C, Kikuchi M. Apoptosis and prognostic factors in myelodysplastic syndromes. *Leuk Lymphoma* 2002; **43**: 257–60.

255. Salih HR, Nuessler V, Denzlinger C, Starling GC, Kiener PA, Schmetzer HM. Serum levels of CD137 ligand and CD178 are prognostic factors for progression of myelodysplastic syndrome. *Leuk Lymphoma* 2004; **45**: 301–8.

256. Gersuk GM, Beckham C, Loken MR, *et al.* A role for tumour necrosis factor-alpha, Fas and Fas-Ligand in marrow failure associated with myelodysplastic syndrome. *Br J Haematol* 1998; **103**: 176–88.

257. Sultana TA, Harada H, Ito K, Tanaka H, Kyo T, Kimura A. Expression and functional analysis of granulocyte colony-stimulating factor receptors on CD34++ cells in patients with myelodysplastic syndrome (MDS) and MDS-acute myeloid leukaemia. *Br J Haematol* 2003; **121**: 63–75.

258. Rigolin GM, Porta MD, Ciccone M, *et al.* In patients with myelodysplastic syndromes response to rHuEPO and G-CSF treatment is related to an increase of cytogenetically normal CD34 cells. *Br J Haematol* 2004; **126**: 501–7.

259. Guidetti F, Grazioli S, Capelli F, *et al.* Primitive hematopoietic stem cells shows a polyclonal pattern in myelodysplastic syndromes. *Haematologica* 2004; **89**: 21–8.

260. Krejcova H, Neuwirtova R, Cermak J, Belickova M, Brdicka R. Cell clonality in myelodysplastic syndrome. *Sb Lek* 2002; **103**: 339–48.

261. Von Hirschhausen R, Saal JG. [Primary myelodysplastic syndrome: prognostic factors and frequent appearance of monoclonal and polyclonal gammopathies.] *Dtsch Med Wochenschr* 1990; **115**: 88–92.

262. Mufti GJ, Figes A, Hamblin TJ, Oscier DG, Copplestone JA. Immunological abnormalities in myelodysplastic syndromes. I. Serum immunoglobulins and autoantibodies. *Br J Haematol* 1986; **63**: 143–7.

263. Gracia A, Lopez F, Perez R, Villegas G. [Immunological changes in chronic myelomonocytic leukemias.] *Sangre (Barc)* 1997; **42**: 429–30.

264. Muller-Sieburg CE, Cho RH, Sieburg HB, Kupriyanov S, Riblet R. Genetic control of hematopoietic stem cell frequency in mice is mostly cell autonomous. *Blood* 2000; **95**: 2446–8.

265. Alexandrakis MG, Passam FH, Kyriakou DS, *et al.* Expression of the proliferation-associated nuclear protein MIB-1 and its relationship with microvascular density in bone marrow biopsies of patients with myelodysplastic syndromes. *J Mol Histol* 2004; **35**: 857–63.

266. Campioni D, Punturieri M, Bardi A, *et al.* In vitro evaluation of bone marrow angiogenesis in myelodysplastic syndromes: a morphological and functional approach. *Leuk Res* 2004; **28**: 9–17.

267. Silver RT, Bennett JM, Deininger M, *et al.* The second international congress on myeloproliferative and myelodysplastic syndromes. *Leuk Res* 2004; **28**: 979–85.

268. Aguayo A. The role of angiogenesis in the biology and therapy of myelodysplastic syndromes. *Curr Hematol Rep* 2004; **3**: 184–91.

269. Bellamy WT, Richter L, Sirjani D, *et al.* Vascular endothelial cell growth factor is an autocrine promoter of abnormal localized immature myeloid precursors

and leukemia progenitor formation in myelodysplastic syndromes. *Blood* 2001; **97**: 1427–34.

270. Estey EH. Modulation of angiogenesis in patients with myelodysplastic syndrome. *Best Pract Res Clin Haematol* 2004; **17**: 623–39.

271. Soenen-Cornu V, Tourino C, Bonnet ML, *et al.* Mesenchymal cells generated from patients with myelodysplastic syndromes are devoid of chromosomal clonal markers and support short- and long-term hematopoiesis in vitro. *Oncogene* 2005; **24**: 2441–8.

272. Flores-Figueroa E, Arana-Trejo RM, Gutierrez-Espindola G, Perez-Cabrera A, Mayani H. Mesenchymal stem cells in myelodysplastic syndromes: phenotypic and cytogenetic characterization. *Leuk Res* 2005; **29**: 215–24.

273. Pagliuca A, Layton DM, Manoharan A, *et al.* Myelofibrosis in primary myelodysplastic syndromes: a clinico-morphological study of 10 cases. *Br J Haematol* 1989; **71**: 499–504.

274. Micheva I, Thanopoulou E, Michalopoulou S, *et al.* Defective tumor necrosis factor alpha-induced maturation of monocyte-derived dendritic cells in patients with myelodysplastic syndromes. *Clin Immunol* 2004; **113**: 310–17.

275. Kikukawa M, Aoki N, Sakamoto Y, Mori M. Study of p53 in elderly patients with myelodysplastic syndromes by immunohistochemistry and DNA analysis. *Am J Pathol* 1999; **155**: 717–21.

276. Krug U, Ganser A, Koeffler HP. Tumor suppressor genes in normal and malignant hematopoiesis. *Oncogene* 2002; **21**: 3475–95.

277. Fidler C, Watkins F, Bowen DT, Littlewood TJ, Wainscoat JS, Boultwood J. NRAS, FLT3 and TP53 mutations in patients with myelodysplastic syndrome and a del(5q). *Haematologica* 2004; **89**: 865–6.

278. Christiansen DH, Andersen MK, Pedersen-Bjergaard J. Mutations with loss of heterozygosity of p53 are common in therapy-related myelodysplasia and acute myeloid leukemia after exposure to alkylating agents and significantly associated with deletion or loss of 5q, a complex karyotype, and a poor prognosis. *J Clin Oncol* 2001; **19**: 1405–13.

279. Imamura N, Abe K, Oguma N. High incidence of point mutations of p53 suppressor oncogene in patients with myelodysplastic syndrome among atomic-bomb survivors: a 10-year follow-up. *Leukemia* 2002; **16**: 154–6.

280. Pedersen-Bjergaard J, Andersen MK, Christiansen DH. Therapy-related acute myeloid leukemia and myelodysplasia after high-dose chemotherapy and autologous stem cell transplantation. *Blood* 2000; **95**: 3273–9.

281. Rund D, Ben-Yehuda D. Therapy-related leukemia and myelodysplasia: evolving concepts of pathogenesis and treatment. *Hematology* 2004; **9**: 179–87.

282. Stone R. Myelodysplastic syndromes after autologous transplantation for lymphoma: the price of progress. *Blood* 1994; **83**: 3437–40.

283. Paquette RL. Diagnosis and management of aplastic anemia and myelodysplastic syndrome. *Oncology* 2002; **16** (Suppl 10): 153–61.

284. Reddy J, Shivapurkar N, Takahashi T, *et al.* Differential methylation of genes that regulate cytokine signaling in lymphoid and hematopoietic tumors. *Oncogene* 2005; **24**: 732–6.

285. Silverman LR. DNA methyltransferase inhibitors in myelodysplastic syndrome. *Best Pract Res Clin Haematol* 2004; **17**: 585–94.

286. Uchida T, Kinoshita T, Nagai H *et al.* Hypermethylation of the p15INK4b gene in myelodysplastic syndromes. *Blood* 1997; **90**: 1403–9.

287. Teofili L, Martini M, Di Mario A, *et al.* Expression of p15 (ink4b) gene during megakaryocytic differentiation of normal and myelodysplastic hematopoietic progenitors. *Blood* 2001; **98**: 495–7.

288. Voso MT, Scardocci A, Guidi F, *et al.* Aberrant methylation of DAP-kinase in therapy-related acute myeloid leukemia and myelodysplastic syndromes. *Blood* 2004; **103**: 698–700.

289. Silverman LR, Holland JF, Weinberg RS, *et al.* Effects of treatment with 5-azacytidine on the in vivo and in vitro hematopoiesis in patients with myelodysplastic syndromes. *Leukemia* 1993; **7** (Suppl 1): 21–9.

290. Issa JP, Gharibyan V, Cortes J, *et al.* Phase II study of low-dose decitabine in patients with chronic myelogenous leukemia resistant to imatinib mesylate. *J Clin Oncol* 2005; **23**: 3948–56.

291. Christman JK. 5-Azacytidine and 5-aza-2'-deoxycytidine as inhibitors of DNA methylation: mechanistic studies and their implications for cancer therapy. *Oncogene* 2002; **21**: 5483–95.

292. Beris P, Samii K, Darbellay R, *et al.* Iron overload in patients with sideroblastic anemia is not related to the presence of the haemochromatosis Cys282Tyr and His63Asp mutations. *Br J Haematol* 1999; **104**: 97–9.

293. Germing U, Gattermann N, Aivado M, Hildebrandt B, Aul C. Two types of acquired idiopathic sideroblastic anemia: a time-tested distinction. *Br J Haematol* 2000; **108**: 724–8.

294. Hahn WC. Role of telomeres and telomerase in the pathogenesis of human cancer. *J Clin Oncol* 2003; **21**: 2034–43.

295. Gilley D, Tanaka H, Herbert BS. Telomere dysfunction in aging and cancer. *Int J Biochem Cell Biol* 2005; **37**: 1000–13.

296. Ohyashiki JH, Sashida G, Tauchi T, Ohyashiki K. Telomeres and telomerase in hematologic neoplasia. *Oncogene* 2002; **21**: 680–7.

297. Rodier F, Kim SH, Nijjar T, Yaswen P, Campisi J. Cancer and aging: the importance of telomeres in genome maintenance. *Int J Biochem Cell Biol* 2005; **37**: 977–90.

298. Deguchi K, Gilliland DG. Cooperativity between mutations in tyrosine kinases and in hematopoietic transcription factors in AML. *Leukemia* 2002; **16**: 740–4.

9

Aging and hematopoietic stress

Lodovico Balducci, Cheryl L. Hardy

Introduction

Aging involves a progressive decline in the functional reserve of multiple organs and systems, which reduces the stress-coping ability of aged individuals. In this chapter we explore the influence of aging on response to hematopoietic stress and the potential mechanisms by which this response may be impaired.

The peripheral blood counts do not appear significantly reduced in the aged [1–3], at least up to age 90, indicating that homeostasis is preserved even in the oldest old, in the absence of stress. In the meantime, incidence and prevalence of diseases that inhibit hematopoiesis, including chronic inflammations, nutritional deficiencies, chronic renal insufficiency, sarcopenia, myelodysplasia, and other hematopoietic malignancies [2,4–8], increase with age. These conditions may be subclinical until revealed by hematopoietic stress, as they prevent the increased production of blood elements required to compensate for accelerated consumption or losses. Even in the absence of specific diseases, hematopoiesis may become progressively exhausted, due to a loss of stem cells and of their self-renewal capacity [9–11]. This exhaustion appears due to a number of mechanisms, including repeated exposure to anoxia/reoxygenation [12–16], epigenetic changes involving loss of DNA-repairing enzymes [11,17] and of negative cell-cycle regulators [18], and increased concentration of substances that may inhibit the self-renewal and the differentiation of hematopoietic progenitors [4,19].

The study of hematopoietic stress has both clinical and biological relevance. The ability of an organism to increase the production of blood elements in response to accelerated losses may mirror an individual's biological age; it may reveal mechanisms that inhibit hematopoiesis and that may be reversed, and it may measure individual tolerance of myelotoxic treatment and indicate the use of supportive care, including transfusions of blood products, hematopoietic growth factors, and antibiotics for the prevention and treatment of infections. These possibilities have never been fully explored due to the difficulty of studying hematopoietic stress in humans:

- Unlike the stress to other systems, such as the cardiovascular or respiratory systems, the study of hematopoietic stress has not been standardized. In particular, there is no information as to the intensity of the stress that should be induced, nor on the response to the stress one should expect.
- Hematopoietic cell lines may be affected to a different extent by aging in different individuals. It is not clear which hematopoietic lineage, if any, is more likely to become compromised with aging.
- The interpretation of the results may be inconclusive, as response to stress may be compromised by mechanisms independent from hematopoietic exhaustion. For example, increased infection-related mortality may be due to decreased ability to produce neutrophils as well as to decreased function of these elements [20–25].

To further complicate the interpretation of the studies, it may be impossible to dissect the influence of

Blood Disorders in the Elderly, ed. Lodovico Balducci, William Ershler, Giovanni de Gaetano.
Published by Cambridge University Press. © Cambridge University Press 2008.

aging and of comorbid diseases on hematopoietic stress. With these reservations in mind we review the current information on hematopoietic stress in the aged, and propose an agenda for future studies.

Hematopoietic stress

The functional reserve capacity of a system is assessed as the ability of that system to increase its performance in conditions of stress. This ability is progressively lost with age. The hematopoietic system is stressed by increased utilization of peripheral blood elements, as in the case of bacterial infections requiring increased neutrophil production, or by the loss of these elements, as may occur with bleeding or hemolysis. Table 9.1 illustrates different forms of experimental and clinical stresses in both animals and humans.

Hematopoietic stress in experimental animals

Chronic exposure to sublethal doses of radiation stresses the self-renewal ability of stem cells and hematopoietic progenitors, by increasing their destruction. In healthy animals of all ages this exposure results in pancytopenia and hematopoietic insufficiency. Recently Zaucha *et al.* [26] submitted a small cohort of young and old dogs to seven sessions of sublethal total body irradiation and found that the recovery of hematopoiesis was compromised in most animals, irrespective of age. These experiments can hardly be considered evidence that age does not affect response to hematopoietic stress, as the dose of radiation had caused substantial and lasting damage in most younger dogs as well. Clearly, the stress was overwhelming irrespective of the animal's age, and a differential effect might have been masked by the intensity of the stress.

The injection of the same dose of gram-negative bacteria or of endotoxins was associated with reduced neutrophilic response and increased incidence of septic shock and mortality in older mice [29] and rats [30], compared with younger animals. It is not clear whether these findings are due to exhausted

hematopoiesis, reduced production of myelopoietic growth factors, decreased neutrophil function, reduced cardiovascular reserve, or a combination of these elements. A number of studies [29,30,57–59] have shown that the production of growth factors by the hematopoietic stroma is reduced with age.

Anoxia [31], bleeding [32], and chronic hemolysis [33] stress erythropoiesis and cause an expansion of the eythropoietic tissue of young mice, but they were not applied to older animals.

Hypothermia is associated with a reversible loss of early pluripotential hematopoietic progenitors (CFU-GM) [34]. This form of stress appears of particular interest for two reasons. First, it seems to affect the viability of the hematopoietic progenitors themselves and so it may provide a reliable estimate of the hematopoietic reserve. Second, it may reproduce the physiologic conditions of advanced aging that are associated with reduced thermoregulation [60]. Unfortunately, data related to hypothermia in older animals are wanting.

For reasons that are not clear, overcrowding is a form of hematopoietic stress, at least for mice [35–37]. More than two decades ago, Boranic and Poljak-Blazi [35] found that the concentration of hematopoietic progenitors was reduced in mice who were caged in groups of five and more. The investigators of the Arkansas Aging Center found that the concentrations of both myeloid progenitors, CFU-C, and pluripotent progenitors, CFU-S, were reduced in the marrow of older (42 months) mice, but not in younger (6 months) or adult (21 months) animals [36,37]. This study has special interest as it indicates that hematopoietic stress may be felt most at the extreme of an animal's lifespan. Also it was suggested that overcrowding may reflect a form of stress particularly germane to the living conditions of human elderly confined in adult living facilities.

Electric shock may also cause a depletion of hematopoietic elements. Malacrida *et al.* [38] found that the application of electric shock caused a decline in hematopoietic progenitors in rats that were restrained, but not in unrestrained rats, suggesting that restraining and shock were synergistic.

Table 9.1. Experimental and clinical hematopoietic stress that may be utilized for the study of hematopoiesis and aging.

(a) Animal studies

Stress	Animal species	Effects of aging
Sublethal chronic irradiation	Dogs [26]	No effect
	Mice [27,28]	Not studied
Infections and injection of endotoxins	Mice [29]	Decreased mobilization of neutrophils following injection of endotoxins or of *Escherichia coli*
	Rats [30]	Decreased mobilization of neutrophils and increased risk of endotoxic shock
Hypoxia/anoxia	Mice [31]	Increased production and distribution of erythropoietic tissue; effects of aging not studied
Bleeding	Mice [32]	Not studied
Chronic hemolysis	Mice [33]	Not studied
Hypothermia	Mice [34]	Cold reduced the concentration of hematopoietic progenitors; effects of aging not studied
Overcrowding	Mice [35–37]	Overcrowding reduced the concentration of stem cells and early hematopoietic progenitors in older but not in younger mice
Electric shock and immobilization	Rats [38]	Electric shock in combination with immobilization caused a loss of hematopoietic elements in the marrow of rats. If rats were allowed to escape shock, no hematopoietic effects were seen. The effects of age were not studied

(b) Human studies

Stress	Influence of aging
Mobilization of neutrophils and hematopoietic progenitors by hydrocortisone, epinephrine, and growth factors [39–44]	Decreased neutrophil response to hydrocortisone, not significantly decreased response to epinephrine and filgrastim. Decreased response of circulating hematopoietic progenitors to sarmograstim
Mobilization of myelopoietic progenitors (CFU-C) with exercise and ACTH [45]	Effects of aging not studied
Mobilization of CD34+ cells in preparation for autologous stem cell rescue in patients with multiple myeloma [46]	Reduced yield of CD34+ cells in patients aged 70 and older
Erythropoietic response to bleeding [47,48]	Reduced with aging
Infection-related morbidity and mortality [20–25,49]	Increased with age, but in part it may be due to decreased neutrophil functions and to immunosenescence that results in inadequate production of hematopoietic growth factors
Risk of myelotoxicity following cytotoxic chemotherapy [41,50–56]	Increased risk of neutropenia and neutropenic infections over ages 65–70. No clear effects on anemia and thrombocytopenia

If confirmed, this observation may be germane to the condition of many elderly individuals, whose inability to transfer results in chronic restraint, which may exacerbate the effects of environmental insults on hematopoiesis.

Hematopoietic stress in humans

A number of substances that cause neutrophilia may be used to assess the ability of older individuals to mobilize neutrophils or to increase their production [39]. Hydrocortisone stimulates the release of mature neutrophils from the bone marrow, and is used to estimate individual neutrophil reserves; epinephrine reduces the margination of neutrophils and provides a measure of total neutrophil counts; in addition to stimulating the release of mature neutrophils, filgrastim stimulates the proliferation and commitment of myelopoietic progenitors, while sarmograstim increases the concentration of pluripotent hematopoietic progenitors in the circulation by stimulating their proliferation. Chatta *et al.* [39] studied the granulocyte reserve of younger (<30) and older (≥ 70) individuals following hydrocortisone, epinephrine, and filgrastim, and found that the increment of neutrophils following epinephrine and filgrastim was unaffected by age, while the neutrophilic response to hydrocortisone was blunted in the elderly. They concluded that aging did not affect the baseline neutrophil count, nor the ability of hematopoietic progenitors to proliferate and differentiate, but was associated with a reduced reserve of neutrophils, which may explain the increased susceptibility to infections and to infection-related morbidity and mortality. These results are consistent with studies in cancer patients demonstrating that the response to filgrastim is well maintained in the elderly [40–43].

In a study performed more than 20 years ago, Balducci *et al.* [61] showed that protein-calorie malnutrition was associated with reduced granulocytic reserve. It is possible that age-associated sarcopenia may explain in part the reduced granulocyte reserve. Increased circulating levels of cortisone caused either by exercise or by injections of ACTH

may elicit the release of hematopoietic progenitors into the circulating blood [45], but this effect was not studied in the aged. This finding is relevant because age is associated with chronically elevated levels of hormones from the adrenal cortex in the circulation, which may hasten hematopoietic exhaustion. Chatta *et al.* also compared the response of pluripotent progenitors CFU-GM in the circulation of younger and older individuals and found that the baseline concentration of these elements was similar, but the increment following sarmograstim was reduced in the elderly [44]. Based on these results, they concluded that age is associated with a reduced reserve of hematopoietic progenitors, or alternatively with a reduced ability of these elements to respond to growth factors. These possibilities were borne as well by studies of stem cell mobilization and autologous stem cell rescue after high-dose chemotherapy for multiple myeloma [46]. Among more than 800 multiple myeloma patients, 105 of whom were aged 70 and older, the yield of CD34+ cells declined linearly with increasing age, and this decline became more rapid after age 70. Yet age was not a poor prognostic factor for treatment outcome, indicating that the concentration of stem cells, though reduced, was adequate to repopulate the bone marrow.

Following bleeding for blood donation the reticulocyte response was lower in older than in younger individuals, suggesting that the reconstitution of the red blood cell mass may take longer in the elderly [47,48]. The mechanism for this reduced erythropoietic response to bleeding is disputed. Some authors found that the production of erythropoietin may be blunted with aging [47,48,62], while others found it increased [63] and ascribed inadequate erythropoietic response to anemia to reduced concentration of erythropoietic progenitors or to increased resistance of these elements to erythropoietin.

As already stated, the incidence of infection and the risk of mortality from infection increases with age [20–25,49]. The role, if any, of reduced granulocyte reserve and granulocyte production remains unknown. Clearly, reduced neutrophil function is partly responsible for increased incidence and severity of bacterial infections in the elderly, while reduced cellular immunity [49] may be responsible for increased risk and lethality of infections from intracellular organisms [64].

By causing a repetitive destruction of hematopoietic progenitors, cytotoxic anti-neoplastic chemotherapy represents a common form of hematopoietic stress. A number of studies have reported that the incidence and severity of neutropenia and neutropenic infections following cytotoxic chemotherapy increased with patient age [58–56,65]. Morrison *et al.* [50] and Chrischilles *et al.* [51] found that the risk of neutropenic infections for patients with large-cell lymphoma treated with CHOP-like combination chemotherapy were 40–45% for individuals aged 65 and older and less that 20% for the younger ones. These studies are particularly relevant because they encompassed a large number of patients treated in the community and reflect the experience in the general population, not just in the selected population of clinical trials. Bastion *et al.* [52] reported that the risk of neutropenia, infections, and infectious deaths increased after age 69 in lymphoma patients also treated with CTVP, a combination chemotherapy similar to CHOP, while Osby *et al.* [41] reported an incidence of grade 3–4 neutropenia of 91% and a risk of neutropenic infections of 48% among individuals 65 and over treated with CHOP or CNOP. In a review of the experience of the South West Oncology Group (SWOG), Kim *et al.* [53] found that age 65 and over was an independent risk factor for neutropenic infections in patients receiving cytotoxic chemotherapy for different types of malignancies [53], and Crivellari *et al.* [54] reported increased incidence of neutropenia and neutropenic infections for women with breast cancer aged 65 and over treated with adjuvant chemotherapy according to the protocols of the International Breast Cancer Study Group (IBCSG). In a review of multiple oncology practices Lyman *et al.* [55] established that age, performance status, and previous exposure to chemotherapy were independent risk factors for chemotherapy-induced neutropenia and neutropenic infections.

The influence of age on chemotherapy-induced anemia and thrombocytopenia is not as well established and deserves more study.

Purposefully, we have not examined the effects of age on the myelosuppression following treatment of acute myeloid leukemia (AML) [56]. While it is well known that the prognosis of AML is poorer in the elderly, that the risk of neutropenic infection is higher, and that the time to bone-marrow recovery is more prolonged, these results may be due to the fact that older individuals develop a disease that is different from that of younger individuals and the disease, rather than the patient's age, is responsible for reduced hematopoietic reserve.

Discussion

The analysis of both animal and human studies indicates that the hematopoietic reserve, that is the ability to cope with increased lost of peripheral blood elements, may become impaired with age. The best established facts include:

- In rodents, very advanced age is associated with a rapid depletion of hematopoietic progenitors in the presence of overcrowding [35–37].
- Endotoxin injection and experimental septicemia are associated with decreased neutrophil mobilization and increased mortality in older animals [29,30].
- Older humans are less able than young ones to mobilize neutrophils after injection of hydrocortisone and to increase the concentration of hematopoietic progenitors in the circulation after injections of sarmograstim and other growth factors [43,44,46].
- Age is an independent risk factor for chemotherapy-induced neutropenia, neutropenic infections, and infectious mortality in the course of neutropenia [41,50–55,65].

Figure 9.1 illustrates the mechanisms by which the response to hematopoietic stress may be compromised in the aged. Some of these mechanisms may be reversible, including drugs, nutritional deficiency (such as cyanocobalamin and iron deficiency), protein-calorie malnutrition, and acute disease. Irreversible compromise of hematopoiesis

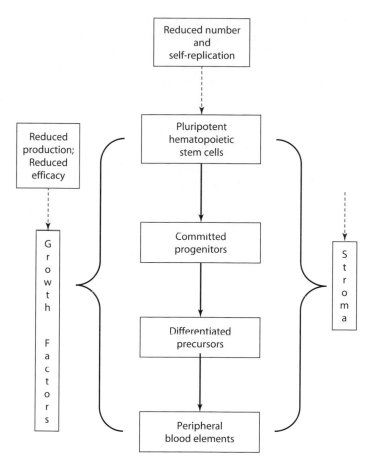

Figure 9.1 Mechanisms by which the hematopoietic reserve may become compromised with aging.

may derive from exposure to cytotoxic agents, such as anti-neoplastic chemotherapy and irradiation, genomic damage to the hematopoietic stem cells as found in myelodysplasia, loss of the ability of the stroma to home hematopoietic progenitors and to produce growth factors. Of special interest is the role of inflammatory cytokines, whose concentration in the circulation increases with age [4], in impairing the hematopoietic response to stress. It is known for example that increased concentrations of interleukin 6 are associated with anemia, decreased production of erythropoietin, decreased response of erythropoietic progenitors to erythropoietin, and increased production of hepcidin, which decreases iron absorption and mobilization (see also Chapter 13) [29,66].

This review also suggests a number of research projects both in experimental animals and in humans. These include the exposure of older animals (or of transgenic animals with accelerated senescence) to well-established forms of hematopoietic stress such as hypothermia, electric shock, restraint, and chronic hemolysis; an investigation of the ability of the aging stroma to home stem cells and to produce growth factors; and a study of the effects of drugs and malnutrition.

In humans a standardized form of clinically assessable hematopoietic stress, such as the response of circulating hematopoietic stem cells to sarmograstim [45] appears desirable, to assess the influence of circulating cytokines and corticosteroids on the response to stress.

REFERENCES

1. Inelmen EM, D'Alessio M, Gatto MR, *et al*. Descriptive analysis of the prevalence of anemia in a randomly selected sample of elderly people living at home: some results of an Italian multicentric study. *Aging (Milano)* 1994; **6**: 81–9.

2. Guralnik JM, Eisenstaedt RS, Ferrucci L, Klein HG, Woodman RC. Prevalence of anemia in persons 65 years and older in the United States: evidence for a high rate of unexplained anemia. *Blood* 2004; **104**: 2263–8.

3. Garry PJ, Goddwin JS, Hunt WC. Iron status and anemia in the elderly: new findings and a review of previous studies. *J Am Geriatr Soc* 1983; **31**: 389–99.

4. Ferrucci L, Corsi A, Lauretani F, *et al*. The origins of age-related proinflammatory state. *Blood* 2005; **105**: 2294–9.

5. Weiss G, Goodnough LT. Anemia of chronic disease. *N Engl J Med* 2005; **352**: 1011–23.

6. Anía BJ, Suman VJ, Fairbanks VF, Rademacher DM, Melton JL. Incidence of anemia in older people: an epidemiologic study in a well defined population. *J Am Geriatr Soc* 1997; **45**: 825–31.

7. Hamerman D. Frailty, cancer cachexia and near death. In Balducci L, Lyman GH, Ershler WB, Extermann M, eds, *Comprehensive Geriatric Oncology*, 2nd edn (London: Taylor and Francis, 2004), 236–49.

8. Lancet JE, Willman CL, Bennett JM. Acute myelogenous leukemia and aging: clinical interactions. *Hematol Oncol Clin North Am* 2000; **16**: 251–67.

9. Globerson A. Hemopoietic stem cells and aging. *Exp Gerontol* 1999; **34**: 137–46.

10. Van Zant G, Liang Y. The role of stem cells in aging. *Exp Hematol* 2003; **31**: 659–72.

11. Van Zant G. Genetic control of stem cells: implications for aging. *Int J Hematol* 2003; **77**: 29–36.

12. Zhang X, Li J, Sejas DP, Pang Q. The ATM/p53/p21 pathway influences cell fate decision between apoptosis and senescence in reoxygenated hematopoietic progenitor cells. *J Biol Chem* 2005; **280**: 19635–40.

13. Ito K, Hirao A, Arai F, *et al*. Regulation of oxidative stress by ATM is required for self-renewal of hemopoietic stem cells. *Nature* 2004; **431**: 997–1002.

14. Stepanova L, Sorrentino BP. A limited role for p16Ink4a and p19Arf in the loss of hematopoietic stem cells during proliferative stress. *Blood* 2005; **106**: 827–32.

15. Spike BT, Dirlam A, Dibling BC, *et al*. The Rb tumor suppressor is required for stress erythropoiesis. *EMBO J* 2004; 23: 4319–29.

16. Spike BT, Macleod KF. The Rb tumor suppressor in stress responses and hemopoietic homeostasis. *Cell Cycle* 2005; **4**: 42–5.

17. Prasher JM, Lalai AS, Heijmans-Antonissen C, *et al*. Reduced hematopoietic reserve in DNA interstrand crosslink repair-deficient Ercc1(-/-)mice. *EMBO J* 2005; **24**: 861–71.

18. Walkley CR, Fero ML, Chien WM, Purton LE, McArthur GA. Negative cell cycle regulators cooperatively control self-renewal and differentiation of haemopoietic stem cells. *Nat Cell Biol* 2005; **7**: 172–8.

19. Henckaerts E, Langer JC, Orenstein J, Snoeck HW. The positive regulatory effect of TGF-beta 2 on primitive human hematopoietic stem and progenitor cells is dependent on age, genetic background, and serum factors. *J Immunol* 2004; **173**: 2486–93.

20. Butcher SK, Killampalli V, Chahal H, Kaya Alpar E, Lord JM. Effect of age on susceptibility to post-traumatic infection in the elderly. *Biochem Soc Trans* 2003; **31**: 449–51.

21. Braga PC, Sala MT, Dal Sasso M, Mancini L, Sandrini MC, Annoni G. Influence of age on oxidative bursts (chemo-illuminescence) of polymorphonuclear neutrophil leukocytes. *Gerontology* 1998; **44**: 192–7.

22. Wenisch C, Patruta S, Daxbock F, Krause R, Horl W. Effect of age on human neutrophil function. *J Leukocyte Biol* 2000; **67**: 40–5.

23. Rossini F. Prognosis of infection in elderly patients with hematological malignancies. *Supp Care Cancer* 1996; **4**: 46–50.

24. Bender BS. Infectious disease risk in the elderly. *Immunol Allergy Clin North Am* 2003; **23**: 57–64.

25. Ruben FL, Dearwater SR, Norden CW, *et al*. Clinical infections in the noninstitutionalized geriatric age groups: methods utilized and incidence of infections: the Pittsburgh Good Health Study. *Am J Epidemiol* 1995; **141**: 145–57.

26. Zaucha GM, Yu C, Mathioudakis G, *et al*. Hematopoietic responses to stress conditions in young dogs comparing with elderly dogs. *Blood* 2001; **98**: 322–7.

27. Seed TM. Hematopoietic tissue repair under chronic low daily irradiation. *Adv Space Res* 1996; **18**: 65–70.

28. Mauch P, Rosenblatt M, Hellman S. Permanent loss in stem cell self-renewal capacity following stress to the marrow. *Blood* 1988; **72**: 1193–6.

29. Baraldi-Junkins CA, Beck AC, Rothstein G. Hematopoiesis and cytokines: relevance to cancer and aging. *Hematol Oncol Clin North Am* 2000; **14**: 45–61.

30. Vollmar B, Pradarutti S, Nickels RM, Menger MD. Age-associated loss of immunomodulatory protection by granulocyte-colony stimulating factor in endotoxic rats. *Shock* 2002; **18**: 348–54.

31. Mide SM, Huygens P, Bozzini CE, Fernandez Pol JA. Effects of human recombinant erythropoietin on differentiation and distribution of erythroid progenitors cells on murine medullary and splenic erythropoiesis during hypoxia and post-hypoxia. *In Vivo* 2001; **15**: 125–32.

32. Godoy HM, Faifer CL, Velazco V. Effects of multiple doses of T2 toxins on the erythroid response capacity of mice following extensive experimental bleeding. *Nat Toxins* 1997; **5**: 152–6.

33. Maggio-Price L, Wolf NS, Priestley GV, Pietrzyk ME, Bernstein SE. Evaluation of stem cell reserve using serial bone marrow transplantation and competitive repopulation in a murine model of chronic hemolytic anemia. *Exp Hematol* 1988; **16**: 653–9.

34. de Souza Queiroz J, Malacrida SA, Justo GZ, Queiroz ML. Myelopoetic response in mice exposed to acute cold/restraint stress. Modulation by Chlorella Vulgaris prophylactic treatment. *Immunopharmacol Immunotoxicol* 2004; **26**: 455–67.

35. Boranic M, Poljak-Blazi M. Effect of the overcrowding stress on hemopoietic colony formation in mice. *Exp Hematol* 1983; **11**: 873–7.

36. Williams LH, Udupa KB, Lipschitz DA: Evaluation of the effect of age on hematopoiesis in the c57bl/6 mouse. *Exp Hematol* 1986; **14**: 827–32.

37. Lipschitz DA. Age-related decline in hemopoietic reserve capacity. *Semin Oncol* 1995; **22** (Suppl 1): 3–6.

38. Malacrida SA, Teixeira NA, Queiroz ML: Hematopoietic changes in rats after inescapable and escapable shocks. *Immunother Immunotoxicol* 1997; **19**: 523–37.

39. Chatta GS, Price TH, Stratton JR, Dale DC. Aging and marrow neutrophil reserves. *J Am Geriatr Soc* 1994; **42**: 77–81.

40. Zinzani PL, Storti S, Zaccaria A, *et al*. Elderly aggressive-histology non-Hodgkin's lymphoma: first-line VNCOP-B regimen experience on 350 patients. *Blood* 1999; **94**: 33–8.

41. Osby E, Hagberg H, Kvaloy S, *et al*. CHOP is superior to CNOP in elderly patients with aggressive lymphoma while outcome is unaffected by filgrastim treatment: results of a Nordic Lymphoma Group randomized trial. *Blood* 2003; **101**: 3840–8.

42. Doorduijn JK, van der Holt B, van der Hem KG, *et al*. Randomized trial of granulocyte-colony stimulating factor (G-CSF) added to CHOP in elderly patients with aggressive non-Hodgkin's lymphoma. *Blood* 2000; **96**: 133a.

43. Chatta DS, Dale DC. Aging and haemopoiesis. Implications for treatment with haemopoietic growth factors. *Drugs Aging* 1996; **9**: 37–47.

44. Chatta GS, Price TH, Allen RC, Dale DC. Effects of in vivo recombinant methionyl human granulocyte colony-stimulating factor on the neutrophil response and peripheral blood colony-forming cells in healthy young and elderly adult volunteers. *Blood* 1994; **84**: 2923–9.

45. Barrett AJ, Longhurst P, Sneath P, Watson JG. Mobilization of CFU-C by exercise and ACTH induced stress in man. *Exp Hematol* 1978; **6**: 590–4.

46. Morris CL, Siegel E, Barlogie B, *et al*. Mobilization of CD34+ cells in elderly patients (≥ 70 years) with multiple myeloma: influence of age, prior therapy, platelet count and mobilization regimen. *Br J Haematol* 2003; **120**: 413–23.

47. Matsuo T, Kario K, Kodoma K, Asada R. An inappropriate erythropoietic response to iron deficiency anaemia in the elderly. *Clin Lab Hematol* 1995; **17**: 317–21.

48. Goodnough LT, Price TH, Parvin CA. The endogenous erythropoietin response and the erythropoietic response to blood loss anemia: the effects of age and gender. *J Lab Clin Med* 1995; **126**: 57–64.

49. Angelis P, Scharf S, Christophidis N. Effects of aging on neutrophil function and its relevance to bacterial infections in the elderly. *J Clin Lab Immunol* 1997; **49**: 33–40.

50. Morrison VA, Picozzi V, Scott S, *et al*. The impact of age on delivered dose-intensity and hospitalizations for febrile neutropenia in patients with intermediate-grade non-Hodgkin's lymphoma receiving initial CHOP chemotherapy: a risk factor analysis. *Clin Lymphoma* 2001; **2**: 47–56.

51. Chrischilles E, Delgado DJ, Stolshek BS, *et al*. Impact of age and colony stimulating factor use in hospital length of stay for febrile neutropenia in CHOP-treated non-Hodgkin's lymphoma patients. *Cancer Control* 2002; **9**: 203–11.

52. Bastion Y, Blay JY, Divine M, *et al*. Elderly patients with aggressive non-Hodgkin's lymphoma: disease presentation, response to treatment and survival. A Groupe d'Etude des Lymphomes de l'Adulte Study on 453 patients older than 69 years. *J Clin Oncol* 1997; **15**: 2945–53.

53. Kim YJ, Rubenstein EB, Rolston KV, *et al*. Colony-stimulating factors (CSFs) may reduce complications

and death in solid tumor patients with fever and neu-tropenia. *Proc ASCO* 2000; **19**: 612a, abstract 2411.

54. Crivellari D, Bonetti M, Castiglione-Gertsch M, *et al.* Burdens and benefits of adjuvant cyclophosphamide, methotrexate and fluorouracil and tamoxifen for eld-erly patients with breast cancer: The international Breast Cancer Study Group Trial vii. *J Clin Oncol* 2000; **18**: 1412–22.

55. Lyman GH, Morrison VA, Dale DC, *et al.* Risk of febrile neutropenia among patients with intermediate-grade non-Hodgkin's lymphoma receiving CHOP chemo-therapy. *Leuk Lymphoma* 2003; **44**: 2069–76.

56. Buchner T. Acute myelogenous leukemia. In Balducci L, Lyman GH, Ershler WB, Extermann M, eds, *Comprehensive Geriatric Oncology*, 2nd edn (London: Taylor and Francis, 2004), 109–34.

57. Lee MA, Segal GM, Bagby JC. The hematopoietic microenvironment in the elderly: defects in IL-1 induced CSF expression in vitro. *Exp Hematol* 1989; 17: 952–6.

58. Kumagai T, Morimoto K, Saitoh T, Tsuboi I, Aikawa S, Horie T. Age-related changes in myelopoietic response to lipopolysaccaride in senescence-accelerated mice. *Mech Ageing Dev* 2000; **112**: 153–7.

59. Cai NS, Li DD, Cheung HT, Richardson A. The expres-sion of granulocyte/macrophage colony-stimulating factor in activated mouse lymphocytes declines with age. *Cell Immunol* 1990; **130**: 311–19.

60. Duthie EH, Physiology of aging: relevance to symp-toms, perceptions, and treatment tolerance. In Balducci L, Lyman GH, Ershler WB, Extermann M, eds, *Comprehensive Geriatric Oncology*, 2nd edn (London: Taylor and Francis, 2004), 207–22.

61. Balducci L, Little DD, Glover NG, Hardy CS, Steinberg MH. Granulocyte reserve in cancer and malnutrition. *Ann Intern Med* 1983; **98**: 610–11.

62. Artz AS, Fergusson D, Drinka PJ, *et al.* Prevalence of anemia in skilled nursing home resident. *Arch Gerontol Geriatr* 2004; **39**: 201–6.

63. Woodman R, Ferrucci L, Guralnik J. Anemia in older adults. *Curr Opin Hematol* 2005; **12**: 123–8.

64. Burns E, Goodwin JS. Immunological changes of aging. In Balducci L, Lyman GH, Ershler WB, Extermann M, eds, *Comprehensive Geriatric Oncology*, 2nd edn (London: Taylor and Francis, 2004), 158–70.

65. Balducci L, Hardy CL, Lyman GH. Hemopoiesis and aging. In Balducci L, Extermann M, eds, *Biological Basis of Geriatric Oncology* (New York, NY: Springer, 2005), 553–60.

66. Rothstein G. Disordered hematopoiesis and myelodys-plasia in the elderly. *J Am Geriatr Soc* 2003; **51** (Suppl 3): S22–S26.

10

Immunoglobulin response and aging

Yuping Deng, Stefan Gravenstein

Introduction

Structure, classes, and functions of immunoglobulins

Immunoglobulins (Igs) are a group of structurally similar proteins produced exclusively by plasma B cells in response to an immunogen – such as a vaccine – and which function as antibodies. Igs are a major serum component, comprising more than 20% of the total plasma proteins. The basic unit of Igs contains two heavy chains (molecular weight of 50–70 kD each) and two light chains (about 23 kD each), forming a "Y" shape, with the light chains attaching to both arms of the Y. The top areas of the arms, termed the variable region, are highly variable and contain the binding domain specific to an antigenic area (antigenic domain) on the immunogen.

It is estimated that there are up to 10^{11} different Igs in the Ig repertoire. This Ig diversity is achieved mainly by gene rearrangement of Ig genes in B cells.

There are five different classes of Ig in human blood, corresponding to the five different classes of Ig heavy chains γ (IgG), α (IgA), μ (IgM), δ (IgD), and ε (IgE). Any one of these heavy chains can pair with two different light chains, κ and λ. Details of these Ig classes, together with their functions, can be found in Table 10.1.

Through direct binding to microbial particles, Igs can neutralize the microbial infectivity, protecting and helping the host to recover. In addition, the binding of Igs can also induce other immunological events, such as killing microbial or infected cells, via NK-cell activation or complement fixation pathways. Many immune cells, including macrophages, platelets, mast cells, and basophils, have Ig receptors.

Table 10.1. Properties of selected classes of immunoglobulins.

Class	Formation	Half-life	Serum concentration (mg/ml)	Function
IgG	Monomer	21 days	0.5–10	Protective and autoimmunity
IgA	Monomer or dimer	7 days	0.05–3	Mucosal immunity
IgM	Pentamer	7 days	1.5	Early immune response
IgD	Monomer (membrane-bound)	2 days	0.03	Activating B cells
IgE	Monomer	2 days	0.0005	Allergic reaction via activating neutrophil and mast cells

Blood Disorders in the Elderly, ed. Lodovico Balducci, William Ershler, Giovanni de Gaetano.
Published by Cambridge University Press. © Cambridge University Press 2008.

Ig-cell receptor binding leads to cell activation and other downstream events. Evidently, Igs play a critical role in the immune response to pathogenic infection and provide protective immunity in response to vaccination. Igs are also involved in the pathogenesis of autoimmune diseases.

Antibody-secreting B cells: origin, lineage, activation, and survival

Antibody-secreting B cells (ASC) are derived from naive B cells which originate in bone marrow. After encountering antigens via the membrane-bound Ig, B cells are activated. With the help of T cells, activated B cells become plasma blast cells that secrete Igs. Some plasma cells are activated in the germinal center (GC), where B cells go through somatic hypermutation leading to the production of high-affinity antibody. In GC, B cells are stimulated by antigens in the form of immune complexes and by costimulatory molecules highly expressed by follicular dendritic cells. Some plasma blast cells then become memory plasma cells, which mostly remain in the bone marrow. In mice, long-lived plasma cells can maintain specific serum antibody levels for the animal's lifetime [1,2]. In the case of people, researchers still debate whether long-lived plasma cells can survive for a lifetime or whether they have a defined half-life, a situation in which their constant replacement is needed at a low rate if antibody levels are to be maintained. There are two lineages of B cells, B1 and B2. B1 cells produce mostly IgM, IgG3, and IgA, with low binding affinity, and thus B1 activation is considered to be a part of the innate immune response. B2 cells produce Igs with high affinity and are considered important for the adaptive immune response.

An overview of the age-related changes in serum immunoglobulins

Igs are present in newborns before infants are faced with any microbial challenge. This is due in part to antibody production from B1 lineage, and in part also to passage from the mother through the placenta, colostrum, and milk. After a drop in the first few months, the Ig levels increase slowly until adulthood, during which they remain relatively stable. Abnormal elevations in Igs have been observed in elderly people, and in patients with autoimmune diseases [3].

Immunoglobulin response and aging

Immunoglobulin response to infections and vaccines

Aging in people is associated with increased incidences of infectious diseases. Infections or reactivation of viral pathogens such as influenza, respiratory syncytial virus (RSV), and herpes zoster are more prominent in elderly people than in their younger counterparts [4,5]. Elderly individuals also experience a higher incidence of bacterial infections such as tuberculosis and pneumococcal pneumonia [6]. In addition to the increase in incidence, elderly people also have greater morbidity and mortality from infectious diseases. Hospitalization due to infection is much more common in older than in younger adults or children. Because antibodies play an important role in preventing and combating infections, the age-related increase in incidence and morbidity and mortality from the infectious diseases suggests that there might be an age-related impaired Ig response to infectious pathogens.

In 1929, Thomsen and Kettel first reported that humoral immunity was affected by aging [7]. These authors reported that the titer of natural serum antibodies to the A and B erythrocyte antigens (isoagglutinins) declined with age. Forty years later, the serum concentration of another natural antibody specific for a foreign antigen, *Salmonella* flagellin, was also reported to decline with age [8]. More direct evidence of the age-related decline in Ig production comes from clinical studies of antibody response to vaccines. Antibody response to virtually all foreign protein, including vaccines against encephalitis, hepatitis, influenza, salmonella, and tetanus toxoid, is lower in older than in younger adults [9]. The decline in Ig reflects not only quantitative but qualitative changes. For instance, sera from elderly patients immunized with pneumococcal vaccine contained high levels of anti-polysaccharide and anti-phosphorylcholine (PC) antibodies (a major epitope on the surface of pneumococcal bacilli), but the antibodies failed to opsonize (kill) pneumococci [10]. The age-related qualitative decline in Ig was also demonstrated in animal studies [11]. In this study, it was demonstrated that purified anti-PC antibody produced by young mice provided better protection than the same amount from old mice, when recipient mice were challenged with a lethal dose of pneumococci.

Age-related decline in Ig production to influenza vaccination

Influenza and pneumonia is the fifth leading cause of death among people aged over 65 years. Influenza also leads as an important cause of catastrophic disability, greatly affecting the quality of life of elderly persons [12,13]. In the USA alone, an estimated $10 billion is spent annually due to the impact of influenza [14]. Thus, influenza vaccination is recommended for elderly adults. Although it is cost-effective [14], influenza vaccination only prevents infection in 30–40% in those aged over 65, compared to 70–90% in those under 65 [15]. It is believed that an age-related decline in antibody response is accountable for the age-reduced vaccine efficacy in elderly people.

The most commonly used influenza vaccine for elderly people is the trivalent inactivated vaccine (TIV) comprising viral subunits from three different influenza strains, A/H3N2, A/H1N1, and influenza B. Compared to healthy young subjects, healthy elderly subjects typically have less antibody response to A/H1N1, and to influenza B in some cases. By contrast, antibody responses to the influenza A/H3N2 strains were comparable between the two age groups [16–18]. These observations have been reported by several independent groups [19,20, Deng *et al.* unpublished]. The reduced antibody response was evident when the antibodies were measured by hemagglutination-inhibition analysis (HIA) or by IgG ELISA [16–18]. In one of the studies, one group of elderly subjects failed to produce antibody to the A/H1N1 vaccine strain, although HI antibody was formed to the closely related A/Singapore/6/86 H1N1 strain, not contained in the vaccine [16]. The antibody produced by this group of elderly also neutralized A/Taiwan/1/86-induced viral cytotoxicity in vitro. Interestingly and unexpectedly, the IgA responses to the H3N2 vaccine strain were higher in the older than in the younger participants [16]. Therefore, the age-related immune-response change appears to be related to influenza strain.

The mechanism for the age-related decline in the Ig response to specific vaccine strains remains poorly understood. Experiments using the ELISA platform for antibody specificity and titer suggest that the age-related decline is confined to the IgG class [16] and IgG1 subtype [21]. It is suggested that the observed age-related differences in antibody responses to A/H1N1 strains are probably not due to aging of the immune system itself, but are determined by differences in immune priming [19,22,23]. Age provides the time-opportunity for A/H1N1 exposure (i.e., greater number of influenza seasons experienced in which to have become infected), leaving older people with a greater likelihood to have experienced a natural A/H1N1 infection than younger ones. Thus age, rather than immunosenescence per se, could skew the specificity of the antibody response through prior priming in life toward antibodies that are directed to the priming virus, thereby producing a reduced Ig response to the vaccine strain of A/H1N1. Nevertheless, the reduction in vaccine-specific response to A/H1N1 may still reflect an immunosenescent marker, although priming provides an alternative, perhaps less dire, explanation. As for the A/H3N2 strain, it is assumed that both elderly and young people have similar exposure history, as this virus, unlike the A/H1N1, is in wide circulation during most seasons. Because influenza vaccination occurs as an annual event, the accumulative effect of repeated vaccination has also been implicated for differences observed between healthy young and healthy elderly subjects. The general consensus has remained that repeated vaccination does not contribute to the observed age-related decline in the vaccine response [18].

The qualitative difference in Ig response with age is also observed in response to influenza vaccination. The IgA to the A/H1N1 strain in the elderly has a significantly lower avidity index than that of younger subjects [18].

The health status of older people also influences the outcome of the antibody response to influenza vaccination. Elderly patients with reduced function as measured by activities of daily living (ADL) had lower Ig response to all influenza vaccine antigens [24]. When health status was instead assessed by Chronic Health Evaluation score, influenza vaccine Ig response was reduced against only one vaccine component [25].

Over the years, scientists have tested several strategies to improve the antibody response in late life, including increasing the vaccine dose, with the addition of adjuvants, or through protein conjugation. In general, a higher dose does improve the Ig response (at the expense of greater reactogenicity). For example [26], at a $10\,\mu$g dose, IgG, IgG1, and HI responses were twofold lower in the elderly than in young volunteers. A $20\,\mu$g dose increased the IgG, IgG1, and HI levels in the elderly to that in the young adults at the $10\,\mu$g dose, while the IgA1 rose to significantly higher levels than in the young. A $60\,\mu$g dose increased antibody levels in the young but did not further increase the response in the elderly participants. In one of the studies where vaccine adjuvants were evaluated, thymosin alpha one or placebo was given twice weekly, beginning with vaccination, over four weeks [27]. HI responses were significantly higher in the group receiving the thymic peptide. Also, Ig responses to influenza vaccine were increased as measured by neutralization and HIA assays where influenza vaccines were conjugated with diphtheria toxoid [28].

Mechanisms for the age-related decline in immunoglobulin production in response to immunologic challenge

Immune system overview

Because Igs are an integral component of the immune system, an overview of the immune system and how

aging impacts the system are discussed briefly below. The immune system can be divided into innate and adaptive components. The innate immunity, through macrophages, dendritic cells, and NK cells, functions as the first line of defense against infections. Adaptive immunity consists of antibody-mediated humoral immunity and cell-mediated immunity (CMI) driven by T cells. Innate immunity is non-specific and thus often inadequate for eliminating microbial invasions. This innate immunity is mostly mediated by a set of toll-like receptors (TLRs) recognizing pathogen-associated molecular patterns (PAMPs) [29,30]. The recognition of pathogens by TLRs triggers a series of events leading to the activation of macrophages and dendritic cells and their secretion of pro-inflammatory cytokines such as TNF-α and type-I interferons [30]. These events, together with the antigen processing and presentation to T and B cells, lead to the downstream activation of the adapted immunity, transitioning the non-specific innate response to a highly specific and efficient one. The innate and adaptive immunity, including the humoral and CMI, are interrelated and function together to fight off infection. For example, although antibodies are secreted exclusively by B cells, T cells play a pivotal role in providing "helps" to B cells via cytokine secretion and cell–cell contact, critical for the differentiation from naive B cells to mature ASC.

Age-related changes in the immune system

Aging has a profound negative impact on the immune system as a whole, while the degree of impact on particular immune cell populations varies. How aging affects the cell populations involved in innate immunity remains relatively less well understood than those of the adaptive T- and B-cell populations. NK cells increase in numbers and in frequency, while cellular function, particularly the cytotoxicity function, declines with age [31]. Emerging evidence indicates that aging coincides with a decline in plasmacytoid dendritic cells [32, Deng *et al.* unpublished]. The most obvious effect of aging on the immune system can be found in T-cell populations. As a result of thymic involution, elderly people and experimental animals have fewer naive T cells and more memory T cells. Moreover, T cells from elderly individuals and aged animals have reduced cellular function compared to their younger counterparts. Both naive and memory T cells from older donors proliferate less and secrete less interleukin 2 and other cytokines in response to stimulation. Aging is also associated with a shift from type 1 to type 2 cytokine production, roughly corresponding to relative type 1 and 2 helper cell activity, respectively. Type 1 cytokines promote CMI while type 2 cytokines facilitate the humoral response. It is still not clear if some of the age-related changes in B cells are due to the impact of aging directly or an indirect consequence of the age-related changes in T cells. However, aging is associated with a decline in the quantity and quality of antibody production to immunological challenge, while the levels of autoantibody increase with age. For more information on the age-related changes of the immune system, please see book chapters by Miller [33] and Murasko & Gardner [34]. Mechanisms underlying these age-related changes in Ig response are also discussed below.

Three schools of thought on the age-related decline in antibody response to foreign antigens

Currently there are three competing schools of thought on the dominant mechanism leading to the age-related decline in antibody production in response to foreign antigens. These lines of thinking have attributed the age-related difference in Ig production to upstream effects of T-cell, B-cell, and follicular dendritic cell (FDC) populations, respectively. Despite the different emphases, these three different points of views are not mutually exclusive.

One line of thinking attributes much of the age-related decline in Ig production to T-cell changes [35]. More specifically, proponents of this theory argue that the age-related decline in Ig production reflects repertoire changes in B cells as a function of T-cell senescence. Experiments supporting this view show that the impaired process of somatic

hypermutation (a process leading to the production of Igs with high affinity) in aged mice can be restored, at least in part, by replacing the T-helper cells of old mice with those from young mice [36]. Hirokawa *et al.* restored antibody levels to those of young mice by transplanting young thymus but not old thymus tissue into young irradiated mice [37]. Later, Szewczuk *et al.* employed transfer studies to demonstrate that the production of high-affinity antibodies correlates inversely with the age of the thymocyte donor [38]. Only those irradiated mice given syngeneic fetal liver cells with thymocytes from 2- to 4-month-old but not with thymocytes from 12- to 24-month-old mice generated high-affinity antibodies.

The second dominant theory to explain the age-related decline in Ig production blames intrinsic defects in B cells, and is bolstered by evidence derived from both aged animals and people [39]. Frasca *et al.* demonstrated that intrinsic changes in B cells developing with age can have a significant impact on antibody production [40]. The ability to undergo class switch recombination (CSR) in aged stimulated B cells is significantly reduced with age, and this has been attributed to the impaired induction of E47, a transcription factor encoded by the *E2A* gene [41,42]. Further studies show that the mRNA levels of the *E2A*-encoded transcripts are lower in activated splenic B cells from old mice than in those from young mice [43]. This difference has been ascribed to higher rates of decay of the *E2A* mRNA in old B cells [43].

The remaining school of thought attributes the bulk of age-related defects in Igs to changes in FDCs [44]. This theory argues against B- and T-cell senescence contributing prominently to the age-related decline in Ig response. Its proponents suggest that neither B nor T cells from aged hosts are limiting factors for three major reasons. First, J11D^{lo} cells – the precursors of GC B memory cells – do not appear to be altered by aging and respond to T-dependent antigen stimulation as vigorously as young B memory cells [45]. Second, when aged B cells were adoptively transferred into young recipient mice, they produced equivalent levels of antigen-specific antibody that underwent affinity maturation and isotype switching [46]. And, third, in in-vitro experiments using antigen-primed old T cells and young memory B cells and young FDCs, the old T cells (22 months) functioned similarly to young T cells, and T-cell help did not appear to be a limiting factor over a broad range of T–B cell ratios [44]. Furthermore, there is evidence supporting the role of FDCs as the most critical causal factor for the age-related decline in Ig response. First, aging leads to FDC atrophy and a reduced number of germinal centers. More importantly, in in-vitro experiments where B cells, T cells, and FDCs from old or young mice were tested, FDCs seemed to be the only limiting factor accountable for the age-related decline in Ig production [44].

Age-related increase in autoantibodies

Antibodies that react with self-antigens are called autoantibodies. Aging in people is associated with an increase in autoantibodies [47]. Autoantibodies can be divided into two groups: organ-specific autoantibodies that bind to organ-specific antigen such as thyroglobulin, and non-organ-specific autoantibodies specific for self-antigens that are not organ-specific, such as DNA and Igs. The proportion of healthy people with organ-specific autoantibodies increases with age, although this trend is not evident in people above 90 years old [48]. In contrast, non-organ-specific autoantibodies increase throughout life, including among the oldest old.

Aging is associated with an increase in the production of autoantibodies as a by-product of the immune response to vaccinations. Some of the autoantibodies are reactive to the variable region of Ig that reacts to the vaccine antigen, called anti-idiotypic autoantibodies. The age-related increase in autoantibody production coincides with the decreased production of antibodies specific for the vaccine antigens. Immunization of elderly individuals with tetanus toxoid resulted in a greater number of autoantibody-producing lymphocytes than in younger subjects [49]. Similar phenomena are observed in mice. Old mice immunized with sheep

erythrocytes (SRBC) had lower levels of anti-SRBC antibody-forming cells/spleen but higher anti-mouse red blood cell (RBC) autoantibody-forming cells/spleen compared to young mice [50]. This age-associated inversion in the production of antibodies specific for self-antigens and vaccine antigen is called "cross-wiring."

There are several factors explaining the underlying mechanism of the age-related increase in autoantibody, which are related to the age-related decline in the antibody response to foreign antigens: (1) the shift in number and activity from B2 to B1 lymphocytes during aging; (2) an increasing frequency of autoantibody-producing plasma cells; (3) the polyclonal B-cell activation, known to stimulate autoantibody production [47]. These factors can be summarized as the age-related changes in B-cell repertoire, which can be eventually attributed to the thymic dysregulation that occurs with age, the same element responsible for the age-related decrease in antibody response to foreign antigens discussed above. Thymectomy in young mice results in autoantibody formation in all of them. Studies by Crisi *et al.* suggest that the failure of negative thymic selection of T cells reactive with self major histocompatibility complex (MHC) class II molecules contributes to the increase in autoantibody [51]. The age-related increase in Th2 response may also contribute to the age-associated polyclonal B-cell activation [52]. Finally, the host environment itself may stimulate production of autoantibodies. Old mice reconstituted with bone marrow produce higher level of autoantibodies than do young mice reconstituted in the same fashion [53]. Health status also relates to autoantibodies: chronically ill individuals are more likely to have non-organ-specific autoantibodies, which is a risk factor predicting shortened survival.

Although aging is associated with an increase in autoantibody, there is no obvious casual relationship between the presence of autoantibody and autoimmune diseases in elderly people. On the other hand, the presence of high levels of autoantibody may contribute to the age-related decline in antibody response to foreign antigen from the homeostatic point of view, i.e., that the total level of Igs or Ig-producing plasma cells remains constant. Presence of plasma cells for autoantibodies might hinder the expansion and existence of plasma cells specific for foreign antigens [54]. In addition, the presence of anti-idiotypic autoantibodies may also inhibit the antibody response to foreign antigen by binding to the BCR on B cells specific for the foreign antigen. The suppressive role of anti-idiotypic antibody has been demonstrated in a clinical study of tetanus toxoid vaccination. Higher levels of serum anti-idiotypic autoantibodies specific for anti-tetanus toxoid antibodies were found in elderly subjects, correlating with a decreased antibody response to tetanus toxoid [55].

ACKNOWLEDGEMENTS

We thank Dr. Nianyong Chen for assisting in the literature search. This work is funded in part by the National Institutes of Health, R2158004.

REFERENCES

1. Slifka MK, Antia R, Whitmire JK, Ahmed R. Humoral immunity due to long-lived plasma cells. *Immunity* 1998; **8**: 363–72.

2. Manz RA, Thiel A, Radbruch A. Lifetime of plasma cells in the bone marrow. *Nature* 1997; **388**: 133–4.

3. Manz RA, Hauser AE, Hiepe F, Radbruch A. Maintenance of serum antibody levels. *Annu Rev Immunol* 2005; **23**: 367–86.

4. Bender BS. Infectious disease risk in the elderly. *Immunol Allergy Clin North Am* 2003; **23**: 57–64.

5. Nicholson KG, Kent J, Hammersley V, Cancio E. Acute viral infections of upper respiratory tract in elderly people living in the community: comparative, prospective, population based study of disease burden. *BMJ* 1997; **315**: 1060–4.

6. Ginaldi L, Loreto MF, Corsi MP, Modesti M, De Martinis M. Immunosenescence and infectious diseases. *Microbes Infect* 2001; **3**: 851–7.

7. Thomsen O, Kettel K. Die starke der menchlichen Isoagglutinine und entsperchenden Blutkorperchenrezeptoren in verchiende Leb ensaltern, *Z Immunitatsforsch* 1929; **63**: 67.

8. Rowley MJ, Buchanan H, Mackay IR. Reciprocal change with age in antibody to extrinsic and intrinsic antigens. *Lancet* 1968; **2**: 24–6.

9. Schwab R, Walters CA, Weksler ME. Host defense mechanisms and aging. *Semin Oncol* 1989; **16**: 20–7.

10. Musher DM, Chapman AJ, Goree A, Jonsson S, Briles D, Baughn RE. Natural and vaccine-related immunity to *Streptococcus pneumoniae*. *J Infect Dis* 1986; **154**: 245–56.

11. Nicoletti C, Yang X, Cerny J. Repertoire diversity of antibody response to bacterial antigens in aged mice. III. Phosphorylcholine antibody from young and aged mice differ in structure and protective activity against infection with *Streptococcus pneumoniae*. *J Immunol* 1993; **150**: 543–9.

12. Gross PA, Hermogenes AW, Sacks HS, Lau J, Levandowski RA. The efficacy of influenza vaccine in elderly persons. A meta-analysis and review of the literature. *Ann Intern Med* 1995; **123**: 518–27.

13. Thompson WW, Shay DK, Weintraub E, *et al.* Mortality associated with influenza and respiratory syncytial virus in the United States. *JAMA* 2003; **289**: 179–86.

14. Nichol KL, Margolis KL, Wuorenma J, Von Sternberg T. The efficacy and cost effectiveness of vaccination against influenza among elderly persons living in the community. *N Engl J Med* 1994; **331**: 778–84.

15. Falsey AR, Cunningham CK, Barker WH, *et al.* Respiratory syncytial virus and influenza A infections in the hospitalized elderly. *J Infect Dis* 1995; **172**: 389–94.

16. Remarque EJ, de Bruijn IA, Boersma WJ, Masurel N, Ligthart GJ. Altered antibody response to influenza H1N1 vaccine in healthy elderly people as determined by HI, ELISA, and neutralization assay. *J Med Virol* 1998; **55**: 82–7.

17. de Bruijn IA, Remarque EJ, Beyer WE, le Cessie S, Masurel N, Ligthart GJ. Annually repeated influenza vaccination improves humoral responses to several influenza virus strains in healthy elderly. *Vaccine* 1997; **15**: 1323–9.

18. de Bruijn IA, Remarque EJ, Jol-van der Zijde CM, van Tol MJ, Westendorp RG, Knook DL. Quality and quantity of the humoral immune response in healthy elderly and young subjects after annually repeated influenza vaccination. *J Infect Dis* 1999; **179**: 31–6.

19. McElhaney JE, Meneilly GS, Lechelt KE, Beattie BL, Bleackley RC. Antibody response to whole-virus and split-virus influenza vaccines in successful ageing. *Vaccine* 1993; **11**: 1055–60.

20. Powers DC, Belshe RB. Effect of age on cytotoxic T lymphocyte memory as well as serum and local antibody responses elicited by inactivated influenza virus vaccine. *J Infect Dis* 1993; **167**: 584–92.
21. Deng Y, Jing Y, Campbell AE, Gravenstein S. Age-related impaired type 1 T cell responses to influenza: reduced activation ex vivo, decreased expansion in CTL culture in vitro, and blunted response to influenza vaccination in vivo in the elderly. *J Immunol* 2004; **172**: 3437–46.
22. Hennessy AV, Davenport FM. 1958. Epidemiologic implications of the distribution by age of antibody response to experimental influenza virus vaccines. *J Immunol* 1958; **80**: 114–21.
23. Pyhala R, Kinnunen L, Kumpulainen V, Ikonen N, Kleemola M, Cantell K. Vaccination-induced HI antibody to influenza A(H1N1) viruses in poorly primed adults under circumstances of low antigenic drift. *Vaccine* 1993; **11**: 1013–17.
24. Remarque EJ, Nijhuis EW, Hinloopen B, Nagelkerken L, van der Velde EA, Ligthart GJ. Correlation between the antibody response to influenza vaccine and helper T cell subsets in healthy aging. *Vaccine* 1996; **14**: 127–30.
25. Gross PA, Quinnan GV Jr, Weksler ME, Setia U, Douglas RG Jr. Relation of chronic disease and immune response to influenza vaccine in the elderly. *Vaccine* 1989; **7**: 303–8.
26. Remarque EJ, van Beek WC, Ligthart GJ, *et al.* Improvement of the immunoglobulin subclass response to influenza vaccine in elderly nursing-home residents by the use of high-dose vaccines. *Vaccine* 1993; **11**: 649–54.
27. Gravenstein S, Duthie EH, Miller BA, *et al.* Augmentation of influenza antibody response in elderly men by thymosin alpha one: a double-blind placebo-controlled clinical study. *J Am Geriatr Soc* 1989; **37**: 1–8.
28. Gravenstein S, Drinka P, Duthie EH, *et al.* Efficacy of an influenza hemagglutinin-diphtheria toxoid conjugate vaccine in elderly nursing home subjects during an influenza outbreak. *J Am Geriatr Soc* 1994; **42**: 245–51.
29. Kopp E, Medzhitov R. Recognition of microbial infection by Toll-like receptors. *Curr Opin Immunol* 2003; **15**: 396–401.
30. Beutler B. The Toll-like receptors: analysis by forward genetic methods. *Immunogenetics* 2005; **57**: 385–92.
31. Kutza J, Murasko DM. Effects of aging on natural killer cell activity and activation by interleukin-2 and IFN-alpha. *Cell Immunol* 1994; **155**: 195–204.
32. Shodell M, Siegal FP. Circulating, interferon-producing plasmacytoid dendritic cells decline during human ageing. *Scand J Immunol* 2002; **56**: 518–21.
33. Miller R. *Fundamental Immunology, Aging and Immune Function* (New York, NY: Lippincott-Raven, 1998).
34. Murasko D, Gardner M. Immunology of aging. In Hazzard WR, ed, *Principles of Geriatric Medicine and Gerontology* (New York: McGraw-Hill, 2003), 35–52.
35. Song H, Price PW, Cerny J. Age-related changes in antibody repertoire: contribution from T cells. *Immunol Rev* 1997; **160**: 55–62.
36. Yang X, Stedra J, Cerny J. Relative contribution of T and B cells to hypermutation and selection of the antibody repertoire in germinal centers of aged mice. *J Exp Med* 1996; **183**: 959–70.
37. Hirokawa K, Albright JW, Makinodan T. Restoration of impaired immune functions in aging animals. II. Effect of syngeneic thymus and bone marrow grafts. *Clin Immunol Immunopathol* 1976; **5**: 371–6.
38. Szewczuk MR, DeKruyff RH, Goidl EA, Weksler ME, Siskind GW. Ontogeny of B lymphocyte function. VIII. Failure of thymus cells from aged donors to induce the functional maturation of B lymphocytes from immature donors. *Eur J Immunol* 1980; **10**: 918–23.
39. Frasca D, Riley RL, Blomberg BB. Humoral immune response and B-cell functions including immunoglobulin class switch are downregulated in aged mice and humans. *Semin Immunol* 2005; **17**: 378–84.
40. Frasca D, Van der Put E, Riley RL, Blomberg BB. Reduced Ig class switch in aged mice correlates with decreased E47 and activation-induced cytidine deaminase. *J Immunol* 2004; **172**: 2155–62.
41. Frasca D, Van Der Put E, Riley RL, Blomberg BB. Age-related differences in the E2A-encoded transcription factor E47 in bone marrow-derived B cell precursors and in splenic B cells. *Exp Gerontol* 2004; **39**: 481–9.
42. Riley RL, Blomberg BB, Frasca D. B cells, E2A, and aging. *Immunol Rev* 2005; **205**: 30–47.
43. Frasca D, Van der Put E, Landin AM, Gong D, Riley RL, Blomberg BB. RNA stability of the E2A-encoded transcription factor E47 is lower in splenic activated B cells from aged mice. *J Immunol* 2005; **175**: 6633–44.
44. Aydar Y, Balogh P, Tew JG, Szakal AK. Follicular dendritic cells in aging, a "bottle-neck" in the humoral immune response. *Ageing Res Rev* 2004; **3**: 15–29.
45. Linton PJ. The status of progenitors of memory B cells in aged mice. *Aging Immunol Infect Dis* 1993; **4**: 35–46.

46. Dailey RW, Eun SY, Russell CE, Vogel LA. B cells of aged mice show decreased expansion in response to antigen, but are normal in effector function. *Cell Immunol* 2001; **214**: 99–109.

47. Weksler ME. Changes in the B-cell repertoire with age. *Vaccine* 2000; **18**: 1624–8.

48. Hallgren HM, Buckley CE 3rd, Gilbertsen VA, Yunis EJ. Lymphocyte phytohemagglutinin responsiveness, immunoglobulins and autoantibodies in aging humans. *J Immunol* 1973; **111**: 1101–7.

49. Welch MJ, Fong S, Vaughan J, Carson D. Increased frequency of rheumatoid factor precursor B lymphocytes after immunization of normal adults with tetanus toxoid. *Clin Exp Immunol* 1983; **51**: 299–304.

50. Bovbjerg DH, Kim YT, Schwab R, Schmitt K, DeBlasio T, Weksler ME. "Cross-wiring" of the immune response in old mice: increased autoantibody response despite reduced antibody response to nominal antigen. *Cell Immunol* 1991; **135**: 519–25.

51. Crisi GM, Tsiagbe VK, Russo C, Basch RS, Thorbecke GJ. Evaluation of presence and functional activity of potentially self-reactive T cells in aged mice. *Int Immunol* 1996; **8**: 387–95.

52. Kirman I, Zhao K, Tschepen I, *et al.* Treatment of old mice with IL-2 corrects dysregulated IL-2 and IL-4 production. *Int Immunol* 1996; **8**: 1009–15.

53. Doria G, Mancini C, Utsuyama M, Frasca D, Hirokawa K. Aging of the recipients but not of the bone marrow donors enhances autoimmunity in syngeneic radiation chimeras. Mech Ageing Dev 1997; **95**: 131–42.

54. Weksler ME, Goodhardt M. Do age-associated changes in "physiologic" autoantibodies contribute to infection, atherosclerosis, and Alzheimer's disease? *Exp Gerontol* 2002; **37**: 971–9.

55. Arreaza EE, Gibbons JJ Jr, Siskind GW, Weksler ME. Lower antibody response to tetanus toxoid associated with higher auto-anti-idiotypic antibody in old compared with young humans. *Clin Exp Immunol* 1993; **92**: 169–73.

11

Biological and clinical significance of monoclonal gammopathy

Arati V. Rao, Harvey Jay Cohen

Introduction

Monoclonal gammopathy of unknown significance (MGUS) affects up to 2% of persons aged 50 years or over, and about 3% of those older than 70 years. The aim of this chapter is to highlight some of the features of this disease process and its relationship to aging. It will focus on (1) epidemiology, (2) biology of MGUS and the role of various cytokines in the pathophysiology, (3) correlation of the biology of MGUS with aging, (4) diagnosis and follow-up of patients with MGUS, and (5) natural history and predictors of progression in patients with MGUS.

Epidemiology

The monoclonal gammopathies are a group of disorders associated with proliferation of a single clone (monoclonal) of plasma cells. They are characterized by the secretion of an immunologically homogenous monoclonal protein (M-protein, M-component, M-spike, or paraprotein). Each M-protein consists of two heavy (H) polypeptide chains of the same class and subclass, and two light (L) chains of the same type. The heavy chains are IgG, IgM, IgA, IgD, and IgE, while the light-chain types are kappa (κ), and lambda (λ). In contrast, a polyclonal gammopathy is characterized by an increase in one or more heavy chains, and in both types of light chains, and is usually associated with an inflammatory or reactive process [1]. The term monoclonal gammopathy of unknown significance (MGUS) was first coined by

Kyle *et al.*, to replace the term benign monoclonal gammopathy, which was misleading because, at diagnosis, it is not known if the disease process will remain stable and asymptomatic, or evolve into symptomatic multiple myeloma (MM) [2].

The International Myeloma Working Group has defined MGUS as the presence of a monoclonal protein in patients without the evidence of multiple myeloma, amyloidosis, Waldenström macroglobulinemia (WM), or any other B-cell lymphoproliferative disorder. More specifically it is defined as an M-spike of $<3.0\,g/dL$ or trace or no light chains in a 24-hour urine collection, less than 10% plasma cells in the bone marrow, and no related organ or tissue impairment, i.e., no lytic bone lesions, and the absence of anemia, hypercalcemia, and renal insufficiency [1]. As for most cancers, especially hematologic malignancies, this condition demonstrates an increased incidence with age and affects up to 2% of persons $\geqslant 50$ years and about 3% of those older than 70 years [3]. A screening study conducted in Sweden demonstrated MGUS in 0.1–0.2% of persons aged 30–49 years, 1.1–2.0% of persons 50–79 years, and in 5.7% of persons 80–89 years [4]. In a cluster of cases of MM, Kyle *et al.* were able to detect an M-protein in 15 of 1200 persons 50 years or older (1.25%) [3], and in France, 303 of 17 968 persons 50 years or older (1.7%) had an M-protein [5]. Crawford *et al.* have reported that 10% of 111 persons older than 80 years had an M-protein ranging in concentration from 0.2 to 1.8 g/dL [6]. This has also been reiterated by Cohen *et al.*, who found that 3.6% of 816 persons 70 years or older had an M-protein [7]. As with

Blood Disorders in the Elderly, ed. Lodovico Balducci, William Ershler, Giovanni de Gaetano. Published by Cambridge University Press. © Cambridge University Press 2008.

MM, the incidence of MGUS is higher in African–Americans than in whites, and in one study the prevalence of an M-protein was 8.4% in 916 African–Americans [7]. In contrast, the incidence of MGUS is only about 2.7% in elderly Japanese patients [8]. The monoclonal protein in MGUS is most commonly IgG (73%), followed by IgM (14%) and IgA (11%). The light chains in MGUS most commonly involve the κ molecules (62%) [9].

MGUS is frequently a single abnormality, but it may be associated with many other diseases, as would be expected in the elderly populations. Most common associations have been with the B-cell lymphoproliferative disorders like chronic lymphocytic leukemia, non-Hodgkin lymphoma, and hairy-cell leukemia [10]. One prospective study showed that MGUS was detected in 1.1% of patients with solid tumors referred for systemic chemotherapy [11]. A third of patients with chronic neutrophilic leukemia, which is a rare disorder characterized by persistent leukocytosis of mature neutrophils, have an elevated M-protein [12]. It has also been seen in Gaucher's disease [13], myelofibrosis, hepatitis C infection, HIV infection [14], rheumatoid arthritis [15], and other related disorders. Interestingly, MGUS has been observed after liver, renal, and bone-marrow transplantation, and in these patients the development of an M-protein correlated with the presence of a viral infection, e.g., cytomegalovirus infection [16,17].

The gammopathies can be further classified as:

- benign (IgG, IgM, IgA, IgD)
- associated with malignancies that are not known to produce monoclonal proteins
- idiopathic Bence-Jones proteinuria [18,19]
- biclonal gammopathies [20]
- triclonal gammopathies [21]

Idiopathic Bence-Jones proteinuria is a condition in which patients excrete large amounts of monoclonal light chains (Bence-Jones protein) and follow a benign course. A small series of seven patients revealed no evidence of malignant plasma-cell disorder, and no serum M-protein, but urine light-chain excretion of >1 g/day [19]. In all these patients the

plasma cell labeling index was low. After a follow-up of 7–28 years, three of the seven patients, developed MM, while two other patients developed asymptomatic MM, and evolving MM. One patient developed primary amyloidosis after 12 years, and two patients continued to have stable levels of Bence-Jones proteins. The authors suggested that patients with idiopathic Bence-Jones proteinuria should be monitored regularly and indefinitely.

Of patients with a gammopathy of unknown significance, 3–4% have a biclonal gammopathy, characterized by the production of two different M-proteins. This may be due to the proliferation of two different clones of plasma cells each producing an unrelated monoclonal protein, or it may result from a single clone of plasma cells producing two M-proteins. In a series of 57 biclonal gammopathy patients, the most common diagnoses were biclonal gammopathy of undetermined significance (65%), multiple myeloma (16%), and lymphoproliferative disease (19%) [20]. The clinical features and response to therapy were similar to patients with monoclonal gammopathy. Of note, serum protein electrophoresis (SPEP) may produce only a single band on the acetate strip, and the biclonal gammopathy may be recognized only by immunofixation.

Triclonal gammopathy has also been reported, and these patients may also have underlying lymphoproliferative disorder, or a nonhematologic condition causing production of three different immunoglobulins [21].

Biology of MGUS and the role of various cytokines

It is well known that germinal-center B cells uniquely modify the DNA of immunoglobulin (Ig) genes through sequential rounds of somatic hypermutation, antigen selection, and IgH switch recombination. Post-germinal-center plasmablasts can generate plasmablasts that have successfully completed somatic hypermutation and IgH switching before migrating to the bone marrow, where stromal cells enable terminal differentiation into plasma cells. MGUS and MM are both characterized by the accumulation of transformed plasmablasts or plasma cells in the bone marrow [22,23]. However, MGUS is less proliferative than MM, with <1% cells synthesizing DNA [24]. Gene expression profiling data has demonstrated a higher level of cyclin D1, D2, or D3 mRNA in patients with MGUS and subsequently with MM, when compared to normal plasma cells [25]. This allows the plasma cells to be more susceptible to proliferative stimuli, with selective expansion, after interacting with bone-marrow stromal cells that produce interleukin 6 (IL-6) and other cytokines. There is also some evidence that the Rb protein which controls the cell-cycle restriction point from G1 to S phase might be dysregulated due to methylation of p16, which can inhibit cyclinD/CDK4 and thus prevent phosphorylation of Rb [26]. This, along with deletion of chromosome 13, may be the earliest change in MGUS that allows progression to MM [24]. In addition, activating mutations of N-ras and K-ras are absent with MGUS but are seen in 30–40% patients with MM [27].

Role of IL-6, IL-6R, IL-1β, and TNF-α

The function, differentiation, and survival of hematopoietic cells are governed by the presence of certain cytokines. These cytokines in turn require expression of an appropriate cellular receptor to exert their many biologic effects. The development of MGUS and MM is dependent upon different cytokines like granulocyte colony-stimulating factor (G-CSF), interferon alpha (IFN-α), leukemia inhibitory factor (LIF), IL-11, tumor necrosis factor alpha (TNF-α), and IL-6. IL-6, a multifunctional cytokine, has been thoroughly investigated in MM and MGUS and may possess the most biologic and clinical significance [28]. The primary function of IL-6 is to stimulate the differentiation of mature B cells into plasma cells and also to allow proliferation of plasmablasts in the bone marrow [29]. In addition, IL-6 is known to inhibit fas- and dexamethesone-induced plasma-cell apoptosis in vitro [30,31].

Initial clinical observations have suggested that high serum IL-6 levels correlate with advanced disease, aggressive disease, and chemotherapy refractoriness [32]. Multiple studies have been performed to demonstrate that IL-6 stimulates proliferation of myeloma cells in vitro, and anti-IL-6 antibodies or IL-6 antisense oligonucleotides can inhibit IL-6-stimulated growth of myeloma cells. The autocrine and paracrine functions of IL-6 in myeloma, along with IL-6 transgenic mouse models, has also been studied. The expression of IL-6 receptors (IL-6R) by myeloma cells, and responses in patients treated with anti-IL-6 antibodies, have also been examined in order to study the role of IL-6 in the pathophysiology of MGUS and MM [33,34]. More recently, similar findings have also been confirmed in patients with MGUS. Sati *et al.* developed a dual-color fluorescence *in-situ* hybridization (FISH) technique to investigate the expression of IL-6 mRNA in bone-marrow cells of patients with MM, with MGUS, and in healthy bone-marrow donors [35]. The IL-6 protein could be detected by direct immunofluorescence in all plasma cells from all patients with MM, and in those with MGUS, with lower levels of expression in patients with MGUS than in those with MM. However, neither the IL-6 mRNA nor protein could be detected in normal plasma cells from healthy subjects. These data demonstrated that patients with MGUS and MM express the IL-6 mRNA, and support the hypothesis of autocrine synthesis of IL-6 in these patients. Most investigators, however, agree that the contribution of autocrine IL-6 is minimal, and there are emerging data that the paracrine secretion of IL-6 is the major factor in the pathogenesis of MGUS, MM, and other monoclonal gammopathies [36].

IL-6 production has been detected by Th2 T cells, monocytes, endothelial cells, fibroblasts, and bone-marrow stromal cells, and the latter is probably the major source of IL-6 in monoclonal gammopathies [37]. This has been confirmed by Klein *et al.*, who attributed the high production of IL-6 to adherent cells of the bone-marrow microenvironment by demonstrating a spontaneous proliferation of myeloma cells in vitro. Recombinant IL-6 was able to amplify this proliferation, and anti-IL-6 antibodies were able to inhibit these cells [28].

Of note, the signaling of IL-6 is mediated via a specific heterodimer receptor made up of an α chain of 80 kD (IL-6R) and a β transducer chain of 130 kD (gp130). A remarkable feature of the IL-6 receptor is the agonist role of its soluble form (sIL-6R), which is able to bind IL-6 with an affinity similar to that of membrane IL-6R. Also, the IL-6/sIL-6R complex is able to bind and activate the gp130 transducer chain [38,39]. Stasi *et al.* investigated the clinical significance of serum sIL-6R in 81 patients with MGUS, and 164 patients with MM, and found higher levels of sIL-6R in the MM patients. In a univariate analysis, sIL-6R was a significant but weak prognostic indicator, and higher levels were associated with shorter survival [40].

The relationship of IL-6 to other cytokines like TNF-α and IL-1β has also been well studied. TNF-α and IL-1β are potent inducers of IL-6 production and play a role in paracrine secretion of IL-6 [41]. These two cytokines, especially IL-1β, are potent osteoclast-activating factors and play a role in the development of lytic lesions (Fig. 11.1). Lacy *et al.* performed in-situ hybridization for IL-1β using bone-marrow aspirates from 51 patients with MM, 7 with smoldering myeloma, 21 with MGUS, and 5 healthy

subjects [42]. IL-1β mRNA was detected in plasma cells from a majority of patients with MM (49 of 51) and smoldering myeloma, but only 5 of 21 patients with MGUS, and none of the normal subjects had any detectable IL-1β mRNA. This contrast in cytokine expression of IL-6 and IL-1β between patients with MGUS and MM has also been demonstrated by Donovan *et al.* [43]. TNF-α plays a role in the production of IL-6 in a dose-dependent fashion. Blade *et al.* measured serum levels of IL-6 and TNF-α in 38 healthy subjects and 100 patients with MGUS. IL-6 levels were significantly higher in MGUS than in healthy controls ($p < 0.0001$). Similarly, TNF-α levels were significantly higher in MGUS than in control populations ($p = 0.015$) [44].

More recently, the role of adhesion molecules in the biology of myeloma has been studied [45]. Normal B cells are able to home to certain tissues due to the presence of surface adhesion molecules. Myeloma cells may express a variety of surface adhesion molecules such as NCAM (CD56), ICAM (CD54), HCAM (CD44), and others. A recent study has also demonstrated impaired osteoblastogenesis in myeloma, thought to be due to increased levels of cytokines like IL-1β, TNF-α, and IL-6 which in

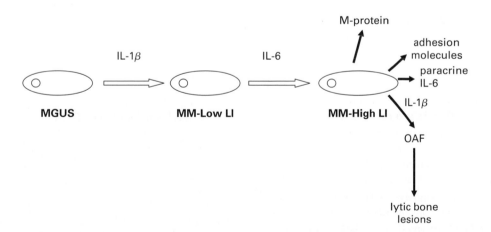

Figure 11.1 Role of IL-1β and IL-6 in the transition of MGUS to MM. MM, multiple myeloma; MGUS, monoclonal gammopathy of unknown significance; LI, labeling index; OAF, osteoclast-activating factor. Adapted from Lacy MQ *et al.*, *Blood* 1999; **93**: 300–5 [42].

turn led to upregulation of ICAM-1 [46]. It has also been hypothesized that acquisition of NCAM expression in myeloma is a malignancy-related phenomenon. NCAM (CD56) is strongly expressed on most myeloma cells but is not found on normal plasma cells. In one study, CD56 expression in high density was present in 43 of 57 patients with untreated MM and in none of 23 patients with MGUS [47]. IL-6 has been shown to increase HCAM (CD44) gene expression and cause overexpression of all CD44 variant exons [48]. It is thought that these adhesion molecules play a role in cell-to-cell contact between myeloma cells and marrow stromal cells, and this maybe leads to the homing of myeloma cells to the bone marrow and to the development of osteolytic bone lesions, and may also play a crucial role in myeloma cell survival.

IL-6 and bone-marrow angiogenesis

There has been a study which demonstrated that vascular endothelial growth factor (VEGF) expressed and secreted by myeloma cells stimulates the expression of IL-6 by microvascular endothelial cells and the bone-marrow stromal cells. In turn, IL-6 stimulates the expression of VEGF, which as we know is a potent stimulator of angiogenesis [49]. Numerous studies have now demonstrated that marrow angiogenesis parallels tumor progression and correlates with tumor growth and metastatic potential in multiple myeloma patients. We also have evidence that bone-marrow angiogenesis progressively increases along the spectrum of plasma-cell disorders, from MGUS to advanced myeloma. This has been studied in the bone-marrow samples of 400 patients (76 with MGUS) by immunohistochemical staining for CD34 to identify microvessels, and compared to normal bone-marrow samples [50]. The median microvessel density per $\times$ 400 high-power field was 1.3 in controls, 3 in MGUS, 11 in newly diagnosed MM, and 20 in relapsed MM. Higher-grade angiogenesis was noted with more advanced disease, and this correlated with the bone-marrow plasma-cell percentage, bone-marrow plasma-cell labeling index, and survival.

Role of HHV-8

Human herpesvirus 8 (HHV-8), also known as Kaposi sarcoma-associated herpesvirus (KSHV), was originally described after isolation from a patient with Kaposi sarcoma [51]. In these patients it has been isolated from primary sarcoma cells as well as B cells, macrophages, and dendritic cells. HHV-8 has also been shown to be associated with systemic Castleman disease, and primary effusion lymphoma where it is localized to just the malignant cells. The viral genome encodes a large number of homologs of cellular genes, including genes functioning in cell regulation (cyclin D), control of apoptosis (bcl-2, death effector domain proteins), cell–cell interaction, immunoregulation, and cytokine signaling, especially IL-6 [52]. IL-6, which is considered an important growth factor for myeloma, and a biologically active homolog to human IL-6, termed vIL-6, has been identified in the HHV-8 genome [53]. This vIL-6 binds to gp130 directly, suggesting that this molecule may directly activate IL-6R signal transduction without binding to the IL-6R α chain. HHV-8 also contains the viral homolog for interferon regulatory factor (vIRF), which has been detected in patients with multiple myeloma. Fibroblasts transfected with vIRF develop into stromal tumors when injected into nude mice, thus suggesting vIRF has properties of a viral oncogene [54]. Rettig *et al.* have demonstrated vIL-6 RNA transcripts in cultured KSHV-infected bone-marrow dendritic cells, thus suggesting a role in producing paracrine stimulation of plasma-cell growth and the possibility of transformation of MGUS to MM [55]. However, a follow-up study refuted these findings by using PCR analysis for multiple regions of the HHV-8 genome and serologic studies on patients with MM and found no role of HHV-8 in the etiology of MM [56]. Ablashi *et al.* performed serologic assays (whole-virus ELISA) to detect IgG antibody to HHV-8 in 362 patients with MGUS and 110 patients with MM. Only 7.8% of the MGUS sera contained HHV-8 antibody to lytic proteins, and no differences were noted in the distribution of antibody to HHV-8 in sera from MGUS patients who progressed to MM. The seroprevalence of HHV-8 in MGUS (7.8%), MM (5.4%), and healthy donors (5.9%) was similar, thus arguing for the lack of epidemiologic evidence of HHV-8 in the pathogenesis of MM. Currently, it is unclear if MGUS patients with HHV-8 infection will progress and go on to develop overt MM.

Relationship between aging and the development of monoclonal gammopathy

The prevalence findings discussed previously in the Epidemiology section suggest that there may be some fundamental changes that occur with the process of aging that make individuals more susceptible to developing a monoclonal gammopathy. Animal models have provided some clues in understanding the pathophysiology of age-related monoclonal gammopathy. In aging C57BL/KaLwRij mice, 80% of aged animals will develop a monoclonal gammopathy that is essentially indistinguishable from an MGUS in humans [57,58]. Also, plasma-cell dyscrasias such as MGUS, MM, or WM are rarely seen in C57BL/KaLwRij mice less than two years old. It is hypothesized that these animals may have a dysregulated immune system that predisposes them to develop a monoclonal gammopathy. Radl has demonstrated his findings in the C57BL/KaLwRij mice as an imbalance between a failing T-cell compartment (due to an involuted thymus) with an otherwise intact B-cell compartment [57]. The loss of a balanced T-cell/B-cell dichotomy in the immune system may lead to a restriction of the B-cell repertoire and thus to excessive B-cell clonal proliferation, excessive immunoglobulin production, and ultimately to the development of a monoclonal gammopathy.

More recently, Ellis *et al.* have demonstrated that the relative numbers of the CD30+ T-cell subset and levels of CD30 expression are elevated in activated lymphocytes from normal aged individuals (⩾60 years) and in MGUS patients, when compared to younger controls [59]. Peripheral blood lymphocytes from MGUS patients and age-matched controls produced comparable levels of IL-6 when activated with anti-CD3 plus IL-2, and costimulation with a soluble form of CD30 ligand (sCD30L/CD8alpha) augmented anti-CD3 inducible IL-6 production similarly in both groups. However, peripheral blood lymphocytes from MGUS patients also produced measurable IL-6 when activated with sCD30L/CD8alpha alone. This capability was associated with the unique presence of CD30+ T cells in the peripheral blood of MGUS patients. Furthermore, a higher percentage of activated MGUS T cells express CD30 when activated by incubation with idiotype-expressing autologous serum than those activated by anti-CD3 plus IL-2. These results indicate that quantitative alterations in CD30+ T cells accompany aging and MGUS, and that these cells may contribute to the chronic activation of B cells though the production of IL-6.

In addition to the above murine data, there is also a wealth of data to indicate that IL-6 gene expression, along with tissue and serum levels of IL-6, all increase with age. As indicated before, IL-6 is the chief cytokine implicated in the development of MM [60–64]. Early observations demonstrated an age-associated rise in IL-6 in autoimmune prone mice [63]. However, subsequent studies have demonstrated a similar age-associated increase in IL-6 in "normal" (without any disease) mice. Similarly, an age-associated increase in IL-6 has been described in healthy older humans and in older adults with coincident age-associated diseases like Alzheimer dementia, osteoporosis, and lymphoproliferative disorders [65]. One proposed mechanism for this age-associated increase in IL-6 is the reduced influence of normally inhibiting sex steroids on endogenous IL-6. The ability of estrogen to repress IL-6 expression has been studied in human endometrial stromal cells and from observations that menopause or oophorectomy resulted in increased IL-6 levels [66,67]. Similarly, dihydrotestosterone also inhibits IL-6, albeit to a lesser extent than estrogen [68]. In one study orchiectomy induced bone-marrow

IL-6 protein and mRNA expression and led to increased replication of bone-marrow osteoclast progenitors, which was prevented by administration of IL-6-neutralizing antibody or implantation of a slow-release form of testosterone [69]. Thus it seems likely that at the time of menopause or andropause, IL-6 gene expression is not that tightly regulated, leading to inappropriate expression in some tissues and a rise in serum levels. This age-associated rise in IL-6 is of physiologic consequence, rendering an individual susceptible to a number of disease processes induced by pro-inflammatory signals, including MM osteoclast stimulation, lymphoproliferative disorders, decreased functional status, and frailty [70]. One might hypothesize that in an older patient with MGUS, the rise in IL-6 levels may potentiate the usual molecular changes seen in an aging individual, like decreased immune surveillance, decreased DNA repair, telomere shortening, and decreased chromosomal stability, and thus lead to development of MM (Fig. 11.2).

Diagnosis and follow-up of patients with MGUS

The initial workup for a patient with MGUS should include a complete history and physical examination, complete blood count, blood film, serum electrolytes, blood urea nitrogen, serum creatinine, and calcium. High-resolution agarose gel serum protein electrophoresis (SPEP) is the recommended method for detection of an M-protein [1]. An M-protein is usually seen as a dense discrete band on the agarose gel electrophorectic strip or as a tall, narrow spike or peak in the beta or gamma regions, or rarely in the $alpha_2$ region of the densitometer tracing (Fig. 11.3). A polyclonal increase in the immunoglobulins will produce a broad band that is limited to the gamma region. An M-protein may be present even when the total protein concentration, beta- and gamma-globulin levels, and quantitative serum immunoglobulin levels are all within normal limits. A small M-protein may be concealed in the normal

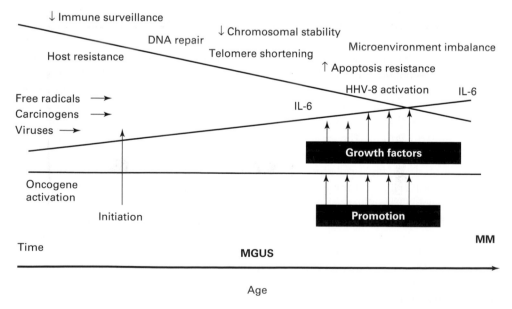

Figure 11.2 Relationship between age, HHV-8, and IL-6 in the pathogenesis of MGUS and MM. Adapted from Cohen HJ *et al.* in Balducci L *et al.*, eds, *Comprehensive Geriatric Oncology* (London: Taylor and Francis, 2004), 194–203 [71].

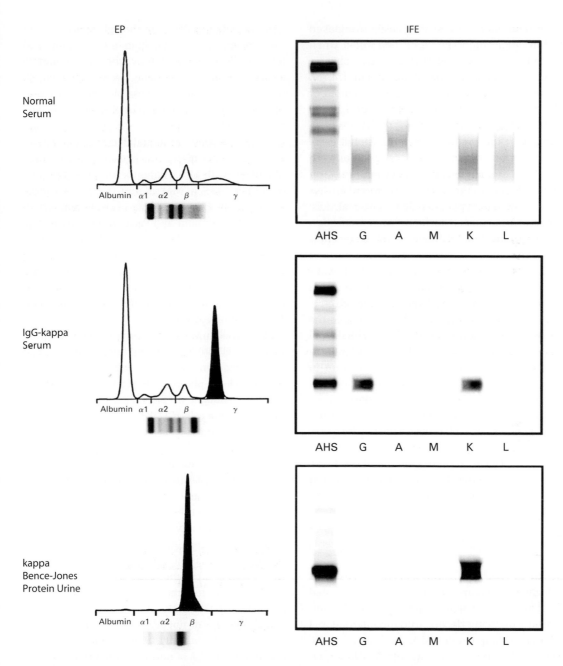

Figure 11.3 Serum and urine monoclonal protein. EP, electrophoresis; IFE, immunofixation. Adapted from Wu J *et al.*, *Clin Geriatr* 2005; **13**: 18–24 [72].

beta or gamma areas and thus easily overlooked [73]. Immunofixation should be performed when a peak or band is seen on SPEP, and this confirms the presence of and type of M-protein [74,75]. Immunofixation can detect a serum M-protein of 0.02 g/dL and a urine M-protein of 0.004 g/dL.

Urine protein electrophoresis (UPEP) is also important in the evaluation of monoclonal gammopathy. Ideally, immunofixation of a 24-hour urine sample is recommended but it can be performed on a random sample or the first morning specimen. It is not uncommon for a patient to have a normal SPEP with no M-protein, but for urine immunofixation to show a monoclonal light chain [76]. Other studies might include a bone-marrow aspiration and biopsy, a radiological skeletal bone survey, quantitative serum immunoglobulins, and 24-hour urine collection for protein quantitation and electrophoresis. Light chains may not be detected in the urine because of reabsorption by the proximal renal tubules. Also, there is variation in glomerular filtration and tubular function, and this is relevant in patients with non-secretory myeloma, solitary plasmacytoma, or primary systemic amyloidosis. These issues may be circumvented by measuring serum free light chains, which has been shown to be a very sensitive method of detecting and monitoring light chains [77]. The quantitative immunoassays can detect less than 0.1 mg/dL κ and λ chains compared to 15–50 mg/dL by immunofixation, and 50–200 mg/dL by SPEP [78].

It is important to differentiate a patient with MGUS from one with MM or WM. Most patients with MGUS are asymptomatic, and may be diagnosed incidentally by their primary-care physicians performing a workup for anemia or other related conditions. The size of the M-protein is helpful, and has been a matter of debate, with the International Myeloma Working Group using the level of 3 g/dL as the cutoff value [1]. Patients with MGUS do not have any signs or symptoms from related organ and tissue damage, as cited above. Most patients with MM or WM have a reduction in polyclonal or background immunoglobulins, while only 30% of patients with MGUS have a decrease in polyclonal

immunoglobulins. The morphologic appearance of the bone marrow might help in differentiation, and this was illustrated in a study where bone-marrow aspirates from 154 patients were examined by blinded cytologists [79]. These patients underwent bone-marrow aspiration as part of a workup for suspected myeloma. The single morphologic characteristic that strongly differentiated MM from MGUS was the presence of large nucleoli in the plasma cells of patients with MM. Higher percentage of plasma cells (mean 48% in MM vs. 10% in MGUS), irregular cytoplasmic contour of plasma cells, presence of cartwheel chromatin and vacuolization, more anisocytosis and plasma cells in clusters were features more prominent with MM bone-marrow specimens. Of note, the popular and commonly used beta-2 microglobulin level is thought not to be useful in differentiating normal individuals from those with MGUS or with early MM [80].

Plasma cells in MM are phenotypically distinct from their normal counterparts, and this has been studied by flow cytometry in patients with MGUS and MM [81]. The clonal plasma cells of patients with MGUS show a phenotypic profile similar to that of myelomatous plasma cells (CD38+, CD56+, and CD19−), although the proportion of phenotypically normal plasma cells is higher in patients with MGUS than in those with myeloma. Thus, there are actually two populations of plasma cells in persons with MGUS: one is normal and polyclonal (CD38+, CD56−, CD19+), and the other is clonal and has an abnormal immunophenotype (CD38+, CD56+, CD19−). This study also demonstrated that the proportion of bone-marrow plasma cells that was polyclonal (as assessed by flow cytometry of bone-marrow aspirate with the use of four monoclonal antibodies – CD38 or CD138, CD56, CD19, and CD45) was the best single factor for distinguishing between MGUS and multiple myeloma. Only 1.5% of patients with MM had more than 3% of normal plasma cells, whereas 98% of patients with MGUS had more than 3%.

Conventional cytogenetics is not very useful in differentiating MGUS from MM, because of the low number of cells in metaphase in MGUS. It is now thought that MGUS patients already have the chromosomal characteristics of a plasma-cell malignancy, and this was confirmed in a study in which interphase FISH was performed on bone-marrow plasma cells of 36 patients with MGUS. Chromosomal abnormalities were identified in 53% patients, with gains in chromosomes 3, 11, 7, and 18 most commonly seen [82]. The deletion of chromosome 13q is a clinically relevant feature in MM, and one study utilized interphase FISH to demonstrate deletion of the 13q14 locus in 45% patients with MGUS [83]. This was confirmed by a long-term follow-up study (median follow-up 30 months) using conventional cytogenetics and interphase/metaphase FISH in 18 asymptomatic, untreated MGUS patients [84]. Deletion of 13q14 was identified in five of these patients, and all five progressed to MM 6 to 12 months after identification of the 13q anomaly. The authors concluded that the extent of 13q deletion does not vary with clinical outcome, and plays a crucial role in the pathogenesis of MM by conferring a proliferative advantage to clonal plasma cells. However, these results must be interpreted with caution since transition from MGUS to MM can also occur in patients with normal karyotype, as suggested by two patients in the same study.

Another tool in distinguishing the two conditions might be the presence and amount of circulating plasma cells that can be seen in MM, MGUS, and smoldering myeloma. However, a recent study of 327 patients with MGUS has suggested that patients who had detectable plasma cells in the peripheral blood had a shorter median progression-free survival, shorter median survival, and shorter time to initiation of any therapy for progressive disease [85].

Finally, the plasma-cell labeling index, which measures the synthesis of DNA, is a useful test for differentiating MGUS from MM. This was evaluated in one study of 80 patients (59 MM, 20 MGUS, 1 plasma-cell leukemia) where plasma-cell proliferation analysis was performed after bromodeoxyuridine (BRD-URD) incorporation and double immunoenzymatic labeling on cytological smears [86]. The BRD-URD is incorporated into the nucleus of cells synthesizing DNA. The plasma-cell labeling index (percentage of cells in S phase) was 0.25 for MGUS, 0.4 for stage I MM, 2.4 for stage III MM, and 3.7 for plasma-cell leukemia. While there was no correlation between the labeling index and beta-2 microglobulin levels between the MGUS and MM patients, there was a correlation of these variables within the different stages of MM.

Thus, making the right diagnosis of MGUS is important, as these patients need regular follow-up in order to detect the development of the malignant form, i.e., MM or other related disorders. It has been suggested by Kyle & Rajkumar that if a patient has a serum M-protein value of <1.5 g/dL and no other features suggestive of a plasma-cell dyscrasia, (i.e., no anemia, hypercalcemia, renal failure) a bone-marrow examination or skeletal bone survey is not required and an SPEP should be repeated annually [87]. Patients with M-protein levels between 1.5 and 2.5 g/dL who are asymptomatic should have additional studies performed, including quantitative immunoglobulins and 24-hour UPEP, but do not need a bone-marrow biopsy or skeletal survey. The SPEP should be repeated every 3–6 months for a year and if stable the duration between the tests can be increased to 6–12 months and then annually or if any symptoms occur. If the M-protein level is >2.5 g/dL, complete workup, including quantitative immunoglobulins, 24-hour UPEP, bone-marrow aspiration and biopsy, and skeletal bone survey, must be performed. Given the data we have from recent studies, it might be useful to check serum free light chains in patients with M-protein >1.5 mg/dL and use it along with the kappa/lambda free light chain ratio to risk-stratify patients with MGUS in order to predict progression to more malignant disease (Table 11.1) [88]. If the M-protein is IgM, a bone-marrow aspiration and biopsy is indicated to rule out WM or any other lymphoproliferative disorder. If all the studies are normal, the SPEP can be repeated every 2–3 months for a year, and if stable can be repeated at 6- to 12-month intervals. It is unusual for a serum monoclonal protein to disappear during long-term follow-up. Formerly, if the M-protein remained stable for 3–5 years, the process was assumed to be benign and additional follow-up was not mandatory. However, the most recent data

Table 11.1. Risk stratification using the size of the serum M-protein and free light chain (FLC) ratio [89].

Risk group	No. of patients	Hazard ratio	Absolute risk of progression at 20 years (%)
Low (serum M-protein <1.5 g/dL and normal FLC ratio [0.26–1.65])	606	1	7
Intermediate (either risk factor present)	373	3.5	26
High (serum M-protein ≥1.5 g/dL and abnormal FLC ratio [<0.26 or >1.65])	169	6.8	46

from Kyle *et al.* have demonstrated an average risk of development of a malignant process of 1% per year [90]. This study found a relative risk of 7.3 for MM, WM, primary amyloidosis, chronic lymphocytic leukmia, IgM lymphoma, and plasmacytoma in the patients with MGUS, as compared to white subjects in the Iowa SEER registry from 1973 to 1997.

Natural history and predictors of progression

There have been multiple studies conducted on the natural history of this relatively indolent disease. This chapter, however, will focus on the most recent studies, with large patient populations and long durations of follow-up. In one study, Baldini *et al.* followed 335 patients with MGUS for a median period of 70 months [91]. The frequency of malignant transformation was 6.8%, and there was no difference in patients with IgM, IgG, or IgA monoclonal protein. In a univariate analysis of the IgG cases, the relative risks for developing multiple myeloma were as follows: 2.4 for each 1 g/dL increase in IgG serum monoclonal component, 3.2 for detectable light chain proteinuria, 4.4 for an increase of one unit log bone-marrow plasma-cell percentage, 6.1 for age >70 years, 3.6 and 13.1 for a reduction in one or two polyclonal immunoglobulins. Patients with an M-spike of ≤1.5 g/dL, bone-marrow plasma cells <5%, and no urinary light chains were at lowest risk, and it was suggested in this paper that patients do not need a skeletal bone survey or bone-marrow examination until there is evidence of progressive disease. In another study by Rajkumar *et al.* [89], 1384 patients with MGUS were

followed for 34 years (median 15.4 years) and during this follow-up MM, lymphoma with an IgM serum monoclonal protein, primary amyloidosis, macroglobulinemia, chronic lymphocytic leukemia, or plasmacytoma developed in 115 (8%) patients. The cumulative probability of progression to one of these disorders was about 10% at 10 years, 21% at 20 years, and 26% at 25 years. The overall risk of progression was about 1% per year, and patients were at risk of progression even after 25 years or more of stable MGUS. Of note, patients with MGUS had shorter median survival than expected for age- and sex-matched controls (8.1 years vs. 11.8 years, $p <$ 0.001). After analysis of all baseline factors only the concentration and type of monoclonal protein were independent predictors of progression. In this study patients with IgM or IgA monoclonal protein had an increased risk of progression as compared to patients with IgG monoclonal protein ($p < 0.001$), and the risk of progression was directly related to the concentration of monoclonal protein in the serum at the time of diagnosis of MGUS ($p < 0.001$). Finally, a study by Cesana *et al.* followed 1104 patients with MGUS for 33 years (median follow-up 65 months) [92]. Cumulative transformation probability at 10 and 15 years was 14% and 30% respectively, with 64 patients (5.8%) evolving to multiple myeloma or other related disorders. Marrow plasmacytosis greater than 5%, detectable Bence-Jones proteinuria, polyclonal serum immunoglobulin reaction, and a high erythrocyte sedimentation rate were independent factors influencing MGUS transformation.

One very elegant study has hypothesized that the presence of free light chains in the serum, with abnormal kappa/lambda ratio, would indicate clonal evolution in the neoplastic plasma cell and thus increased risk of progression in MGUS [93]. These investigators utilized a novel, highly sensitive serum free light chain assay that has recently been introduced into clinical practice. It enables the quantification of free kappa and lambda chains secreted by plasma cells, i.e., those not bound to intact immunoglobulin. Monoclonal elevations can be reliably distinguished from polyclonal elevations using the kappa/lambda ratio. The free light chain ratios were determined in 47 patients with MGUS who had documented progression to MM or related malignancy, and compared to 50 patients with MGUS who had no evidence of progression. The presence of higher kappa/lambda free light chain ratio was associated with a higher risk of MGUS progression (relative risk 2.5, 95% CI 1.6–4.0, $p < 0.001$). The same group has now utilized the kappa/lambda free light chain ratio along with the serum M-protein level in 1384 patients with MGUS to risk-stratify these patients and thus predict the absolute risk of progression at 20 years (Table 11.1). An abnormal kappa/lambda free light chain ratio of <0.26 or >1.65 was considered a major independent risk factor for progression of MGUS to MM or other related malignancy.

Thus, in general MGUS can be characterized as a pre-malignant condition with a limited and controlled lymphoplasmacytic expansion and a benign course. However, transformation to a more malignant condition like MM can occur, and generally is associated with higher tumor burden and a progressively downward course.

Summary

Monoclonal gammopathy of unknown significance, a pre-malignant condition, is the most common plasma-cell dyscrasia, and its incidence increases with age. It is characterized by a serum M-protein of <3.0 g/dL or trace or no light chains in a 24-hour urine collection, less than 10% plasma cells in the bone marrow, and the absence of lytic bone lesions, anemia, hypercalcemia, and renal insufficiency.

There is a clear association between aging and the development of monoclonal gammopathy, and this may be due to increased levels of IL-6 and other related cytokines. Long-term follow-up studies have demonstrated the rate of transformation of MGUS to MM or related disorder to be 1% per year. Risk factors for progression have been studied by multiple groups, and those that place the patient at high risk include size of M-protein, presence of urinary light chains, and bone-marrow plasmacytosis. More sophisticated tests like the plasma-cell labeling index, and FISH to detect 13q deletion, might also be helpful in determining risk of transformation. More recently, very sensitive assays for serum free light chains have been developed, enabling us to calculate the kappa/lambda chain ratio and use this to predict progression of MGUS to more serious MM. While there are no absolute findings at the time of diagnosis of MGUS that allow us to distinguish patients who will remain stable from those who will develop more malignant disease, we do have many diagnostic tests in our armamentarium to help follow these patients.

REFERENCES

1. International Myeloma Working Group. Criteria for the classification of monoclonal gammopathies, multiple myeloma and related disorders: a report of the International Myeloma Working Group. *Br J Haematol* 2003; **121**: 749–57.

2. Kyle RA. Monoclonal gammopathy of undetermined significance: natural history in 241 cases. *Am J Med* 1978; **64**: 814–26.

3. Kyle RA, Finkelstein S, Elveback LR, Kurland LT. Incidence of monoclonal proteins in a Minnesota community with a cluster of multiple myeloma. *Blood* 1972; **40**: 719–24.

4. Axelsson U, Bachmann R, Hallen J. Frequency of pathological proteins (M-components) from 6,995 sera from an adult population. *Acta Med Scand* 1966; **179**: 235–47.

5. Saleun JP, Vicariot M, Deroff P, Morin JF. Monoclonal gammopathies in the adult population of Finistere, France. *J Clin Pathol* 1982; **35**: 63–8.

6. Crawford J, Eye MK, Cohen HJ. Evaluation of monoclonal gammopathies in the "well" elderly. *Am J Med* 1987; **82**: 39–45.

7. Cohen HJ, Crawford J, Rao MK, Pieper CF, Currie MS. Racial differences in the prevalence of monoclonal gammopathy in a community-based sample of the elderly. *Am J Med* 1998; **104**: 439–44.

8. Bowden M, Crawford J, Cohen HJ, Noyama O. A comparative study of monoclonal gammopathies and immunoglobulin levels in Japanese and United States elderly. *J Am Geriatr Soc* 1993; **41**: 11–14.

9. Kyle RA. Monoclonal gammopathy of undetermined significance and solitary plasmacytoma. Implications for progression to overt multiple myeloma. *Hematol Oncol Clin North Am* 1997; **11**: 71–87.

10. Hansen DA, Robbins BA, Bylund DJ, Piro LD, Saven A, Ellison DJ. Identification of monoclonal immunoglobulins and quantitative immunoglobulin abnormalities in hairy cell leukemia and chronic lymphocytic leukemia. *Am J Clin Pathol* 1994; **102**: 580–5.

11. Anagnostopoulos A, Galani E, Gika D, Sotou D, Evangelopoulou A, Dimopoulos MA. Monoclonal gammopathy of undetermined significance (MGUS) in patients with solid tumors: effects of chemotherapy on the monoclonal protein. *Ann Hematol* 2004; **83**: 658–60.

12. Rovira M, Cervantes F, Nomdedeu B, Rozman C. Chronic neutrophilic leukaemia preceding for seven years the development of multiple myeloma. *Acta Haematol* 1990; **83**: 94–5.

13. Shoenfeld Y, Berliner S, Pinkhas J, Beutler E. The association of Gaucher's disease and dysproteinemias. *Acta Haematol* 1980; **64**: 241–3.

14. Hamazaki K, Baba M, Hasegawa H, *et al.* Chronic hepatitis C associated with monoclonal gammopathy of undetermined significance. *J Gastroenterol Hepatol* 2003; **18**: 459–60.

15. Youinou P, Le Goff P, Renier JC, Hurez D, Miossec P, Morrow WJ. Relationship between rheumatoid arthritis and monoclonal gammopathy. *J Rheumatol* 1983; **10**: 210–15.

16. Hashino S, Imamura M, Kobayashi S, Kobayashi H, Kasai M, Miyazaki T. Monoclonal gammopathy (IgA: lambda) after autologous T-cell-depleted bone marrow transplantation in a patient with non-Hodgkin's lymphoma. *Ann Hematol* 1993; **67**: 135–7.

17. Passweg J, Thiel G, Bock HA. Monoclonal gammopathy after intense induction immunosuppression in renal transplant patients. *Nephrol Dial Transplant* 1996; **11**: 2461–5.

18. Kyle RA, Maldonado JE, Bayrd ED. Idiopathic Bence Jones proteinuria: a distinct entity? *Am J Med* 1973; **55**: 222–6.

19. Kyle RA, Greipp PR. "Idiopathic" Bence Jones proteinuria: long-term follow-up in seven patients. *N Engl J Med* 1982; **306**: 564–7.

20. Kyle RA, Robinson RA, Katzmann JA. The clinical aspects of biclonal gammopathies. Review of 57 cases. *Am J Med* 1981; **71**: 999–1008.

21. Ray RA, Schotters SB, Jacobs A, Rodgerson DO. Triclonal gammopathy in a patient with plasma cell dyscrasia. *Clin Chem* 1986; **32**: 205–6.

22. Hideshima T, Bergsagel PL, Kuehl WM, Anderson KC. Advances in biology of multiple myeloma: clinical applications. *Blood* 2004; **104**: 607–18.

23. Kuehl WM, Bergsagel PL. Multiple myeloma: evolving genetic events and host interactions. *Nat Rev Cancer* 2002; **2**: 175–87.

24. Fonseca R, Barlogie B, Bataille R, *et al.* Genetics and cytogenetics of multiple myeloma: a workshop report. *Cancer Res* 2004; **64**: 1546–58.

25. Bergsagel PL, Kuehl WM. Critical roles for immunoglobulin translocations and cyclin D dysregulation in multiple myeloma. *Immunol Rev* 2003; **194**: 96–104.

26. Guillerm G, Gyan E, Wolowiec D, *et al.* p16(INK4a) and p15(INK4b) gene methylations in plasma cells from monoclonal gammopathy of undetermined significance. *Blood* 2001; **98**: 244–6.

27. Liu P, Leong T, Quam L, *et al.* Activating mutations of N- and K-ras in multiple myeloma show different clinical associations: analysis of the Eastern Co-operative Oncology Group Phase III Trial. *Blood* 1996; **88**: 2699–706.

28. Klein B, Zhang XG, Lu ZY, Bataille R. Interleukin-6 in human multiple myeloma. *Blood* 1995; **85**: 863–72.

29. Lotz M. Interleukin-6: a comprehensive review. *Cancer Treat Res* 1995; **80**: 209–33.

30. Chauhan D, Pandey P, Ogata A, *et al.* Dexamethasone induces apoptosis of multiple myeloma cells in a JNK/SAP kinase independent mechanism. *Oncogene* 1997; **15**: 837–43.

31. Chauhan D, Kharbanda S, Ogata A, *et al.* Interleukin-6 inhibits Fas-induced apoptosis and stress-activated protein kinase activation in multiple myeloma cells. *Blood* 1997; **89**: 227–34.

32. Zhang XG, Klein B, Bataille R. Interleukin-6 is a potent myeloma-cell growth factor in patients with aggressive multiple myeloma. *Blood* 1989; **74**: 11–13.

33. Hallek M, Bergsagel PL, Anderson KC. Multiple myeloma: increasing evidence for a multistep transformation process. *Blood* 1998; **91**: 3–21.

34. Chen YH, Shiao RT, Labayog JM, Modi S, Lavelle D. Modulation of interleukin-6/interleukin-6 receptor cytokine loop in the treatment of multiple myeloma. *Leuk Lymphoma* 1997; **27**: 11–23.

35. Sati HI, Apperley JF, Greaves M, *et al*. Interleukin-6 is expressed by plasma cells from patients with multiple myeloma and monoclonal gammopathy of undetermined significance. *Br J Haematol* 1998; **101**: 287–95.

36. Klein B, Zhang XG, Jourdan M, *et al*. Paracrine rather than autocrine regulation of myeloma-cell growth and differentiation by interleukin-6. *Blood* 1989; **73**: 517–26.

37. Treon SP, Anderson KC. Interleukin-6 in multiple myeloma and related plasma cell dyscrasias. *Curr Opin Hematol* 1998; **5**: 42–8.

38. Gaillard JP, Mani JC, Liautard J, Klein B, Brochier J. Interleukin-6 receptor signaling, gp80 and gp130 receptor interaction in the absence of interleukin-6. *Eur Cytokine Netw* 1999; **10**: 43–8.

39. Gaillard JP, Liautard J, Klein B, Brochier J. Major role of the soluble interleukin-6/interleukin-6 receptor complex for the proliferation of interleukin-6-dependent human myeloma cell lines. *Eur J Immunol* 1997; **27**: 3332–40.

40. Stasi R, Brunetti M, Parma A, Di Giulio C, Terzoli E, Pagano A. The prognostic value of soluble interleukin-6 receptor in patients with multiple myeloma. *Cancer* 1998; **82**: 1860–6.

41. Sati HI, Greaves M, Apperley JF, Russell RG, Croucher PI. Expression of interleukin-1 beta and tumour necrosis factor-alpha in plasma cells from patients with multiple myeloma. *Br J Haematol* 1999; **104**: 350–7.

42. Lacy MQ, Donovan KA, Heimbach JK, Ahmann GJ, Lust JA. Comparison of interleukin-1 beta expression by in situ hybridization in monoclonal gammopathy of undetermined significance and multiple myeloma. *Blood* 1999; **93**: 300–5.

43. Donovan KA, Lacy MQ, Kline MP, *et al*. Contrast in cytokine expression between patients with monoclonal gammopathy of undetermined significance or multiple myeloma. *Leukemia* 1998; **12**: 593–600.

44. Blade J, Filella X, Montoto S, *et al*. Interleukin 6 and tumour necrosis factor alpha serum levels in monoclonal gammopathy of undetermined significance. *Br J Haematol* 2002; **117**: 387–9.

45. Van Riet I, Van Camp B. The involvement of adhesion molecules in the biology of multiple myeloma. *Leuk Lymphoma* 1993; **9**: 441–52.

46. Silvestris F, Cafforio P, Calvani N, Dammacco F. Impaired osteoblastogenesis in myeloma bone disease: role of upregulated apoptosis by cytokines and malignant plasma cells. *Br J Haematol* 2004; **126**: 475–86.

47. Sonneveld P, Durie BG, Lokhorst HM, Frutiger Y, Schoester M, Vela EE. Analysis of multidrug-resistance (MDR-1) glycoprotein and CD56 expression to separate monoclonal gammopathy from multiple myeloma. *Br J Haematol* 1993; **83**: 63–7.

48. Vincent T, Mechti N. IL-6 regulates CD44 cell surface expression on human myeloma cells. *Leukemia* 2004; **18**: 967–75.

49. Dankbar B, Padro T, Leo R, *et al*. Vascular endothelial growth factor and interleukin-6 in paracrine tumor-stromal cell interactions in multiple myeloma. *Blood* 2000; **95**: 2630–6.

50. Rajkumar SV, Mesa RA, Fonseca R, *et al*. Bone marrow angiogenesis in 400 patients with monoclonal gammopathy of undetermined significance, multiple myeloma, and primary amyloidosis. *Clin Cancer Res* 2002; **8**: 2210–16.

51. Moore PS, Chang Y. Detection of herpesvirus-like DNA sequences in Kaposi's sarcoma in patients with and without HIV infection. *N Engl J Med* 1995; **332**: 1181–5.

52. Ganem D. KSHV and Kaposi's sarcoma: the end of the beginning? *Cell* 1997; **91**: 157–60.

53. Moore PS, Boshoff C, Weiss RA, Chang Y. Molecular mimicry of human cytokine and cytokine response pathway genes by KSHV. *Science* 1996; **274**: 1739–44.

54. Gao SJ, Boshoff C, Jayachandra S, Weiss RA, Chang Y, Moore PS. KSHV ORF K9 (vIRF) is an oncogene which inhibits the interferon signaling pathway. *Oncogene* 1997; **15**: 1979–85.

55. Rettig MB, Ma HJ, Vescio RA, *et al*. Kaposi's sarcoma-associated herpesvirus infection of bone marrow dendritic cells from multiple myeloma patients. *Science* 1997; **276**: 1851–4.

56. Ablashi DV, Chatlynne L, Thomas D, *et al*. Lack of serologic association of human herpesvirus-8 (KSHV) in patients with monoclonal gammopathy of undetermined significance with and without progression to multiple myeloma. *Blood* 2000; **96**: 2304–6.

57. Radl J. Age-related monoclonal gammapathies: clinical lessons from the aging C57BL mouse. *Immunol Today* 1990; **11**: 234–6.

58. Radl J. Aging and proliferative homeostasis: monoclonal gammapathies in mice and men. *Lab Anim Sci* 1992; **42**: 138–41.

59. Ellis TM, Le PT, DeVries G, Stubbs E, Fisher M, Bhoopalam N. Alterations in CD30(+) T cells in monoclonal gammopathy of undetermined significance. *Clin Immunol* 2001; **98**: 301–7.

60. Ershler WB. Interleukin-6: a cytokine for gerontologists. *J Am Geriatr Soc* 1993; **41**: 176–81.

61. Ershler WB, Sun WH, Binkley N, *et al.* Interleukin-6 and aging: blood levels and mononuclear cell production increase with advancing age and in vitro production is modifiable by dietary restriction. *Lymphokine Cytokine Res* 1993; **12**: 225–30.

62. Suzuki H, Yasukawa K, Saito T, *et al.* Serum soluble interleukin-6 receptor in MRL/lpr mice is elevated with age and mediates the interleukin-6 signal. *Eur J Immunol* 1993; **23**: 1078–82.

63. Tang B, Matsuda T, Akira S, *et al.* Age-associated increase in interleukin 6 in MRL/lpr mice. *Int Immunol* 1991; **3**: 273–8.

64. Wei J, Xu H, Davies JL, Hemmings GP. Increase of plasma IL-6 concentration with age in healthy subjects. *Life Sci* 1992; **51**: 1953–6.

65. Ershler WB, Sun WH, Binkley N. The role of interleukin-6 in certain age-related diseases. *Drugs Aging* 1994; **5**: 358–65.

66. Kania DM, Binkley N, Checovich M, Havighurst T, Schilling M, Ershler WB. Elevated plasma levels of interleukin-6 in postmenopausal women do not correlate with bone density. *J Am Geriatr Soc* 1995; **43**: 236–9.

67. Tabibzadeh SS, Poubouridis D, May LT, Sehgal PB. Interleukin-6 immunoreactivity in human tumors. *Am J Pathol* 1989; **135**: 427–33.

68. Daynes RA, Araneo BA, Ershler WB, Maloney C, Li GZ, Ryu SY. Altered regulation of IL-6 production with normal aging: possible linkage to the age-associated decline in dehydroepiandrosterone and its sulfated derivative. *J Immunol* 1993; **150**: 5219–30.

69. Zhang J, Pugh TD, Stebler B, Ershler WB, Keller ET. Orchiectomy increases bone marrow interleukin-6 levels in mice. *Calcif Tissue Int* 1998; **62**: 219–26.

70. Ershler WB, Keller ET. Age-associated increased interleukin-6 gene expression, late-life diseases, and frailty. *Ann Rev Med* 2000; **51**: 245–70.

71. Cohen HJ, Nikcevich D. Natural history and epidemiology of monoclonal gammopathies. In Balducci L, Lyman GH, Ershler WB, Extermann M, eds, *Comprehensive Geriatric Oncology*, 2nd edn (London: Taylor and Francis, 2004), 194–203.

72. Wu J, Seo PH, Cohen HJ. Approach to monoclonal gammopathy of unknown significance in the older patient. *Clin Geriatr* 2005; **13**: 18–24.

73. O'Connell TX, Horita TJ, Kasravi B. Understanding and interpreting serum protein electrophoresis. *Am Fam Physician* 2005; **71**: 105–12.

74. Attaelmannan M, Levinson SS. Understanding and identifying monoclonal gammopathies. *Clin Chem* 2000; **46**: 1230–8.

75. Keren DF, Warren JS, Lowe JB. Strategy to diagnose monoclonal gammopathies in serum: high-resolution electrophoresis, immunofixation, and kappa/lambda quantification. *Clin Chem* 1988; **34**: 2196–201.

76. Keren DF, Alexanian R, Goeken JA, Gorevic PD, Kyle RA, Tomar RH. Guidelines for clinical and laboratory evaluation patients with monoclonal gammopathies. *Arch Pathol Lab Med* 1999; **123**: 106–7.

77. Drayson M, Tang LX, Drew R, Mead GP, Carr-Smith H, Bradwell AR. Serum free light-chain measurements for identifying and monitoring patients with nonsecretory multiple myeloma. *Blood* 2001; **97**: 2900–2.

78. Bradwell AR, Carr-Smith HD, Mead GP, *et al.* Highly sensitive, automated immunoassay for immunoglobulin free light chains in serum and urine. *Clin Chem* 2001; **47**: 673–80.

79. Milla F, Oriol A, Aguilar J, *et al.* Usefulness and reproducibility of cytomorphologic evaluations to differentiate myeloma from monoclonal gammopathies of unknown significance. *Am J Clin Pathol* 2001; **115**: 127–35.

80. Bataille R, Grenier J, Sany J. Beta-2-microglobulin in myeloma: optimal use for staging, prognosis, and treatment. A prospective study of 160 patients. *Blood* 1984; **63**: 468–76.

81. Ocqueteau M, Orfao A, Almeida J, *et al.* Immunophenotypic characterization of plasma cells from monoclonal gammopathy of undetermined significance patients: implications for the differential diagnosis between MGUS and multiple myeloma. *Am J Pathol* 1998; **152**: 1655–65.

82. Drach J, Angerler J, Schuster J, *et al.* Interphase fluorescence in situ hybridization identifies chromosomal abnormalities in plasma cells from patients with monoclonal gammopathy of undetermined significance. *Blood* 1995; **86**: 3915–21.

83. Konigsberg R, Ackermann J, Kaufmann H, *et al.* Deletions of chromosome 13q in monoclonal gammopathy of undetermined significance. *Leukemia* 2000; **14**: 1975–9.

84. Bernasconi P, Cavigliano PM, Boni M, *et al.* Long-term follow up with conventional cytogenetics and band 13q14 interphase/metaphase in situ hybridization monitoring in monoclonal gammopathies of undetermined significance. *Br J Haematol* 2002; **118**: 545–9.

85. Kumar S, Rajkumar SV, Kyle RA, *et al.* Prognostic value of circulating plasma cells in monoclonal gammopathy of undetermined significance. *J Clin Oncol* 2005; **23**: 5668–74.

86. Ffrench M, Ffrench P, Remy F, *et al.* Plasma cell proliferation in monoclonal gammopathy: relations with other biologic variables: diagnostic and prognostic significance. *Am J Med* 1995; **98**: 60–6.

87. Kyle RA, Rajkumar SV. Monoclonal gammopathies of undetermined significance. *Hematol Oncol Clin North Am* 1999; **13**: 1181–202.

88. Rajkumar SV, Kyle RA, Therneau TM, *et al.* Serum free light chain ratio is an independent risk factor for progression in monoclonal gammopathy of undetermined significance. *Blood* 2005; **106**: 812–17.

89. Rajkumar SV, Kyle RA, Therneau TM, *et al.* Presence of an abnormal serum free light ratio is an independent risk factor for progression in monoclonal gammopathy of undetermined significance. *Blood* (ASH Annual Meeting Abstracts), Nov 2004; **104**: 3647.

90. Kyle RA, Therneau TM, Rajkumar SV, *et al.* A long-term study of prognosis in monoclonal gammopathy of undetermined significance. *N Engl J Med* 2002; **346**: 564–9.

91. Baldini L, Guffanti A, Cesana BM, *et al.* Role of different hematologic variables in defining the risk of malignant transformation in monoclonal gammopathy. *Blood* 1996; **87**: 912–18.

92. Cesana C, Klersy C, Barbarano L, *et al.* Prognostic factors for malignant transformation in monoclonal gammopathy of undetermined significance and smoldering multiple myeloma. *J Clin Oncol* 2002; **20**: 1625–34.

93. Rajkumar SV, Kyle RA, Therneau TM, *et al.* Presence of monoclonal free light chains in the serum predicts risk of progression in monoclonal gammopathy of undetermined significance. *Br J Haematol* 2004; **127**: 308–10.

PART III

Anemia of aging

12

Erythropoietin and aging

Andrew S. Artz

Introduction

Anemia represents a common problem among the elderly, with a prevalence of 5–10% for the community-dwelling elderly between 65 and 74 years, and over 20% for seniors 85 years and over. In hospitalized elderly patients and in skilled nursing facilities, anemia prevalence ranges from 40 to 50%. The recent appreciation of the numerous adverse consequences of anemia has generated interest in a more complete understanding of anemia in the elderly. Erythropoietin (EPO) is a hormone central to the regulation of red-blood-cell production that increases in response to falling hemoglobin concentration. Paradoxically, although EPO levels rise slightly with age in non-anemic elderly people, the expected EPO response to anemia appears significantly blunted in the elderly, supporting a relative endogenous EPO deficiency. This relative EPO deficiency, possibly attributable to occult renal insufficiency, may play a central role in the rising prevalence of anemia with advancing age and unexplained anemia in the elderly.

Erythropoiesis

Hematopoiesis, the production of blood elements, occurs in an orderly hierarchical fashion. Maintenance of mature peripheral blood cells (i.e., platelets, red blood cells or erythrocytes, neutrophils, eosinophils, basophils, monocytes, lymphocytes, natural killer cells, and dendritic cells) demands ongoing production to meet losses and respond to stresses. A pluripotent hematopoietic stem cell produces committed progenitors of myeloid, erythroid, and megakaryocytic lineages. Erythropoiesis denotes the process of forming mature red blood cells. The earliest erythroid lineage progenitors include the BFU-E (burst-forming unit, erythroid), which later give rise to CFU-E (colony-forming unit, erythroid). Normal erythropoiesis in adults occurs exclusively in the bone marrow.

Erythropoietin physiology

Various hematopoietic growth factors support proliferation, differentiation, and survival of stem cells. Erythropoietin, a glycoprotein hematopoietic growth factor composed of 165 amino acids after modification from the 193-amino-acid molecule encoded by mRNA, serves as a primary regulator of red-cell production [1,2]. The markedly elevated circulating EPO levels in patients with aplastic anemia allowed initial EPO isolation from the urine [3]. The glycosylation present on EPO delays clearance of the molecule, but is not necessary for biologic activity [4]. Synthesis and EPO regulation occur primarily through the kidney, from interstitial fibroblasts and/or from proximal tubular cells, with a smaller contribution by liver hepatocytes [5–9]. As a consequence, renal failure inexorably leads to anemia from impaired EPO production.

Under normal homeostasis, suppressed transcription of EPO leads to a minimal constitutive production. Reduced tissue oxygenation (rather than diminished red-cell production), typically from anemia or hypoxia, potently stimulates synthesis with logarithmically elevated serum EPO levels [10]. Hypoxic conditions promote activation of the hypoxia inducible factor 1 (HIF-1) pathway, with expression of the alpha and beta subunits, and eventual downstream EPO gene transcription [11]. With reduced oxygen delivery, the number of renal cells producing EPO may also increase [9]. Elevated serum EPO levels enhance erythrocyte production primarily by inhibiting apoptosis of erythroid progenitor cells, although EPO also promotes erythroid progenitor proliferation and differentiation [12].

Erythropoiesis with aging

Early laboratory models helped guide subsequent human studies describing EPO kinetics with aging. Basal erythropoiesis and red-cell mass in aged mice appears similar to younger mice, although measured hematocrit may be slightly lower secondary to dilution [13,14]. In response to stressors, such as hypoxia, bleeding, or environmental perturbation, aged mice have an impaired erythropoietic response [13,15,16]. Human studies in older subjects with unexplained anemia have shown normal BFU-E cells but diminished CFU-E, the erythroid precursors most replete with EPO receptors, suggesting a block in differentiation possibly mediated by inadequate endogenous EPO levels. Further, CFU-E viability requires EPO [17].

Erythropoietin receptors

Hematopoietic growth factors in general bind with high affinity to specific receptors on target cells. EPO activity necessitates binding to erythropoietin receptors (EPO-R). Within the marrow compartment, EPO receptors (EPO-R) occur on the two classes of committed erythroid precursors, the BFU-E and CFU-E [18]. While BFU-E cells have a high proliferative capacity, they only have low EPO-R expression. The CFU-E cells, progeny of the BFU-E cells, have a lower proliferative capacity but increased EPO-R density. After EPO attaches to EPO-R, signal transduction permits cell survival. The heterogeneity

of EPO sensitivity at the molecular level of such cells may also facilitate erythropoietic regulation [19].

Non-marrow activity of erythropoietin and erythropoietin receptors

Recognition of EPO in non-hematopoietic tissue has pointed to the potentially pleiotropic effects of the hormone. The presence of EPO-R on vascular endothelial cells [20], various renal cells [21,22], human tumor cells [23], and the central nervous system (CNS) reflect a multiplicity of non-hematopoietic roles for EPO, and possibly therapeutic implications. Research into the understanding of EPO in CNS development and homeostasis has been particularly fruitful. Similar to the bone-marrow compartment, hypoxia-regulated EPO and EPO-R expression occur within the central nervous system [24–27]. Endogenous EPO does not significantly cross the blood–brain barrier [28], although large pharmacologic doses may penetrate the CNS. EPO may protect the CNS after hypoxic injury [29], motivating studies of pharmacologic EPO as neuroprotective therapy after strokes, with promising preliminary results [30]. Changes with advancing age have not been studied.

Normal erythropoietin response to anemia

Serum endogenous EPO levels typically remain within a narrow reference range for young healthy patients at normal hemoglobin concentrations. Isolation of extremely high concentrations of EPO from the urine of patients with aplastic anemia helped uncover the dynamic nature of EPO regulation in response to anemia. The advent of immunoassays to measure serum EPO further promoted research clarifying serum EPO kinetics [31].

Relative erythropoietin deficiency

Determining the expected rise in serum EPO to anemia remains problematic and complicates both clinical and research data interpretation. Reference ranges reported by laboratories describe serum EPO levels from non-anemic healthy populations and do not reflect the dynamic nature of EPO responses. Interpretation of these values may result in confusion, as a serum EPO level within the reference range (approximately 4–28 mIU/mL, depending on the laboratory) for an anemic patient often signifies a relative EPO deficiency. Multiple methods of quantifying EPO responsiveness have further complicated evaluating studies, including mean and median EPO levels, with and without adjustment for hemoglobin concentration. Generating a standard curve documenting the expected serum EPO for a given hemoglobin concentration enables appropriate statistical modeling but also requires logarithmic transformation of EPO levels. Such transformations further complicate clinical interpretation.

Among younger subjects with significant anemia, a normal EPO response has been characterized as a semilogarithmic increase. In general, serum EPO levels inversely correlate with hemoglobin, at least with significant degrees of anemia in younger subjects experiencing blood loss, iron deficiency, hemolysis, or erythroid marrow aplasia. Assuming this represents the normal kinetics of serum EPO in response to anemia, a curve of the appropriate EPO concentration for the degree of anemia has been proposed [32,33]. Lack of precision represents a major obstacle to comparing EPO levels to this "normal curve." For example, it remains unknown what EPO concentration below the predicted level should be considered low. Nevertheless, the predicted EPO level for a given hemoglobin concentration may approximate an appropriate EPO response and permit defining a relative EPO deficiency.

Renal failure exemplifies the prototypical anemia from impaired EPO production. In many other conditions, EPO levels are elevated above the reference range for non-anemic controls but remain significantly below the expected concentration. For example, an EPO level of 50 mIU/mL at a hemoglobin of 9.0 g/dL, although far above the reference range, would still be considered a suboptimal EPO response. This inadequate EPO response for the degree of anemia commonly occurs with conditions such as cancer, HIV, and rheumatoid arthritis [34–36]. The mechanism may be multifactorial, but it is likely that there is a contribution from reduced renal EPO secretion and impaired marrow responsiveness.

Erythropoietin levels in the elderly

Non-anemic elderly

Multiple studies have assessed endogenous serum EPO levels in older subjects without anemia (Table 12.1).

Japanese older subjects living in a "home for aged" were compared to younger healthy controls [37]. The non-anemic older subjects had numerically but statistically non-significant higher mean EPO levels (mean EPO of 20.4 mIU/mL and 15.7 mIU/mL for older and younger, respectively). In a study of older adults with a mean age of 77.8 years residing in a home for the elderly, Kario and colleagues ascertained serum EPO levels [39]. An elevated mean EPO level of 26.9 mIU/mL (±15.2) was observed among the 116 non-anemic elderly, compared to a mean of 15.8 mIU/mL in younger controls. Kario *et al.* subsequently reported higher EPO levels among non-anemic elderly (mean EPO of 24.3 mIU/mL) compared to younger subjects (mean EPO of 14.8 mIU/mL) [40]. Also, they showed a significant inverse relationship between EPO and hemoglobin (Hb) concentrations in non-anemic elderly subjects ($r = -0.302$, $p < 0.001$). Further, a significant association existed between advancing age and rising EPO ($r = 0.220$, $p < 0.01$). These studies provided early evidence for mildly increased EPO occurring with advancing age and/or slight reductions of hemoglobin concentration, even within the normal range.

Powers and colleagues found EPO levels in 25 healthy elderly people, with an age range of 60–82 years, to be similar to those in younger controls (means of 10.8 and 13.1 mIU/mL, respectively) [38]. In a larger cohort, the same author showed similar EPO levels in younger and older subjects, after adjusting for hematocrit [41]. Joosten and

Table 12.1. EPO levels in non-anemic elderly adults compared to younger adults.

Study	Population	Control	Result (mean ± SD)
Mori *et al.* 1988 [37]	$n = 78$ (13 with chronic disease, 16 with cancer, 10 without etiology), home for the aged Age 70–89 years	$n = 127$ Age 22–46 years	Elderly mean EPO 20.4 ± 10.4 Younger 15.7 ± 1.3
Powers *et al.* 1989 [38]	$n = 25$ Age 60–82 years	$n = 30$ Age < 65 years	Elderly mean EPO 10.8 ± 6.4 Younger 13.1 ± 5.5
Kario *et al.* 1991 [39]	$n = 116$ Mean age 77.8 years for all elderly	$n = 26$, volunteers Mean age 42.4	Elderly mean EPO 26.9 ± 15.2 Younger 15.8 EPO rose with age
Kario *et al.* 1992 [40]	$n = 150$, ambulatory Age > 60 years	$n = 111$ Mean age 46 years	Elderly mean EPO 24.3 (17.2–34.5) Younger 14.8 Age-related increase in EPO
Nafziger *et al.* 1993 [41]	$n = 30$	Not provided	Elderly mean EPO 11 ± 3.5 Levels "similar" to non-anemic young
Joosten *et al.* 1993 [42]	$n = 27$, hospitalized Mean age 81.5 years	$n = 30$, hospital staff Mean age 32.5 years	Elderly mean EPO 7.5 Younger mean EPO 9.5
Goodnough *et al.* 1995 [43]	$n = 31$, autologous blood donors prior to surgery Mean age 71.1 years	$n = 40$, from same population Age < 65 years, mean 47.6 years	Elderly with higher EPO using Log EPO and age No difference in EPO in subset of 18 patients
Ershler *et al.* 2005 [44]	$n = 143$, healthy elderly Mean age 62 years	None	Mean EPO 13.0 and rose with advancing age

EPO, serum endogenous erythropoietin level (mIU/mL).

colleagues quantified endogenous EPO levels in hospitalized non-anemic elderly patients with a mean age of 81.5 years and mean hemoglobin of 14.2 g/dL, and compared them to young controls with a mean hemoglobin of 14.6 g/dL [42]. They showed mean EPO levels did not differ by age cohort, with levels of 7.5 and 9.5 mIU/mL for older and younger subjects, respectively. These studies by Powers and Joosten appear contradictory to earlier data on rising EPO levels with age in those without anemia. However, Powers' subjects primarily carried a diagnosis of rheumatoid arthritis, a condition known to blunt EPO responses, and the participants in the study by Joosten were hospitalized patients, presumably having other comorbid conditions also

blunting EPO responsiveness. Thus, one could not isolate age-related changes in EPO responsiveness.

To identify the diurnal variations in endogenous EPO, Pasqualetti and colleagues measured serum EPO in 20 younger adults with a mean age of 45 years and mean hemoglobin of 13.9 g/dL and compared them to older adults with a mean age of 65 years and mean hemoglobin of 13.5 g/dL [46]. In general, EPO levels peaked around 6 pm and were at their lowest around midnight. Young and old subjects exhibited a similar diurnal variation, although younger subjects had higher mean daily levels ($p < 0.05$) and more diurnal variation ($p < 0.05$) in EPO relative to older subjects. The significance of these findings remains unclear, although one may postulate that more tightly regulated EPO in the young resulted in stronger temporal changes.

Endogenous EPO response to anemia in the elderly

As previously stated, determining a normal EPO response to hemoglobin changes represents a major challenge in accurate characterization of EPO kinetics. Clearly, young subjects with hemolytic anemia or subjected to phlebotomy have a brisk rise in serum EPO levels. An absolute EPO deficiency causes anemia in renal failure, and a relative EPO deficiency contributes to anemia in various conditions such as cancer, autoimmune conditions, prematurity, and human immunodeficiency. Studies evaluating serum endogenous EPO in anemic elderly subjects have allowed a better understanding of changes in serum EPO and erythropoiesis with aging.

Studies in anemic elderly

Mori *et al.* examined iron-deficient anemic older subjects from ages 70 to 89 years, and found elevated endogenous EPO levels with lower hemoglobin concentrations [37]. The preserved EPO responsiveness in elderly iron-deficient anemic subjects indicated that age does not necessarily confer an absolute EPO deficiency.

In one of the earliest studies describing a relative EPO deficiency in the elderly, Carpenter and colleagues detailed hematologic parameters and EPO concentration for a large group of younger and older subjects (aged 70 years and over) [47]. EPO levels rose among the iron-deficient elderly with worsening anemia. In contrast, for the elderly with normocytic anemia ($n = 375$), the EPO response to anemia was reduced relative to the elderly with microcytic or macrocytic anemia and relative to all iron-deficient anemic subjects. Similarly, Kario and others reported an inverse semilogarithmic relationship between EPO and Hb concentrations in subjects with Hb concentrations less than 12.0 g/dL ($r = -0.559, p < 0.001$). EPO concentrations in the elderly were lower than those in young subjects with iron-deficiency anemia with the same Hb level [39]. In a follow-up study, the

same group showed elevated EPO levels with falling hemoglobin, but this was restricted to the elderly with iron-deficiency anemia. The authors suggested that while elderly subjects with iron deficiency may have a degree of preserved EPO responsiveness to falling hemoglobin, anemia of advancing age is characterized by a relative EPO deficiency, and they hypothesized that pharmacologic EPO replacement may reverse the deficit [40].

Joosten and others investigated hospitalized older subjects and found that among 24 iron-deficient anemic older persons with a mean age of 83 years and mean hemoglobin of 10.0 g/dL, lower hemoglobin correlated with higher EPO levels [42]. However, in the older subjects with anemia due to chronic disease or acute infection, the lack of correlation between EPO and hemoglobin concentration suggested a blunted EPO response. Whether conditions characterized by inflammation or aging in this hospitalized cohort blunted the EPO response could not be determined.

Among 31 iron-deficient elderly subjects, Nafziger and colleagues observed the expected inverse correlation, with lower hemoglobin and higher EPO concentrations [41]. However, compared to 33 subjects less than 60 years of age, the correlation of rising EPO with lower hemoglobin values was less pronounced. Moreover, there was a trend towards lower EPO levels in older iron-deficient anemic patients relative to younger anemic subjects, reaching significance when hemoglobin concentration fell below 10 g/dL, suggesting that iron deficiency and severe anemia represent additional stimuli to EPO secretion that remain suboptimal in the elderly.

In a study of older Japanese subjects compared to patients under 60 years of age, Matsuo and colleagues enumerated EPO levels and the immature reticulocyte count, a measure of marrow erythropoietic response, among iron-deficient subjects [48]. Higher reticulocyte counts reflect more brisk erythropoiesis. Although median EPO levels did not differ in the young and old, the reticulocyte count/log EPO concentration ratio was 3.3 for older and 8.1 for younger subjects ($p < 0.01$), suggesting a diminished marrow response to circulating endogenous EPO levels among the elderly. The lack of adequate iron for red-cell synthesis confounds a reliable determination of the marrow erythropoietic responsiveness to endogenous EPO secretion. Alternatively, fewer iron stores or reduced capacity with aging to mobilize iron may have accounted for reduced erythropoiesis.

Pieroni and colleagues studied anemia of chronic inflammation in 56 older subjects with cancer, infection, or another inflammatory disorder, and compared them to a control group of older subjects. In general, they observed blunted EPO responsiveness to anemia, until moderate to severe anemia of $<8.5\,g/dL$ [49]. The underlying conditions may also have impaired EPO responsiveness, resulting in blunted EPO levels. Nevertheless, these data, in concert with the study by Joosten and colleagues [42], demonstrate that markedly low hemoglobin levels provide a stronger EPO stimulus.

Kamenetz and colleagues evaluated 17 elderly subjects with unexplained anemia, ranging in age from 65 to 90 years, and compared them to older non-anemic controls and subjects with anemia and recent stroke [50]. Anemia was defined as a hemoglobin concentration $<12\,g/dL$. EPO levels did not significantly differ across the three different groups, reflecting impaired EPO responsiveness in the anemic patients, as one would expect elevated EPO levels in anemic subjects.

In a study of 71 healthy blood donors undergoing aggressive phlebotomy, Goodnough and colleagues characterized the endogenous EPO response [43]. Older subjects had similar EPO responsiveness to phlebotomy. Red-cell expansion in response to phlebotomy showed a non-significant trend for being reduced in the elderly ($p = 0.10$).

In a case series of patients referred to a hematology practice, seven patients were described with unexplained anemia who later received pharmacologic therapy for the anemia. At baseline, hemoglobin and endogenous EPO were $10.0\,g/dL$ and $10.8\,mIU/mL$, respectively, providing evidence for a blunted EPO response in patients primarily with unexplained anemia [51].

We analyzed 900 elderly subjects drawn from five nursing homes to determine anemia prevalence [52]. Eighty-one subjects with anemia or borderline low hemoglobin from the cohort were randomly selected for further characterization [53]. Among 60 patients with confirmed anemia, iron deficiency and unexplained anemia accounted for 23% and 45% of cases, respectively (Table 12.2). Correlating serum EPO levels to hemoglobin concentration revealed increased EPO levels with iron deficiency but no correlation for seniors with unexplained anemia (Fig. 12.1). The rise in EPO among those with iron deficiency appeared less than expected, suggesting that a blunted EPO response, albeit to a lesser degree than in unexplained anemia, existed with iron deficiency. In the anemic residents with adequate renal function (glomerular filtration rate $>30\,mL/minute$ and serum creatinine $<2.0\,g/dL$), calculated creatinine clearance remained independently associated with lower EPO levels when controlling for age, gender, and Hb value ($p = 0.008$), suggesting that even mild renal insufficiency promotes impaired EPO responsiveness.

Although a relative EPO deficiency for the degree of anemia has been described for numerous conditions, such as cancer, prematurity, human immunodeficiency, autoimmune conditions, and the intensive care unit, limited data assess the impact of older age in these diseases on endogenous EPO responsiveness. In a small cohort of 20 cancer patients aged 70 years and over undergoing platinum-based chemotherapy, Cascinu and others reported mean endogenous EPO levels similar to those in patients younger than 70 years (51 and $62\,mIU/mL$, respectively) [54]. Absent correlations of serum EPO for hemoglobin, limited inferences regarding age can be made.

EPO responsiveness in the elderly with anemia: conclusions

The studies of anemic older patients permit several conclusions. A relative EPO deficiency characterizes the anemia associated with aging (unexplained anemia). Chronic disease does not adequately explain the blunted responses, suggesting EPO deficiency may be a feature of advancing age and/or occult

Table 12.2. Hematologic parameters and serum EPO for older nursing-home patients by anemia etiology [53].

Type	Hb (g/dL)	EPO (mIU/mL)	MCV (fL)	Ferritin (ng/mL)	IL-6 (pg/mL)	Alb (g/dL)	CRP (mg/dL)
Reference range	11.5–15.0	4.2–27.8	80–98	10–291		3.5–4.8	0–4.9
Iron-deficiency anemia (n = 14)	10.6 ± 1.1	29.0 ± 16.2	85.4 ± 7.0	22.5 ± 14.5	6.6 ± 2.7	3.7 ± 0.5	10.1 ± 15.4
Anemia of chronic disease (n = 8)	11.0 ± 1.5	20.3 ± 7.6	93.1 ± 3.4	167.4 ± 79.1	44.3 ± 72.4	3.6 ± 0.4	36.9 ± 35.5
Idiopathic anemia (n = 27)	10.8 ± 1.0	14.6 ± 7.3	92.3 ± 5.9	201.6 ± 195.6	8.5 ± 7.8	3.6 ± 0.3	6.0 ± 5.0
Chronic renal insufficiency (n = 6)	11.5 ± 0.8	12.5 ± 4.2	89.5 ± 6.5	177.8 ± 215.9	7.5 ± 1.4	3.9 ± 0.3	8.3 ± 5.6
Other (n = 5)	10.0 ± 1.2	13.4 ± 1.6	87.0 ± 9.3	356.0 ± 577.1	98.0 ± 106.8	3.6 ± 0.3	41.1 ± 68.7
Total (n = 60)	10.7 ± 1.1	18.6 ± 11.6	90.1 ± 6.7	166.9 ± 233.6	19.0 ± 41.0	3.7 ± 0.4	13.6 ± 25.7

Values shown are means ± standard deviation.

Hb, hemoglobin; EPO, erythropoietin; MCV, mean corpuscular volume; IL-6, interleukin 6; Alb, albumin; CRP, c-reactive protein.

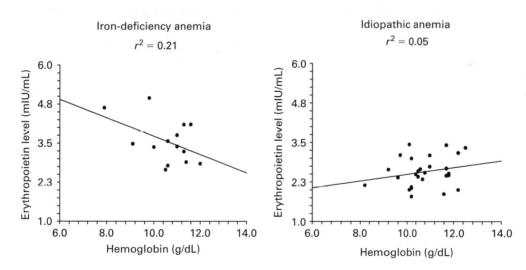

Figure 12.1 Correlations between natural log-transformed erythropoietin levels and hemoglobin, comparing variances (r^2) of patients with iron-deficiency anemia and idiopathic anemia.

renal dysfunction. In the elderly with iron defi- ciency, a degree of EPO responsiveness is preserved. However, iron deficiency, independent of anemia, also raises endogenous EPO levels [55]. Erythroid proliferation may further elevate serum EPO, inde- pendent of hemoglobin concentration [56]. The additional stimulus of iron deficiency for the eld- erly with iron-deficiency anemia enables a degree of preserved EPO responsiveness, but serum EPO levels remain suboptimal.

Serum EPO and hemoglobin changes with aging

Emerging data in large datasets of older patients comprising the spectrum of hemoglobin concentrations have significantly clarified the relationship with advancing age to serum EPO and hemoglobin concentration.

In a large cohort of 641 community-dwelling women 65 years of age and over, Chaves *et al.* correlated serum EPO and hemoglobin concentration [57]. Rising serum EPO levels correlated with lower hemoglobin concentration, even limiting the analysis to those above the World Health Organization anemia threshold of 12 g/dL for women. For example, the mean serum EPO level for a hemoglobin of 12.0 g/dL was 28% (95% CI 15–44%) higher than for woman with a hemoglobin of 13.9 g/dL. The difference persisted even after adjustment for age, renal function, and race. Although the EPO levels rose with declining hemoglobin, the mean EPO level remained within the stated EPO reference range for young healthy controls, even at hemoglobin concentrations of 11 g/dL. For hemoglobin concentration above 14.3 g/dL, the slope of the EPO/hemoglobin curve was zero, reflecting no correlation or EPO responsiveness at this hemoglobin concentration. These data suggest that the EPO secretion mechanism is active to maintain hemoglobin concentration

at minimally reduced concentrations between 12 and 14 g/dL in these women. While it remains unclear to what extent if any the elevated EPO ameliorates the falling hemoglobin, the data challenge traditional notions of abnormal hemoglobin concentration, as homeostatic mechanisms react to very mild reductions in red blood cells.

Ferrucci and colleagues explored EPO levels from the InCHIANTI study, a large cohort (*n* = 1453) of prospectively followed community-dwelling elderly Italians [58]. Higher EPO levels were associated with both older age and inflammatory markers in non-anemic subjects. Higher EPO also correlated with declining hemoglobin below 13 g/dL. Paradoxically, among anemic patients, inflammation resulted in reduced EPO levels.

The lack of longitudinal EPO data has limited inferences about EPO changes with aging. Ershler and colleagues reported longitudinal serum EPO levels among 143 participants in the Baltimore Longitudinal Study in Aging with at least eight years of study follow-up [44]. In general, healthy volunteers participated in this study, with frequent and intensive follow-up, facilitating the documentation of age-related changes independent of serious comorbid conditions. Using sera frozen every 1–2 years, EPO changes with age for individuals were determined. Baseline characteristics at study entry included a median age of 62 years, median hemoglobin of 14.7 g/dL, and median

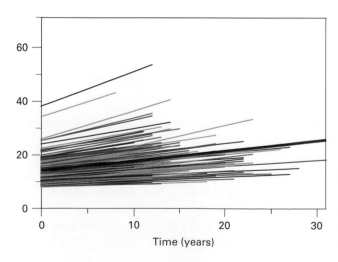

Figure 12.2 Predicted erythropoietin levels over time. Baltimore Longitudinal Study in Aging [44]. *See color plate section.*

EPO level of 13.0 mIU/mL (range 6.0 to 47.1). EPO levels varied inversely with hemoglobin concentration and increased with time (and thus advancing age) (Fig. 12.2). The authors stratified groups by separating 59 subjects with hypertension or diabetes,

hypothesizing that diseases impairing renal function would exacerbate any age-related EPO deficiency. For each hemoglobin concentration, the hypertension/diabetes group had a significantly higher EPO level for the baseline measurement than subjects

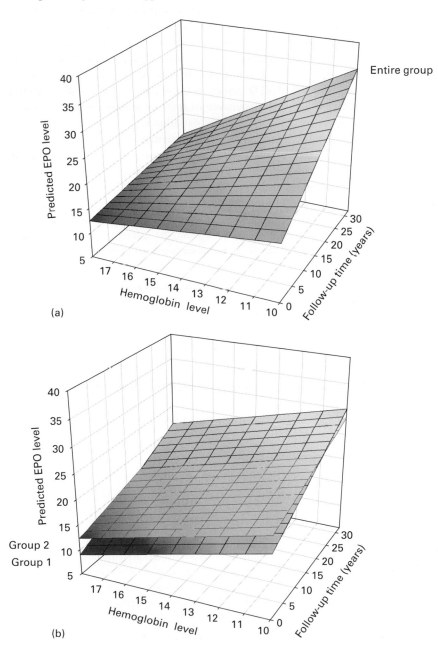

(a)

(b)

Figure 12.3 Predicted hemoglobin and serum erythropoietin level: (a) for the entire group; (b) for subjects with diabetes or hypertension (group 2) compared to subjects with these conditions (group 1). Baltimore Longitudinal Study in Aging [44]. *See color plate section.*

without a predisposition to renal disease (Fig. 12.3). Interestingly, EPO levels rose less steeply for a given hemoglobin decline with time in the hypertension/diabetes group ($p = 0.03$), potentially reflecting an occult defect in EPO responsiveness in subjects predisposed to renal impairment. In subjects later developing anemia, a significant rise occurred in EPO levels with time (and aging), suggesting that rising EPO represents a compensatory response to erythron loss.

The studies by Chaves *et al.* [57], Ferruci *et al.* [58], and Ershler [44] in different populations, using different statistical analyses, lead to similar conclusions regarding endogenous EPO regulation in the elderly. First, EPO levels rise with advancing age, possibly as a mechanism to maintain red-blood-cell mass. With reduced EPO responsiveness with age, possibly exacerbated by inflammation and/or renal disease, hemoglobin concentration falls and may even lead to anemia. Whether reduced red-cell survival, a latent stem-cell defect, or other factors result in the need for enhanced erythropoiesis remains unclear. Second, although moderately severe anemia with hemoglobin concentration below 10 g/dL provokes a stronger endogenous EPO response, minimally reduced hemoglobin may also promote increased EPO, albeit to a lesser degree. Because older patients with unexplained anemia rarely have severe anemia, the EPO stimulus may function adequately to prevent serious anemia, in the absence of other coexisting conditions.

Understanding the relative EPO deficiency in the elderly

Several mechanisms may account for an inadequate erythropoietin response in older persons. Cytokine dysregulation may reduce EPO secretion or marrow responsiveness, or mild renal disease without a change in glomerular filtration may diminish production [44]. Age-related regulations could also impair EPO responsiveness through attenuated transcription or translation.

There is a sound rationale supporting the theory that the relative EPO deficiency in the elderly is primarily due to renal insufficiency. In the prototypical model of complete renal failure, inadequate EPO responsiveness rather than a primary marrow problem causes anemia [59]. Even in renal conditions without overt renal glomerular filtration abnormalities, endocrine function as measured by EPO response to anemia may be impaired. Children with nephritic syndrome, prior to significant renal clearance impairment, have a blunted endogenous EPO response to anemia [60]. A similar blunted EPO response occurs in patients with diabetes, independent of reduced glomerular filtration [61]. Finally, administration of angiotensin-converting-enzyme medication may suppress EPO secretion and precipitate anemia [62,63]. The longitudinal data from Ershler and colleagues support a blunted EPO response in patients with normal serum creatinine but conditions predisposing to renal dysfunction (i.e. diabetes and hypertension). A decline in renal function may be a feature of aging accentuated by hypertension and diabetes [64]. One may hypothesize that impaired endocrine function of the kidney in older adults represents an early marker of renal damage. Alternatively, renal endocrine function may be more prone to age-related decline than renal exocrine function.

Exogenous (pharmacologic) therapy with erythropoiesis-stimulating proteins

Pharmacologic erythropoietin

Biochemical characterization of endogenous EPO quickly led to successful efforts to synthesize EPO for pharmacologic therapy, with the cloned recombinant human EPO showing in-vivo activity [65].

Several therapeutic formulations of erythropoiesis-stimulating proteins (ESP) are available, including epoetin beta, epoetin alpha, and most recently darbepoetin alpha, with new formulations under active investigation. Epoetin alpha, similar to endogenous erythropoietin, has most commonly been used. Darbepoetin alpha contains additional N-linked carbohydrate chains compared to epoetin alpha, with up to 22 sialic acid residues [66]. The increased sialic acid content of darbepoetin alpha prolongs the serum half-life two to three times by reduced drug clearance. Darbepoetin and epoetin alpha formulations appear to have similar efficacy.

Response of elderly to ESPs

No prospective randomized trials correcting anemia of aging have been published, although some trials are ongoing. The literature on treating older anemic patients with ESPs primarily has focused on disease-specific indications, such as cancer, renal failure, and preoperative autologous blood donation. Most analyses of age consist of retrospective reviews comparing older to younger subjects treated for a specific disease. Reduced allogeneic red-cell transfusion and quality of life represent the primary endpoints for most trials.

One case series details treatment for seven outpatient elderly anemic subjects with apparent unexplained anemia [51]. The mean baseline hemoglobin was 10.0 g/dL, and mean serum endogenous EPO level was 10.8 mIU/mL. The initial starting dose of epoetin alpha of 20 000 units enabled a response in all subjects, with a mean hemoglobin rise of 3.5 mg/dL (Fig. 12.4).

Disease-specific indications

Adjunct for autologous red-blood-cell donation

In patients undergoing transuretheral resection of the prostate (TURP) for benign prostatic hypertrophy, Goya and colleagues reported that adjuvant epoetin alpha or epoetin beta with iron support promoted autologous blood donation for 68 patients ranging from 60 to 77 years of age. All subjects achieved the desired autologous blood donation [67].

Goodnough and colleagues assessed healthy blood donors after aggressive phlebotomy given various doses of recombinant EPO [43]. No correlation existed between red-cell expansion in older and younger subjects, using age 65 years as a cutoff point. Moreover, studying red-cell response to the ESP as a function of age showed no association ($p = 0.74$).

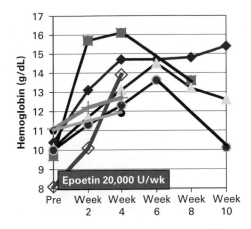

Figure 12.4 Hemoglobin response for epoetin alpha treatment of elderly with unexplained anemia [51]. *See color plate section.*

Renal insufficiency

Renal impairment commonly occurs among the elderly, and may be under-recognized as an etiology in anemia. A large literature on treatment of renal insufficiency and renal failure with ESPs has been published. Fink and colleagues characterized the age-related response to anemia therapy by re-examining a large trial of patients with chronic kidney disease not undergoing dialysis treated with epoetin alpha [68]. The three age cohorts compared included subjects 80 years ($n = 186$), 65–79 years ($n = 531$), and <65 years ($n = 621$). In addition to a similar mean hemoglobin change across groups of 2.4 g/dL, very similar mean weekly epoetin alpha doses were required.

Cancer-related anemia

Shank and Balducci reviewed studies employing colony-stimulating factors, including ESPs [69]. Among 204 subjects, mostly with malignancy, 33% of those aged 65 years and older responded to ESP granulocyte-stimulating-factor therapy as well as younger subjects.

Demetri and colleagues pooled data from three studies employing various dosing schemes of epoetin alpha in 4572 cancer patient 60 years and over and compared them with 2541 younger cancer patients [70]. A rise of 2 gm/dL or more in hemoglobin, independent of transfusion, was experienced by 65.5% of older patients and 64.9% of younger subjects. Elderly patients also demonstrated significant quality-of-life improvements (using the linear analog scale assessment), although slightly less than younger patients. Increasingly, higher hemoglobin area under the curve (AUC) over the course of the study has shown enhanced quality of life. In subset analysis, older subjects derive similar benefit to younger subjects from higher AUC measurements.

Additionally, multiple randomized studies employing ESPs for cancer-related anemia have indicated that age does not predict hematologic response [71,72].

Conclusions

Studies of disease-specific indications demonstrate that older subjects respond as well as younger subjects to pharmacologic therapy. Thus, adequate marrow erythroid responsiveness exists in older subjects, offering further evidence that in anemia associated with aging, a relative endogenous EPO deficiency plays a pathogenic role. Guidelines specific for the treatment of anemia associated with aging await randomized controlled trials. At present, clinical judgment and inferences guide treatment decisions on the use of red-blood-cell transfusions and/or pharmacologic therapy. Use of an ESP, however, would be appropriate at least to obviate red-blood-cell transfusion.

REFERENCES

1. Recny MA, Scoble HA, Kim Y. Structural characterization of natural human urinary and recombinant DNA-derived erythropoietin. Identification of des-arginine 166 erythropoietin. *J Biol Chem* 1987; **262**: 17156–63.
2. Sasaki R, Masuda S, Nagao M. Erythropoietin: multiple physiological functions and regulation of biosynthesis. *Biosci Biotechnol Biochem* 2000; **64**: 1775–93.
3. Miyake T, Kung CK, Goldwasser E. Purification of human erythropoietin. *J Biol Chem* 1977; **252**: 5558–64.
4. Dordal MS, Wang FF, Goldwasser E. The role of carbohydrate in erythropoietin action. *Endocrinology* 1985; **116**: 2293–9.
5. Koury ST, Bondurant MC, Koury MJ. Localization of erythropoietin synthesizing cells in murine kidneys by in situ hybridization. *Blood* 1988; **71**: 524–7.
6. Lacombe C, Da Silva JL, Bruneval P, *et al.* Peritubular cells are the site of erythropoietin synthesis in the murine hypoxic kidney. *J Clin Invest* 1988; **81**: 620–3.
7. Koury ST, Bondurant MC, Koury MJ, Semenza GL. Localization of cells producing erythropoietin in murine liver by in situ hybridization. *Blood* 1991; **77**: 2497–503.
8. Bachmann S, Le Hir M, Eckardt KU. Co-localization of erythropoietin mRNA and ecto-5'-nucleotidase immunoreactivity in peritubular cells of rat renal cortex indicates that fibroblasts produce erythropoietin. *J Histochem Cytochem* 1993; **41**: 335–41.
9. Loya F, Yang Y, Lin H, Goldwasser E, Albitar M. Transgenic mice carrying the erythropoietin gene promoter linked to lacZ express the reporter in proximal convoluted tubule cells after hypoxia. *Blood* 1994; **84**: 1831–6.
10. Erslev AJ. Erythropoietin. *N Engl J Med* 1991; **324**: 1339–44.
11. Porter DL, Goldberg MA. Regulation of erythropoietin production. *Exp Hematol* 1993; **21**: 399–404.
12. Liboi E, Carroll M, D'Andrea AD, Mathey-Prevot B. Erythropoietin receptor signals both proliferation and erythroid-specific differentiation. *Proc Natl Acad Sci USA* 1993; **90**: 11351–5.
13. Boggs DR. Hematopoiesis and aging: IV. Mass and distribution of erythroid marrow in aged mice. *Exp Hematol* 1985; **13**: 1044–7.
14. Boggs DR, Patrene KD. Hematopoiesis and aging III: Anemia and a blunted erythropoietic response to hemorrhage in aged mice. *Am J Hematol* 1985; **19**: 327–38.
15. Udupa KB, Lipschitz DA. Erythropoiesis in the aged mouse: I. Response to stimulation in vivo. *J Lab Clin Med* 1984; **103**: 574–80.
16. Udupa KB, Lipschitz DA. Erythropoiesis in the aged mouse: II. Response to stimulation in vitro. *J Lab Clin Med* 1984; **103**: 581–8.
17. Koury MJ, Bondurant MC. Maintenance by erythropoietin of viability and maturation of murine erythroid precursor cells. *J Cell Physiol* 1988; **137**: 65–74.
18. Krantz SB. Erythropoietin. *Blood* 1991; **77**: 419–34.
19. Kelley LL, Koury MJ, Bondurant MC, Koury ST, Sawyer ST, Wickrema A. Survival or death of individual proerythroblasts results from differing erythropoietin sensitivities: a mechanism for controlled rates of erythrocyte production. *Blood* 1993; **82**: 2340–52.

20. Carlini RG, Dusso AS, Obialo CI, Alvarez UM, Rothstein M. Recombinant human erythropoietin (rHuEPO) increases endothelin-1 release by endothelial cells. *Kidney Int* 1993; **43**: 1010–14.

21. Morakkabati N, Gollnick F, Meyer R, Fandrey J, Jelkmann W. Erythropoietin induces Ca2+ mobilization and contraction in rat mesangial and aortic smooth muscle cultures. *Exp Hematol* 1996; **24**: 392–7.

22. Westenfelder C, Biddle DL, Baranowski RL. Human, rat, and mouse kidney cells express functional erythropoietin receptors. *Kidney Int* 1999; **55**: 808–20.

23. Acs G, Acs P, Beckwith SM, *et al.* Erythropoietin and erythropoietin receptor expression in human cancer. *Cancer Res* 2001; **61**: 3561–5.

24. Masuda S, Nagao M, Takahata K, *et al.* Functional erythropoietin receptor of the cells with neural characteristics. Comparison with receptor properties of erythroid cells. *J Biol Chem* 1993; **268**: 11208–16.

25. Juul SE, Anderson DK, Li Y, Christensen RD. Erythropoietin and erythropoietin receptor in the developing human central nervous system. *Pediatr Res* 1998; **43**: 40–9.

26. Juul SE, Yachnis AT, Christensen RD. Tissue distribution of erythropoietin and erythropoietin receptor in the developing human fetus. *Early Hum Dev* 1998; **52**: 235–49.

27. Juul SE, Yachnis AT, Rojiani AM, Christensen RD. Immunohistochemical localization of erythropoietin and its receptor in the developing human brain. *Pediatr Dev Pathol* 1999; **2**: 148–58.

28. Juul SE, Stallings SA, Christensen RD. Erythropoietin in the cerebrospinal fluid of neonates who sustained CNS injury. *Pediatr Res* 1999; **46**: 543–7.

29. Lewczuk P, Hasselblatt M, Kamrowski-Kruck H, *et al.* Survival of hippocampal neurons in culture upon hypoxia: effect of erythropoietin. *Neuroreport* 2000; **11**: 3485–8.

30. Ehrenreich H, Hasselblatt M, Dembowski C, *et al.* Erythropoietin therapy for acute stroke is both safe and beneficial. *Mol Med* 2002; **8**: 495–505.

31. Garcia JF, Ebbe SN, Hollander L, Cutting HO, Miller ME, Cronkite EP. Radioimmunoassay of erythropoietin: circulating levels in normal and polycythemic human beings. *J Lab Clin Med* 1982; **99**: 624–35.

32. Cazzola M, Guarnone R, Cerani P, Centenara E, Rovati A, Beguin Y. Red blood cell precursor mass as an independent determinant of serum erythropoietin level. *Blood* 1998; **91**: 2139–45.

33. Barosi G. Inadequate erythropoietin response to anemia: definition and clinical relevance. *Ann Hematol* 1994; **68**: 215–23.

34. Baer AN, Dessypris EN, Goldwasser E, Krantz SB. Blunted erythropoietin response to anaemia in rheumatoid arthritis. *Br J Haematol* 1987; **66**: 559–64.

35. Spivak JL, Barnes DC, Fuchs E, Quinn TC. Serum immunoreactive erythropoietin in HIV-infected patients. *JAMA* 1989; **261**: 3104–7.

36. Miller CB, Jones RJ, Piantadosi S, Abeloff MD, Spivak JL. Decreased erythropoietin response in patients with the anemia of cancer. *N Engl J Med* 1990; **322**: 1689–92.

37. Mori M, Murai Y, Hirai M, *et al.* Serum erythropoietin titers in the aged. *Mech Ageing Dev* 1988; **46**: 105–9.

38. Powers JS, Lichtenstein MJ, Collins JC, Krantz SB, Greene HL, Buchholz T. Serum erythropoietin in healthy older persons. *J Am Geriatr Soc* 1989; **37**: 388–9.

39. Kario K, Matsuo T, Nakao K. Serum erythropoietin levels in the elderly. *Gerontology* 1991; **37**: 345–8.

40. Kario K, Matsuo T, Kodama K, Nakao K, Asada R. Reduced erythropoietin secretion in senile anemia. *Am J Hematol* 1992; **41**: 252–7.

41. Nafziger J, Pailla K, Luciani L, Andreux JP, Saint-Jean O, Casadevall N. Decreased erythropoietin responsiveness to iron deficiency anemia in the elderly. *Am J Hematol* 1993; **43**: 172–6.

42. Joosten E, Van Hove L, Lesaffre E, *et al.* Serum erythropoietin levels in elderly inpatients with anemia of chronic disorders and iron deficiency anemia. *J Am Geriatr Soc* 1993; **41**: 1301–4.

43. Goodnough LT, Price TH, Parvin CA. The endogenous erythropoietin response and the erythropoietic response to blood loss anemia: the effects of age and gender. *J Lab Clin Med* 1995; **126**: 57–64.

44. Ershler WB, Sheng S, McKelvey J, *et al.* Serum erythropoietin and aging: a longitudinal analysis. *J Am Geriatr Soc* 2005; **53**: 1360–5.

45. Powers JS, Krantz SB, Collins JC, *et al.* Erythropoietin response to anemia as a function of age. *J Am Geriatr Soc* 1991; **39**: 30–2.

46. Pasqualetti P, Casale R. No influence of aging on the circadian rhythm of erythropoietin in healthy subjects. *Gerontology* 1997; **43**: 206–9.

47. Carpenter MA, Kendall RG, O'Brien AE, *et al.* Reduced erythropoietin response to anaemia in elderly patients with normocytic anaemia. *Eur J Haematol* 1992; **49**: 119–21.

48. Matsuo T, Kario K, Kodoma K, Asada R. An inappropriate erythropoietic response to iron deficiency anaemia in the elderly. *Clin Lab Haematol* 1995; **17**: 317–21.

49. Pieroni L, Foglietti MJ, Andreux JP, Albou D, Nafziger J. Factors involved in the anaemia of chronic disorders in elderly patients. *Gerontology* 1997; **43**: 326–34.

50. Kamenetz Y, Beloosesky Y, Zeltzer C, *et al.* Relationship between routine hematological parameters, serum IL-3, IL-6 and erythropoietin and mild anemia and degree of function in the elderly. *Aging (Milano)* 1998; **10**: 32–8.

51. Ershler WB, Artz AS, Kandahari MM. Recombinant erythropoietin treatment of anemia in older adults. *J Am Geriatr Soc* 2001; **49**: 1396–7.

52. Artz AS, Fergusson D, Drinka PJ, *et al.* Prevalence of anemia in skilled-nursing home residents. *Arch Gerontol Geriatr* 2004; **39**: 201–6.

53. Artz AS, Fergusson D, Drinka PJ, *et al.* Mechanisms of unexplained anemia in the nursing home. *J Am Geriatr Soc* 2004; **52**: 423–7.

54. Cascinu S, Del Ferro E, Fedeli A, Ligi M, Alessandroni P, Catalano G. Recombinant human erythropoietin treatment in elderly cancer patients with cisplatin-associated anemia. *Oncology* 1995; **52**: 422–6.

55. Teruel JL, Marcen R, Navarro JF, *et al.* Influence of body iron stores on the serum erythropoietin concentration in hemodialyzed patients. *Am J Nephrol* 1994; **14**: 95–8.

56. Cazzola M, Beguin Y. New tools for clinical evaluation of erythron function in man. *Br J Haematol* 1992; **80**: 278–84.

57. Chaves PH, Xue QL, Guralnik JM, Ferrucci L, Volpato S, Fried LP. What constitutes normal hemoglobin concentration in community-dwelling disabled older women? *J Am Geriatr Soc* 2004; **52**: 1811–16.

58. Ferrucci L, Guralnik JM, Woodman RC, *et al.* Circulating erythropoietin (EPO) and pro-inflammatory markers in elderly (≥65) persons with and without anemia. *Blood* 2004; **104**: Abstract 1629.

59. McGonigle RJ, Wallin JD, Shadduck RK, Fisher JW. Erythropoietin deficiency and inhibition of erythropoiesis in renal insufficiency. *Kidney Int* 1984; **25**: 437–44.

60. Feinstein S, Becker-Cohen R, Algur N, *et al.* Erythropoietin deficiency causes anemia in nephrotic children with normal kidney function. *Am J Kidney Dis* 2001; **37**: 736–42.

61. Thomas MC, Cooper ME, Tsalamandris C, MacIsaac R, Jerums G. Anemia with impaired erythropoietin response in diabetic patients. *Arch Intern Med* 2005; **165**: 466–9.

62. Onoyama K, Sanai T, Motomura K, Fujishima M. Worsening of anemia by angiotensin converting enzyme inhibitors and its prevention by antiestrogenic steroid in chronic hemodialysis patients. *J Cardiovasc Pharmacol* 1989; **13** (Suppl 3): S27–S30.

63. Akpolat T, Gumus T, Bedir A, Adam B. Acute effect of trandolapril on serum erythropoietin in uremic and hypertensive patients. *J Nephrol* 1998; **11**: 94–7.

64. Lindeman RD, Tobin JD, Shock NW. Association between blood pressure and the rate of decline in renal function with age. *Kidney Int* 1984; **26**: 861–8.

65. Lin FC, Yeh SJ, Wu D. Determinants of simultaneous fast and slow pathway conduction in patients with dual atrioventricular nodal pathways. *Am Heart J* 1985; **109**: 963–70.

66. Egrie JC, Browne JK. Development and characterization of novel erythropoiesis stimulating protein (NESP). *Nephrol Dial Transplant* 2001; **16** (Suppl 3): 3–13.

67. Goya N, Toda F, Nishino S, *et al.* Autotransfusion supported by erythropoietin therapy in transurethral resection of the prostate. *Scand J Urol Nephrol* 1998; **32**: 383–7.

68. Fink JC, Yektashenas BH, Blasi MV, Klausner MA, Woodman RC, Provenzano R. Treatment of CKD anemia in octogenarians: a comparison of epoetin alfa (EPO) in elderly (65–79; ≥80) and non-elderly (<65 years) patients. *Blood* 2004; **104**: Abstract 3724.

69. Shank WA Jr, Balducci L. Recombinant hemopoietic growth factors: comparative hemopoietic response in younger and older subjects. *J Am Geriatr Soc* 1992; **40**: 151–4.

70. Demetri GD, Dale DC, Aapro MS. Epoetin alpha improves hemoglobin and quality of life in anemic geriatric cancer patients over 60 years receiving chemotherapy. *Blood* 2003; **102**: Abstract 4368.

71. Gonzalez-Baron M, Ordonez A, Franquesa R, *et al.* Response predicting factors to recombinant human erythropoietin in cancer patients undergoing platinum-based chemotherapy. *Cancer* 2002; **95**: 2408–13.

72. Osterborg A, Brandberg Y, Molostova V, *et al.* Randomized, double-blind, placebo-controlled trial of recombinant human erythropoietin, epoetin beta, in hematologic malignancies. *J Clin Oncol* 2002; **20**: 2486–94.

13

Iron and aging

Elizabeta Nemeth, Tomas Ganz

Iron is an essential trace element

Iron is required by almost all living organisms [1]. In mammals, iron is a component of heme in oxygen-transporting and storage proteins (hemoglobin and myoglobin), and a component of heme or iron–sulfur clusters in many redox enzymes, including enzymes of the mitochondrial respiratory chain and the ribonucleotide reductase, involved in deoxyribonucleotide synthesis. As these enzymes have a vital role in cell proliferation and cell viability, iron deficiency results in inhibition of cell proliferation and eventually in cell death [2]. On a systemic level, mild iron deficiency can produce subtle deficits in endurance, work capacity, and possibly neuropsychological performance [3–5]. More severe iron deficits cause iron-deficiency anemia, which impairs oxygen delivery to tissues and has adverse effects on cardiopulmonary function.

In response to infection, humans and animals sequester iron into iron-binding proteins (e.g., lacto-ferrin, siderocalin) and locations less accessible to most invading microbes (cytoplasm of macrophages and hepatocytes) [6]. This is an important innate host defense mechanism, as most microbes require iron for their growth. However, this response also impairs the delivery of iron to the nascent erythrocytes in the bone marrow and results in anemia of inflammation (anemia of chronic disease). Although anemia of inflammation is usually mild to moderate, it too can exacerbate concurrent cardiopulmonary deficits.

Iron excess also has deleterious consequences [7]. As a transition metal, free iron promotes generation of oxygen radicals by catalyzing the Fenton reaction in which Fe^{2+} reacts with H_2O_2 or lipid peroxides. The result is formation of highly reactive $OH^\bullet$ or $LO^\bullet$ and $LOO^\bullet$ radicals, which can cause damage to the lipid membranes, proteins and nucleic acids. Although the evidence is still controversial, it has been postulated that excess iron contributes to the aging process and to the development of disorders associated with aging.

The toxic effects of iron are minimized through mechanisms that assure that little or no free iron is found in the body under normal circumstances. Any iron that is not incorporated in heme-containing or iron–sulfur cluster proteins is bound to transport or storage proteins from which it can be mobilized for use. In plasma, iron is tightly bound to transferrin (Tf), an abundant plasma glycoprotein that delivers iron to most cells via a ubiquitously expressed transferrin receptor (TfR1). Inside the cells, iron is deposited in ferritin, a spherical protein cage which can store up to 4500 iron atoms. The ferritin molecule is assembled from 24 polypeptide subunits. Serum ferritin is a molecule related to the L-subunit of cytoplasmic ferritin, and its serum concentrations increase with iron stores and inflammation [8].

Iron homeostasis in humans

Complex mechanisms have evolved to maintain extracellular iron concentrations in a relatively narrow range, and to provide cells with adequate but not excessive iron for their metabolic needs.

Blood Disorders in the Elderly, ed. Lodovico Balducci, William Ershler, Giovanni de Gaetano.
Published by Cambridge University Press. © Cambridge University Press 2008.

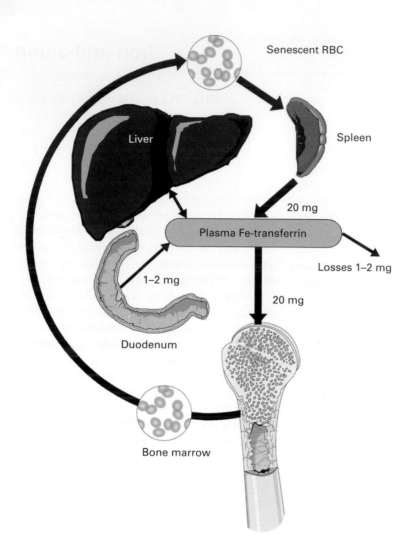

Figure 13.1 Major iron flows during normal iron homeostasis. Most iron enters plasma from macrophages that recycle senescent erythrocytes (RBC), with smaller amounts coming from hepatocyte stores and dietary absorption in the duodenum. Most plasma iron is destined for the hemoglobin in developing erythrocytes in the bone marrow. In the absence of bleeding, iron losses from desquamation of intestinal epithelia and skin are relatively minor. *See color plate section.*

Extracellular iron concentration and distribution of iron to cells depends on iron absorption, recycling, storage, and utilization. Iron is excreted by shedding of intestinal and skin cells, and through minor blood loss in the intestine. In principle, the iron content of shed epithelial cells could be subject to regulation [9], but this has not been systematically examined.

Total body iron in adults amounts to approximately 3–4 g. Two-thirds of that is incorporated in the heme moiety of hemoglobin found in erythroid precursors and mature erythrocytes. Normal erythrocytes live on average 120 days, and under average circumstance 20 mL of erythrocytes (packed volume) containing a total of 20 mg iron are destroyed each day. Thus, to maintain homeostasis, 20 mg of iron is required daily for production of hemoglobin for new erythrocytes (Fig. 13.1). Iron absorption from the diet, however, supplies only 1–2 mg daily. The rest is derived by recycling iron from senescent red blood cells. The process occurs in reticuloendothelial macrophages, which phagocytose and lyse old and damaged red blood cells. Heme is degraded by heme oxygenase and iron is recovered and exported into plasma, ready for utilization by the erythron.

Smaller amounts of iron from myoglobin and various redox enzymes are also recycled.

Even though recycled iron accounts for most of the daily iron supply, the rate of intestinal iron absorption is important in the long term. Over many months, inadequate dietary supply results in iron deficiency and anemia, whereas chronically increased iron absorption, due to genetic defects affecting iron regulatory circuits, leads to iron-overload diseases.

A quarter of the total body iron (0.5–1.0 g) is stored in macrophages and hepatocytes as a reserve which can be easily mobilized for erythropoiesis. The stores, however, can become depleted when iron uptake is less than iron usage and loss, such as with decreased dietary iron uptake or excessive blood loss. With stores depleted, erythropoiesis becomes iron-restricted, eventually resulting in the development of iron-deficiency anemia. Iron-overload disorders develop when iron uptake (through diet, parenteral delivery, or erythrocyte transfusions) exceeds iron utilization and loss. Excess iron is deposited in the liver and eventually in other organs, such as the heart, pancreas, and pituitary gland. If untreated, tissue injury due to excess iron will eventually lead to organ dysfunction. In general, liver damage (hepatic fibrosis, cirrhosis) is unlikely to occur when liver iron concentration is increased to less than ten times normal, an iron content associated with serum ferritin below 1000 ng/mL [10]. It is much less clear whether these lesser degrees of iron overload cause any clinical disease or accelerate coexisting disease processes.

Molecular mechanisms of iron transport

Beginning with absorption from the diet, to reaching its sites of utilization, iron needs to be transported across multiple cell membranes. Specific transmembrane proteins mediate iron import into and export out of the cells. Duodenal absorptive cells take up both heme and non-heme iron from the diet. Heme transport is less well understood, but candidate intestinal heme transporters have been described

[11]. Inside the enterocyte, iron is released from the heme and is thought to be exported out of the cell by a common pathway together with non-heme iron. Non-heme dietary iron is in the insoluble Fe^{3+} form, and is first reduced to Fe^{2+} by duodenal cytochrome b-like ferrireductase (Dcytb) and then transported across the membrane by divalent metal transporter 1 (DMT-1), a proton/metal symporter. Selective inactivation of DMT-1 in intestine of mice results in severe anemia [12].

Most cells meet their iron needs by taking up TF-bound iron from plasma. Binding of diferric or monoferric TF to transferrin receptor 1 (TfR1) initiates endocytosis of the complex. Early endosomes undergo acidification by a proton pump, resulting in the release of iron from the complex. Iron is transferred across endosomal membrane into the cytoplasm by DMT-1, while apo-Tf and TfR1 are recycled back to the cell surface. Although the Tf/TfR1 pathway is of particular importance for iron uptake by erythroid precursors, it is likely used by most cell types since TfR1 is ubiquitously expressed and inactivation of TfR1 results in embryonic death [13].

Certain cell types can take up iron by Tf-independent mechanisms. Mice deficient in functional Tf develop severe iron overload in non-hematopoietic tissues, such as liver and pancreas [14], indicating that these tissues can take up iron by an alternative mechanism. In addition, monocytes and macrophages can take up hemoglobin by haptoglobin-mediated binding to hemoglobin scavenger receptor (CD163). This pathway is particularly prominent in diseases with intravascular hemolysis such as sickle-cell anemia and thalassemia. Additional uptake mechanisms may exist for iron sequestered in ferritin or hemopexin, but the mechanisms have not been well characterized. Finally, phagocytosis of senescent erythrocyte by specialized macrophages constitutes an important indirect iron uptake mechanism.

In contrast with multiple iron uptake mechanisms, only one pathway for cellular iron export has been described to date. A membrane multispanning channel ferroportin is found in all the cell types exporting iron into plasma: duodenal enterocytes, macrophages, hepatocytes, placental trophoblasts, and cells of the central nervous system (CNS). Total ferroportin deficiency in mice or zebrafish is embryonic lethal, due to the lack of iron transfer across the maternal–fetal interface [9]. Selective inactivation of ferroportin that spares the maternal–fetal interface allows survival to birth but leads to iron-trapping in enterocytes, hepatocytes, and macrophages in the face of severe systemic iron deficiency, indicating the unique and non-redundant function of ferroportin in cellular iron export.

Iron export by ferroportin and subsequent loading onto TF also requires presence of multicopper oxidases, which convert Fe^{2+} to Fe^{3+}. An abundant plasma protein, ceruloplasmin, is involved in iron export from non-intestinal cells and its homolog hephaestin aids iron export from intestinal cells. Deficiency of ceruloplasmin in patients and mice also leads to iron accumulation in macrophages and hepatocytes, as well as in cells of the CNS, resulting in iron-restricted erythropoiesis and neurodegeneration [15]. Hephaestin deficiency results in severe iron-deficiency anemia [16].

Molecular mechanisms of systemic iron homeostasis

The recently discovered peptide hormone hepcidin is the key regulator of systemic iron homeostasis. Hepcidin is produced in the liver, circulates in plasma, and is excreted in urine [17,18]. The active form of the peptide is a 25-amino-acid β-sheet hairpin stabilized by four disulfide bonds. In mice, hepcidin deficiency due to disruption of a neighboring gene resulted in iron overload similar to human hereditary hemochromatosis [19], and in humans disruption of hepcidin gene causes the most severe form of iron overload – juvenile hemochromatosis [20]. Conversely, overexpression of hepcidin in transgenic mice resulted in severe iron-deficiency anemia [21]. Similarly, overproduction of hepcidin by liver tumors in patients with type 1a glycogen storage disease caused iron-refractory anemia which resolved only after resection of the tumor, or after

liver transplantation [22]. Hepcidin is thus a negative regulator of iron homeostasis, and the production of hepcidin is in turn homeostatically regulated by iron and anemia. Both dietary and parenteral iron load induced hepcidin mRNA in mice [23,24], and in humans ingestion of a single dose of 65 mg of iron resulted in an increase in urinary hepcidin within several hours [24]. It is not yet clear how iron (presumably through TF saturation) regulates hepcidin production and release. The best available information comes from genetic lesions in patients and animal models where hepcidin production is deficient in spite of iron overload. It now appears that almost all hereditary hemochromatoses are due to absolute or relative hepcidin deficiency, but only a handful of reported cases involve lesions in the hepcidin gene itself. Homozygous or compound heterozygous mutations in three other genes, *HFE*, *HJV*, and *TfR2*, result in partial or complete hepcidin deficiency [25–31], indicating that these genes probably function as modulators or regulators of hepcidin synthesis and release. Of these, *HJV* appears to have the closest relationship to hepcidin because homozygous *HJV* disruption phenotypically mimics the disruption of hepcidin gene itself and both result in juvenile hemochromatosis [31], whereas mutations in *HFE* and *TfR2* result in a milder adult form of the disease. The details of the pathway by which iron regulates hepcidin production, however, remain to be worked out.

Molecular mechanisms of hepcidin regulation by anemia are also unknown. Anemia and hypoxemia suppress hepcidin production. In animal models, bleeding or PHZ-induced hemolysis in mice caused a decrease in hepcidin mRNA level [32–35], as did the exposure of mice and rats to a hypoxic atmosphere [32,36]. Anemia could be regulating hepcidin through tissue hypoxia (possibly through involvement of hypoxia-inducible factor, HIF, which could directly regulate hepcidin gene expression) or indirectly by stimulation of erythropoiesis and increased demand for iron, resulting in decreased TF saturation, which would suppress hepcidin synthesis. Whichever the pathway, hepcidin was found to be decreased in diseases with ineffective erythropoiesis such as thalassemias [37] despite the concomitant iron overload, indicating a strong and dominant effect of anemia over iron on hepcidin production. The consequent low levels of hepcidin in these patients may be responsible for the hyperabsorption of iron with resulting organ damage.

The principal bioactivity of hepcidin is the rapid induction of hypoferremia. Injection of a single dose of synthetic hepcidin in mice caused a dramatic drop in serum iron within one hour, and the effect persisted for up to 72 hours [38]. In mice, and presumably also in humans, the effective concentrations of hepcidin are in the 100–1000 nM range [38,39]. Hepcidin acts by binding to the sole cellular iron exporter, ferroportin, and causing its internalization and degradation [39], with effective concentrations of hepcidin in the same 100–1000 nM range as those required for the induction of hypoferremia in vivo. As pointed out earlier, ferroportin is found in all the tissues that export iron into plasma: basolateral membranes of duodenal enterocytes and the cell membranes of placental cells, hepatocytes, and macrophages [9]. In these locations, ferroportin is in a unique position to regulate the inflow into plasma of iron from dietary or maternal sources, from hepatic stores, and from macrophages engaged in recycling senescent erythrocytes. The homeostatic loop involving hepcidin and ferroportin maintains normal extracellular iron concentrations. When plasma TF saturation rises as a result of dietary iron intake, it acts as a stimulus for hepcidin release. Under the influence of increased hepcidin, ferroportin is internalized from the cell membrane and degraded (Fig. 13.2). The influx of iron into plasma is decreased and the small plasma iron pool is restored to normal by continued utilization of iron, mainly for erythropoiesis. The same regulatory circuitry is responsible for inflammation-related hypoferremia and anemia.

Inflammation and iron

It has been known for many decades that inflammation alters iron metabolism by decreasing the iron content of plasma (hypoferremia of inflammation). If inflammation is sufficiently severe or chronic, a normocytic normochromic anemia (anemia of chronic disease, anemia of inflammation) eventually develops. Although this anemia resembles iron-deficiency anemia by developing in the setting of low plasma iron, it differs from iron-deficiency anemia by the presence of stainable iron in bone-marrow macrophages, and by elevated serum ferritin – both indicative of adequate iron stores. The molecular basis of these changes was only recently elucidated, and it centers on the regulation of hepcidin by inflammation [40]. Hepcidin production increases in inflammation, and injections of turpentine, Freund's adjuvant, or lipopolysaccharide (LPS) were all shown to increase hepatic hepcidin mRNA expression in mice and rats [24,32,41]. In addition, increased urinary hepcidin levels were seen in patients with infection and inflammatory disorders [42], and infusion of LPS in healthy subjects also resulted in a rapid increase in urinary hepcidin [43]. Unlike iron and hypoxia, molecular pathways of hepcidin regulation by inflammation are better understood and primarily involve the inflammatory cytokine interleukin 6 (IL-6). Treatment of primary hepatocytes with IL-6 in vitro, or injection of IL-6 in mice or humans, increased hepcidin production within hours [24,42]. IL-1 also induced hepcidin in human hepatocytes, but this effect was dependent on the intermediate production of IL-6. Tumor necrosis factor alpha (TNF-α) suppressed hepcidin synthesis in human hepatocyte cell lines [24]. Experiments in mice lacking IL-6 show that other cytokines, including IL-1, may contribute to hepcidin induction during inflammation, but it is not certain whether the specific hepcidin-stimulatory cytokines are the same in mice and humans [44].

Increased plasma hepcidin induces the internalization and degradation of ferroportin in macrophages, hepatocytes, and duodenal enterocytes, thus trapping iron in these cells and preventing the efflux of iron into plasma (Fig. 13.3). Within hours, the continued utilization of iron by developing erythrocytes depletes the plasma iron compartment, causing hypoferremia. Erythropoiesis, and more specifically heme and hemoglobin synthesis, become iron-limited,

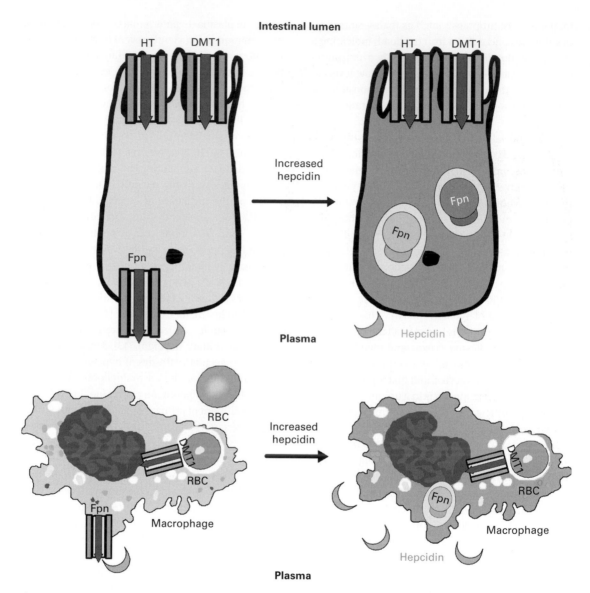

Figure 13.2 Hepcidin–ferroportin interaction regulates the flow of iron into plasma. Absorptive enterocytes acquire iron from the diet through the DMT-1 iron transporter, and as heme, using apical heme transporters (HT) (top panel). DMT-1 is also involved in the translocation of iron across the phagosomal membrane of macrophages (bottom panel). The red arrows indicate iron flows through channels. Cytoplasmic iron from duodenal enterocytes and macrophages is exported into plasma through the iron channel ferroportin (Fpn). Hepcidin binds to ferroportin, and induces its internalization and degradation. The loss of ferroportin results in decreased efflux of iron from cells into plasma and accumulation of iron in cytoplasmic ferritin (blue color). *See color plate section.*

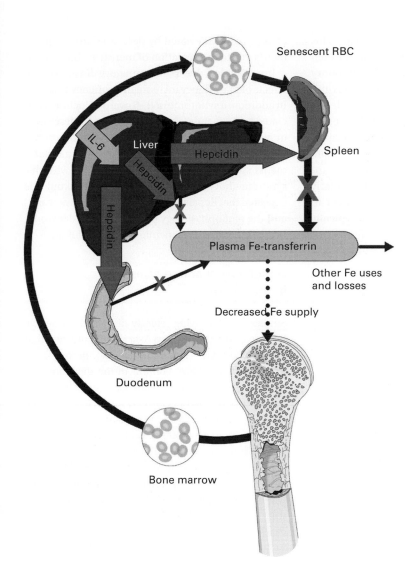

Figure 13.3 Changes of iron flows during inflammation. IL-6 and other cytokines induce hepcidin production and increased concentrations of hepcidin inhibit iron efflux from erythrocyte-recycling macrophages (predominantly in the spleen), from hepatic storage, and from the duodenum into plasma. Hypoferremia develops, and erythropoiesis becomes iron-limited. *See color plate section.*

as evidenced by increased substitution of zinc for iron during heme synthesis (zinc protoporphyrin). By apparently unrelated mechanisms, inflammation also shortens erythrocyte lifespan, and the decreased erythrocyte supply and increased erythrocyte loss lead to anemia. The hypoferremia and anemia eventually turn off hepcidin production so that a new setpoint is reached at a lower serum iron and blood hemoglobin concentration.

Hereditary hemochromatosis

Hereditary hemochromatosis encompasses a genetically and clinically heterogeneous group of disorders characterized by increased and dysregulated iron absorption in the small intestine [45]. A common form of the disorder in populations of northern European ancestry is due to mutations in the *HFE* gene (predominantly Cys282Tyr homozygotes but also compound heterozygotes with His63Asp). This form has a low clinical penetrance (higher in men than in women) but commonly causes laboratory abnormalities including elevated serum ferritin, elevated TF saturation, and elevated serum levels of hepatic enzymes. Less commonly the disorder progresses to cirrhosis, and can affect other organs including the pancreas, the joints, and the skin. The prevalence of HFE-related hereditary hemochromatosis does not diminish among the elderly because the disease does not shorten lifespan in most affected individuals [46]. A phenotypically similar disorder is due to homozygous mutations in *TfR2*, the gene encoding the transferrin receptor 2 [47]. Recently, a patient with a very severe early-onset form of hemochromatosis was found to have mutations that disrupted both the *HFE* and *TfR2* genes [48], indicating that these genes may provide additive signals to the iron regulatory pathway. The clinically most severe form of hemochromatosis is referred to as juvenile hemochromatosis because of its early age of onset in adolescents. Juvenile hemochromatosis is most often due to homozygous or compound heterozygous mutations in the *HJV* gene (encoding hemojuvelin) and less commonly due to homozygous mutations in the *HAMP* gene (encoding hepcidin). Based on the phenotypes of these disorders in humans and in mice, hepcidin and hemojuvelin appear to be non-redundant components of the iron regulatory pathway.

Disorders of iron metabolism in the elderly

In the simplest terms, a disorder of iron metabolism can arise from the altered iron uptake through changes in diet or iron absorption, the maldistribution of iron due to primary or secondary changes in hepcidin production, or the loss of iron due to known or occult blood loss. The aging process increases the prevalence of specific disorders affecting each of these phases of iron metabolism. Due to social, physical, and sometimes psychological factors, diets often become more restricted as people age. In elderly women, any decrease of iron intake is

at least partly alleviated by decreased iron requirements due to the cessation of menstrual blood loss.

Iron disorders due to inflammatory diseases or the effects of malignancy increase in frequency with age. In addition, a syndrome of IL-6 overproduction associated with anemia and frailty has been described, in which no specific inflammatory stimulus has been discerned [49]. Although hepcidin measurements specifically focusing on the elderly with this syndrome have not yet been reported, it would be expected that hepcidin excretion would be increased and the pathophysiology of the iron disorder would be similar to classical anemia of inflammation.

Epidemiology of iron disorders in the elderly

Studies of free-living elderly in North America, Europe, and industrialized Asia [50–52] indicate that iron deficiency is uncommon (<5%), perhaps due to relatively high iron content of the diets and low prevalence of diseases causing excessive blood loss. Iron excess, defined as elevated serum ferritin in the absence of laboratory evidence of inflammation (e.g., normal C-reactive protein), is more common (about 8–13%) but its clinical significance is uncertain.

Anemia is a common clinical finding among the elderly: its reported prevalence above the age of 65 was 11.0% in men and 10.2% in women, and more than 20% above the age of 85 [53]. However, most cases of anemia in older adults develop without a clearly identifiable cause, and the treatment is empiric and often ineffective. Improved understanding of and treatment for anemia in the elderly is an important goal because anemia is associated with reduced survival and increased risk of functional decline and cognitive impairment.

Conclusion

Iron disorders are very common among the elderly but the currently available options for the diagnosis and therapy of these disorders are limited. A remarkable progress in fundamental understanding of the regulation of iron flows in health and disease has been made in the last few years, with hepcidin emerging as the key regulator of iron homeostasis and the pathogenic factor in most iron diseases. These advances should provide important opportunities for the development of improved diagnostics and treatments for iron disorders.

REFERENCES

1. Andrews NC. Molecular control of iron metabolism. *Best Pract Res Clin Haematol* 2005; **18**: 159–69.

2. Le NT, Richardson DR. The role of iron in cell cycle progression and the proliferation of neoplastic cells. *Biochim Biophys Acta* 2002; **1603**: 31–46.

3. Brownlie T, Utermohlen V, Hinton PS, Haas JD. Tissue iron deficiency without anemia impairs adaptation in endurance capacity after aerobic training in previously untrained women. *Am J Clin Nutr* 2004; **79**: 437–43.

4. Zhu YI, Haas JD. Iron depletion without anemia and physical performance in young women. *Am J Clin Nutr* 1997; **66**: 334–41.

5. Beard JL, Connor JR. Iron status and neural functioning. *Annu Rev Nutr* 2003; **23**: 41–58.

6. Laham N, Ehrlich R. Manipulation of iron to determine survival: competition between host and pathogen. *Immunol Res* 2004; **30**: 15–28.

7. Papanikolaou G, Pantopoulos K. Iron metabolism and toxicity. *Toxicol Appl Pharmacol* 2005; **202**: 199–211.

8. Torti FM, Torti SV. Regulation of ferritin genes and protein. *Blood* 2002; **99**: 3505–16.

9. Donovan A, Lima CA, Pinkus JL, *et al.* The iron exporter ferroportin/Slc40a1 is essential for iron homeostasis. *Cell Metab* 2005; **1**: 191–200.

10. Tavill AS. Diagnosis and management of hemochromatosis. *Hepatology* 2001; **33**: 1321–8.

11. Shayeghi M, Latunde-Dada GO, Oakhill JS, *et al.* Identification of an intestinal heme transporter. *Cell* 2005; **122**: 789–801.

12. Gunshin H, Fujiwara Y, Custodio AO, Direnzo C, Robine S, Andrews NC. Slc11a2 is required for intestinal iron absorption and erythropoiesis but dispensable in placenta and liver. *J Clin Invest* 2005; **115**: 1258–66.

13. Levy JE, Jin O, Fujiwara Y, Kuo F, Andrews NC. Transferrin receptor is necessary for development of erythrocytes and the nervous system. *Nat Genet* 1999; **21**: 396–9.

14. Trenor CC 3rd, Campagna DR, Sellers VM, Andrews NC, Fleming MD. The molecular defect in hypotransferrinemic mice. *Blood* 2000; **96**: 1113–18.

15. Xu X, Pin S, Gathinji M, Fuchs R, Harris ZL. Aceruloplasminemia: an inherited neurodegenerative disease with impairment of iron homeostasis. *Ann NY Acad Sci* 2004; **1012**: 299–305.

16. Anderson GJ, Frazer DM, McKie AT, Vulpe CD. The ceruloplasmin homolog hephaestin and the control of intestinal iron absorption. *Blood Cells Mol Dis* 2002; **29**: 367–75.

17. Park CH, Valore EV, Waring AJ, Ganz T. Hepcidin, a urinary antimicrobial peptide synthesized in the liver. *J Biol Chem* 2001; **276**: 7806–10.

18. Krause A, Neitz S, Magert HJ, *et al.* LEAP-1, a novel highly disulfide-bonded human peptide, exhibits antimicrobial activity. *FEBS Lett* 2000; **480**: 147–50.

19. Nicolas G, Bennoun M, Devaux I, *et al.* Lack of hepcidin gene expression and severe tissue iron overload in upstream stimulatory factor 2 (USF2) knockout mice. *Proc Natl Acad Sci USA* 2001; **98**: 8780–5.

20. Roetto A, Papanikolaou G, Politou M, *et al.* Mutant antimicrobial peptide hepcidin is associated with severe juvenile hemochromatosis. *Nat Genet* 2003; **33**: 21–2.

21. Nicolas G, Bennoun M, Porteu A, *et al.* Severe iron deficiency anemia in transgenic mice expressing liver hepcidin. *Proc Natl Acad Sci USA* 2002; **99**: 4596–601.

22. Weinstein DA, Roy CN, Fleming MD, Loda MF, Wolfsdorf JI, Andrews NC. Inappropriate expression of hepcidin is associated with iron refractory anemia: implications for the anemia of chronic disease. *Blood* 2002; **100**: 3776–81.

23. Pigeon C, Ilyin G, Courselaud B, *et al.* A new mouse liver-specific gene, encoding a protein homologous to human antimicrobial peptide hepcidin, is overexpressed during iron overload. *J Biol Chem* 2001; **276**: 7811–19.

24. Nemeth E, Rivera S, Gabayan V, *et al.* IL-6 mediates hypoferremia of inflammation by inducing the synthesis of the iron regulatory hormone hepcidin. J Clin Invest 2004; **113**: 1271–6.

25. Ahmad KA, Ahmann JR, Migas MC, *et al.* Decreased liver hepcidin expression in the hfe knockout mouse. *Blood Cells Mol Dis* 2002; **29**: 361–6.

26. Bridle KR, Frazer DM, Wilkins SJ, *et al.* Disrupted hepcidin regulation in HFE-associated haemochromatosis and the liver as a regulator of body iron homoeostasis. *Lancet* 2003; **361**: 669–73.

27. Kawabata H, Fleming RE, Gui D, *et al.* Expression of hepcidin is down-regulated in TfR2 mutant mice

manifesting a phenotype of hereditary hemochromatosis. *Blood* 2005; **105**: 376–81.

28. Nemeth E, Roetto A, Garozzo G, Ganz T, Camaschella C. Hepcidin is decreased in TFR2 hemochromatosis. *Blood* 2005; **105**: 1803–6.

29. Huang FW, Pinkus JL, Pinkus GS, Fleming MD, Andrews NC. A mouse model of juvenile hemochromatosis. *J Clin Invest* 2005; **115**: 2187–91.

30. Niederkofler V, Salie R, Arber S. Hemojuvelin is essential for dietary iron sensing, and its mutation leads to severe iron overload. *J Clin Invest* 2005; **115**: 2180–6.

31. Papanikolaou G, Samuels ME, Ludwig EH, *et al.* Mutations in HFE2 cause iron overload in chromosome 1q-linked juvenile hemochromatosis. *Nat Genet* 2004; **36**: 77–82.

32. Nicolas G, Chauvet C, Viatte L, *et al.* The gene encoding the iron regulatory peptide hepcidin is regulated by anemia, hypoxia, and inflammation. *J Clin Invest* 2002; **110**: 1037–44.

33. Frazer DM, Inglis HR, Wilkins SJ, *et al.* Delayed hepcidin response explains the lag period in iron absorption following a stimulus to increase erythropoiesis. *Gut* 2004; **53**: 1509–15.

34. Latunde-Dada GO, Vulpe CD, Anderson GJ, Simpson RJ, McKie AT. Tissue-specific changes in iron metabolism genes in mice following phenylhydrazine-induced haemolysis. *Biochim Biophys Acta* 2004; **1690**: 169–76.

35. Bondi A, Valentino P, Daraio F, *et al.* Hepatic expression of hemochromatosis genes in two mouse strains after phlebotomy and iron overload. *Haematologica* 2005; **90**: 1161–7.

36. Leung PS, Srai SK, Mascarenhas M, Churchill LJ, Debnam ES. Increased duodenal iron uptake and transfer in a rat model of chronic hypoxia is accompanied by reduced hepcidin expression. *Gut* 2005; **54**: 1391–5.

37. Papanikolaou G, Tzilianos M, Christakis JI, *et al.* Hepcidin in iron overload disorders. *Blood* 2005; **105**: 4103–5.

38. Rivera S, Nemeth E, Gabayan V, Lopez MA, Farshidi D, Ganz T. Synthetic hepcidin causes rapid dose-dependent hypoferremia and is concentrated in ferroportin-containing organs. *Blood* 2005; **106**: 2196–9.

39. Nemeth E, Tuttle MS, Powelson J, *et al.* Hepcidin regulates cellular iron efflux by binding to ferroportin and inducing its internalization. *Science* 2004; **306**: 2090–3.

40. Ganz T. Hepcidin: a regulator of intestinal iron absorption and iron recycling by macrophages. *Best Pract Res Clin Haematol* 2005; **18**: 171–82.

41. Frazer DM, Wilkins SJ, Millard KN, McKie AT, Vulpe CD, Anderson GJ. Increased hepcidin expression and hypoferraemia associated with an acute phase response are not affected by inactivation of HFE. *Br J Haematol* 2004; **126**: 434–6.

42. Nemeth E, Valore EV, Territo M, Schiller G, Lichtenstein A, Ganz T. Hepcidin, a putative mediator of anemia of inflammation, is a type II acute-phase protein. *Blood* 2003; **101**: 2461–3.

43. Kemna E, Pickkers P, Nemeth E, van der Hoeven H, Swinkels D. Time-course analysis of hepcidin, serum iron, and plasma cytokine levels in humans injected with LPS. *Blood* 2005; **106**: 1864–6.

44. Lee P, Peng H, Gelbart T, Wang L, Beutler E. Regulation of hepcidin transcription by interleukin-1 and interleukin-6. *Proc Natl Acad Sci USA* 2005; **102**: 1906–10.

45. Pietrangelo A. Hereditary hemochromatosis: a new look at an old disease. *N Engl J Med* 2004; **350**: 2383–97.

46. Beutler E, Felitti VJ, Koziol JA, Ho NJ, Gelbart T. Penetrance of 845G--> A (C282Y) HFE hereditary haemochromatosis mutation in the USA. *Lancet* 2002; **359**: 211–18.

47. Camaschella C, Roetto A, Cali A, *et al.* The gene TFR2 is mutated in a new type of haemochromatosis mapping to 7q22. *Nat Genet* 2000; **25**: 14–15.

48. Pietrangelo A, Caleffi A, Henrion J, *et al.* Juvenile hemochromatosis associated with pathogenic mutations of adult hemochromatosis genes. *Gastroenterology* 2005; **128**: 470–9.

49. Ershler WB. Biological interactions of aging and anemia: a focus on cytokines. *J Am Geriatr Soc* 2003; **51** (3 Suppl): S18–S21.

50. Fleming DJ, Jacques PF, Tucker KL, *et al.* Iron status of the free-living, elderly Framingham Heart Study cohort: an iron-replete population with a high prevalence of elevated iron stores. *Am J Clin Nutr* 2001; **73**: 638–46.

51. Milman N, Pedersen AN, Ovesen L, Schroll M. Iron status in 358 apparently healthy 80-year-old Danish men and women: relation to food composition and dietary and supplemental iron intake. *Ann Hematol* 2004; **83**: 423–9.

52. Wang JL, Shaw NS. Iron status of the Taiwanese elderly: the prevalence of iron deficiency and elevated iron stores. *Asia Pac J Clin Nutr* 2005; **14**: 278–84.

53. Guralnik JM, Eisenstaedt RS, Ferrucci L, Klein HG, Woodman RC. Prevalence of anemia in persons 65 years and older in the United States: evidence for a high rate of unexplained anemia. *Blood* 2004; **104**: 2263–8.

14

Prevalence and mechanisms of B$_{12}$ deficiency

Sally P. Stabler

Introduction

Vitamin B$_{12}$ (cobalamin) is a scarce nutrient found mainly in foods of animal origin which is necessary for both hematopoiesis and myelination of the central and peripheral nervous system [1]. It is widely recognized that seniors are at highest risk for vitamin B$_{12}$ deficiency, and since vitamin B$_{12}$ replacement is generally effective, inexpensive, and non-toxic, there is great incentive to find and correct deficiency. However, there are occasional difficulties diagnosing vitamin B$_{12}$ deficiency, as will be outlined in this chapter.

Vitamin B$_{12}$ is required for only two enzymes (see Table 14.1). As a cofactor for methionine synthase, methyl B$_{12}$ participates in a reaction that converts homocysteine to methionine, producing the tetrahydrofolate needed for reactions of DNA and RNA synthesis [2]. The other B$_{12}$-dependent reaction salvages energy in the form of propionyl-CoA, which is converted to L-methylmalonyl-CoA. The adenosyl-B$_{12}$-dependent enzyme L-methylmalonyl CoA mutase supplies succinyl-CoA to the Krebs cycle [3]. The measurement of the substrates, homocysteine, and a product of methylmalonyl CoA, methylmalonic acid (MMA), have proved extremely useful in the diagnosis of vitamin B$_{12}$ and folate deficiency. MMA and/or total homocysteine values are always (>95%) elevated in clinical B$_{12}$ deficiency and are the first abnormality when B$_{12}$ is withdrawn [4,5].

A complex mechanism for absorption and distribution of vitamin B$_{12}$ has evolved in higher organisms in order to conserve this nutrient [6]. Food

Table 14.1. Vitamin B$_{12}$-dependent enzymes and substrates.

L-Methylmalonyl-CoA mutase
Inhibition causes increased methylmalonic acid and +/−2 methylcitric acid
Methionine synthase
Inhibition causes increased total homocysteine and +/− cystathionine

vitamin B$_{12}$ is generally protein-bound and must be released in the stomach, by acid and peptic digestion, and the released vitamin B$_{12}$ is then bound to haptocorrin and carried into the duodenum. The gastric parietal cells produce an intrinsic factor (IF) that binds to vitamin B$_{12}$ after it is released from haptocorrin in the duodenum by the action of pancreatic enzymes and bicarbonate. The vitamin B$_{12}$-IF complex is bound to a specific receptor in the ileum, cubulin, which is internalized with other proteins such as amnionless and possibly megalin playing a role [7]. The vitamin B$_{12}$-IF complex is then sequestered in a lysosome and by unknown means is released and eventually is found in the circulation bound to one of three binding proteins [3]. Transcobalamin II (TCII) is the specific vitamin B$_{12}$ delivery protein, and all cells have specific TCII receptors for vitamin B$_{12}$ uptake. However, most of the vitamin B$_{12}$ in the circulation is bound to haptocorrins of unknown function. This may be why serum B$_{12}$ levels have limited sensitivity and specificity in documenting clinical deficiency. The enterohepatic circulation plays an important role in conserving vitamin B_{12} since 2–9 µg of vitamin B_{12} is released into bile per day and must be reabsorbed using the IF/ileal absorption system or it is lost in the stool [6].

Causes of vitamin B_{12} deficiency

Vitamin B_{12} is readily available in an omnivorous diet, with particularly rich sources being beef, pork, eggs, shellfish, and organ meats [8]. Therefore, it has generally been assumed that symptomatic vitamin B_{12} deficiency is due to malabsorption of the vitamin, although recent studies of vegetarians show that dietary vitamin B_{12} deficiency is more common than previously realized [8,9]. A study of seniors from rural Georgia showed that elevated MMA correlated with a lack of daily meat or dairy intake [10]. It is likely, however, that most cases of symptomatic vitamin B_{12} deficiency result from the malabsorption syndromes that are listed in Table 14.2. Pernicious anemia is the term applied to an autoimmune disease that causes type A atrophic gastritis (antral sparing) and the loss of IF. Antibodies appear to be targeting the gastric $H+/K+/-$ ATPase in the parietal cells, resulting in achlorhydria and lack of intrinsic factor, causing both malabsorption and loss of B_{12} in the bile [11].

Pernicious anemia is found in all populations but is most common in persons of African and northern European origin [8]. Patients and/or their families are frequently found to have other autoimmune disorders, which are listed in Table 14.3 [12]. The most common association is with autoimmune thyroid disease. The incidence of pernicious anemia increases with each decade of life, and the peak age was between 70 and 80 years in a study from Sweden [13]. Undiagnosed pernicious anemia could be as high as 4% in seniors [14,15]. Reported incidence of pernicious anemia ranges from 1 to 50 per 100 000, with lower numbers reported from Asia and higher numbers from the USA and Europe [1].

Pernicious anemia may be the end result of lifelong atrophic gastritis, which initially causes iron deficiency and dyspepsia. Some evidence exists that

Table 14.2. Causes of vitamin B_{12} deficiency in seniors.

Dietary	Limited intake of animal protein
Malabsorption	Pernicious anemia – lack of intrinsic factor
	Food-cobalamin malabsorption – lack of acid, pepsin
	Gastric resection or bypass
	Jejunal bacterial overgrowth
	Ileal disease or resection
	Chronic pancreatitis
Drugs	Nitrous oxide anesthesia
	Metformin
	Gastric-acid blocking drugs

Table 14.3. Autoimmune disorders associated with pernicious anemia.

Autoimmune thyroid disease
Vitiligo
Insulin-dependent diabetes mellitus
Autoimmune cytopenias
Collagen vascular disease
Myasthenia gravis
Addison's disease
Premature ovarian failure

Helicobacter pylori plays a causal or contributing role in the production of the pathologic antibodies that target the parietal cells [16,17].

A milder form of vitamin B_{12} malabsorption, often termed "food-cobalamin malabsorption," is also very common in seniors [18]. Despite extensive investigation of patients with this syndrome, the underlying pathology is not clear. The Schilling test usually shows normal absorption of crystalline vitamin B_{12}, but testing involving protein-bound vitamin B_{12} may show a decrease in absorption [19,20]. These findings correlate to some extent with the presence of atrophic gastritis on upper gastrointestinal endoscopy and with low values for pepsinogen I [21]. However, there are significant numbers of subjects found in well-investigated cohorts who have low serum B_{12} and elevated MMA despite apparently normal gastric findings and vice versa [22,23]. African-Americans may have lower prevalence of mild B$_{12}$ malabsorption than white Americans [24,25].

Gastric and ileal resections, but also bariatric surgery or urinary diversion procedures involving these organs, are all associated with the development of vitamin B$_{12}$ deficiency [26,27]. Most patients who have had vagotomy and pyloroplasty for peptic ulcer will be in the older age range, and they should be prospectively screened for vitamin B$_{12}$ deficiency, which may occur combined with iron deficiency [27]. Metformin [28] and stomach acid-blocking drugs [29,30] have been said to cause vitamin B$_{12}$ deficiency in seniors. Recently a clinical situation of fairly rapid onset of vitamin B$_{12}$-deficient myelopathy developing after anesthesia with nitrous oxide has been described, since nitrous oxide inactivates methionine synthase. These patients may have had underlying subclinical vitamin B$_{12}$ deficiency unmasked by the nitrous oxide challenge [31,32].

Megaloblastic anemia due to vitamin B$_{12}$ deficiency

The findings of severe megaloblastic anemia due to pernicious anemia are shown in Table 14.4; patients may have all, some, or a few of these abnormalities [33,34]. The classically described syndrome of megaloblastic anemia due to pernicious anemia can be easy to recognize with extremely high mean red-cell volume (MCV) and pancytopenia [35]. If the patient also had positive anti-intrinsic factor antibodies and a very low serum vitamin B$_{12}$ value then most clinicians would readily make a diagnosis. Patients as described above are the rarest presentation of vitamin B$_{12}$ deficiency [36], and mixed anemias are extremely common in seniors [10]. Seniors frequently have multiple medical problems such as renal insufficiency with erythropoietin deficiency, occult gastrointestinal bleeding with iron deficiency, and chronic inflammation due to arthritis and other rheumatologic conditions. For these reasons, no value of MCV should prevent evaluation for potential vitamin B$_{12}$ deficiency. Serial MCV values from

Table 14.4. Hematologic abnormalities in vitamin B$_{12}$ deficiency.

Megaloblastic anemia	Macrocytes, ovalocytes
	Hypersegmented neutrophils
	Anemia ± pancytopenia
	Basophilic stippling
	Leukoerythroblastic change
Megaloblastic bone marrow	Hypercellularity
	Immature nuclear chromatin pattern
	Nuclear-cytoplasmic dyssyncrony
	Giant bands and metamyelocytes
	Increased erythroblasts
	Karyorrhexis of nuclei
Clinical chemistry	Low haptoglobin
	High LDH
	High indirect bilirubin

previous years may show a subtle rise, which can be informative. An increased red-cell distribution width (RDW), which suggests that macrocytes are present, can be a useful clue. *Hyper*segmentation of granulocytes can help differentiate B$_{12}$ deficiency from myelodysplastic syndrome, where *hypo*segmentation is more likely. Anemia is usually present and moderately severe before neutropenia or thrombocytopenia is seen, in contrast to the primary bone-marrow disorders, such as myelodysplasia [35]. The serum LDH can be extremely high in severe anemia and with the elevated indirect bilirubin and low haptoglobin may suggest hemolysis as the diagnosis. This intramedullary hemolysis of red-blood-cell precursors is termed "ineffective erythropoiesis." In anemic patients the bone-marrow aspirate and biopsy are usually hypercellular and show nuclear-cytoplasmic dyssynchrony such that the nuclei appear open and immature compared to the cytoplasm. There may also be giant bands and metamyelocytes. Occasionally the expansion of extremely megaloblastic erythroblasts raises the suspicion of acute leukemia, and flow cytometry of these cells can be described as compatible with erythroleukemia [8].

Vitamin B$_{12}$ deficiency of the nervous system

There is a strong inverse correlation between the neurologic manifestations of vitamin B$_{12}$ deficiency and the severity of hematologic abnormalities, which is unexplained [37–39]. It is also unknown why vitamin B$_{12}$ deficiency causes demyelination of the spinal cord, peripheral nerves, and occasionally cranial nerves and the brain. Approximately 30% of subjects with pernicious anemia develop neurologic problems, some of which are listed in Table 14.5. Paresthesias were found to be the most common symptom in the largest series of subjects with B$_{12}$-deficient neurologic disease ever reported, but the symptoms can be quite variable [38]. Generally, there is loss of proprioception and gait abnormalities prior to loss of sensation and actual motor weakness, but individual patients vary widely. Serum MMA and homocysteine are elevated in patients with neurologic signs even when hematologic findings are normal [5,37]. In the last 10 years, many reports of spinal and brain magnetic resonance imaging findings in vitamin B$_{12}$ deficiency have been described [39–41]. The demyelinated regions show a symmetric hyperintense signal on T2-weighted imaging. These findings decrease or correct after B$_{12}$ replacement. Motor and sensory nerve conduction studies are abnormal [39]. The more severe the neurologic abnormalities are at diagnosis, and the longer they have been present, the less chance that they will resolve completely with treatment [38,39]. Ongoing damage can always be arrested, however, so early diagnosis is imperative.

Just as there are multifactoral causes of anemia in seniors, the situation is if anything worse for neurologic abnormalities in seniors. Diabetic neuropathy, claudication, joint abnormalities, spinal abnormalities, paraproteinemias, toxic medications, and cerebral vascular disease may coexist with vitamin B$_{12}$ deficiency in the elderly population. The loss of vibration sense is extremely common in seniors and rarely responds to vitamin B$_{12}$ treatment. The psychiatric abnormalities seen with vitamin B$_{12}$ deficiency include depression, paranoia, mania,

Table 14.5. Neurologic symptoms and abnormalities in vitamin B$_{12}$ deficiency.

Paresthesias
Numbness
Gait ataxia
Loss of proprioception and vibration sense
Leg weakness
Loss of special senses
Optic atrophy
Lhermitte's syndrome
Incontinence and impotence
Memory loss
Personality change
Depression

irritability, and personality change [37,38]. Memory loss has been noted, and patients have sometimes even been diagnosed as Alzheimer dementia, although it has been difficult to show improvement in cognition after vitamin B$_{12}$ treatment. The psychiatric abnormalities respond readily, however [38]. Further discussion of the central nervous system effects of hyperhomocysteinemia and vitamin B$_{12}$ deficiency is found below.

Diagnosis of vitamin B$_{12}$ deficiency

Serum vitamin B$_{12}$ has been the time-honored screening test for vitamin B$_{12}$ deficiency. There are many assays in clinical use, with many labs now moving away from the radiodilution assays to newer methods such as those using chemiluminescence. At present it is not clear whether different assays will have the same sensitivity and specificity in detecting deficient patients, and certainly the normal range with different assays varies widely [42,43]. Newer assays for holotranscobalamin II also have limited sensitivity and specificity and may be affected by renal status [44–46]. The clinical dilemma is that not all patients with symptomatic vitamin B$_{12}$ deficiency will have a level below a laboratory predetermined lower range and that at least as many as 50% of those with a low level will have no reversible clinical abnormalities, and normal MMA and homocysteine values [4,36,37]. In general, very low serum values (<100 pg/mL) or those in the upper half of the normal range generally correlate with the presence or absence of significant vitamin B_{12} deficiency, respectively. However, the physician will encounter values frequently in the equivocal range of 100–400 pg/mL, and depending on the age and health of a population studied approximately 10–50% of such individuals will have elevation of MMA and/or homocysteine [10,47–49]. Thus, many experts recommend assaying MMA and/or homocysteine in order to improve both sensitivity and specificity of diagnosis [49–52].

Use of methylmalonic acid in the diagnosis of B_{12} deficiency

More than 95% of patients with megaloblastic anemia due to B_{12} deficiency (largely pernicious anemia), and 95% of those with neurologic defects due to B_{12} deficiency (largely without hematologic abnormalities), were found to have elevated MMA and total homocysteine in a study of over 300 patients [5]. Both MMA and total homocysteine values can range as high as the values seen in inborn errors of metabolism in patients who have severe clinical B_{12} deficiency [5, 53–58]. Most of these clinically affected subjects had serum MMA > 500 nmol/L. Another investigation showed that in subjects with serum vitamin B_{12} < 200 pg/mL elevated MMA and/or total homocysteine predicted a fall in MCV, rise in hematocrit, or improvement in neurologic abnormalities, after treatment [36]. The clinician can use these data to predict whether clinical abnormalities seen in a patient with a low or low-normal serum vitamin B_{12} value will respond to treatment with vitamin B_{12}. This is particularly important when evaluating clinical syndromes in seniors because of the multiple disease conditions often present and confusing multifactorial causes of anemia and neurological syndromes.

A practical approach to assessing vitamin B_{12} status in seniors would be as follows, starting from the screening serum vitamin B_{12} value. If <100 pg/ml

then treat with vitamin B_{12} and monitor for response. If the B_{12} value is between 100 and 400 pg/ml then it may be prudent to measure serum MMA and/or serum total homocysteine *before* deciding whether to treat with B_{12}. If the serum MMA is higher than the normal range then it is likely the subject has vitamin B_{12} deficiency. If only serum homocysteine is elevated then it not known whether the subject has B_{12} deficiency, folate deficiency, or both. Renal insufficiency causes mild elevations of both MMA [57] and total homocysteine [59], but of course renal insufficiency and serum vitamin B_{12} deficiency will frequently coexist in seniors [24]. In such patients, a markedly elevated 2-methylcitric acid or cystathionine (available in many lab panels with MMA and total homocysteine) may help with the specific diagnosis of B_{12} deficiency [60,61]. Since the latter two metabolites are highly dependent on renal excretion, they will often be quite elevated when MMA and total homocysteine are only slightly above a normal range, indicating that impaired renal excretion is the more likely cause of the elevated metabolites. MMA and/or homocysteine must be measured before treatment since within hours to days they will normalize [54,55].

The cause of vitamin B_{12} deficiency can sometimes be determined using ancillary tests. The Schilling test is no longer easily available in most hospitals and is plagued with problems of sensitivity [62]. High fasting serum gastrin and low pepsinogen I are seen with atrophic gastritis and point to malabsorption of B_{12} [18,21]. Anti-intrinsic-factor antibodies are highly specific but much less sensitive in diagnosing pernicious anemia. Blood for these antibodies must not be drawn immediately after a B_{12} injection, because of false-positive results. Endoscopy is reserved for patients with appropriate symptoms only.

Vitamin B_{12} replacement therapy

Vitamin B_{12} deficiency may be treated with either intramuscular (IM) injections or high-dose oral formulations [63–66]. There are fewer data available about the efficacy of nasal gels or sublingual preparations of B_{12}. An effective initial parenteral treatment in the patient with severe clinical abnormalities is vitamin B_{12} 1000 μg IM daily if the patient is hospitalized with severe anemia, then weekly for approximately eight weeks. Subjects with severe demyelinating disease of the spinal cord may benefit by having weekly or biweekly injections for up to six months. Stable patients can then receive 1000 μg IM per month. Approximately 10–20% of patients with severe malabsorption of B_{12} will not have normal serum MMA with injections spaced at four weeks, however [64]. The injections can often be accomplished by family members, etc., so that the patient does not need monthly visits to a healthcare facility.

A high-dose oral B_{12} randomized trial showed higher serum B_{12} values and lower MMA values at four months [64]. In addition, high-dose vitamin B_{12} tablets, usually 1000 μg per day, have been used in Sweden for 40 years with great success [63]. Thus, a reasonable alternative to injections is 1000–2000 μg orally daily. It is controversial whether the patient is better served by IM or oral replacement [67,68]. An advantage of parenteral treatment is that the patient remains under observation and thus there will be better compliance with treatment. The opponents of the parenteral approach note that vitamin B_{12} replacement is incorrectly discontinued by physicians frequently [69], and/or that changing medical providers may cause lapses in treatment. In addition, IM injections are painful and cause bleeding in very frail, debilitated individuals. An advantage of oral treatment in the USA is that the high-dose tablets are obtainable from all grocery stores and pharmacies without a prescription so the patient will always have access to the therapy.

Ironically, the cost of the daily tablets is considerably higher than self-administered injections or those obtained at a medical facility for most senior US patients. There may also be problems with the bioavailability of some preparations, and food decreases absorption [63,64]. Daily therapy in a patient who may be taking 5–10 other medications may also be a problem. The common lay perception that vitamins are an optional therapy could also be dangerous in the patient with pernicious anemia, since cessation of therapy will eventually cause relapse of the original clinical syndrome within six months to two years [69]. Complete correction of anemia can be expected if adequate erythropoietin and iron are available. However, mixed anemias are to be expected in seniors and it is not uncommon that the primary marrow disorders coexist with mild B_{12} deficiency. Patients with pretreatment serum MMA 500–1000 nmol/L rarely have correction of anemia since there is usually an additional underlying cause [10]. Likewise, only neurological symptoms due to B_{12} deficiency will respond. In contrast, MMA and homocysteine (especially in folate-fortified populations) will correct, often dropping into the low-normal range [10,47,66,70].

Prevention of vitamin B_{12} deficiency in seniors

Many screening studies during the 1990s show that senior populations throughout the world have a fairly high prevalence (10–30%) of vitamin B_{12} deficiency as shown by low serum vitamin B_{12} levels and/or elevated MMA and/or homocysteine [8,10,22,24,47,48,71–74]. Most studies of dietary intake show that vitamin B_{12} intake is adequate in developed countries [72]. Thus, it is assumed that malabsorption of food cobalamin is the probable cause of deficiency in most seniors, and speculated that small doses of crystalline (not food protein-bound) B_{12} would prevent or treat deficiency. The recently revised US food pyramid scheme noted that seniors should obtain their vitamin B_{12} from a crystalline source but the dose required was not specified [75]. Supplemental vitamin B_{12} in multivitamins or other forms (not food-bound) in doses greater than approximately 25 μg/day decreases the prevalence of elevated MMA and low serum B_{12} values in seniors in a number of studies [48,71]. In contrast, when subjects with elevated MMA were treated (some already on multivitamins) with increasing oral doses, a 25 μg and 100 μg daily dose corrected MMA in only 10% and 25% of the group [76]. After treatment with

$1000\,\mu g$ the subjects corrected, including the one subject with pernicious anemia. In summary, smaller oral doses may prevent deficiency, but this study and others show that those who are found to have metabolic deficiency require higher doses to correct metabolites [77]. Individualizing the B_{12} dose needed by repeated serologic testing is more expensive and time-consuming, as compared to recommending a minimum of $1000\,\mu g/day$. Most multivitamins in the USA contain only small amounts of B_{12} combined with $400\,\mu g$ of folic acid, which added to a folate-fortified diet may mean that some vitamin B_{12}-deficient seniors are receiving enough folate to potentially mask megaloblastic anemia due to pernicious anemia, leading to untreated and neglected neurologic deficits.

Health effects of hyperhomocysteinemia and vitamin B_{12} deficiency

Deficiency of and inborn errors in B_{12}, folate, or B_6 vitamin-dependent pathways can cause hyperhomocysteinemia [2]. The serum total homocysteine is a sensitive indicator of folate status only if vitamin B_{12} status is adequate [10,58,78–81]. In fact, the folate status of a population can be inferred by the population mean total homocysteine values. However, the high prevalence of metabolic B_{12} deficiency in seniors is a major cause of hyperhomocysteinemia [10,73,78]. Since folate fortification in 1998 in the USA and Canada, mean serum homocysteine values have fallen [71,81–83]. However, the causal contribution of vitamin B_{12} deficiency to hyperhomocysteinemia now is much greater [80].

It has been difficult to determine whether the ill effects of hyperhomocysteinemia are attributable to the amino acid itself or to vitamin B_{12} or folate (or both) deficiency. See Table 14.6 for associations. Many studies use the nonspecific and insensitive serum vitamin B_{12} value instead of MMA values to assess B_{12} status. Inadequate oral B_{12} doses have often been combined with folic acid, which results in suboptimal homocysteine lowering in seniors. The food folate fortification program in the USA and

Table 14.6. Conditions associated with hyperhomocysteinemia.

Venous thrombosis
Cerebral and cardiovascular disease
Dementing syndromes
Depression and other psychiatric syndromes
Osteoporosis

Canada starting in 1998 has compromised the power of long-term and interventional studies [79,84].

Since hyperhomocysteinemia due to inborn errors of metabolism causes thrombotic vascular disease, it has been speculated, and widely studied, as to whether milder hyperhomocysteinemia, largely due to vitamin deficiency, would also be implicated [85–89]. There are case reports of venous thrombosis in patients with pernicious anemia with extremely high values of total homocysteine [90]. However, it is not clear whether the mild increases in homocysteine seen with subclinical vitamin B_{12} deficiency, especially in senior populations, are direct causes of vascular disease or just markers of unhealthy conditions such as renal insufficiency or an unhealthy lifestyle. Prospective randomized trials of treatment with combinations of vitamin B_{12} and folate in recurrent stroke, cardiac, and cerebral vascular disease show mixed results [84,91–92]. Currently, large prospective trials of combination vitamin therapy are in progress and may provide more definitive results [93]. Whatever the trial results the clinician will still need to decide whether it is wise to treat the asymptomatic senior patient with elevated MMA and homocysteine with vitamin B_{12}.

Many studies show that elevated homocysteine is associated with poor cognition and psychiatric abnormalities [46,94–96]. A recent report showed that the diagnosis of Alzheimer disease was increased after 11 years in those who had the highest baseline homocysteine values from a Framingham population [97], who had a high prevalence of B_{12} deficiency in another study [48]. More studies are needed to determine the benefit of treatment [98].

Recent investigations have shown that hyperhomocysteinemia is a risk factor for osteoporosis and fractures [99,100] and combination vitamin replacement in stroke patients resulted in fewer fractures [101].

REFERENCES

1. Stabler SP, Allen RH. Megaloblastic anemias. In Goldman L, Ausiello D, eds, *Cecil Textbook of Medicine*, 22nd edn (Philadelphia, PA: Saunders, 2004), 1050–7.

2. Mudd SH, Levy HL, Kraus JP. Disorders of transsulfuration. In Scriver CS, Beaudet AL, Sly WS, Valle D, eds, *The Metabolic & Molecular Bases of Inherited Disease*, 8th edn (New York, NY: McGraw Hill, 2001), Vol. 1: 2007–56.

3. Rosenblatt DS, Fenton WA. Inherited disorders of folate and cobalamin transport and metabolism. In Scriver CS, Beaudet AL, Sly WS, Valle D, eds, *The Metabolic & Molecular Bases of Inherited Disease*, 8th edn (New York, NY: McGraw-Hill, 2001), Vol. 1: 3897–934.

4. Lindenbaum J, Savage DG, Stabler SP, Allen RH. Diagnosis of cobalamin deficiency: II. Relative sensitivities of serum cobalamin, methylmalonic acid, and total homocysteine concentrations. *Am J Hematol* 1990; **34**: 99–107.

5. Savage DG, Lindenbaum J, Stabler SP, Allen RH. Sensitivity of serum methylmalonic acid and total homocysteine determinations for diagnosing cobalamin and folate deficiencies. *Am J Med* 1994; **96**: 239–46.

6. Allen RH. Cobalamin (vitamin B12) absorption and malabsorption. *View Dig Dis* 1982; **14**: 17–20.

7. Alpers DH. What is new in vitamin B(12)? *Curr Opin Gastroenterol* 2005; **21**: 183–6.

8. Stabler SP, Allen RH. Vitamin B12 deficiency as a worldwide problem. *Ann Rev Nutr* 2004; **24**: 299–326.

9. Herrmann W, Geisel J. Vegetarian lifestyle and monitoring of vitamin B-12 status. *Clin Chim Acta* 2002; **326**: 47–59.

10. Johnson MA, Hawthorne NA, Brackett WR, *et al.* Hyperhomocysteinemia and vitamin B-12 deficiency in elderly using Title IIIc nutrition services. *Am J Clin Nutr* 2003; **77**: 211–20.

11. Toh BH, van Driel IR, Gleeson PA. Pernicious anemia. *N Engl J Med* 1997; **337**: 1441–8.

12. Eisenbarth GS. Autoimmune polyendocrine syndromes. *Adv Exp Med Biol* 2004; **552**: 204–18.

13. Borch K, Liedberg G. Prevalence and incidence of pernicious anemia. An evaluation for gastric screening. *Scand J Gastroenterol* 1984; **19**: 154–60.

14. Carmel R. Prevalence of undiagnosed pernicious anemia in the elderly. *Arch Intern Med* 1996; **156**: 1097–100.

15. Krasinski SD, Russell RM, Samloff IM, *et al.* Fundic atrophic gastritis in an elderly population. Effect on hemoglobin and several serum nutritional indicators. *J Am Geriatr Soc* 1986; **34**: 800–6.

16. Annibale B, Lahner E, Negrini R, *et al.* Lack of specific association between gastric autoimmunity hallmarks and clinical presentations of atrophic body gastritis. *World J Gastroenterol* 2005; **11**: 5351–7.

17. Hershko C, Ronson A, Souroujon M, *et al.* Variable hematological presentation of autoimmune gastritis: age-related progression from iron deficiency to cobalamin depletion. *Blood* 2006; **107**: 1673–9.

18. Carmel R. Cobalamin, the stomach, and aging. *Am J Clin Nutr* 1997; **66**: 750–9.

19. Dawson DW, Sawers AH, Sharma RK. Malabsorption of protein bound vitamin B12. *Br Med J* 1984; **288**: 675–8.

20. Scarlett JD, Read H, O'Dea K. Protein-bound cobalamin absorption declines in the elderly. *Am J Hematol* 1992; **39**: 79–83.

21. Mardh E, Mardh S, Mardh B, Borch K. Diagnosis of gastritis by means of a combination of serological analyses. *Clin Chim Acta* 2002; **320**: 17–27.

22. Joosten E, Pelemans W, Devos P, *et al.* Cobalamin absorption and serum homocysteine and methylmalonic acid in elderly subjects with low serum cobalamin. *Eur J Haematol* 1993; **51**: 25–30.

23. Lindgren A, Swolin B, Nilsson O, *et al.* Serum methylmalonic acid and total homocysteine in patients with suspected cobalamin deficiency: a clinical study based on gastrointestinal histopathological findings. *Am J Hematol* 1997; **56**: 230–8.

24. Stabler SP, Allen RH, Fried LP, *et al.* Racial differences in prevalence of cobalamin and folate deficiencies in disabled elderly women. *Am J Clin Nutr* 1999; **70**: 911–19.

25. Carmel R, Green R, Jacobsen DW, *et al.* Serum cobalamin, homocysteine, and methylmalonic acid concentrations in a multiethnic elderly population: ethnic and sex differences in cobalamin and metabolite abnormalities. *Am J Clin Nutr* 1999; **70**: 904–10.

26. Yale CE, Gohdes PN, Schilling RF. Cobalamin absorption and hematologic status after two types of gastric surgery for obesity. *Am J Hematol* 1993; **42**: 63–6.

27. Sumner AE, Chin MM, Abrahm JL, *et al.* Elevated methylmalonic acid and total homocysteine levels show high prevalence of vitamin B$_{12}$ deficiency after gastric surgery. *Ann Intern Med* 1996; **124**: 469–76.

28. Wulffele MG, Kooy A, Lehert P, *et al.* Effects of short-term treatment with metformin on serum concentrations of homocysteine, folate and vitamin B$_{12}$ in type 2 diabetes mellitus: a randomized, placebo-controlled trial. *J Intern Med* 2003; **254**: 455–63.

29. Marcuard SP, Albernaz L, Khazanie PG. Omeprazole therapy causes malabsorption of cyanocobalamin (vitamin B$_{12}$). *Ann Intern Med* 1994; **120**, 211–15.

30. Ruscin JM, Page RL 2nd, Valuck RJ. Vitamin B(12) deficiency associated with histamine(2)-receptor antagonists and a proton-pump inhibitor. *Ann Pharmacother* 2002; **36**: 812–16.

31. Kinsella LJ, Green R. "Anesthesia paresthetica": nitrous oxide-induced cobalamin deficiency. *Neurology* 1995; **45**, 1608–10.

32. Marie RM, Le Biez E, Busson P, *et al.* Nitrous oxide anesthesia-associated myelopathy. *Arch Neurol* 2000; **57**: 380–2.

33. Lindenbaum J, Nath BJ. Megaloblastic anaemia and neutrophil hypersegmentation. *Br J Haematol* 1980; **44**: 511–13.

34. Koury MJ, Ponka P. New insights into erythropoiesis: the roles of folate, vitamin B$_{12}$, and iron. *Annu Rev Nutr* 2004; **24**: 105–31.

35. Savage DG, Ogundipe A, Allen RH, *et al.* Etiology and diagnostic evaluation of macrocytosis. *Am J Med Sci* 2000; **319**: 343–52.

36. Stabler SP, Allen RH, Savage DG, Lindenbaum J. Clinical spectrum and diagnosis of cobalamin deficiency. *Blood* 1990; **76**: 871–81.

37. Lindenbaum J, Healton EB, Savage DG, *et al.* Neuropsychiatric disorders caused by cobalamin deficiency in the absence of anemia or macrocytosis. *N Engl J Med* 1988; **318**: 1720–8.

38. Healton EB, Savage DG, Brust JC, *et al.* Neurologic aspects of cobalamin deficiency. *Medicine* 1991; **70**: 229–45.

39. Puri V, Chaudhry N, Goel S, *et al.* Vitamin B$_{12}$ deficiency: a clinical and electrophysiological profile. *Electromyogr Clin Neurophysiol* 2005; **45**: 273–84.

40. Tracey JP, Schiffman FJ. Magnetic resonance imaging in cobalamin deficiency. *Lancet* 1992; **339**: 1172–3.

41. Pittock SJ, Payne TA, Harper CM. Reversible myelopathy in a 34-year-old man with vitamin B12 deficiency. *Mayo Clin Proc* 2002; **77**: 291–4.

42. Steijns LS, Braams-Wiatrowska JK, Luiting HJ, van der Weide J. Evaluation of nonisotopic binding assays for measuring vitamin B$_{12}$ and folate in serum. *Clin Chim Acta* 1996; **248**: 135–41.

43. Carmel R, Brar S, Agrawal A, Penha PD. Failure of assay to identify low cobalamin concentrations. *Clin Chem* 2000; **46**: 2017–18.

44. Herrmann W, Obeid R, Schorr H, Geisel J. The usefulness of holotranscobalamin in predicting vitamin B12 status in different clinical settings. *Curr Drug Metab* 2005; **6**: 47–53.

45. Hvas AM, Nexo E. Holotranscobalamin: a first choice assay for diagnosing early vitamin B deficiency? *J Intern Med* 2005; **257**: 289–98.

46. Miller JW, Garrod MG, Rockwood AL, *et al.* Measurement of total vitamin B$_{12}$ and holotranscobalamin, singly and in combination, in screening for metabolic vitamin B12 deficiency. *Clin Chem* 2006; **52**: 278–85.

47. Pennypacker LC, Allen RH, Kelly JP, *et al.* High prevalence of cobalamin deficiency in elderly outpatients. *J Am Geriatr Soc* 1992; **40**: 1197–204.

48. Lindenbaum J, Rosenberg IH, Wilson PW, *et al.* Prevalence of cobalamin deficiency in the Framingham elderly population. *Am J Clin Nutr* 1994; **60**: 2–11.

49. Bolann BJ, Solli JD, Schneede J, *et al.* Evaluation of indicators of cobalamin deficiency defined as cobalamin-induced reduction in increased serum methylmalonic acid. *Clin Chem* 2000; **46**: 1744–50.

50. Snow CF. Laboratory diagnosis of vitamin B$_{12}$ and folate deficiency: a guide for the primary care physician. *Arch Intern Med* 1999; **159**: 1289–98.

51. Holleland G, Schneede J, Ueland PM, *et al.* Cobalamin deficiency in general practice. Assessment of the diagnostic utility and cost-benefit analysis of methylmalonic acid determination in relation to current diagnostic strategies. *Clin Chem* 1999; **45**: 189–98.

52. Klee GG. Cobalamin and folate evaluation: measurement of methylmalonic acid and homocysteine vs. vitamin B(12) and folate. *Clin Chem* 2000; **46**: 1277–83.

53. Norman EJ, Martelo OJ, Denton MD. Cobalamin (vitamin B12) deficiency detection by urinary methylmalonic acid quantitation. *Blood* 1982; **59**: 1128–31.

54. Stabler SP, Marcell PD, Podell ER, *et al.* Assay of methylmalonic acid in the serum of patients with cobalamin deficiency using capillary gas chromatography-mass spectrometry. *J Clin Invest* 1986; **77**: 1606–12.

55. Stabler SP, Marcell PD, Podell ER, *et al.* Elevation of total homocysteine in the serum of patients with cobalamin

or folate deficiency detected by capillary gas chromatography-mass spectrometry. *J Clin Invest* 1988; **81**: 466–74.

56. Brattstrom L, Israelsson B, Lindgarde F, Hultberg B. Higher total plasma homocysteine in vitamin B12 deficiency than in heterozygosity for homocystinuria due to cystathionine beta-synthase deficiency. *Metabolism* 1988; **37**: 175–8.

57. Moelby L, Rasmussen K, Jensen MK, Pedersen KO. The relationship between clinically confirmed cobalamin deficiency and serum methylmalonic acid. *J Intern Med* 1990; **228**: 373–8.

58. Refsum H, Smith AD, Ueland PM, *et al*. Facts and recommendations about total homocysteine determinations: an expert opinion. *Clin Chem* 2004; **50**: 3–32.

59. Hultberg B, Andersson A, Sterner G. Plasma homocysteine in renal failure. *Clin Neph* 1993; **40**: 230–5.

60. Allen RH, Stabler SP, Savage DG, Lindenbaum J. Elevation of 2-methylcitric acid I and II levels in serum, urine, and cerebrospinal fluid of patients with cobalamin deficiency. *Metabolism* 1993; **42**: 978–88.

61. Stabler SP, Lindenbaum J, Savage DG, Allen RH. Elevation of serum cystathionine levels in patients with cobalamin and folate deficiency. *Blood* 1993; **81**: 3404–13.

62. Krynyckyi BR, Zuckier LS. Accuracy of measurement of dual-isotope Schilling test urine samples: a multicenter study. *J Nucl Med* 1995; **36**: 1659–65.

63. Berlin H, Berlin R, Brante G. Oral treatment of pernicious anemia with high doses of vitamin B12 without intrinsic factor. *Acta Med Scand* 1968; **184**: 247–58.

64. Kuzminski AM, Del Giacco EJ, Allen RH, *et al*. Effective treatment of cobalamin deficiency with oral cobalamin. *Blood* 1998; **92**: 1191–8.

65. Kondo H. Haematological effects of oral cobalamin preparations on patients with megaloblastic anaemia. *Acta Haematol* 1998; **99**: 200–5.

66. Bjorkegren K, Svardsudd K. Elevated serum levels of methylmalonic acid and homocysteine in elderly people. A population-based intervention study. *J Intern Med* 1999; **246**: 317–24.

67. Lederle FA. Oral cobalamin for pernicious anemia. Medicine's best kept secret? *JAMA* 1991; **265**: 94–5.

68. Hathcock JN, Troendle GJ. Oral cobalamin for treatment of pernicious anemia? *JAMA* 1991; **265**: 96–7.

69. Savage D, Lindenbaum J. Relapses after interruption of cyanocobalamin therapy in patients with pernicious anemia. *Am J Med* 1983; **74**: 765–72.

70. Naurath HJ, Joosten E, Riezler R, *et al*. Effects of vitamin B12, folate, and vitamin B6 supplements in elderly people with normal serum vitamin concentrations. *Lancet* 1995; **346**: 85–9.

71. Rajan S, Wallace JI, Beresford SA, *et al*. Screening for cobalamin deficiency in geriatric outpatients: prevalence and influence of synthetic cobalamin intake. *J Am Geriatr Soc* 2002; **50**: 624–30.

72. Howard JM, Azen C, Jacobsen DW, *et al*. Dietary intake of cobalamin in elderly people who have abnormal serum cobalamin, methylmalonic acid and homocysteine levels. *Eur J Clin Nutr* 1998; **52**: 582–7.

73. Clarke R, Refsum H, Birks J, *et al*. Screening for vitamin B-12 and folate deficiency in older persons. *Am J Clin Nutr* 2003; **77**: 1241–7.

74. Wolters M, Hermann S, Hahn A. B vitamin status and concentrations of homocysteine and methylmalonic acid in elderly German women. *Am J Clin Nutr* 2003; **78**: 765–72.

75. Russell RM, Rasmussen H, Lichtenstein AH. Modified food guide pyramid for people over seventy years of age. *J Nutr* 1999; **129**: 751–3.

76. Rajan S, Wallace JI, Brodkin KI, *et al*. Response of elevated methylmalonic acid to three dose levels of oral cobalamin in older adults. *J Am Geriatr Soc* 2002; **50**: 1789–95.

77. Seal EC, Metz J, Flicker L, Melny J. A randomized, double-blind, placebo-controlled study of oral vitamin B_{12} supplementation in older patients with subnormal or borderline serum vitamin B12 concentrations. *J Am Geriatr Soc* 2002; **50**: 146–51.

78. Stabler SP, Lindenbaum J, Allen RH. The use of homocysteine and other metabolites in the specific diagnosis of vitamin B-12 deficiency. *J Nutr* 1996; **126**: 1266S–1272S.

79. Ray JG, Cole DE, Boss SC. An Ontario-wide study of vitamin B12, serum folate, and red cell folate levels in relation to plasma homocysteine: is a preventable public health issue on the rise? *Clin Biochem* 2000; **33**: 337–43.

80. Liaugaudas G, Jacques PF, Selhub J, *et al*. Renal insufficiency, vitamin B(12) status, and population attributable risk for mild hyperhomocysteinemia among coronary artery disease patients in the era of folic acid-fortified cereal grain flour. *Arterioscler Thromb Vasc Biol* 2001; **21**: 849–51.

81. Ganji V, Kafai MR. Trends in serum folate, RBC folate, and circulating total homocysteine concentrations in the United States: analysis of data from National Health and Nutrition Examination Surveys, 1988–1994, 1999–2000, and 2001–2002. *J Nutr* 2006; **136**: 153–8.

82. Jacques PF, Selhub J, Bostom AG, Wilson PW, Rosenberg IH. The effect of folic acid fortification on plasma folate and total homocysteine concentrations. *N Engl J Med* 1999; **340**: 1449–54.

83. Rader JI. Folic acid fortification, folate status and plasma homocysteine. *J Nutr* 2002; **132**: 2466S–2470S.

84. Spence JD, Bang H, Chambless LE, Stampfer MJ. Vitamin Intervention for Stroke Prevention trial: an efficacy analysis. *Stroke* 2005; **36**: 2404–9.

85. Nygard O, Nordrehaug JE, Refsum H, *et al.* Plasma homocysteine levels and mortality in patients with coronary artery disease. *N Engl J Med* 1997; **337**: 230–6.

86. Refsum H, Ueland PM, Nygard O, Vollset SE. Homocysteine and cardiovascular disease. *Ann Rev Med* 1998; **49**: 31–62.

87. Ueland PM, Refsum H, Beresford SA, Vollset SE. The controversy over homocysteine and cardiovascular risk. *Am J Clin Nutr* 2000; **72**: 324–32.

88. Vollset SE, Refsum H, Tverdal A, *et al.* Plasma total homocysteine and cardiovascular and noncardiovascular mortality: the Hordaland Homocysteine Study. *Am J Clin Nutr* 2001; **74**: 130–6.

89. Moat SJ, Lang D, McDowell IF, *et al.* Folate, homocysteine, endothelial function and cardiovascular disease. *J Nutr Biochem* 2004; **15**: 64–79.

90. Gradman WS, Daniel J, Miller B, Haji-Aghaii M. Homocysteine-associated acute mesenteric artery occlusion treated with thrombectomy and bowel resection. *Ann Vasc Surg* 2001; **15**: 247–50.

91. Schnyder G, Rouvinez G. Total plasma homocysteine and restenosis after percutaneous coronary angioplasty: current evidence. *Ann Med* 2003; **35**: 156–63.

92. Lange H, Suryapranata H, De Luca G, *et al.* Folate therapy and in-stent restenosis after coronary stenting. *N Engl J Med* 2004; **350**: 2673–81.

93. B-Vitamin Treatment Trialists' Collaboration. Homocysteine-lowering trials for prevention of cardiovascular events: a review of the design and power of the large randomized trials. *Am Heart J* 2006; **151**: 282–7.

94. Bottiglieri T. Folate, vitamin B$_{12}$, and neuropsychiatric disorders. *Nutr Rev* 1996; **54**: 382–90.

95. Stabler SP. Vitamins, homocysteine, and cognition. *Am J Clin Nutr* 2003; **78**: 359–60.

96. Nurk E, Refsum H, Tell GS, *et al.* Plasma total homocysteine and memory in the elderly: the Hordaland Homocysteine Study. *Ann Neurol* 2005; **58**: 847–57.

97. Seshadri S, Beiser A, Selhub J, *et al.* Plasma homocysteine as a risk factor for dementia and Alzheimer's disease. *N Engl J Med* 2002; **346**: 476–83.

98. van Asselt DZ, Pasman JW, van Lier HJ, *et al.* Cobalamin supplementation improves cognitive and cerebral function in older, cobalamin-deficient persons. *J Gerontol A Biol Sci Med Sci* 2001; **56**: M775–M779.

99. McLean RR, Jacques PF, Selhub J, *et al.* Homocysteine as a predictive factor for hip fracture in older persons. *N Engl J Med* 2004; **350**: 2042–9.

100. van Meurs JB, Dhonukshe-Rutten RA, Pluijm SM, *et al.* Homocysteine levels and the risk of osteoporotic fracture. *N Engl J Med* 2004; **350**: 2033–41.

101. Sato Y, Honda Y, Iwamoto J, *et al.* Effect of folate and mecobalamin on hip fractures in patients with stroke: a randomized controlled trial. *JAMA* 2005; **293**: 1082–8.

15

Consequences of chronic anemia in the older person

Lodovico Balducci

Introduction

Anemia, whose prevalence and incidence increase with age, has been associated with a number of adverse outcomes in older individuals [1]. It is attractive to hypothesize that the reversal of anemia may effect compression of morbidity, which is the main goal of geriatric medicine [2,3]. More prolonged health and independence may improve the quality of life and reduce the management cost of the older aged person.

After studying the epidemiology of anemia and aging, this chapter explores the adverse consequences of anemia in the elderly and the outcomes of anemia management.

Epidemiology and causes of anemia in older age

Definition of anemia

The World Health Organization (WHO) defines anemia as hemoglobin levels lower than $12\,g/dL$ in women and $13.5\,g/dL$ in men [4]. In older people, however, this definition should be revised based on two types of findings:

- People of different ethnic origins may have different levels of hemoglobin in homeostatic conditions. In the NHANES III study, the prevalence of anemia was much higher among older African-Americans than among white, Asian, or Hispanic elderly (Fig. 15.1) [4]. In the same database Patel

et al. [5] demonstrated that mild anemia was not associated with adverse outcomes in blacks. These findings suggest that hemoglobin levels may be lower in black individuals than in other ethnic groups in normal conditions.

- For women aged 65 and older followed prospectively in the Women's Health and Aging Studies (WHAS), the risk of mortality, disability, and functional impairment increased inversely with hemoglobin levels, when these dropped below $13\,g/dL$ [6,7]. The EPESE [8] and the InCHIANTI [9] studies demonstrated the best level of physical performance in the elderly when hemoglobin levels were between 13 and $14.5\,g/dL$, in both men and women. These findings indicate that the WHO definition of anemia is too restrictive, at least for post-menopausal white women.

Prevalence and incidence of anemia in the older aged person

For the following discussion, the WHO definition of anemia is adopted, and the data that contradict this definition in different studies will be mentioned.

In the NHANES III study [4] the prevalence of anemia was approximately 9.5% in individuals aged 65 and older, and it increased with age. Anemia was more common in older men than in older women, but the difference between the sexes disappeared if one considered anemic the women whose hemoglobin levels were lower than $13\,g/dL$. In the Olmsted County studies, which involved 95% of the

Blood Disorders in the Elderly, ed. Lodovico Balducci, William Ershler, Giovanni de Gaetano.
Published by Cambridge University Press. © Cambridge University Press 2008.

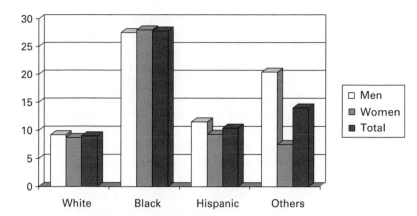

Figure 15.1 Prevalence of anemia among different populations aged 65 and older.

population of that county, the prevalence of anemia was somewhat higher than in NHANES III. This discrepancy might have been due to the fact that the whole population of the county, including the sickest individuals, was accounted for. The Olmsted County studies reported an increase in both prevalence and incidence of anemia with age [10,11].

An Italian cross-sectional study showed that the prevalence of anemia was 9.2% for individuals aged 65 and over [12]. While the prevalence of anemia increased with age, the mean levels of hemoglobin were maintained remarkably constant at least up to age 85, suggesting that anemia, even mild anemia, is not a consequence of age. Other studies contradict this conclusion, however. In a cohort study of Japanese aging individuals the levels of hemoglobin decreased by an average 0.036 g/dL per year for women and by 0.04 g/dL for men between the ages of 70 and 80, in the absence of any disease [13]. Similar findings were reported among Swedish healthy individuals aged 70–88 [14]. Clearly, even if there is a drop in the hemoglobin levels in normal aging, this decline is modest. The increased prevalence and incidence of anemia with age cannot be accounted for by aging itself, and is best explained by increased prevalence of chronic diseases that may cause anemia.

Not surprisingly, the prevalence of anemia was higher among older individuals living in an adult living facility than among home-dwelling elders [15–17].

Table 15.1. Causes of anemia, as reported in two cross-sectional studies.

Cause	Olmsted County [10] (%)	NHANES III [4] (%)
Infection	23	—
Anemia of chronic disease (anemia of chronic inflammation)	17	20
Iron deficiency	8	20
Nutritional	8	14
Chronic kidney disease	8	12
Unexplained	36	34

Causes of anemia in the aged

The most common causes of anemia in older individuals in the NHANES III [4] and the Olmsted county [10] studies are shown in Table 15.1. Anemia of unknown cause accounted for approximately 30% of cases. Undoubtedly, more causes might have been unearthed by more complete diagnostic investigations. Aging is associated with an almost universal decline in glomerular filtration rate (GFR), which may not be associated with increased serum creatinine levels, due to age-related sarcopenia [18]. Renal insufficiency may explain many of these cases, as the production of erythropoietin declines for GFR <60 mL/minute [19]. As aging is a chronic

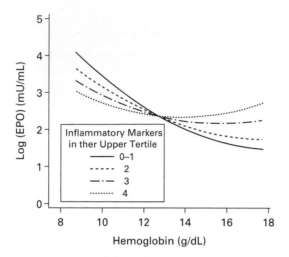

Figure 15.2 Relationship between the levels of hemoglobin, circulating erythropoietin (EPO), and circulating inflammatory marker in the InCHIANTI study. From Ferrucci *et al.* (2005) [20], with permission.

and progressive inflammation, anemia of chronic inflammation may also account for unexplained causes of anemia. Ferrucci *et al.* demonstrated a condition of relative erythropoietin insufficiency in older individuals [20] (Fig. 15.2). When the circulating levels of erythropoietin were plotted against the levels of hemoglobin and the levels of inflammatory cytokines one could observe that:

- In the absence of inflammation, erythropoietin levels were lowest for normal hemoglobin levels and increased proportionally with the drop in hemoglobin. This inverse relation of circulating levels of erythropoietin and hemoglobin is commonly seen in patients with iron deficiency.
- In the presence of inflammation, the circulating levels of erythropoietin were abnormally high for normal levels of hemoglobin, but failed to increase in the presence of anemia. These data suggest that the sensitivity of erythropoietic precursors to erythropoietin is decreased and that the maximal capacity to produce erythropoietin is also decreased. Both effects may be mediated by the inflammatory cytokines.

Early myelodysplasia may also have accounted for a small number of cases of anemia of unknown cause [4].

It is important to notice that many causes of anemia in older individuals are reversible.

When a source of bleeding is not immediately recognized, the diagnosis of iron deficiency should always trigger investigations of chronic occult bleeding from the gastrointestinal tract. In addition to cancer and ulcers, chronic bleeding in older individuals may be due to diverticuli or angiodysplasia of the large bowel. Iron deficiency secondary to *Helicobacter pylori* has been recently described [21], but its prevalence in older individuals is unknown. The absorption of food iron decreases with age due to gastric achylia and also to increased circulating levels of hepcidin [22]. This is an enzyme that destroys ferroportin, a protein responsible for carrying the iron from the gastrointestinal tract into the circulation.

Incidence and prevalence of cobalamin deficiency increase with age [23,24], due to inability to digest food-bound vitamin. The gastric secretion of both hydrochloric acid and pepsin, which are essential to the digestion of vitamin B_{12}, decline with age. When the concentration of red blood cell folates is normal, anemia may not be present and the main consequences of cobalamin deficiency are neurological, including dementia and posterior column lesions.

Not surprisingly, anemia of chronic inflammation is a common form of anemia in the elderly, as the prevalence of chronic diseases increases with age. As mentioned before, anemia of chronic inflammation may be present even in the absence of detectable diseases, as aging itself is associated with increased concentration of inflammatory markers in the circulation [25]. Inflammation portends the two mechanisms of this form of anemia: relative erythropoietin deficiency and decreased iron mobilization, due to increased concentration of hepcidin in the circulation [26]. At least some forms of anemia of chronic inflammation, such as cancer-related anemia, may be reversed by a combination of pharmacological doses of erythropoietin and intravenous iron [27,28]. This treatment strategy is controversial, however, as it has been associated with increased mortality, whose causes include thromboembolic phenomena and possibly stimulation of cancer growth [29–31].

The role of hypogonadism in the pathogenesis of anemia of older individuals has been highlighted by Ferrucci *et al.* in the InCHIANTI study. These investigators found low levels of circulating testosterone in three-quarters of older men and women with anemia [32]. In addition, low testosterone levels were highly predictive of future development of anemia in non-anemic subjects. The possibility of preventing or reversing anemia with testosterone replacement needs to be studied.

Even anemia of myelodysplasia may be reversed in some cases. Lenalidomide induces a complete hematologic and cytogenetic response in 80% of patients with refractory anemia and 5q(−) cytogenetic abnormalities [33]. Transfusion independence and more prolonged survival result from this treatment. Lenalidomide may also be active in a smaller portion of patients with different forms of refractory anemia. Transfusion independence may also be achieved in more advanced forms of myelodysplasia with the nucleotide analogs azacytidine and decitabin [34].

Consequences of anemia

The clinical consequences of anemia are listed in Table 15.2.

Anemia and mortality

Anemia was an independent risk factor for mortality in older individuals, according to seven cohort studies (Table 15.3) [6,10,35–39]. The results of two studies are particularly provocative, as they suggest a revision of the WHO definition of anemia in older women. The WHAS reported an increased risk of mortality for hemoglobin levels <13.4 g/dL in home-dwelling women aged 65 and over followed for an average of 11 years [6]. Zakai *et al.* found that mortality was increased for hemoglobin levels lower than 12.7 g/dL for women and 13.5 g/dL for men [37]. In all studies the risk of mortality appeared to

Table 15.2. Consequences of anemia.

Increased risk of mortality
Increased risk of functional dependence
Increased risk of dementia
Increased risk of delirium
Increased risk of chemotherapy-related toxicity
Increased risk of congestive heart failure and coronary
  death
Increased risk of falls

Table 15.3. Studies reporting an association of anemia and mortality in the older aged person.

Author	Age of subjects	Hb level used to define anemia
Ania *et al.* 1997 [10]	>70	<12
Izaks *et al.* 1999 [35]	>85	<12
Kikuchi *et al.* 2001 [36]	>70	<12
Chaves *et al.* 2002 [6]	>65	<13.4
Zakai *et al.* 2005 [37]	>65	<13.7 men
		<12.6 women
Penninx *et al.* 2006 [38]	>65	WHO criteria
Culleton *et al.* 2006 [39]	>65	WHO criteria

be independent of coexisting diseases causing anemia. Anemia could be interpreted as a marker of frailty, a condition associated with critically reduced functional reserve and increased vulnerability to environmental injury [40].

Anemia and functional dependence

Preservation of function (prolongation of active life expectancy) is a major goal of geriatric medicine, and the identification of reversible causes and mechanisms of functional dependence is a research priority. Is anemia a cause of functional dependence? Several studies seem to indicate that this is the case. The WHAS, EPESE, and InCHIANTI studies demonstrated that among elderly people living at home anemia was associated with mobility impairment and with dependence in instrumental activities of daily living (IADLs) [7–9]. Of special interest, the risk of mobility and functional decline increased inversely with hemoglobin levels lower than 13 g/dL, in both men and women. Again, these findings emphasize the inadequacy of the WHO definition of anemia, at least for older women.

In cancer patients Luciani *et al.* demonstrated that anemia was associated with dependence in activities of daily living (ADL) and IADL [41], and in assisted living facilities a strong correlation of anemia and functional dependence was also observed [17,42]. In hospitalized elderly patients, anemia has been associated with delayed rehabilitation [43]. It is not clear whether anemia is itself a cause of functional dependence or is a marker of more advanced aging and of frailty. Reversal of anemia of chronic inflammation with erythropoietic growth factors has been shown to lead to improved quality of life and reduced fatigue [44–46]. The effects of anemia correction on functional dependence have never been studied, however. Reversal of anemia of chronic inflammation in older individuals should not be attempted outside the context of well-controlled randomized clinical trials, in view of the potential adverse effects of erythropoietic growth factors.

Anemia and therapeutic complications

Anemia has been associated with increased risk of medical and surgical complications. In five studies conducted in cancer patients anemia was associated with increased risk of myelotoxicity and non-myelotoxic complications [47–51]. One possible explanation is that the concentration of circulating free drugs increases in the presence of anemia, as the majority of anti-neoplastic agents are bound to red blood cells. Seemingly, hypoxia may also enhance the susceptibility of normal tissues to the toxicity of chemotherapy. At present, there is no proof that correction of anemia with erythropoietic growth factors or transfusions prevents the complications of anti-neoplastic treatment. Once more, anemia may represent a marker of frailty in older cancer patients rather than a cause of increased toxicity. In hospitalized older patients anemia has been associated

with increased incidence of delirium [52,53]. Brain hypoxia as well as increased circulating free drugs may have been responsible, at least in part, for this complication.

Of special interest in older patients is the influence of anemia on the outcome of hip fractures. Anemia was present in approximately 30% of patients who suffered a hip fracture [54,55], and many more patients became anemic during hospitalization. In a consecutive cohort of 550 patients who underwent surgery for hip fracture and survived to discharge between 1997 and 1998, Halm *et al.* [55] reported an average drop in hemoglobin of 2.8 g/dL, after surgery. Seemingly surgical bleeding, hemodilution from intravenous fluids, repeated phlebotomies, and inadequate nutrition were responsible for this change. The influence of anemia on surgical outcome is controversial, however. Some authors have reported that postoperative anemia was associated with increased risk of death and hospital readmission [54–56], and with delayed and incomplete walking rehabilitation [57,58]. Other authors failed to find an association between anemia at discharge, death, functional dependence, and walking impairment [59].

The effects of blood transfusions on outcome are also unclear. According to one study, postoperative blood transfusions reduced the readmission rate to the hospital, especially for patients whose hemoglobin levels had dropped below 10 g/dL [55], but had little effect on mortality and recovery of mobility. Other authors expressed concern that blood transfusion might impair the immune system and delay recovery [60–62].

Anemia and heart disease

The influence of anemia on the pathogenesis and outcome of congestive heart failure (CHF), and on the outcome of coronary artery disease, has been studied – as has the role of CHF in the pathogenesis of anemia.

The association of chronic anemia and CHF is well known [63–67]. Of interest, the prevalence of anemia increases with the severity of symptoms [68] and of diastolic dysfunction [69].

In patients undergoing hemodialysis, anemia has been associated with increased risk of left ventricular hypertrophy and CHF that may be prevented when anemia is corrected with erythropoietin [65–67,70]. The influence of heart failure in the pathogenesis of anemia is less clear. It may include fluid retention and hemodilution, bone marrow hypoxia, increased level of inflammatory cytokines in the circulation, reduced production of erythropoietin from declining GFR, and sarcopenia [71]. Iron deficiency may also occur due to decreased absorption from edema of the bowel wall. In addition, some of the drugs used to manage CHF can cause anemia. For example, ACE inhibitors may inhibit the synthesis of erythropoietin [72] and may increase the concentration in the circulation of the tetrapeptide Ac-SDKP, which inhibits erythropoiesis [73].

Irrespective of its causes, anemia in patients with CHF is associated with increased mortality, increased risk and duration of hospitalization [68–70,74–77], and reduced tolerance of exercise [78]. In at least one study [79], a decline of hemoglobin over a 12-month period was associated with increased morbidity and mortality in patients with CHF.

Anemia may worsen CHF through a number of mechanisms, including increased ventricular preload, myocardial hypoxia, increased cardiac work. Of particular interest is the release of neurohormones and cytokines that are toxic to the myocardium.

It remains unclear whether the association between anemia and poor outcomes in CHF patients is causal, or whether anemia is merely a marker of risk. It cannot be excluded that hemoglobin is the marker of some other adverse factors among CHF patients, such as higher circulating cytokines and chemokines, which are associated with greater disease severity. However, anemia could aggravate CHF through a number of mechanisms, including exacerbation of myocardial and peripheral hypoxia, increased venous return and cardiac work, and consequent left ventricular hypertrophy [80]. Of interest, increased levels of circulating erythropoietin portend a poor prognosis in patients with CHF,

seemingly because they reflect the level of tissue hypoxia [20].

The role of anemia in the pathogenesis of CHF is well documented by clinical trials. In patients undergoing hemodialysis, correction of anemia with erythropoietin prevented the development of left ventricular hypertrophy and CHF [70]. In patients with CHF, correction of anemia with erythropoietin improved symptoms and functional class and reduced the risk of hospitalization [68]. In a small randomized controlled study a three-month treatment with erythropoietin was associated with improvement in submaximal and maximal exercise capacity [81]. It is unknown whether correction of anemia may lead to improved survival and other long-term outcomes. It should be underlined that the beneficial effects of erythropoietin may be partly independent from the correction of anemia, as erythropoietin may have a free-radical scavenging effect that protects the vascular endothelium, an anti-inflammatory effect, and it may improve the myocardial trophism [81–83].

The benefits of red-blood-cell transfusions in patients with CHF are controversial. Though widely broadcast, the recommendation to transfuse CHF patients with hemoglobin levels lower than 10 g/dL is not evidence-based [84].

The interaction of anemia with coronary heart disease (CHD) is not clear. In general, patients with CHD are more likely to be anemic than age- and sex-matched controls. The pathogenesis of anemia may be related in part to increased concentration of circulating inflammatory cytokines in acute coronary syndrome. The average prevalence of anemia in patients with myocardial infarction is 15%, and 50% among those 75 and older [85]. For percutaneous coronary angioplasty patients, the prevalence of anemia varies between 15 and 31% [86,87].

In patients with acute coronary syndrome anemia is an independent risk factor for mortality [85]: in the presence of ST elevation in the electrocardiogram the mortality risk is inversely related to the levels of hemoglobin below 14 g/dL. In addition, anemia is an independent risk factor for mortality, procedural complications, more prolonged hospitalization, and contrast nephropathy for patients undergoing percutaneous coronary interventions [86–92].

The role of blood transfusions in patients with acute coronary syndromes is controversial. Raising hematocrit levels above 25% has led to increased risk of death and reinfarction in patients with myocardial infarction [93,94]. In individuals aged 65 and older, however, decreased mortality was observed when the hematocrit was kept between 30 and 33% [95]. The interpretation of these studies is unclear, as they included patients with different comorbidity and functional reserve. It is very possible that blood transfusion was simply a marker of individuals with more serious comorbidity. The guidelines from the American College of Cardiology/American Heart Association recommend correction of anemia in patients with acute coronary syndrome, but do not specify the level of hemoglobin that should be achieved.

Anemia and geriatric syndromes

In patients with chronic renal failure the risk of dementia was increased if anemia had not been corrected with erythropoietin [96]. Among older patients, Atti *et al.* reported that the prevalence of dementia was higher among anemic than among non-anemic individuals [97]. Among elders with normal mental status, those who were anemic were at higher risk of developing dementia over the following five years. In addition, anemia predicted dementia in hospitalized patients with normal mental status [98]. In the WHAS, Chaves *et al.* reported decline in executive function in the presence of mild anemia [99].

Anemia has also been associated with an increased risk of falls, both in institutions and in the community [100].

Should anemia always be treated?

Clearly anemia, even mild anemia, may be associated with adverse outcomes in older individuals. Does that mean that reversal of anemia may prevent these adverse outcomes?

The weight of evidence indicates that:

- Patients with iron deficiency, cobalamin deficiency, and other reversible causes of anemia should receive appropriate treatment.

As far as the use of erythropoiesis-stimulating agents (ESA) is concerned:

- The use of epoetin or darbepoetin to maintain hemoglobin levels around 12 g/dL is beneficial to patients with chronic renal failure. This strategy prevents left ventricular hypertrophy, CHF, and possibly cognitive decline [68–70,96]. Higher levels of hemoglobin have been associated with increased risk of thromboembolism, hypertension, and mortality [101]. It is reasonable to assume that the same correction of anemia may be beneficial to patients with renal insufficiency and decreased production of erythropoietin.
- In cancer patients, correction of chemotherapy-induced anemia with erythropoietic growth factors reduces the need for blood transfusion and improves the energy levels. All studies seem to indicate that hemoglobin levels up to 12 g/dL are safe. The use of ESA in patients with cancer-related anemia is controversial [102].
- In all other forms of anemia of chronic inflammation, the benefit of using ESA is unproven. This strategy should not be deployed outside of randomized clinical trials.

REFERENCES

1. Balducci L, Aapro M. Anemia and aging or anemia of aging. *Cancer Treat Res* 2007; in press.
2. Mor V. The compression of morbidity hypothesis: a review of research and prospects for the future. *J Am Geriatr Soc* 2005; **53** (9 Suppl): S308–S309.
3. Fries GF. Frailty, heart disease, and stroke: the compression of morbidity paradigm. *Am J Prev Med* 2005; **29** (5 Suppl 1): 164–8.
4. Guralnik JM, Eisenstaedt RS, Ferrucci L, Klein HG, Woodman RC. Prevalence of anemia in persons 65 years and older in the United States: evidence for a high rate of unexplained anemia. *Blood* 2004; **104**: 2263–8.

5. Patel KV, Harris TB, Faulhaber M, *et al.* Racial variation in the relationship of anemia with mortality and mobility disability among older adults. *Blood* 2007; **109**: 4663–70.

6. Chaves PH, Ashar B, Guralnik JM, Fried LP. Looking at the relationship between hemoglobin concentration and prevalent mobility difficulty in older women. Should the criteria currently used to define anemia in older people be reevaluated? *J Am Geriatr Soc* 2002; **50**: 1257–64.

7. Chaves PH, Semba RD, Leng SX, *et al.* Impact of anemia and cardiovascular diseases on frailty status of community dwelling women. The Women's Health and Aging Studies I and II. *J Gerontol A Biol Sci Med Sci* 2005; **60**: 729–35.

8. Penninx BW, Pahor M, Cesari M, *et al.* Anemia is associated with disability and decreased physical performance and muscle strength in the elderly. *J Am Geriatr Soc* 2004; **52**: 719–24.

9. Cesari M, Penninx BW, Lauretani F, *et al.* Hemoglobin levels and skeletal muscle: results from the InCHIANTI study. *J Gerontol A Biol Sci Med Sci* 2004; **59**: 238–41.

10. Ania BJ, Suman VJ, Fairbanks VF, Rademacher DM, Melton LJ 3rd. Incidence of anemia in older people: an epidemiologic study in a well defined population. *J Am Geriatr Soc* 1997; **45**: 825–31.

11. Ania BJ, Suman VJ, Fairbanks VF, *et al.* Prevalence of anemia in medical practice: community versus referral patients. *Mayo Clin Proc* 1994; **69**: 730–5.

12. Inelmen EM, Alessio MD, Gatto MRA, *et al.* Descriptive analysis of the prevalence of anemia in a randomly selected sample of elderly people at home: some results of an Italian multicentric study. *Aging Clin Exp Res* 1994; **6**: 81–9.

13. Yamada M, Wong FL, Suzuki G, *et al.* Longitudinal trends of hemoglobin levels in a Japanese population: RERF's Adult Health Study subjects. *Eur J Haematol* 2003; **70**: 129–35.

14. Nilsson-Ehle H, Jagenburg R, Landahl S, *et al.* Blood hemoglobin declines in the elderly: implications for reference intervals for age 70 to 88. *Eur J Haematol* 2000; **65**: 297–305.

15. Artz AS, Fergusson D, Drinka PJ, *et al.* Prevalence of anemia in skilled-nursing home residents. *Arch Gerontol Geriatr* 2004; **39**: 201–6.

16. Kalchataler T, Tan ME. Anemia in institutionalized elderly patients. *J Am Geriatr Soc* 1980; **28**: 108–13.

17. Ania Lafuente BJ, Fernandez-Burriel Tercero M, Suarez Almenara JL, *et al.* [Anemia and functional incapacity at admission to a geriatric home.] *An Med Interna* 2001; **18**: 9–12.

18. Duthie EH. Physiology of aging: relevance to symptom perception and treatment tolerance. In Balducci L, Lyman GH, Ershler WB, Extermann M, eds, *Comprehensive Geriatric Oncology*, 2nd edn (London: Taylor and Francis, 2004), 207–22.

19. Ble A, Fink J, Woodman R, *et al.* Renal function, erythropoietin and anemia of older persons: the InCHIANTI study. *Arch Intern Med* 2005; **165**: 2222–7.

20. Ferrucci L, Guralnik JM, Woodman RC, *et al.* Proinflammatory state and circulating erythropoietin in persons with and without anemia. *Am J Med* 2005; **118**: 1288.

21. Choi JW. Serum-soluble transferrin receptor concentrations in *Helicobacter pylori*-associated iron-deficiency anemia. *Ann Hematol* 2006; **85**: 735–7.

22. Lin L, Valore EV, Nemeth D, *et al.* Iron transferrin regulates hepcidin synthesis in primary hepatocyte culture through hemojuvelin and BMP2/4. *Blood* 2007; **110**: 2182–9.

23. Sipponen P, Laxen F, Huotari K, *et al.* Prevalence of low vitamin B12 and high homocysteine in serum of an elderly male population: association with atrophic gastritis and *Helicobacter pylori* infection. *Scand J Gastroenterol* 2003; **38**: 1209–16.

24. Selhub J, Jacques PF, Roenberg IH, *et al.* Serum total homocysteine concentrations in the third National Health and Nutrition Examination Survey (1991–1994): population reference ranges and contribution of vitamin status to high serum concentrations. *Ann Intern Med* 1999; **131**: 331–9.

25. Ferrucci L, Corsi A, Lauretani F, *et al.* The origins of age-related proinflammatory state. *Blood* 2005; **105**: 2294–9.

26. Weiss G, Goodnough LT. Anemia of chronic disease. *N Engl J Med* 2005; **352**: 1011–23.

27. Goodnough LT. Erythropoietin and iron-restricted erythropoiesis. *Exp Hematol* 2007; **35** (4 Suppl 1): 167–72.

28. Auerbach M, Ballard H, Trout JR, *et al.* Intravenous iron optimizes the response to recombinant human erythropoietin in cancer patients with chemotherapy-related anemia: a multicenter, open-label, randomized trial. *J Clin Oncol* 2004; **22**: 1301–7.

29. Leyland-Jones B, Semiglazov V, Pawlicki M, *et al.* Maintaining normal hemoglobin levels with epoetin alfa in mainly nonanemic patients with metastatic breast cancer receiving first-line chemotherapy: a survival study. *J Clin Oncol* 2005; **23**: 2606–17.

30. Wright JR, Ung YC, Julian JA, *et al.* Randomized, double-blind, placebo-controlled trial of erythropoietin in non-small-cell lung cancer with disease-related anemia. *J Clin Oncol* 2007; **26**: 1027–32.

31. Henke M, Mattern D, Pepe M, *et al.* Do erythropoietin receptors on cancer cells explain unexpected clinical findings? *J Clin Oncol* 2006; **24**: 4708–13.

32. Ferrucci L, Maggio M, Brandinelli S, *et al.* Low testosterone levels and the risk of anemia in older men and women. *Arch Intern Med* 2006; **166**: 1380–8.

33. List A, Dewald G, Bennett J, *et al.* Lenalidomide in the myelodysplastic syndrome with chromosome 5q deletion. *N Engl J Med* 2006; **355**: 1456–65.

34. Estey E. Acute myeloid leukemia and myelodysplastic syndromes in older patients. *J Clin Oncol* 2007; **25**: 1908–15.

35. Izaks GJ, Westendorp RGJ, Knook DL. The definition of anemia in older persons. *JAMA* 1999; **281**: 1714–19.

36. Kikuchi M, Inagaki T, Shinagawa N. Five-year survival of older people with anemia: variation with hemoglobin concentration. *J Am Geriatr Soc* 2001; **49**: 1226–8.

37. Zakai NA, Katz R, Hirsch C, *et al.* A prospective study of anemia status, hemoglobin concentration, and mortality in an elderly cohort: the Cardiovascular Health Study. *Arch Intern Med* 2005; **165**: 2214–20.

38. Penninx BW, Pahor M, Woodman RC, *et al.* Anemia in old age is associated with increased mortality and hospitalization. *J Gerontol Med Sci* 2006; **61**: 474–9.

39. Culleton BF, Manns BJ, Zhang J, *et al.* Impact of anemia on hospitalization and mortality in older adults. *Blood* 2006; **107**: 3841–6.

40. Walston A, Headley EC, Ferrucci L, *et al.* Research agenda for frailty in older adults: toward a better understanding of physiology and etiology. Summary from the American Geriatrics Society/National Institute on Aging Research Conference on Frailty in Older Adults. *J Am Geriatr Soc* 2006; **54**: 991–1001.

41. Luciani A, Balducci L, Extermann M, *et al.* Fatigue may be a cause of functional dependence in older cancer patients. *Crit Rev Oncol Hematol* 2007; in press.

42. Maraldi C, Ble A, Zuliani G, *et al.* Association between anemia and physical disability in older patients: role of comorbidity. *Aging Clin Exp Res* 2006; **18**: 485–92.

43. Maraldi C, Volpato S, Cesari L, *et al.* Anemia and recovery from disability in activities of daily living in hospitalized older persons. *J Am Geriatr Soc* 2006; **54**: 632–6.

44. Gabrilove JL, Cleeland CS, Livingston RB, *et al.* Clinical evaluation of once-weekly dosing of epoetin alfa in chemotherapy patients: improvements in hemoglobin and quality of life are similar to three-times-weekly dosing. *J Clin Oncol* 2001; **19**: 2875–82.

45. Littlewood TJ, Bajett E, Nortier JW, *et al.* Effects of epoetin alfa on hematologic parameters and quality of life in cancer patients receiving nonplatinum chemotherapy: results of a randomized, double-blind, placebo-controlled trial. *J Clin Oncol* 2001; **19**: 2865–74.

46. Crawford J. Erythropoiesis-stimulating protein support and survival. *Oncology* 2006; **20** (8 Suppl 6): 39–43.

47. Extermann M, Chen A, Cantor AB, *et al.* Predictors of tolerance from chemotherapy in older patients: a prospective pilot study. *Eur J Cancer* 2002; **38**: 1466–73.

48. Schrijvers D, Highley M, DeBruyn E, Van Oosterom AT, Vermorken JB. Role of red blood cells in pharmacokinetics of chemotherapeutic agents. *Anticancer Drugs* 1999; **10**: 147–53.

49. Ratain MJ, Schilsky RL, Choi KE, *et al.* Adaptive control of etoposide administration: impact of interpatient pharmacodynamic variability. *Clin Pharmacol Ther* 1989; **45**: 226–33.

50. Silber JH, Fridman M, Di Paola RS, *et al.* First-cycle blood counts and subsequent neutropenia, dose reduction, or delay in early stage breast cancer therapy. *J Clin Oncol* 1998; **16**: 2392–400.

51. Wolff D, Culakova E, Poniewierski MS, *et al.* Predictors of chemotherapy-induced neutropenia and its complications: results from a prospective nationwide registry. *J Support Oncol* 2005; **3** (6 Suppl 4): 24–5.

52. Joosten E, Lemiengre J, Nelis T, *et al.* Is anaemia a risk factor for delirium in acute geriatric population? *Gerontology* 2006; **52**: 382–5.

53. Marcantonio ER, Goldman I, Oray EJ, *et al.* The association of intraoperative factors with the development of postoperative delirium. *Am J Med* 1998; **105**: 380–4.

54. Marks R, Allegrante JP, Ronald MacKenzie C, Lane JM. Hip fractures among the elderly: causes, consequences and control. *Ageing Res Rev* 2003; **2**: 57–93.

55. Halm EA, Wang JJ, Boockvar K, *et al.* The effect of perioperative anemia on clinical and functional outcomes in patients with hip fracture. *J Orthop Trauma* 2004; **18**: 369–74.

56. Gruson KI, Aharonoff GB, Egol KA, Zuckerman JD, Koval KJ. The relationship between admission hemoglobin level and outcome after hip fracture. *J Orthop Trauma* 2002; **16**: 39–44.

57. Lawrence VA, Silverstein JH, Cornell JE, Pederson T, Noveck H, Carson JL. Higher Hb level is associated

with better early functional recovery after hip fracture repair. *Transfusion* 2003; **43**: 1717–22.

58. Hagino T, Sato E, Tonotsuka H, Ochiai S, Tokai M, Hamada Y. Prediction of ambulation prognosis in the elderly after hip fracture. *Int Orthop* 2006; **30**: 315–19.

59. Su H, Aharonoff GB, Zuckerman JD, Egol KA, Koval KJ. The relation between discharge hemoglobin and outcome after hip fracture. *Am J Orthop* 2004; **33**: 576–80.

60. Carson JL, Noveck H, Berlin JA, Gould SA. Mortality and morbidity in patients with very low postoperative Hb levels who decline blood transfusion. *Transfusion* 2002; **42**: 812–18.

61. Hill GE, Frawley WH, Griffith KE, Forestner JE, Minei JP. Allogeneic blood transfusion increases the risk of postoperative bacterial infection: a meta-analysis. *J Trauma* 2003; **54**: 908–14.

62. Carson JL, Altman DG, Duff A, *et al.* Risk of bacterial infection associated with allogeneic blood transfusion among patients undergoing hip fracture repair. *Transfusion* 1999; **39**: 694–700.

63. Maraldi C, Volpato S, Cesari M, *et al.* Anemia, physical disability and survival in older patients with heart failure. *J Card Fail* 2006; **12**: 533–9.

64. Lewis BS, Karkabi B, Jaffe R, *et al.* Anemia and heart failure: statement of the problem. *Nephrol Dial Transplant*, 2005; **20** (Suppl 7): 3–6.

65. Phillips S, Olimann H, Schink T, *et al.* The impact of anaemia and kidney function in congestive heart failure and preserved systolic function. *Nephrol Dial Transplant* 2005; **20**: 915–19.

66. Elabassi W, Fraser M, Williams K, *et al.* Prevalence and clinical complications of anemia in congestive heart failure patients followed at a specialized heart function clinic. *Congest Heart Fail* 2006; **12**: 258–64.

67. Vasu S, Kelly P, Lawson WE. Anemia in heart failure: a concise review. *Clin Cardiol* 2005; **28**: 454–8.

68. Silverberg DS, Wexler D, Iaina A. The role of anemia in congestive heart failure and chronic kidney insufficiency: the cardio renal anemia syndrome. *Perspect Biol Med* 2004; **47**: 575–89.

69. Brucks S, Little WC, Chao T, *et al.* Relation of anemia to diastolic heart failure and the effect on outcome. *Am J Cardiol* 2004; **93**: 1055–7.

70. Silverberg DS, Wexler D, Iaina A, *et al.* Anemia, chronic renal disease and congestive heart failure: the cardio renal anemia syndrome. The need for cooperation between cardiologists and nephrologists. *Int Urol Nephrol* 2006; **38**: 295–310.

71. Felker GM, Adams KF, Jr, Gattis WA, O'Connor CM. Anemia as a risk factor and therapeutic target in heart failure. *J Am Coll Cardiol* 2004; **44**: 959–66.

72. van der Meer P, Lipsic E, Westenbrink BD, *et al.* Levels of hematopoiesis inhibitor N-acetyl-seryl-aspartyl-lysyl-proline partially explain the occurrence of anemia in heart failure. *Circulation* 2005; **112**: 1743–7.

73. Wang AY, Yu AW, Lam CW, *et al.* Effects of losartan or enalapril on hemoglobin, circulating erythropoietin, and insulin-like growth factor-1 in patients with and without posttransplant erythrocytosis. *Am J Kidney Dis* 2002; **39**: 600–8.

74. Lindenfeld J. Prevalence of anemia and effects on mortality in patients with heart failure. *Am Heart J* 2005; **149**: 391–401.

75. Mozaffarian D, Nye R, Levy WC. Anemia predicts mortality in severe heart failure: the prospective randomized amlodipine survival evaluation (PRAISE). *J Am Coll Cardiol* 2003; **41**: 1933–9.

76. Kosiborod M, Smith GL, Radford MJ, Foody JM, Krumholz HM. The prognostic importance of anemia in patients with heart failure. *Am J Med* 2003; **114**: 112–19.

77. O'Meara E, Clayton T, McEntegart MB, *et al.* Clinical correlates and consequences of anemia in a broad spectrum of patients with heart failure: results of the Candesartan in Heart Failure: Assessment of Reduction in Mortality and Morbidity (CHARM) Program. *Circulation* 2006; **113**: 986–94.

78. Kalra PR, Bolger AP, Francis DP, *et al.* Effect of anemia on exercise tolerance in chronic heart failure in men. *Am J Cardiol* 2003; **91**: 888–91.

79. Anand IS, Kuskowski MA, Rector TS, *et al.* Anemia and change in hemoglobin over time related to mortality and morbidity in patients with chronic heart failure: results from Val-HeFT. *Circulation* 2005; **112**: 1121–7.

80. van der Meer P, Voors AA, Lipsic E, Smilde TD, van Gilst WH, van Veldhuisen DJ. Prognostic value of plasma erythropoietin on mortality in patients with chronic heart failure. *J Am Coll Cardiol* 2004; **44**: 63–7.

81. Masuda S, Nagao M, Sasaki R. Erythropoietic, neurotrophic, and angiogenic functions of erythropoietin and regulation of erythropoietin production. *Int J Hematol* 1999; **70**: 1–6.

82. Sasaki R, Masuda S, Nagao M. Erythropoietin: multiple physiological functions and regulation of biosynthesis. *Biosci Biotechnol Biochem* 2000; **64**: 1775–93.

83. Calvillo L, Latini R, Kajstura J, *et al.* Recombinant human erythropoietin protects the myocardium from ischemia-reperfusion injury and promotes

beneficial remodeling. *Proc Natl Acad Sci USA* 2003; **100**: 4802–6.

84. Welch HG, Meehan KR, Goodnough LT. Prudent strategies for elective red blood cell transfusion. *Ann Intern Med* 1992; **116**: 393–402.

85. Sabatine MS, Morrow DA, Giugliano RP, *et al*. Association of hemoglobin levels with clinical outcomes in acute coronary syndromes. *Circulation* 2005; **111**: 2042–9.

86. Nikolsky E, Aymong ED, Halkin A, *et al*. Impact of anemia in patients with acute myocardial infarction undergoing primary percutaneous coronary intervention: analysis from the Controlled Abciximab and Device Investigation to Lower Late Angioplasty Complications (CADILLAC) Trial. *J Am Coll Cardiol* 2004; **44**: 547–53.

87. Nikolsky E, Mehran R, Aymong ED, *et al*. Impact of anemia on outcomes of patients undergoing percutaneous coronary interventions. *Am J Cardiol* 2004; **94**: 1023–7.

88. Reinecke H, Trey T, Wellmann J, *et al*. Haemoglobin-related mortality in patients undergoing percutaneous coronary interventions. *Eur Heart J* 2003; **24**: 2142–50.

89. McKechnie RS, Smith D, Montoye C, *et al*. Prognostic implication of anemia on in-hospital outcomes after percutaneous coronary intervention. *Circulation* 2004; **110**: 271–7.

90. Lee PC, Kini AS, Ahsan C, Fisher E, Sharma SK. Anemia is an independent predictor of mortality after percutaneous coronary intervention. *J Am Coll Cardiol* 2004; **44**: 541–6.

91. Halkin A, Singh M, Nikolsky E, *et al*. Prediction of mortality after primary percutaneous coronary intervention for acute myocardial infarction: the CADILLAC risk score. *J Am Coll Cardiol* 2005; **45**: 1397–405.

92. Mehran R, Aymong ED, Nikolsky E, *et al*. A simple risk score for prediction of contrast-induced nephropathy after percutaneous coronary intervention: development and initial validation. *J Am Coll Cardiol* 2004; **44**: 1393–9.

93. Rao SV, Jollis JG, Harrington RA, *et al*. Relationship of blood transfusion and clinical outcomes in patients with acute coronary syndromes. *JAMA* 2004; **292**: 1555–62.

94. Yang X, Alexander KP, Chen AY, *et al*. The implications of blood transfusions for patients with non-ST-segment elevation acute coronary syndromes: results from the CRUSADE National Quality Improvement Initiative. *J Am Coll Cardiol* 2005; **46**: 1490–5.

95. Wu WC, Rathore SS, Wang Y, Radford MJ, Krumholz HM. Blood transfusion in elderly patients with acute myocardial infarction. *N Engl J Med* 2001; **345**: 1230–6.

96. Pickett JL, Theberge DC, Brown WS, Schweitzer SU, Nissenson AR. Normalizing hematocrit in dialysis patients improves brain function. *Am J Kidney Dis* 1999; **33**: 1122–30.

97. Atti AR, Palmer K, Volpato S, *et al*. Anemia increases the risk of dementia in cognitively intact elderly. *Neurobiol Aging* 2006; **27**: 278–84.

98. Zamboni V, Cesari M, Zuccala G, *et al*. Anemia and cognitive performance in hospitalized older patients: results from the GIFA study. *Int J Geriatr Psychiatry* 2006; **21**: 529–34.

99. Chaves PH, Carlson MC, Ferrucci L, *et al*. Association between mild anemia and executive function impairment in community dwelling older women: the Women's Health and Aging Study II. *J Am Geriatr Soc* 2006; **54**: 1429–35.

100. Penninx BW, Pluijm SM, Lips P, *et al*. Late-life anemia is associated with increased risk of recurrent falls. *J Am Geriatr Soc* 2005; **53**: 2106–11.

101. Singh AK, Szczech L, Tang KL, *et al*. Correction of anemia with epoetin alfa in chronic kidney disease. *N Engl J Med* 2006; **355**: 2085–98.

102. Wilson J, Yao GL, Raftery J, *et al*. A systematic review and economic evaluation of epoetin alfa, epoetin beta and darbepoetin alfa in anaemia associated with cancer, especially that attributable to cancer treatment. *Health Technol Assess* 2007; **11**: 1–220.

16

The pathogenesis of late-life anemia

Bindu Kanapuru, William B. Ershler

Introduction

As detailed elsewhere in this volume, anemia is often overlooked in the geriatric population. Historically, a decrease in hemoglobin concentration was accepted either as a part of "normal aging" or as a composite reflection of an underlying disease process. Currently, however, there is an evolving literature indicating the importance of anemia in older individuals with regard to physical and cognitive function, severity of comorbidities, and survival. For example, anemia may increase the risk for and severity of a number of age-associated diseases, including atherosclerosis, diabetes, Alzheimer disease, and osteoporosis. Furthermore, anemia is now considered an important component of the phenotype of frailty [1,2]. Thus anemia has become a topic of increasing interest among investigators and clinicians in geriatric medicine. It has also become a focal point in hematology, as a precise explanation for the commonly observed normocytic anemia associated with advanced age (and especially frailty) has yet to be clarified.

Upon careful analysis, the occurrence of anemia may often be explained by any one of the well-understood mechanisms that result in anemia at all ages. However, in older patients, frequently more than one process is involved (e.g., iron deficiency and inflammatory disease). In fact, in 15–50% of the cases, a single prominent cause of anemia can not be identified, and this condition has been termed "anemia unspecified" [3] or "anemia unexplained" [4] (Table 16.1).

Table 16.1. Features of anemia unexplained (AU).

Hemoglobin	10.5–12 g/dL
Reticulocyte index	Low
MCV	80–95 fL
Serum iron	Low–normal
TIBC	Normal
% iron saturation	Low–normal
Vitamin B_{12}, folate, ESR, TSH	Normal
Platelet and white blood counts	Normal
Creatinine clearance	>30 mL/min

MCV, mean corpuscular volume; TIBC, total iron-binding capacity; ESR, erythrocyte sedimentation rate; TSH, thyroid-stimulating hormone.

The levels of certain pro-inflammatory cytokines have been shown to be inappropriately increased to a varying extent in elderly populations, and this has been causally linked to the development of physiologic alterations that may result in the development of frailty (e.g., decreased lean body mass, osteopenia, and low-grade anemia) [5]. Indeed, certain findings in anemic elderly individuals bear close resemblance to those of anemia of inflammation, suggesting that similar pathologic processes may be operating in the elderly.

Definition and prevalence of anemia in the elderly

Many investigators have relied on the established World Health Organization (WHO) criteria for

Blood Disorders in the Elderly, ed. Lodovico Balducci, William Ershler, Giovanni de Gaetano.
Published by Cambridge University Press. © Cambridge University Press 2008.

Table 16.2. Prevalence of anemia and anemia unexplained (AU) in the elderly.

	Population	% Anemic	% AU
Guralnik *et al.* [4]	Community (NHANES III)	11	33
Ble *et al.* [11]	Community (InCHIANTI)	10	37
Tecson *et al.* IASIA, unpublished	Community, internal medicine practices	21	N/A
Artz *et al.* [10]	Nursing home (NGRC)	49	43
Narayanan [12]	Nursing home	53	N/A

IASIA, Institute for Advanced Studies in Aging; NGRC, National Geriatrics Research Consortium; N/A, not available.

anemia (hemoglobin concentration < 12 g/dL in women and <13 g/dL in men) [6]. These criteria, however, have recently come into question [7] inasmuch as the primary WHO survey described the distribution of hemoglobin levels in a young population of subjects included in a nutrition study and is likely not reflective of the population as a whole. Yet this arbitrary definition has proven of some value. For example, in one recent survey, concentrations below these levels were associated with a two-fold increase in mortality independent of baseline diseases [8]. Using the WHO definition, the prevalence of anemia in a community-dwelling geriatric population (i.e., 65 years or older) was greater than 11.0% in men and 10.2% in women and rose steadily from the age of 50 years, reaching almost 20% in ages 80 and older [4]. The prevalence of anemia had previously been shown to vary on residential status and race, with higher values found in individuals residing at nursing homes and in older African-Americans [4,9]. In the frail elderly, anemia is often more prevalent. Artz and colleagues recently found that approximately 50% of long-term care residents met WHO criteria for anemia, and in almost one-half of these, the anemia was "unexplained" (Table 16.2) [10].

Older patients with anemia have been shown to have reduced physical function [13], sarcopenia [14], osteoporosis [15], less strength [16], more falls [17], more severe comorbidities [18–22], more frequent hospitalizations [23], and shorter survival

[8,23,24] when compared to those of the same age without anemia.

Defining a specific cause for anemia in the aging population is associated with a number of confounding factors. The high prevalence of comorbidity, including arthritis, renal disease, and malignancies, certainly accounts for some of the anemia, as well as iron deficiency from occult blood loss. According to the NHANES data [4], the major causes of anemia in the aging population were nutrient deficiency and anemia of chronic inflammation. Further studies were able to elucidate myelodysplastic syndrome as a cause in a certain percentage of people with unexplained anemia. Yet no specific cause of anemia was identified in more than a third of the population. It is most likely that the unspecified anemia is multifactorial, due to a combination of renal insufficiency, androgen deficiency, and occult inflammatory processes (described below).

"Explained" anemia in the elderly

Table 16.3 shows the clinical and laboratory features of different categories of "explained" anemia.

Iron, B$_{12}$, and folic acid (nutritional anemias)

Approximately one-third of anemia in the NHANES analysis [4] appeared related to a nutrient deficiency, with more than half the subjects in this category

Table 16.3. Features of anemia by classification.

	MCV	Iron/TIBC	Ferritin	ESR/CRP	EPO	CrCl	Misc.
IDA	Small	Low/high	Low	WNL	High	WNL	
ACI	Small	Low/low	Low–high	High	High	WNL	
CKD	WNL	WNL	WNL	WNL	Low	<30 mL/min	
B_{12}/folate	Large	WNL	WNL	WNL	High	WNL	levels
Hypothyroid	Large	WNL	WNL	WNL	High	WNL	TSH up
MDS	WNL–large	WNL	WNL	WNL	High	WNL	marrow
AU	WNL	WNL	WNL	WNL	Low	>30 mL/min	

IDA, iron-deficiency anemia; ACI, anemia of chronic inflammation; CKD, chronic kidney disease; B_{12}, vitamin B_{12}; MDS, myelodysplastic syndrome; AU, Anemia unexplained; CRP, C-reactive protein; EPO, erythropoietin; CrCl, creatinine clearance; WNL, within normal limits. Other abbreviations as in Table 16.1.

deficient in iron, either alone or in combination with folate or B_{12} deficiency. For this group, uncovering the cause of the nutrient deficiency may also lead to important prevention opportunities beyond correction of the anemia. Most older adults with iron deficiency have excess gastrointestinal blood loss, and endoscopic evaluation is likely to find an underlying abnormality. In a study of 100 consecutive older patients with iron-deficiency anemia, Rockey and Cello [25] found 16% with underlying colon cancer or pre-malignant polyps. Folate deficiency may be a clue to underlying malnutrition or alcohol abuse. Catastrophic neurologic complications from B_{12} deficiency may occur despite modest anemia, and are readily prevented by timely diagnosis and treatment with supplemental B_{12} [26].

Anemia of chronic inflammation (ACI)

Anemia of chronic inflammation (also sometimes referred to as the "anemia of chronic disease") is a designation with imprecise boundaries. Typically, ACI refers to the anemia in persons with a high burden of chronic disease without a clearly defined etiology. The current association of this type of anemia with underlying inflammatory disease is an effort to correlate its occurrence with the underlying pathophysiology. The mechanism has much overlap with iron deficiency, but typically iron stores are within normal limits or elevated [27,28]. In those conditions

with elevated inflammatory cytokines, liver production of hepcidin is increased, resulting in reduced intestinal iron absorption and decreased release of iron by the macrophages [29,30].

Distinguishing ACI from iron deficiency can be difficult [31]. A serum ferritin concentration ranging from 20 to 100 μg/dL can be present in iron deficiency when there is an associated inflammatory process [32]. Bone-marrow assessment of stainable iron, or new assays such as serum transferrin receptor [33] or hepcidin [34], might improve differentiation of ACI and iron deficiency.

Renal insufficiency and anemia

Renal function declines with age even in the absence of clinically recognized disease [35]. In those with underlying conditions, such as diabetes mellitus [36] or hypertension [37], the decline is more pronounced. In addition to the exocrine function, the kidney is the major source of erythropoietin, and although not directly linear, erythropoietin production is known to be less than adequate in those with renal insufficiency [38], accounting in large part for the anemia associated with kidney failure. Furthermore, the erythropoietin response has been shown to be less than expected in elderly anemic patients, even without overt renal dysfunction [3,39–41]. In a recently reported survey of 6220 nursing-home residents, 43% were found to

Table 16.4. Component factors of "anemia unexplained" (AU).

	Aging?	Disease
Erythropoietin insufficiency	There is an age-associated decline in GFR and presumably a corresponding reduction in erythropoietin response	Both diabetes and hypertension have been associated with reduction in erythropoietin response and anemia
Cytokine inhibition of erythropoiesis	Certain pro-inflammatory cytokines, most notably interleukin 6 (IL-6), are elevated in serum and tissue sections with advancing age	Inflammatory diseases, including atherosclerosis and cancer, are associated with the presence of increased pro-inflammatory cytokines
Androgen decline (both males and females)	Androgens support erythropoiesis, and levels decline with advancing age	Orchiectomy (as treatment for prostate cancer) is associated with a drop in hemoglobin of 1 g/dL
Myelodysplasia		A disease process and *not* a component of normal aging. To the extent that it may present with anemia (without the other features such as neutropenia or thrombocytopenia), it will account for some component of AU

have a glomerular filtration rate (GFR) of less than 60 mL/min/1.73 m^2 [12], raising the suggestion that chronic renal insufficiency is a major contributor to the high prevalence of anemia in that setting.

Myelodysplasia

Myelodysplastic syndrome (MDS) occurs most commonly in older age groups [42,43]. It is a heterogenous group of disorders that are manifest typically by trilineage marrow dysplasia. Anemia is common and, particularly early in the disease, may be difficult to classify. Usually the anemia associated with myelodysplasia is macrocytic and the peripheral blood smear may indicate abnormalities (qualitative or quantitative) in the white blood cells or platelets. However, bone-marrow examination including cytogenetic studies may be required for accurate diagnosis.

"Anemia unexplained" (AU)

With advancing age, and particularly in the frail elderly, not only is there an increase in the prevalence

of anemia, but there is also an increase in that type of anemia for which a solitary mechanism can be held accountable. However, for most of these patients it is likely that a combination of "normal" age-associated physiologic changes with or without associated pathologic alterations (as above) can, in composite, be explanatory (Table 16.4). Accordingly, to the extent that disease or nutritional factors can be ruled out, some component of the observed anemia is a result of aging per se.

Androgens and aging

Androgens have long been known to stimulate erythropoiesis [44], and hormonal treatment remains effective for some patients with hypoplastic or aplastic anemia [45]. Androgen deficiency, such as observed in patients after orchiectomy or pharmacologic androgen ablation for prostate cancer, typically is associated with a drop in hemoglobin level of approximately 1 g/dL [46,47]. Thus, it is likely that an age-associated decline in androgen contributes to some extent to a decline in erythroid mass and would thereby be one component feature of unexplained anemia.

Cytokines and aging

There is great heterogeneity in cytokine expression with age. Nonetheless, there is consensus that independent of disease, certain cytokines are either qualitatively or quantitatively diminished with age (e.g., interleukin 2[IL-2] and granulocyte-macrophage colony-stimulating factor) whereas others appear to be present at higher levels (ILs 6 and 10). Although IL-1, IL-4, tumor necrosis factor α (TNF-α), and interferon gamma have been studied, the data have been inconsistent in the absence of a definable inflammatory focus [48]. This may be because of variation in technique or cell type investigated.

That cytokines may be involved in the pathogenesis of late-life anemia is suggested by a number of experimental observations. T cells from poor responders to erythropoietin therapy were found to produce increased interferon gamma and TNF-α when compared with those who had responded to treatment or with normal controls [49]. Furthermore, bone-marrow cell cultures treated with serum from patients with inflammation exhibited suppression of colony-forming units (CFU-E), and this effect was reversed by using antibodies against TNF-α and or interferon gamma [50].

Interleukin 6 (IL-6): a prototype mediator of age-associated anemia

IL-6 is a 26 kDa inflammatory cytokine that exhibits marked pleiotropy. It plays a role in the regulation of inflammation, and in endocrine and metabolic functions including osteoclastogenesis, spermatogenesis, stimulation of the endometrial vasculature during the menstrual cycle, and neural cell differentiation and proliferation [5,51]. IL-6 has been implicated in the pathogenesis of several chronic diseases associated with aging, including osteoporosis, Alzheimer disease, atherosclerosis, and neoplasia. Elevations in serum levels of IL-6 have been associated with greater functional impairment [52], depression [53], and death [54,55].

In response to inflammatory stimuli, TNF-α and IL-1 induce the production of IL-6. This in turn inhibits the secretion of IL-1 and TNF-α, activates the production of acute-phase reactants from the liver, and stimulates the hypothalamic–pituitary–adrenal axis to control inflammation [51]. IL-6 plays a role in both the innate and acquired immune response. It is a critical component of the acute-phase inflammatory response, stimulating the production of acute-phase proteins such as C-reactive protein (CRP), serum amyloid A, fibrinogen, complement, and α_1-antitrypsin. In addition, it induces the proliferation and maturation of activated B cells (culminating in the production of antibody), is involved in the proliferation of thymic and peripheral T lymphocytes, induces T-lymphocyte proliferation to cytolytic T lymphocytes (in conjunction with IL-1), and activates natural killer cells [5,56].

Although it is accepted that the expression of the IL-6 protein is tightly regulated under physiologic conditions, the stringent regulatory mechanism is not completely understood. It appears that the gene has multiple regulatory sites, and that different mechanisms may be involved in activation of IL-6 expression in different tissues. It has been shown that under normal circumstances, the expression of IL-6 is tightly regulated by several transcription factors (including NF-κB and NFIL-6), hormonal factors (androgens and estrogens), and glucocorticoids [57,58]. Although the mechanism underlying an age-related increase in IL-6 production has not been fully elucidated, it has been suggested that relaxation of the normally stringent IL-6 gene expression may be attributed to a loss of secondary sex hormones following menopause or andropause [5].

Age-associated changes in IL-6

In young healthy subjects (i.e., those without inflammatory disease or trauma), IL-6 production is tightly regulated as noted above. Thus, IL-6 is generally undetectable in the serum of young subjects, except during inflammation, trauma, or stress. However, a number of studies have demonstrated changes in IL-6 expression following menopause or andropause, even in the absence of illness or inflammation. For example, a study by McKane *et al.* [59] in

80 healthy women aged 24–87 years demonstrated that serum IL-6 levels increased threefold during life and were highly correlated with age ($p < 0.001$). This finding was corroborated by another cross-sectional survey of healthy women, which found that IL-6 plasma levels increased with advancing age ($p < 0.0001$) and positively correlated with postmenopausal status ($p < 0.0001$) [60]. In another large series, serum IL-6 was found to rise exponentially with age ($r = 0.74$, $p < 0.0001$). The median level of IL-6 increased almost tenfold, from 1.16 pg/mL in premenopausal women to 10.27 pg/mL in centenarians [61].

In an analysis of the Framingham Heart Study [62], the production of inflammatory cytokines in elderly subjects was compared with young healthy residents of Framingham. As in other studies [63,64], the investigators found that IL-6 production was increased in the elderly (mean age 78 years) compared with the younger controls (mean age 39.3 years). In this study, inflammation was assessed by measuring CRP. Although production of IL-6 was greatest in elderly patients with elevated CRP, IL-6 was still higher in elderly subjects without elevated CRP levels compared with younger controls. This supports the hypothesis that elevation of IL-6 in the elderly is not solely caused by inflammation, and that age itself may be a contributing factor.

The effect of elevated plasma IL-6 on functional disability, mortality, and depression has been studied in the Established Populations for Epidemiologic Studies of the Elderly (EPESE), which is a large epidemiologic study initiated by the National Institute of Aging involving elderly people living in several different areas of the USA. As with other studies, IL-6 levels were higher in an elderly population aged over 70 years than in younger subjects. The elevated IL-6 levels were associated with declines typical of frailty, such as in overall functional status ($p < 0.0001$) [52], mobility and activities of daily living disability [65], depression [53], and mortality [54].

IL-6 and anemia

In a pilot study, Leng and colleagues [66] reported that the frailty phenotype (as defined by their screening criteria) is associated with high IL-6 and low hemoglobin levels. This intriguing finding lends support to the emerging hypothesis regarding the importance of this particular cytokine in the pathogenesis of AU.

The exact pathophysiology of cytokine-associated anemia remains unclear, although several mechanisms have been proposed. One possibility relates to the negative effects of pro-inflammatory cytokines on erythropoietin synthesis and response [39,40,49,50,67–72]. Serum erythropoietin levels, although higher in this condition compared with non-anemic subjects, are still inappropriately lower than those found in patients with a similar degree of anemia due to iron deficiency [73,74]. A second proposed mechanism involves the stimulatory effects of these same pro-inflammatory cytokines, particularly IL-6, on hepcidin level and activity [28,75,76]. The critical role for hepcidin in producing the anemia of inflammation has recently been elucidated, and engages the inhibitory effects of this molecule on intestinal iron absorption and mobilization [27,77,78].

Cytokines and iron transport

Iron transport begins with the uptake of dietary iron in the ferrous form by the intestinal cells with the help of DMT-1 (divalent metal transporter), and it is transported in blood by transferrin, which delivers iron for erythropoiesis in bone marrow by binding to the transferrin receptor (TfR).

The interactions of these proteins regulate transferrin uptake and ferritin translation based on intracellular iron [79]. Much of the iron is also derived by the recycling of heme upon destruction of senescent erythrocytes and catabolism of hemoglobin. Iron thus formed is taken up by macrophages through the TfR or through non-TfR-mediated uptake through DMT-1, and either stored as ferritin or transported by macrophage ferroportin present in the plasma. Cytokines appear to affect iron transport in every step of the pathway.

As mentioned, hepcidin inhibits iron uptake at the enterocyte by decreasing the expression of DMT-1 [80]. It has been speculated that hepcidin also inhibits iron release from macrophages and enterocytes by interacting with ferroportin 1 [75]. Hepcidin expression by the liver is suppressed by anemia and hypoxia, but strong inflammatory stimuli have been known to induce hepcidin even in the setting of anemia [81]. IL-6 has been found to be a major regulator of hepcidin production [76]. After infusion of IL-6, the urinary concentrations of hepcidin increased dramatically in human volunteers [82]. In IL-6 knockout mice no increase in hepcidin expression was detected, even under conditions of iron overload. The transcription of hepcidin by endotoxin-treated macrophages was also found to be blocked by an antibody to IL-6 [28]. In cell models TNF-α reduced the induction of DMT-1 in the enterocytes, thereby causing reduction in intestinal iron transport [83].

As mentioned above, cytokines also play a major role in regulating iron transport in monocytic cells. Cytokines increase both TfR-mediated and non-TfR-mediated iron uptake by macrophages. Inflammatory cytokines also downregulate ferroportin expression and prevent iron export from the macrophages [84]. This, coupled with the IL-6-mediated hepcidin effect, effectively paralyzes the reticuloendothelial system as a source of usable iron. Furthermore, ferritin is inducible by TNF-α, IL-6 and IL-1. Thus, in the presence of inflammatory cytokines, cellular iron intake increases, but not efflux. The net result is less iron available for erythropoiesis and a resultant hypoproliferative anemia.

Cytokines and hematopoiesis

The earliest recognizable erythroid progenitors are the burst-forming unit-erythroid (BFU-E) and colony-forming unit-erythroid (CFU-E). Growth factors that are involved in erythropoiesis include SCF (stem cell factor), IL-3, IL-6, and erythropoietin. SCF and IL-3 act primarily on the pluripotent stem cell and effect differentiation into myeloid stem cell and early colony-forming units. The site of action of erythropoietin in the bone marrow is mainly on the late colony-forming unit (CFU-E) and through interaction with SCF and IL-3 on the burst-forming unit (BFU-E). Erythropoietin inhibits

apoptosis of committed erythroid progenitors and thereby expands red cell mass by preventing apoptosis of erythroid precursors [85–87].

Aging populations usually have normal erythropoiesis under basal conditions but have a diminished capacity to mount an adequate response to stress [84]. Various mechanisms have been postulated by which this dysregulation occurs, including cytokine inhibition of erythropoietin gene expression [1] and erythropoietin resistance. Interferon gamma has been shown to inhibit the growth of erythroid precursors, possibly through its action on the TNF family of proteins [88]. The receptor TRAIL (TNF-related apoptosis-inducing ligand) induced by TNF-α was shown to significantly reduce differentiation of erythroblasts in culture, an effect which was overcome when the culture was supplemented with stem cells, IL-3, and erythropoietin [89]. A similar mechanism has been proposed as a cause for anemia in myelodysplastic syndromes [90]. TNF-α has been shown to reduce the incorporation of tagged iron into erythrocytes, thereby causing a reduction both in erythrocyte number and in survival [91]. Thus it is possible (but unproven) that similar mechanisms may contribute to the anemia observed in elderly individuals with inappropriate levels of pro-inflammatory cytokines.

Erythropoietin is regulated primarily by hypoxia and anemia. In the presence of these stimuli interstitial cells of the kidney increase the secretion of erythropoietin, resulting in an expansion of the red cell mass. As mentioned above, cytokines can cause anemia through their effects on erythropoietin. Serum erythropoietin levels are known to increase with age in healthy adults [72]. In the InCHIANTI study an increase in CRP, IL-6, and other inflammatory markers was associated with higher erythropoietin levels in non-anemic individuals but lower levels in anemic participants [69]. In older iron-deficient individuals, erythropoietin levels were shown to inversely correlate with the hemoglobin levels, but the heightened level of erythropoietin was still significantly lower than that of younger individuals with comparable levels of iron-deficiency anemia [40]. Thus, with advancing age, erythropoietin levels rise, and under healthy circumstances this is sufficient to maintain red cell mass. However, for individuals with reduced capacity to produce erythropoietin (e.g., those with kidney disease), or for those with increased demand (e.g., those with iron deficiency), erythropoietin production capacity is insufficient to meet the demand and anemia occurs.

Decreased erythropoietin response to anemia has also been implicated as a cause in many chronic inflammatory disorders. In-vitro evidence from human hepatoma cell lines shows that IL-1, IL-1β, and TNF-α may directly inhibit erythropoietin production [70,71]. Although the exact mechanism is not known, it is postulated that it is through production of reactive oxygen molecules. IL-6 was also found to have an inhibitory effect on the production of erythropoietin from the kidney, although there have been conflicting reports from liver cell lines [71].

Summary

It is our current belief that AU is not as mysterious as it is complex. There are four age-associated contributing factors that in composite might be explanatory. These are:

(1) An age-associated decline in renal function, which to some extent contributes to a lower than optimal erythropoietin response [39,72,74,11].
(2) An age-associated reduction in androgen levels, in both males and females, which may account for a decline in hemoglobin level of up to 1 g/dL [45,46].
(3) Bone-marrow myelodysplasia, which occurs more frequently with advancing age and may present as refractory anemia without associated white blood cell or platelet features [42,92].
(4) Anemia attributable to age-associated cytokine dysregulation. Pro-inflammatory cytokines, most notably IL-6, have been shown to increase in tissue and in serum with advancing age [56,63,93], and this may occur in the absence of known inflammatory disease [94]. The presence of these pro-inflammatory cytokines has been shown to correlate with the advent of several features of frailty [5] including anemia [66,69] and to have negative prognostic importance with regard to symptoms [52], comorbidities [54,65,66], and survival [54,65]. Elevated cytokine levels may contribute to AU by mechanisms noted above for inflammation (inhibition of erythropoietin and induction of hepcidin).

Thus, we conceptualize AU as occurring as a result of the common age-associated mild/moderate renal insufficiency (low erythropoietin) coupled with the effects of inappropriately raised pro-inflammatory cytokines (low erythropoietin, hepcidin), androgen deficiency, and in some, early myelodysplasia.

REFERENCES

1. Ershler WB. Biological interactions of aging and anemia: a focus on cytokines. *J Am Geriatr Soc* 2003; **51** (3 Suppl): S18–S21.
2. Gabrilove J. Anemia and the elderly: clinical considerations. *Best Pract Res Clin Haematol* 2005; **18**: 417–22.
3. Artz AS, Fergusson D, Drinka PJ, *et al.* Mechanisms of unexplained anemia in the nursing home. *J Am Geriatr Soc* 2004; **52**: 423–7.
4. Guralnik JM, Eisenstaedt RS, Ferrucci L, Klein HG, Woodman RC. Prevalence of anemia in persons 65 years and older in the United States: evidence for a high rate of unexplained anemia. *Blood* 2004; **104**: 2263–8.
5. Ershler WB, Keller ET. Age-associated increased interleukin-6 gene expression, late-life diseases, and frailty. *Annu Rev Med* 2000; **51**: 245–70.
6. Blanc B, Finch CA, Hallberg L. Nutritional anaemias. Report of a WHO Scientific Group. *WHO Tech Rep Ser* 1968; **405**: 1–40.
7. Beutler E, Waalen J. The definition of anemia: what is the lower limit of normal of the blood hemoglobin concentration? *Blood* 2006; **107**: 1747–50.
8. Zakai NA, Katz R, Hirsch C, *et al.* A prospective study of anemia status, hemoglobin concentration, and mortality in an elderly cohort: the Cardiovascular Health Study. *Arch Intern Med* 2005; **165**: 2214–20.
9. Salive ME, Cornoni-Huntley J, Guralnik JM, *et al.* Anemia and hemoglobin levels in older persons: relationship

with age, gender, and health status. *J Am Geriatr Soc* 1992; **40**: 489–96.

10. Artz AS, Fergusson D, Drinka PJ, *et al.* Prevalence of anemia in skilled-nursing home residents. *Arch Gerontol Geriatr* 2004; **39**: 201–6.

11. Ble A, Fink JC, Woodman RC, *et al.* Renal function, erythropoietin, and anemia of older persons: the InCHIANTI study. *Arch Intern Med* 2005; **165**: 2222–7.

12. Narayanan S. Resource utilization and treatment trends of anemia in long term care residents. *J Am Soc Nephrol* 2005; **16**: 549a.

13. Penninx BW, Guralnik JM, Onder G, Ferrucci L, Wallace RB, Pahor M. Anemia and decline in physical performance among older persons. *Am J Med* 2003; **115**: 104–10.

14. Cesari M, Penninx BW, Lauretani F, *et al.* Hemoglobin levels and skeletal muscle: results from the InCHIANTI study. *J Gerontol A Biol Sci Med Sci* 2004; **59**: 249–54.

15. Cesari M, Pahor M, Lauretani F, *et al.* Bone density and hemoglobin levels in older persons: results from the InCHIANTI study. *Osteoporos Int* 2005; **16**: 691–9.

16. Penninx BW, Pahor M, Cesari M, *et al.* Anemia is associated with disability and decreased physical performance and muscle strength in the elderly. *J Am Geriatr Soc* 2004; **52**: 719–24.

17. Penninx BW, Pluijm SM, Lips P, *et al.* Late-life anemia is associated with increased risk of recurrent falls. *J Am Geriatr Soc* 2005; **53**: 2106–11.

18. Beard CM, Kokmen E, O'Brien PC, Ania BJ, Melton LJ, 3rd. Risk of Alzheimer's disease among elderly patients with anemia: population-based investigations in Olmsted County, Minnesota. *Ann Epidemiol* 1997; **7**: 219–24.

19. Besarab A, Bolton WK, Browne JK, *et al.* The effects of normal as compared with low hematocrit values in patients with cardiac disease who are receiving hemodialysis and epoetin. *N Engl J Med* 1998; **339**: 584–90.

20. Cumming RG, Mitchell P, Craig JC, Knight JF. Renal impairment and anaemia in a population-based study of older people. *Intern Med J* 2004; **34**: 20–3.

21. Kosiborod M, Curtis JP, Wang Y, *et al.* Anemia and outcomes in patients with heart failure: a study from the National Heart Care Project. *Arch Intern Med* 2005; **165**: 2237–44.

22. Nissenson AR, Goodnough LT, Dubois RW. Anemia: not just an innocent bystander? *Arch Intern Med* 2003; **163**: 1400–4.

23. Culleton BF, Manns BJ, Zhang J, Tonelli M, Klarenbach S, Hemmelgarn BR. Impact of anemia on hospitalization and mortality in older adults. *Blood* 2006; **107**: 3841–6.

24. Chaves PH, Xue QL, Guralnik JM, Ferrucci L, Volpato S, Fried LP. What constitutes normal hemoglobin concentration in community-dwelling disabled older women? *J Am Geriatr Soc* 2004; **52**: 1811–16.

25. Rockey DC, Cello JP. Evaluation of the gastrointestinal tract in patients with iron-deficiency anemia. *N Engl J Med* 1993; **329**: 1691–5.

26. Lindenbaum J, Healton EB, Savage DG, *et al.* Neuropsychiatric disorders caused by cobalamin deficiency in the absence of anemia or macrocytosis. *N Engl J Med* 1988; **318**: 1720–8.

27. Sears DA. Anemia of chronic disease. *Med Clin North Am* 1992; **76**: 567–79.

28. Weiss G. Pathogenesis and treatment of anaemia of chronic disease. *Blood Rev* 2002; **16**: 87–96.

29. Ganz T. Hepcidin, a key regulator of iron metabolism and mediator of anemia of inflammation. *Blood* 2003; **102**: 783–8.

30. Nemeth E, Rivera S, Gabayan V, *et al.* IL-6 mediates hypoferremia of inflammation by inducing the synthesis of the iron regulatory hormone hepcidin. *J Clin Invest* 2004; **113**: 1271–6.

31. Smith D. Management and treatment of anemia in the elderly. *Clin Geriatr Med* 2002; **10**: 47–53.

32. Chatta GS, Lipschitz D. Anemia. In Hazzard WR, Blass JP, Ettinger WH, Halter JB, Ouslander JG, eds, *Principles of Geriatric Medicine and Gerontology*, 4th edn (New York, NY: McGraw-Hill, 1999), 899–906.

33. Chua E, Clague JE, Sharma AK, Horan MA, Lombard M. Serum transferrin receptor assay in iron deficiency anaemia and anaemia of chronic disease in the elderly. *QJM* 1999; **92**: 587–94.

34. Weinstein DA, Roy CN, Fleming MD, Loda MF, Wolfsdorf JI, Andrews NC. Inappropriate expression of hepcidin is associated with iron refractory anemia: implications for the anemia of chronic disease. *Blood* 2002; **100**: 3776–81.

35. Baylis C, Schmidt R. The aging glomerulus. *Semin Nephrol* 1996; **16**: 265–76.

36. Shumway JT, Gambert SR. Diabetic nephropathy: pathophysiology and management. *Int Urol Nephrol* 2002; **34**: 257–64.

37. Clark B. Biology of renal aging in humans. *Adv Ren Replace Ther* 2000; **7**: 11–21.

38. Spivak JL. Serum immunoreactive erythropoietin in health and disease. *J Perinat Med* 1995; **23**: 13–7.

39. Kario K, Matsuo T, Kodama K, Nakao K, Asada R. Reduced erythropoietin secretion in senile anemia. *Am J Hematol* 1992; **41**: 252–7.

40. Kario K, Matsuo T, Nakao K. Serum erythropoietin levels in the elderly. *Gerontology* 1991; **37**: 345–8.

41. Powers JS, Krantz SB, Collins JC, *et al*. Erythropoietin response to anemia as a function of age. *J Am Geriatr Soc* 1991; **39**: 30–2.

42. Bennett JM, Kouides PA, Forman SJ. The myelodysplastic syndromes: morphology, risk assessment, and clinical management (2002). *Int J Hematol* 2002; **76** (Suppl 2): 228–38.

43. Steensma DP, Bennett JM. The myelodysplastic syndromes: diagnosis and treatment. *Mayo Clin Proc* 2006; **81**: 104–30.

44. Shahidi NT. Androgens and erythropoiesis. *N Engl J Med* 1973; **289**: 72–80.

45. Nissen C, Gratwohl A, Speck B. Management of aplastic anemia. *Eur J Haematol* 1991; **46**: 193–7.

46. Schubert M, Jockenhovel F. Late-onset hypogonadism in the aging male (LOH): definition, diagnostic and clinical aspects. *J Endocrinol Invest* 2005; **28** (3 Suppl): 23–7.

47. Voegeli TA, Kurtz A, Grimm MO, Effert P, Eckardt KU. Anemia under androgen deprivation: influence of flutamide, cyproteroneacetate and orchiectomy on the erythropoietin system. *Horm Metab Res* 2005; **37**: 89–93.

48. Visser M, Pahor M, Taaffe DR, *et al*. Relationship of interleukin-6 and tumor necrosis factor-alpha with muscle mass and muscle strength in elderly men and women: the Health ABC Study. *J Gerontol A Biol Sci Med Sci* 2002; **57**: M326–M332.

49. Cooper AC, Mikhail A, Lethbridge MW, Kemeny DM, Macdougall IC. Increased expression of erythropoiesis inhibiting cytokines (IFN-gamma, TNF-alpha, IL-10, and IL-13) by T cells in patients exhibiting a poor response to erythropoietin therapy. *J Am Soc Nephrol* 2003; **14**: 1776–84.

50. Macdougall IC, Cooper AC. Erythropoietin resistance: the role of inflammation and pro-inflammatory cytokines. *Nephrol Dial Transplant* 2002; **17** (Suppl 11): 39–43.

51. Papanicolaou DA, Wilder RL, Manolagas SC, Chrousos GP. The pathophysiologic roles of interleukin-6 in human disease. *Ann Intern Med* 1998; **128**: 127–37.

52. Cohen HJ, Pieper CF, Harris T, Rao KM, Currie MS. The association of plasma IL-6 levels with functional disability in community-dwelling elderly. *J Gerontol A Biol Sci Med Sci* 1997; **52**: M201–M208.

53. Dentino AN, Pieper CF, Rao MK, *et al*. Association of interleukin-6 and other biologic variables with depression in

older people living in the community. *J Am Geriatr Soc* 1999; **47**: 6–11.

54. Harris TB, Ferrucci L, Tracy RP, *et al*. Associations of elevated interleukin-6 and C-reactive protein levels with mortality in the elderly. *Am J Med* 1999; **106**: 506–12.

55. Volpato S, Guralnik JM, Ferrucci L, *et al*. Cardiovascular disease, interleukin-6, and risk of mortality in older women: the women's health and aging study. *Circulation* 2001; **103**: 947–53.

56. Ershler WB. Interleukin-6: a cytokine for gerontologists. *J Am Geriatr Soc* 1993; **41**: 176–81.

57. Keller ET, Chang C, Ershler WB. Inhibition of NFkappaB activity through maintenance of IkappaBalpha levels contributes to dihydrotestosterone-mediated repression of the interleukin-6 promoter. *J Biol Chem* 1996; **271**: 26267–75.

58. Keller ET, Wanagat J, Ershler WB. Molecular and cellular biology of interleukin-6 and its receptor. *Front Biosci* 1996; **1**: d340–d357.

59. McKane WR, Khosla S, Peterson JM, Egan K, Riggs BL. Circulating levels of cytokines that modulate bone resorption: effects of age and menopause in women. *J Bone Miner Res* 1994; **9**: 1313–18.

60. Kania DM, Binkley N, Checovich M, Havighurst T, Schilling M, Ershler WB. Elevated plasma levels of interleukin-6 in postmenopausal women do not correlate with bone density. *J Am Geriatr Soc* 1995; **43**: 236–9.

61. Giuliani N, Sansoni P, Girasole G, *et al*. Serum interleukin-6, soluble interleukin-6 receptor and soluble gp130 exhibit different patterns of age- and menopause-related changes. *Exp Gerontol* 2001; **36**: 547–57.

62. Roubenoff R, Harris TB, Abad LW, Wilson PW, Dallal GE, Dinarello CA. Monocyte cytokine production in an elderly population: effect of age and inflammation. *J Gerontol A Biol Sci Med Sci* 1998; **53**: M20–M26.

63. Daynes RA, Araneo BA, Ershler WB, Maloney C, Li GZ, Ryu SY. Altered regulation of IL-6 production with normal aging. Possible linkage to the age-associated decline in dehydroepiandrosterone and its sulfated derivative. *J Immunol* 1993; **150**: 5219–30.

64. Eisenhauer EA, Vermorken JB, van Glabbeke M. Predictors of response to subsequent chemotherapy in platinum pretreated ovarian cancer: a multivariate analysis of 704 patients. *Ann Oncol* 1997; **8**: 963–8.

65. Ferrucci L, Harris TB, Guralnik JM, *et al*. Serum IL-6 level and the development of disability in older persons. *J Am Geriatr Soc* 1999; **47**: 639–46.

66. Leng S, Chaves P, Koenig K, Walston J. Serum interleukin-6 and hemoglobin as physiological correlates

in the geriatric syndrome of frailty: a pilot study. *J Am Geriatr Soc* 2002; **50**: 1268–71.

67. Baraldi-Junkins CA, Beck AC, Rothstein G. Hematopoiesis and cytokines. Relevance to cancer and aging. *Hematol Oncol Clin North Am* 2000; **14**: 45–61, viii.

68. Dai C, Krantz SB. Interferon gamma induces upregulation and activation of caspases 1, 3, and 8 to produce apoptosis in human erythroid progenitor cells. *Blood* 1999; **93**: 3309–16.

69. Ferrucci L, Guralnik JM, Woodman RC, *et al.* Proinflammatory state and circulating erythropoietin in persons with and without anemia. *Am J Med* 2005; **118**: 1288.

70. Jelkmann W. Proinflammatory cytokines lowering erythropoietin production. *J Interferon Cytokine Res* 1998; **18**: 555–9.

71. Jelkmann W, Pagel H, Wolff M, Fandrey J. Monokines inhibiting erythropoietin production in human hepatoma cultures and in isolated perfused rat kidneys. *Life Sci* 1992; **50**: 301–8.

72. Ershler WB, Sheng S, McKelvey J, *et al.* Serum erythropoietin and aging: a longitudinal analysis. *J Am Geriatr Soc* 2005; **53**: 1360–5.

73. Bertero MT, Caligaris-Cappio F. Anemia of chronic disorders in systemic autoimmune diseases. *Haematologica* 1997; **82**: 375–81.

74. Goodnough LT, Price TH, Parvin CA. The endogenous erythropoietin response and the erythropoietic response to blood loss anemia: the effects of age and gender. *J Lab Clin Med* 1995; **126**: 57–64.

75. Andrews NC. Anemia of inflammation: the cytokine hepcidin link. *J Clin Invest* 2004; **113**: 1251–3.

76. Lee P, Peng H, Gelbart T, Wang L, Beutler E. Regulation of hepcidin transcription by interleukin-1 and interleukin-6. *Proc Natl Acad Sci USA* 2005; **102**: 1906–10.

77. Ganz T, Nemeth E. Iron imports. IV. Hepcidin and regulation of body iron metabolism. *Am J Physiol Gastrointest Liver Physiol* 2006; **290**: G199–G203.

78. Roy CN, Andrews NC. Anemia of inflammation: the hepcidin link. *Curr Opin Hematol* 2005; **12**: 107–11.

79. Roy CN, Enns CA. Iron homeostasis: new tales from the crypt. *Blood* 2000; **96**: 4020–7.

80. Deicher R, Horl WH. Hepcidin: a molecular link between inflammation and anaemia. *Nephrol Dial Transplant* 2004; **19**: 521–4.

81. Nicolas G, Chauvet C, Viatte L, *et al.* The gene encoding the iron regulatory peptide hepcidin is regulated by anemia, hypoxia, and inflammation. *J Clin Invest* 2002; **110**: 1037–44.

82. Kemna E, Pickkers P, Nemeth E, van der Hoeven H, Swinkels D. Time-course analysis of hepcidin, serum iron, and plasma cytokine levels in humans injected with LPS. *Blood* 2005; **106**: 1864–6.

83. Sharma N, Laftah AH, Brookes MJ, Cooper B, Iqbal T, Tselepis C. A role for tumour necrosis factor alpha in human small bowel iron transport. *Biochem J* 2005; **390**: 437–46.

84. Williams LH, Udupa KB, Lipshitz DA. Evaluation of the effect of age on hematopoiesis in the C57BL/6 mouse. *Exp Hematol* 1986; **14**: 827–32.

85. Boyer SH, Bishop TR, Rogers OC, Noyes AN, Frelin LP, Hobbs S. Roles of erythropoietin, insulin-like growth factor 1, and unidentified serum factors in promoting maturation of purified murine erythroid colony-forming units. *Blood* 1992; **80**: 2503–12.

86. Koury MJ, Bondurant MC. Maintenance by erythropoietin of viability and maturation of murine erythroid precursor cells. *J Cell Physiol* 1988; **137**: 65–74.

87. Koury MJ, Bondurant MC. Erythropoietin retards DNA breakdown and prevents programmed death in erythroid progenitor cells. *Science* 1990; **248**: 378–81.

88. Felli N, Pedini F, Zeuner A, *et al.* Multiple members of the TNF superfamily contribute to IFN-gamma-mediated inhibition of erythropoiesis. *J Immunol* 2005; **175**: 1464–72.

89. Zamai L, Secchiero P, Pierpaoli S, *et al.* TNF-related apoptosis-inducing ligand (TRAIL) as a negative regulator of normal human erythropoiesis. *Blood* 2000; **95**: 3716–24.

90. Campioni D, Secchiero P, Corallini F, *et al.* Evidence for a role of TNF-related apoptosis-inducing ligand (TRAIL) in the anemia of myelodysplastic syndromes. *Am J Pathol* 2005; **166**: 557–63.

91. Moldawer LL, Marano MA, Wei H, *et al.* Cachectin/tumor necrosis factor-alpha alters red blood cell kinetics and induces anemia in vivo. *Faseb J* 1989; **3**: 1637–43.

92. Rothstein G. Disordered hematopoiesis and myelodysplasia in the elderly. *J Am Geriatr Soc* 2003; **51** (3 Suppl): S22–S26.

93. Ershler WB, Sun WH, Binkley N, *et al.* Interleukin-6 and aging: blood levels and mononuclear cell production increase with advancing age and in vitro production is modifiable by dietary restriction. *Lymphokine Cytokine Res* 1993; **12**: 225–30.

94. Ershler WB. Inflammation gone awry: aging or disease. *Blood* 2005; **105**: 2247.

17

Treatment of late-life anemia

William B. Ershler

Anemia in geriatric populations

Common among goals in geriatric medicine is to preserve functional independence and active life. In so doing, it becomes important to recognize and manage conditions that precipitate functional dependence and aggravate coexisting disease. Recent research has identified anemia as one of these contributory conditions, as its presence alone has been associated with diminished physical [1,2] and cognitive function [3], greater likelihood of falling [4], aggravated comorbidities [5–9], and decreased survival [10–12]. Thus the presence of anemia has become a target of clinical investigation in geriatric medicine [13,14].

In general, older community-dwelling individuals appreciate autonomy and have significant negative concerns regarding nursing-home placement [15]. Yet with functional decline, especially if this includes an impairment of one or more of the basic activities of daily living (ADL: bathing, dressing, feeding, transferring, toileting, continence), nursing-home placement becomes increasingly common. For example, rates of nursing-home placement for older individuals with one impaired ADL have ranged from 20% to 70% depending on circumstances, such as caregiver availability, economic factors, and whether or not the impairment was acute or chronic [16,17]. Although not studied in the context of ADLs or nursing-home placement, it is likely that the presence of anemia is a contributing factor to the rate of institutionalization. It has been our premise that a sustained normalization of hemoglobin level will result in sufficient improved function over time to be associated with reduced rates of admission to either nursing home or hospital. Yet data in this regard have been slow to develop and it remains to be proven whether the correction of anemia, particularly the unexplained anemia that occurs late in life [18–21], is of value in terms of physical or cognitive function, quality of life, comorbidity severity, or survival.

Treatment of anemia in the elderly: general concepts

The majority of adults with anemia have a recognizable cause of anemia for which treatment is specific and usually effective (Table 17.1). For those with iron deficiency, oral or parenteral iron is currently of proven value and successful. Of course, clinicians can not be satisfied with a diagnosis of iron deficiency without defining its cause, as it typically is the result of gastrointestinal blood loss and prompt diagnosis can have profound survival implications. In a study of 100 consecutive older patients with iron-deficiency anemia, Rockey and Cello [22] found a bleeding source in 36 patients by upper endoscopy and underlying colon cancer or pre-malignant polyps in 16. The discovery of iron deficiency may also be an early sign of celiac sprue [23].

Similarly, catastrophic neurologic complications from vitamin B_{12} deficiency may occur despite modest anemia and are readily prevented by timely diagnosis and treatment with supplemental B_{12} [24].

Blood Disorders in the Elderly, ed. Lodovico Balducci, William Ershler, Giovanni de Gaetano.
Published by Cambridge University Press. © Cambridge University Press 2008.

Table 17.1. Anemia treatment.

Cause of anemia	Therapy
Iron deficiency	Iron
Inflammatory disease	ESP/transfusion
B_{12}, folate deficiency	Vitamin B_{12}, folic acid
Renal insufficiency	ESP
Myelodysplasia	ESP+G-CSF, azacytidine, halidomide
Anemia unspecified	? ESP

ESP, erythropoiesis-stimulating protein; G-CSF, granulocyte colony-stimulating factor.

Table 17.2. Some risks of allogeneic blood transfusion.

Blood transfusion risk	Estimated frequency per actual unit
Viruses	
Hepatitis B	$1/60\,000-1/200\,000$
Hepatitis C	$1/800\,000-1/1.6 \times 10^6$
HIV	$1/1.4 \times 10^6-1/2.4 \times 10^6$
Bacteria	
Red cells	$1/500\,000$
Platelets	$1/2000$
Acute hemolytic reactions	$1/250\,000-1/1\,000\,000$
Delayed hemolytic reactions	$1/1000$
Transfusion-related acute lung injury	$1/8000$
ABO clerical error	$1/16\,000$

Folic acid deficiency is readily treated, but may be an indication of alcoholism or gastrointestinal disease. Although currently the most common cause of macrocytic anemia is the use of DNA synthesis-inhibiting chemotherapy, if vitamin B_{12} and folic acid are replete, other considerations would be hypothyroidism [25] and myelodysplastic syndrome [26,27], both of which have implications beyond the presence of a reduced hemoglobin concentration.

Chronic kidney disease results in anemia primarily because of diminished capacity for endogenous erythropoietin production. Accordingly, recombinant human erythropoietin and other erythropoiesis-stimulating proteins (ESPs) such as darbepoetin have been successful in restoring hemoglobin levels to normal or near-normal levels, as well as improving aspects of renal, cognitive, and cardiac function [28–34].

Allogeneic red cell transfusion

In patients with acute blood loss, transfusion can be life-saving. However, with the expense of transfusion and the inherent risks (Table 17.2), this procedure should be reserved for life-threatening anemia and would not currently be recommended for the majority of patients with anemia unexplained (AU), in whom the anemia is generally more mild or moderate (not severe), and for whom correction of hemoglobin concentration has not been demonstrated to be efficacious with regard to physical or cognitive function. Although the safety of the blood supply in regard to infectious disease transmission has been improved, some risks, such as bacterial infection of platelets, delayed hemolytic reaction, and transfusion-related acute lung injury, are still relatively common. Also, new viruses are emerging and some may be transmissible through the blood supply. Human error resulting in compatibility mismatches is also notable. Accordingly, in a joint statement from the American Association of Blood Banks, America's Blood Centers, and the American Red Cross, the current guideline for allogeneic transfusion includes the following statement: "Except when the patient's symptoms require immediate enhancement of oxygen-carrying capacity, red cell-containing components should not be used to treat anemia that can be corrected with specific medications such as iron, vitamin B_{12}, folic acid, or recombinant erythropoietin" [35].

Erythropoietin

Erythropoietin, a glycoprotein hormone, plays a critical role in the regulation of hematopoiesis. In response to anemia or hypoxia, erythropoietin is secreted by the kidney [36–39], and to a lesser extent the liver [37,38]. In the bone marrow, erythropoietin receptors are found in lower density on the burst-forming unit-erythroid (BFU-E) and in much higher density on its progeny, the colony-forming unit-erythroid (CFU-E) [40,41]. Erythropoietin bound to its receptor promotes the viability of CFU-E by inhibiting apoptosis [38,42], resulting in increased production of red blood cells.

Recombinant human erythropoietin (rHuEPO) has the identical amino-acid sequence of endogenous erythropoietin and demonstrates the same biologic effects [43]. Darbepoetin is a modified erythropoietin molecule that was designed by introducing five amino-acid changes into the primary sequence of erythropoietin to create two extra consensus N-linked carbohydrate addition sites for a total of five. Endogenous erythropoietin and rHuEPO have only three such sites. Because of its increased carbohydrate content, darbepoetin has a threefold longer serum half-life compared with rHuEPO [44]. More recently, a third-generation molecule, Continuous Erythropoietin Receptor Activator (CERA), incorporating a large polymer chain, has been developed. CERA has an elimination half-life in humans that is considerably longer than the half-life of either recombinant erythropoietin or darbepoetin alpha. CERA is currently in phase III clinical trials [45].

Erythropoietin responsiveness

Numerous studies have examined the endogenous erythropoietin response to anemia with advanced age. Initial animal studies pointed to a blunted erythropoietin response in aged animals [46–49]. Most studies [18,50–54], but not all [55], of older subjects with anemia of chronic disease demonstrate lower serum erythropoietin levels when compared to patients with anemia due to iron deficiency. While the glomerular filtration rate (GFR) is known to decline with age in general [56,57], one study did not demonstrate a tight correlation of blunted erythropoietin response and GFR [54]. An inherent dysregulation of hematopoiesis that commonly occurs in older adults [58] coupled with a suboptimal erythropoietin response, may be central to the pathogenesis of anemia in geriatric populations (see Chapter 16). A reduced endogenous erythropoietin response to anemia in other conditions such as cancer [59,60], rheumatoid arthritis [59,61–63], premature neonates [64], inflammatory bowel disease [65], and advanced human immunodeficiency disease [66,67] has been well described. We suspect that advanced age alone (i.e., without an underlying disease process) is also associated with reduced erythropoietin responsiveness [18].

rHuEPO for the treatment of anemia

With FDA approval in 1989, rHuEPO became an option for treating anemia without the risks and untoward effects of transfusions. rHuEPO is now FDA-approved to treat anemia associated with cancer chemotherapy, myelodysplasia, chronic renal failure, zidovudine treatment of human immunodeficiency, and preoperatively in patients anticipated to require significant allogeneic blood transfusions. rHuEPO has not been approved for the treatment of the unexplained anemia of late life (i.e., for those patients who meet the AU criteria as defined in Table 16.1).

rHuEPO treatment for patients with end-stage renal disease has led to improved quality of life and longer survival [68–80]. The improved quality of life is not isolated to renal-failure patients. Other anemic patients with diseases characterized by inappropriately low erythropoietin level, such as cancer [81–83], human immunodeficiency [79], and rheumatoid arthritis [84], also demonstrate an improved quality of life in addition to raised hemoglobin values.

The high prevalence of anemia and associated comorbidities in nursing-home residents provides a rationale for a clinical trial in this population. To date, there are no published data available on the use of rHuEPO in this setting. Subanalyses in previous studies that included older patients reveal no correlation between age and hemoglobin response [72,78,85,86], suggesting advanced age does not abrogate the benefits of treatment. However, in one report, two elderly patients (93 and 98 years old) were treated with rHuEPO [87], and one of the two developed hyperkalemia and confusion, thereby limiting treatment.

Erythropoietin in the central nervous system

The improved quality of life associated with rHuEPO treatment may be due, at least in part, to factors other than improved red blood cell mass. Recent studies of erythropoietin activity in the central nervous system support a provocative hypothesis: rHuEPO may exert a direct effect on the brain. Synthesis of erythropoietin was originally thought to be limited to the kidney and liver, but discovery of erythropoietin and the erythropoietin receptor (EPO-R) in other human tissue [88] has revised that notion. There is now convincing evidence that erythropoietin and EPO-R are present in human brain cells [89–91]. Further, in animals, hypoxia and anemia induce erythropoietin and possibly EPO-R expression in brain cells [89,91–94]. In animal models, a neuroprotective effect of rHuEPO has been shown to counter experimental hypoxic injury [92,95–97]. Thus, erythropoietin may have an important homeostatic role in the brain.

The presence of EPO-R in brain capillary endothelial cells [96] suggests that renally secreted erythropoietin and exogenously administered rHuEPO may have a direct central nervous system effect. In one study, infants and children treated with recombinant erythropoietin had no measurable CSF levels of erythropoietin [98]. However, in another study, intraperitoneal recombinant erythropoietin in mice elevated CSF levels of erythropoietin and protected against experimentally induced neurologic ischemia [99]. In general, the data support the hypothesis that systemically administered rHuEPO improves quality of life and/or physical and cognitive function, at least in part, by a direct central nervous system mechanism.

Erythropoietin safety

Over a decade and a half of experience with rHuEPO has proven it to be safe, with the primary adverse event being hypertension in renal-failure patients [100]. Seizures and thrombotic complications [101] have been reported, mostly in patients with end-stage renal disease, but also in patients with malignancy [102]. We (IASIA) recently completed a small phase I study of rHuEPO in the nursing home. One patient briefly developed hyperkalemia but no other toxicity was reported or observed. Recently, concerns regarding the widespread use of ESPs have been raised because of the observation of erythropoietin receptors on certain tumor cells. However, there remains no established evidence that rHuEPO or other ESPs promote tumor growth [103]. In general, with adherence to guidelines regarding dose, schedule, and monitoring, ESP treatment is a safe and effective therapy. Adverse consequences are more likely to occur when hemoglobin levels rise too quickly and to levels that exceed the therapeutic goal (i.e., 12 g/dL).

Treatment of "anemia unexplained"

In geriatric medicine, a specific mechanism is often not apparent ("anemia unexplained" [Au]), but the consequences are becoming rapidly described. These are perhaps best documented in the cardiology literature. Anemia acts as a contributory factor to volume and flow overload in the heart and vessels, and has been implicated in the pathophysiology of cardiovascular structural and functional alterations [104,105]. Clinical symptoms are more or less severe depending on the rate at which anemia develops and whether underlying cardiovascular disorders are present. In the presence of cardiovascular conditions, in particular coronary artery disease, acute or short-lasting anemia has been reported to worsen angina and increase the incidence of cardiovascular complications [106]. In chronic situations, anemia leads to progressive cardiac enlargement and left ventricular hypertrophy [107–110]. A decrease in hemoglobin concentration of 1 g/dL has been associated with an increased risk of left ventricular dilatation, systolic dysfunction, chronic heart failure, and also death [104,108,109,111,112]. Other organs/organ systems are similarly affected. Neurological effects of anemia include symptoms such as headaches, loss of concentration, fatigue, reduced performance status, and depression [113,114]. Other studies have suggested that anemia may cause an impairment of cognitive function [29,30,115] and possibly accelerate the progression of Alzheimer disease [5].

Anemia has been shown to be an independent risk factor for death [116,117]. In one study, the mortality risk for individuals aged 85 years and older was approximately twofold higher for those who met World Health Organization anemia criteria [117]. However, this association between anemia and mortality is not limited to the oldest old, as it is also apparent for all those over the age of 65 [116]. Recent data have also indicated that, in women older than 65 years, the inflection point where increased mortality begins to be observed is approximately 13 g/dL [10].

Independent of disease, the presence of anemia has an effect on muscle strength, mobility, and falls, among a number of other performance measures [1,2,4,118,119]. These functional impairments are thought to be the immediate antecedents to impaired ADLs and subsequent loss of autonomy.

Despite the apparent plethora of adverse consequences there is no published evidence (with exception of anemia associated with kidney disease or cancer) that correction of the chronic anemia of late life (AU) is of clinical value. It remains to be seen whether the anemia is contributing to the functional decline or whether it reflects more significant physiological impairments. If treatment were inexpensive and proven to be safe, it is likely we would have the answer to these questions by now, but available treatments are neither inexpensive nor proven safe in this population. Thus judicious clinical investigation is warranted prior to adopting a policy of treating late-life anemia, particularly AU.

Summary

Severe anemia in older people is not often missed or untreated. However, the great majority of anemia in this age group is mild to moderate, and, unless nutritionally related, often undiagnosed and undertreated. With the availability of ESPs, it is tempting to proceed directly to treatment. However, these agents are not completely without adverse consequences, and they are expensive. Currently, there are at least two trials under way to assess the value of correcting late-life anemia, anemia unexplained, in terms of functional outcomes as well as quality of life. Clinicians will soon have sufficient data to decide whether such treatments are warranted.

REFERENCES

1. Penninx BW, Guralnik JM, Onder G, Ferrucci L, Wallace RB, Pahor M. Anemia and decline in physical performance among older persons. *Am J Med* 2003; **115**: 104–10.

2. Penninx BW, Pahor M, Cesari M, *et al.* Anemia is associated with disability and decreased physical performance and muscle strength in the elderly. *J Am Geriatr Soc* 2004; **52**: 719–24.

3. Jacobsen PB, Garland LL, Booth-Jones M, *et al.* Relationship of hemoglobin levels to fatigue and cognitive functioning among cancer patients receiving chemotherapy. *J Pain Symptom Manage* 2004; **28**: 7–18.

4. Penninx BW, Pluijm SM, Lips P, *et al.* Late-life anemia is associated with increased risk of recurrent falls. *J Am Geriatr Soc* 2005; **53**: 2106–11.

5. Beard CM, Kokmen E, O'Brien PC, Ania BJ, Melton LJ, 3rd. Risk of Alzheimer's disease among elderly patients with anemia: population-based investigations in Olmsted County, Minnesota. *Ann Epidemiol* 1997; **7**: 219–24.

6. Besarab A, Bolton WK, Browne JK, *et al.* The effects of normal as compared with low hematocrit values in patients with cardiac disease who are receiving hemodialysis and epoetin. *N Engl J Med* 1998; **339**: 584–90.

7. Cumming RG, Mitchell P, Craig JC, Knight JF. Renal impairment and anaemia in a population-based study of older people. *Intern Med J* 2004; **34**: 20–3.

8. Kosiborod M, Curtis JP, Wang Y, *et al.* Anemia and outcomes in patients with heart failure: a study from the National Heart Care Project. *Arch Intern Med* 2005; **165**: 2237–44.

9. Nissenson AR, Goodnough LT, Dubois RW. Anemia: not just an innocent bystander? *Arch Intern Med* 2003; **163**: 1400–4.

10. Chaves PH, Xue QL, Guralnik JM, Ferrucci L, Volpato S, Fried LP. What constitutes normal hemoglobin concentration in community-dwelling disabled older women? *J Am Geriatr Soc* 2004; **52**: 1811–16.

11. Culleton BF, Manns BJ, Zhang J, Tonelli M, Klarenbach S, Hemmelgarn BR. Impact of anemia on hospitalization and mortality in older adults. *Blood* 2006; **107**: 3841–6.

12. Zakai NA, Katz R, Hirsch C, *et al*. A prospective study of anemia status, hemoglobin concentration, and mortality in an elderly cohort: the Cardiovascular Health Study. *Arch Intern Med* 2005; **165**: 2214–20.

13. Longo DL. Closing in on a killer: anemia in elderly people. *J Gerontol A Biol Sci Med Sci* 2005; **60**: 727–8.

14. Spivak JL. Anemia in the elderly: time for new blood in old vessels? *Arch Intern Med* 2005; **165**: 2187–9.

15. Eckert JK, Morgan LA, Swamy N. Preferences for receipt of care among community-dwelling adults. *J Aging Soc Policy* 2004; **16**: 49–65.

16. Ferrucci L, Guralnik JM, Pahor M, Corti MC, Havlik RJ. Hospital diagnoses, Medicare charges, and nursing home admissions in the year when older persons become severely disabled. *JAMA* 1997; **277**: 728–34.

17. Foley DJ, Ostfeld AM, Branch LG, Wallace RB, McGloin J, Cornoni-Huntley JC. The risk of nursing home admission in three communities. *J Aging Health* 1992; **4**: 155–73.

18. Artz AS, Fergusson D, Drinka PJ, *et al*. Mechanisms of unexplained anemia in the nursing home. *J Am Geriatr Soc* 2004; **52**: 423–7.

19. Ble A, Fink JC, Woodman RC, *et al*. Renal function, erythropoietin, and anemia of older persons: the InCHIANTI study. *Arch Intern Med* 2005; **165**: 2222–7.

20. Guralnik JM, Ershler WB, Schrier SL, Picozzi VJ. Anemia in the elderly: a public health crisis in hematology. *Hematology (Am Soc Hematol Educ Program)* 2005: 528–32.

21. Jelkmann W, Pagel H, Wolff M, Fandrey J. Monokines inhibiting erythropoietin production in human hepatoma cultures and in isolated perfused rat kidneys. *Life Sci* 1992; **50**: 301–8.

22. Rockey DC, Cello JP. Evaluation of the gastrointestinal tract in patients with iron-deficiency anemia. *N Engl J Med* 1993; **329**: 1691–5.

23. Waldo RT. Iron-deficiency anemia due to silent celiac sprue. *Proc (Bayl Univ Med Cent)* 2002; **15**: 16–17.

24. Lindenbaum J, Healton EB, Savage DG, *et al*. Neuropsychiatric disorders caused by cobalamin deficiency in the absence of anemia or macrocytosis. *N Engl J Med* 1988; **318**: 1720–8.

25. Davenport J. Macrocytic anemia. *Am Fam Physician* 1996; **53**: 155–62.

26. Bennett JM, Kouides PA, Forman SJ. The myelodysplastic syndromes: morphology, risk assessment, and clinical management (2002). *Int J Hematol* 2002; **76** (Suppl 2): 228–38.

27. Steensma DP, Bennett JM. The myelodysplastic syndromes: diagnosis and treatment. *Mayo Clin Proc* 2006; **81**: 104–30.

28. Collins AJ. Anaemia management prior to dialysis: cardiovascular and cost-benefit observations. *Nephrol Dial Transplant* 2003; **18** (Suppl 2): ii2–6.

29. Marsh JT, Brown WS, Wolcott D, *et al*. rHuEPO treatment improves brain and cognitive function of anemic dialysis patients. *Kidney Int* 1991; **39**: 155–63.

30. Pickett JL, Theberge DC, Brown WS, Schweitzer SU, Nissenson AR. Normalizing hematocrit in dialysis patients improves brain function. *Am J Kidney Dis* 1999; **33**: 1122–30.

31. Silverberg D. Outcomes of anaemia management in renal insufficiency and cardiac disease. *Nephrol Dial Transplant* 2003; **18** (Suppl 2): ii7–12.

32. Silverberg DS, Wexler D, Blum M, *et al*. The use of subcutaneous erythropoietin and intravenous iron for the treatment of the anemia of severe, resistant congestive heart failure improves cardiac and renal function and functional cardiac class, and markedly reduces hospitalizations. *J Am Coll Cardiol* 2000; **35**: 1737–44.

33. Silverberg DS, Wexler D, Blum M, *et al*. The effect of correction of anaemia in diabetics and non-diabetics with severe resistant congestive heart failure and chronic renal failure by subcutaneous erythropoietin and intravenous iron. *Nephrol Dial Transplant* 2003; **18**: 141–6.

34. Valderrabano F, Jofre R, Lopez-Gomez JM. Quality of life in end-stage renal disease patients. *Am J Kidney Dis* 2001; **38**: 443–64.

35. American Association of Blood Banks, America's Blood Centers, and the American Red Cross. *Circular of Information for the Use of Human Blood and Blood Components* (Bethesda, MD: AABB, 2006).

36. Beru N, McDonald J, Lacombe C, Goldwasser E. Expression of the erythropoietin gene. *Mol Cell Biol* 1986; **6**: 2571–5.

37. Bondurant MC, Koury MJ. Anemia induces accumulation of erythropoietin mRNA in the kidney and liver. *Mol Cell Biol* 1986; **6**: 2731–3.

38. Koury MJ, Bondurant MC. Maintenance by erythropoietin of viability and maturation of murine erythroid precursor cells. *J Cell Physiol* 1988; **137**: 65–74.

39. Lacombe C, Da Silva JL, Bruneval P, *et al*. Peritubular cells are the site of erythropoietin synthesis in the murine hypoxic kidney. *J Clin Invest* 1988; **81**: 620–3.

40. Krantz SB. Erythropoietin. *Blood* 1991; **77**: 419–34.

41. Sawada K, Krantz SB, Dessypris EN, Koury ST, Sawyer ST. Human colony-forming units-erythroid do not require accessory cells, but do require direct interaction with insulin-like growth factor I and/or insulin for erythroid development. *J Clin Invest* 1989; **83**: 1701–9.

42. Koury MJ, Bondurant MC. Erythropoietin retards DNA breakdown and prevents programmed death in erythroid progenitor cells. *Science* 1990; **248**: 378–81.

43. Egrie JC, Strickland TW, Lane J, *et al.* Characterization and biological effects of recombinant human erythropoietin. *Immunobiology* 1986; **172**: 213–24.

44. Cases A. Darbepoetin alfa: a novel erythropoiesis-stimulating protein. *Drugs Today (Barc)* 2003; **39**: 477–95.

45. Macdougall IC. CERA (Continuous Erythropoietin Receptor Activator): a new erythropoiesis-stimulating agent for the treatment of anemia. *Curr Hematol Rep* 2005; **4**: 436–40.

46. Boggs DR, Patrene KD. Hematopoiesis and aging III: Anemia and a blunted erythropoietic response to hemorrhage in aged mice. *Am J Hematol* 1985; **19**: 327–38.

47. Refino CJ, Dallman PR. Rate of repair of iron deficiency anemia and blood loss anemia in young and mature rats. *Am J Clin Nutr* 1983; **37**: 904–9.

48. Udupa KB, Lipschitz DA. Erythropoiesis in the aged mouse: I. Response to stimulation in vivo. *J Lab Clin Med* 1984; **103**: 574–80.

49. Udupa KB, Lipschitz DA. Erythropoiesis in the aged mouse: II. Response to stimulation in vitro. *J Lab Clin Med* 1984; **103**: 581–8.

50. Carpenter MA, Kendall RG, O'Brien AE, *et al.* Reduced erythropoietin response to anaemia in elderly patients with normocytic anaemia. *Eur J Haematol* 1992; **49**: 119–21.

51. Joosten E, Pelemans W, Hiele M, Noyen J, Verhaeghe R, Boogaerts MA. Prevalence and causes of anaemia in a geriatric hospitalized population. *Gerontology* 1992; **38**: 111–17.

52. Kario K, Matsuo T, Kodama K, Nakao K, Asada R. Reduced erythropoietin secretion in senile anemia. *Am J Hematol* 1992; **41**: 252–7.

53. Kario K, Matsuo T, Nakao K. Serum erythropoietin levels in the elderly. *Gerontology* 1991; **37**: 345–8.

54. Nafziger J, Pailla K, Luciani L, Andreux JP, Saint-Jean O, Casadevall N. Decreased erythropoietin responsiveness to iron deficiency anemia in the elderly. *Am J Hematol* 1993; **43**: 172–6.

55. Powers JS, Krantz SB, Collins JC, *et al.* Erythropoietin response to anemia as a function of age. *J Am Geriatr Soc* 1991; **39**: 30–2.

56. Lindeman RD. Overview: renal physiology and pathophysiology of aging. *Am J Kidney Dis* 1990; **16**: 275–82.

57. Rowe JW, Andres R, Tobin JD, Norris AH, Shock NW. The effect of age on creatinine clearance in men: a cross-sectional and longitudinal study. *J Gerontol* 1976; **31**: 155–63.

58. Baraldi-Junkins CA, Beck AC, Rothstein G. Hematopoiesis and cytokines. Relevance to cancer and aging. *Hematol Oncol Clin North Am* 2000; **14**: 45–61.

59. Boyd HK, Lappin TR. Erythropoietin deficiency in the anaemia of chronic disorders. *Eur J Haematol* 1991; **46**: 198–201.

60. Miller CB, Jones RJ, Piantadosi S, Abeloff MD, Spivak JL. Decreased erythropoietin response in patients with the anemia of cancer. *N Engl J Med* 1990; **322**: 1689–92.

61. Baer AN, Dessypris EN, Goldwasser E, Krantz SB. Blunted erythropoietin response to anaemia in rheumatoid arthritis. *Br J Haematol* 1987; **66**: 559–64.

62. Boyd HK, Lappin TR, Bell AL. Evidence for impaired erythropoietin response to anaemia in rheumatoid disease. *Br J Rheumatol* 1991; **30**: 255–9.

63. Hochberg MC, Arnold CM, Hogans BB, Spivak JL. Serum immunoreactive erythropoietin in rheumatoid arthritis: impaired response to anemia. *Arthritis Rheum* 1988; **31**: 1318–21.

64. Brown MS, Garcia JF, Phibbs RH, Dallman PR. Decreased response of plasma immunoreactive erythropoietin to "available oxygen" in anemia of prematurity. *J Pediatr* 1984; **105**: 793–8.

65. Schreiber S, Howaldt S, Schnoor M, *et al.* Recombinant erythropoietin for the treatment of anemia in inflammatory bowel disease. *N Engl J Med* 1996; **334**: 619–23.

66. Camacho J, Poveda F, Zamorano AF, Valencia ME, Vazquez JJ, Arnalich F. Serum erythropoietin levels in anaemic patients with advanced human immunodeficiency virus infection. *Br J Haematol* 1992; **82**: 608–14.

67. Spivak JL, Barnes DC, Fuchs E, Quinn TC. Serum immunoreactive erythropoietin in HIV-infected patients. *JAMA* 1989; **261**: 3104–7.

68. Association between recombinant human erythropoietin and quality of life and exercise capacity of patients receiving haemodialysis. Canadian Erythropoietin Study Group. *BMJ* 1990; **300**: 573–8.

69. Auer J, Simon G, Stevens J, *et al.* Quality of life improvements in CAPD patients treated with subcutaneously administered erythropoietin for anemia. *Perit Dial Int* 1992; **12**: 40–2.

70. Barany P, Pettersson E, Konarski-Svensson JK. Long-term effects on quality of life in haemodialysis patients

of correction of anaemia with erythropoietin. *Nephrol Dial Transplant* 1993; **8**: 426–32.

71. Beusterien KM, Nissenson AR, Port FK, Kelly M, Steinwald B, Ware JE Jr. The effects of recombinant human erythropoietin on functional health and well-being in chronic dialysis patients. *J Am Soc Nephrol* 1996; **7**: 763–73.

72. Delano BG. Improvements in quality of life following treatment with r-HuEPO in anemic hemodialysis patients. *Am J Kidney Dis* 1989; **14** (2 Suppl 1): 14–18.

73. Evans RW. Recombinant human erythropoietin and the quality of life of end-stage renal disease patients: a comparative analysis. *Am J Kidney Dis* 1991; **18** (4 Suppl 1): 62–70.

74. Evans RW, Rader B, Manninen DL. The quality of life of hemodialysis recipients treated with recombinant human erythropoietin. Cooperative Multicenter EPO Clinical Trial Group. *JAMA* 1990; **263**: 825–30.

75. Hosokawa S, Yoshida O. Effect of erythropoietin (rHuEPO) on trace elements and quality of life (Qol) in chronic hemodialysis patients. *Int J Clin Pharmacol Ther* 1994; **32**: 415–21.

76. Levin NW, Lazarus JM, Nissenson AR. National Cooperative rHu Erythropoietin Study in patients with chronic renal failure: an interim report. The National Cooperative rHu Erythropoietin Study Group. *Am J Kidney Dis* 1993; **22** (2 Suppl 1): 3–12.

77. Lundin AP, Delano BG, Quinn-Cefaro R. Perspectives on the improvement of quality of life with epoetin alfa therapy. *Pharmacotherapy* 1990; **10**: 22S–26S.

78. Moreno F, Sanz-Guajardo D, Lopez-Gomez JM, Jofre R, Valderrabano F. Increasing the hematocrit has a beneficial effect on quality of life and is safe in selected hemodialysis patients. Spanish Cooperative Renal Patients Quality of Life Study Group of the Spanish Society of Nephrology. *J Am Soc Nephrol* 2000; **11**: 335–42.

79. Revicki DA, Brown RE, Feeny DH, *et al*. Health-related quality of life associated with recombinant human erythropoietin therapy for predialysis chronic renal disease patients. *Am J Kidney Dis* 1995; **25**: 548–54.

80. Tsakiris D. Morbidity and mortality reduction associated with the use of erythropoietin. *Nephron* 2000; **85** (Suppl 1): 2–8.

81. Demetri GD, Kris M, Wade J, Degos L, Cella D. Quality-of-life benefit in chemotherapy patients treated with epoetin alfa is independent of disease response or tumor type: results from a prospective community oncology study. Procrit Study Group. *J Clin Oncol* 1998; **16**: 3412–25.

82. Glaspy J, Bukowski R, Steinberg D, Taylor C, Tchekmedyian S, Vadhan-Raj S. Impact of therapy with epoetin alfa on clinical outcomes in patients with non-myeloid malignancies during cancer chemotherapy in community oncology practice. Procrit Study Group. *J Clin Oncol* 1997; **15**: 1218–34.

83. Leitgeb C, Pecherstorfer M, Fritz E, Ludwig H. Quality of life in chronic anemia of cancer during treatment with recombinant human erythropoietin. *Cancer* 1994; **73**: 2535–42.

84. Peeters HR, Jongen-Lavrencic M, Bakker CH, Vreugdenhil G, Breedveld FC, Swaak AJ. Recombinant human erythropoietin improves health-related quality of life in patients with rheumatoid arthritis and anaemia of chronic disease; utility measures correlate strongly with disease activity measures. *Rheumatol Int* 1999; **18**: 201–6.

85. Cascinu S, Del Ferro E, Fedeli A, Ligi M, Alessandroni P, Catalano G. Recombinant human erythropoietin treatment in elderly cancer patients with cisplatin-associated anemia. *Oncology* 1995; **52**: 422–6.

86. Shank WA, Jr., Balducci L. Recombinant hemopoietic growth factors: comparative hemopoietic response in younger and older subjects. *J Am Geriatr Soc* 1992; **40**: 151–4.

87. Reilly RB, Polsen JA, Luchi RJ. Erythropoietin therapy for anemia in two nonagenarians. *J Am Geriatr Soc* 1994; **42**: 114–15.

88. Juul SE, Yachnis AT, Christensen RD. Tissue distribution of erythropoietin and erythropoietin receptor in the developing human fetus. *Early Hum Dev* 1998; **52**: 235–49.

89. Juul SE, Anderson DK, Li Y, Christensen RD. Erythropoietin and erythropoietin receptor in the developing human central nervous system. *Pediatr Res* 1998; **43**: 40–9.

90. Juul SE, Yachnis AT, Rojiani AM, Christensen RD. Immunohistochemical localization of erythropoietin and its receptor in the developing human brain. *Pediatr Dev Pathol* 1999; **2**: 148–58.

91. Marti HH, Wenger RH, Rivas LA, *et al*. Erythropoietin gene expression in human, monkey and murine brain. *Eur J Neurosci* 1996; **8**: 666–76.

92. Bernaudin M, Marti HH, Roussel S, *et al*. A potential role for erythropoietin in focal permanent cerebral ischemia in mice. *J Cereb Blood Flow Metab* 1999; **19**: 643–51.

93. Digicaylioglu M, Bichet S, Marti HH, *et al*. Localization of specific erythropoietin binding sites in defined

areas of the mouse brain. *Proc Natl Acad Sci USA* 1995; **92**: 3717–20.

94. Tan CC, Eckardt KU, Firth JD, Ratcliffe PJ. Feedback modulation of renal and hepatic erythropoietin mRNA in response to graded anemia and hypoxia. *Am J Physiol* 1992; **263**: F474–F481.

95. Morishita E, Masuda S, Nagao M, Yasuda Y, Sasaki R. Erythropoietin receptor is expressed in rat hippocampal and cerebral cortical neurons, and erythropoietin prevents in vitro glutamate-induced neuronal death. *Neuroscience* 1997; **76**: 105–16.

96. Sadamoto Y, Igase K, Sakanaka M, *et al.* Erythropoietin prevents place navigation disability and cortical infarction in rats with permanent occlusion of the middle cerebral artery. *Biochem Biophys Res Commun* 1998; **253**: 26–32.

97. Sakanaka M, Wen TC, Matsuda S, *et al.* In vivo evidence that erythropoietin protects neurons from ischemic damage. *Proc Natl Acad Sci USA* 1998; **95**: 4635–40.

98. Juul SE, Stallings SA, Christensen RD. Erythropoietin in the cerebrospinal fluid of neonates who sustained CNS injury. *Pediatr Res* 1999; **46**: 543–7.

99. Brines ML, Ghezzi P, Keenan S, *et al.* Erythropoietin crosses the blood–brain barrier to protect against experimental brain injury. *Proc Natl Acad Sci USA* 2000; **97**: 10526–31.

100. Dunn CJ, Wagstaff AJ. Epoetin alfa. A review of its clinical efficacy in the management of anaemia associated with renal failure and chronic disease and its use in surgical patients. *Drugs Aging* 1995; **7**: 131–56.

101. Churchill DN, Muirhead N, Goldstein M, *et al.* Probability of thrombosis of vascular access among hemodialysis patients treated with recombinant human erythropoietin. *J Am Soc Nephrol* 1994; **4**: 1809–13.

102. Wun T, Law L, Harvey D, Sieracki B, Scudder SA, Ryu JK. Increased incidence of symptomatic venous thrombosis in patients with cervical carcinoma treated with concurrent chemotherapy, radiation, and erythropoietin. *Cancer* 2003; **98**: 1514–20.

103. Stasi R, Amadori S, Littlewood TJ, Terzoli E, Newland AC, Provan D. Management of cancer-related anemia with erythropoietic agents: doubts, certainties, and concerns. *Oncologist* 2005; **10**: 539–54.

104. Foley RN, Parfrey PS, Harnett JD, Kent GM, Murray DC, Barre PE. The impact of anemia on cardiomyopathy, morbidity, and mortality in end-stage renal disease. *Am J Kidney Dis* 1996; **28**: 53–61.

105. London GM, Marchais SJ, Guerin AP, Fabiani F, Metivier F. Cardiovascular function in hemodialysis patients. *Adv Nephrol Necker Hosp* 1991; **20**: 249–73.

106. Metivier F, Marchais SJ, Guerin AP, Pannier B, London GM. Pathophysiology of anaemia: focus on the heart and blood vessels. *Nephrol Dial Transplant* 2000; **15** (Suppl 3): 14–18.

107. Lester LA, Sodt PC, Hutcheon N, Arcilla RA. Cardiac abnormalities in children with sickle cell anemia. *Chest* 1990; **98**: 1169–74.

108. London GM, Fabiani F, Marchais SJ, *et al.* Uremic cardiomyopathy: an inadequate left ventricular hypertrophy. *Kidney Int* 1987; **31**: 973–80.

109. London GM, Parfrey PS. Cardiac disease in chronic uremia: pathogenesis. *Adv Ren Replace Ther* 1997; **4**: 194–211.

110. Parfrey PS, Harnett JD, Barre PE. The natural history of myocardial disease in dialysis patients. *J Am Soc Nephrol* 1991; **2**: 2–12.

111. Silberberg JS, Rahal DP, Patton DR, Sniderman AD. Role of anemia in the pathogenesis of left ventricular hypertrophy in end-stage renal disease. *Am J Cardiol* 1989; **64**: 222–4.

112. Wu WC, Rathore SS, Wang Y, Radford MJ, Krumholz HM. Blood transfusion in elderly patients with acute myocardial infarction. *N Engl J Med* 2001; **345**: 1230–6.

113. Murphy PT, Hutchinson RM. Identification and treatment of anaemia in older patients. *Drugs Aging* 1994; **4**: 113–27.

114. Salive ME, Cornoni-Huntley J, Guralnik JM, *et al.* Anemia and hemoglobin levels in older persons: relationship with age, gender, and health status. *J Am Geriatr Soc* 1992; **40**: 489–96.

115. Nissenson AR. Epoetin and cognitive function. *Am J Kidney Dis* 1992; **20** (1 Suppl 1): 21–4.

116. Ania BJ, Suman VJ, Fairbanks VF, Rademacher DM, Melton LJ, 3rd. Incidence of anemia in older people: an epidemiologic study in a well defined population. *J Am Geriatr Soc* 1997; **45**: 825–31.

117. Izaks GJ, Westendorp RG, Knook DL. The definition of anemia in older persons. *JAMA* 1999; **281**: 1714–17.

118. Cesari M, Pahor M, Lauretani F, *et al.* Bone density and hemoglobin levels in older persons: results from the InCHIANTI study. *Osteoporos Int* 2005; **16**: 691–9.

119. Cesari M, Penninx BW, Lauretani F, *et al.* Hemoglobin levels and skeletal muscle: results from the InCHIANTI study. *J Gerontol A Biol Sci Med Sci* 2004; **59**: 249–54.

Part IV

Hematologic malignancies and aging

18

Cancer chemotherapy in the older person

Lodovico Balducci

Introduction

The incidence and prevalence of cancer increases with age [1]. In the year 2000, more than 50% of all malignancies occurred in the 12% of the population aged 65 and older. In the year 2030, the older population will account for 20% of the whole population and for 70% of all cancers [1]. The number of older individuals receiving cytotoxic chemotherapy is progressively increasing, and it is legitimate to ask whether age may influence efficacy and toxicity of chemotherapy, especially the incidence of myelosuppression, which is the most common complication. In this chapter we will review the pharmacology of cytotoxic chemotherapy in the older aged person and explore methods to ameliorate the risk of toxicity.

Pharmacologic changes of aging

Pharmacokinetics

Most pharmacokinetic parameters may be influenced by age (Fig. 18.1). The absorption of nutrients decreases progressively due to reduced splanchnic circulation and absorbing surface, and reduced gastric motility and secretions [2]. It is not clear whether bioavailability and efficacy of oral drugs may also be compromised. This is a practical issue as more oral cytotoxic agents are emerging [3]. Oral agents are particularly suitable for the management of the older aged person, as they may be administered at home, and the dose may be adjusted on a daily basis.

The volume of distribution (Vd) of hydrosoluble drugs decreases, and that of liposoluble ones increases, due to progressive loss of total body water and accumulation of fat. In addition to body composition, the Vd of hydrosoluble agents is also determined by albumin and hemoglobin concentration, as many of these agents are bound to circulating proteins and red blood cells. While the area under the curve (AUC) does not change with the Vd, its shape does. The peak drug concentration, which in most cases is associated with more toxicity, increases when the Vd is reduced. Anemia reduces the Vd of hydrosoluble agents and is associated with increased risk of chemotherapy-related toxicity [4].

The hepatic uptake of drugs decreases with age because of reduced splanchnic circulation and hepatocyte number, and the hepatic metabolism through P450 cytochrome-dependent reactions (type 1 reactions) decreases as well, while the activity of type 2 reactions does not appear to be influenced by aging [2,4]. Type 1 reactions are oxidoreductive, are responsible for the activation and deactivation of many agents, and are catalyzed by the P450 cytochrome enzyme system [4]. Polypharmacy, which is common among older individuals, may affect the activity of type 1 reactions in the aged. Type 2 reactions involve glucuronation, sulfation, and acetylation and are responsible for deactivating drugs. Not all products of type 2 reactions should be considered inactive, however. For example morphine 6-glucuronide is ten times more active and morphine 3-glucuronide more toxic than the parent compound [5].

Blood Disorders in the Elderly, ed. Lodovico Balducci, William Ershler, Giovanni de Gaetano.
Published by Cambridge University Press. © Cambridge University Press 2008.

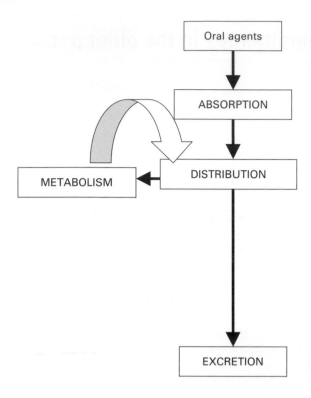

Figure 18.1 Pharmacokinetic parameters that may be influenced by age.

Renal excretion of drugs is almost always reduced, as a decline in glomerular filtration rate (GFR) is almost universal with aging. In addition to drugs whose parent compound is excreted by the kidney, such as methotrexate, bleomycin, and carboplatin, a decline of GFR may increase activity and toxicity of compounds that give rise to active metabolite excreted by the kidneys, such as daunorubicin or idarubicin [4].

Pharmacodynamics

Changes in pharmacodynamics may be responsible for reduced effectiveness and increased toxicity of cancer chemotherapy. Increased resistance may be due to:

- Increased prevalence of tumors that express the multidrug resistance (*MDR1*) gene, responsible for encoding the P-glycoprotein, which pumps natural agents (antibiotics, plant derivatives) outside the cells. This increased prevalence is well documented in the case of acute myeloid leukemia [6].
- Resistance to apoptosis, as is the case in follicular lymphoma with overexpression of *Bcl-2* [4].
- Overexpression of enzymes that are the target of specific agents (dihydrofolate reductase and topoisomerase I and II), or alternatively production of aberrant forms of the enzyme, with reduced sensitivity to pharmacologic inhibition. This possibility is mainly theoretical [4].
- Decreased tumor vascularization and oxygenation, with reduced sensitivity to drugs that damage the tumor cells by production of free radicals, such as the alkylating agents. This possibility has been demonstrated in experimental tumor systems [4].
- Decreased proliferation rate of the neoplasm. This may be the reason why cytotoxic chemotherapy may not be as effective in older women with breast cancer as it is in younger women [4].

Table 18.1. Age and myelotoxicity of cancer chemotherapy: results of six retrospective trials.

Authors	Patients (n)	Percentage of patients ≥65 and/or ≥70	Source
Begg & Carbone 1983 [8]	5459	≥70: 13%	ECOG database
Gelman & Taylor 1984 [9]	231	≥70: 13%	Dana Farber Cancer Center. Patients over 65 had been treated prospectively with dose-adjustment for cyclophosphamide and methotrexate and 2/3 FU dose, and results compared with 161 fully evaluable younger patients. Patients over 80 experienced shortened survival.
Christman *et al.* 1992 [10]	170	≥70: 42%	Piedmont Oncology Group database; high degree of patient selection
Giovanazzi-Bannon *et al.* 1994 [11]	672	≥65: 40% ≥70: 25%	Illinois Cancer Center phase II trials
Ibrahim *et al.* 1996 [12]	1011	≥65: 24% ≥70: 20%	M. D. Anderson Hospital patients with metastatic breast cancer aged 50 and older
Ibrahim *et al.* 2000 [13]	390	≥65: 18% ≥70: <10%	M. D. Anderson Hospital patients with breast cancer receiving anthracycline-containing adjuvant chemotherapy

Pharmacodynamic changes underlying increased toxicity may include:

- Reduced effectiveness of DNA repair by normal cells. This possibility was demonstrated in patients treated with cisplatin. In the circulating monocytes of individuals younger than 50, the presence of DNA adducts lasted an average of 20 hours; in those of individuals aged 70 and older, it lasted longer than 80 hours [7].
- Reduced ability of aging cells to catabolize cytotoxic drugs. This possibility is only theoretical in humans [4].

Decreased functional reserve of normal organ systems

Age is a risk factor for myelotoxicity, mucositis, peripheral and central neurotoxicity, and cardiotoxicity from cytotoxic chemotherapy.

Myelotoxicity

Six retrospective studies (Table 18.1) have reported that the risk of myelotoxicity was not increased with the patient's age [8–13]. These studies are important, as they demonstrate that chemotherapy may be safely administered to individuals over 70, but they are not representative of the general older population for the following reasons:

- The population was highly selected. As few as 10% of patients included in these studies were 70 and older, while 35–40% of individuals affected by those neoplasms are 70 and over. Likewise, individuals over 80 were virtually absent.
- All studies were conducted in major referral centers, where the patients are generally self-selected, or by major cooperative groups that have highly exacting eligibility criteria.
- In the experience of the Eastern Cooperative Oncology Group (ECOG), patients 70 and older treated with a number of agents, including

Table 18. 2. Incidence of life-threatening neutropenia, neutropenic infections, and death in older individuals with large-cell non-Hodgkin lymphomas treated with CHOP-like regimens.

Authors	Patients (n)	Regimen	Age	Neutropenia (%)	Neutropenic fever (%)	Treatment-related deaths (%)	Growth factor
Zinzani et al. 1999 [20]	161	VNCOP-B	60+	44	32	1.3	—
Sonneveld et al. 1995 [21]	148	CHOP	60+	not reported	not reported	14	—
		CNOP	60+	not reported	not reported	13	—
Gomez et al. 1998 [22]	26	CHOP	60+	24	8	0	GM-CSF
			70+	73	42	20	GM-CSF
Tirelli et al. 1998 [23]	119	VMP	70+	50	21	7	—
		CHOP	70+	48	21	5	—
Bastion et al. 1997 [24]	444	CVP	70+	9	7	12	—
		CTVP	70+	29	13	15	—
Doorduijn et al. 2000 [25]	152	CHOP	65+	21	10	5	—
Osby et al. 2003 [26]	455	CHOP	60+	91	47	not reported	—
		CNOP					

methotrexate, nitrosurea, and doxorubicin, did indeed experience increased risk of myelodepression [8].

A number of other studies have reported an increased risk of chemotherapy myelotoxicity with age. Kim et al. [14] reviewed the experience of the South West Oncology Group, and Crivellari et al. [15] the experience of the International Breast Cancer Study Group, and both reported increased risk of myelotoxicity after age 65. Crivellari also reported that approximately 40% of older women with breast cancer received a total dose of chemotherapy lower than two-thirds of the planned dose, as a result of myelotoxicity. Chrischilles et al. [16] reviewed cases of patients with non-Hodgkin lymphoma (NHL) treated in the community and found that the incidence of neutropenic infections in the absence of growth factors was approximately 20% for those younger than 65 and 45% for older patients. Of particular interest, hospitalization for neutropenic infection was prolonged by 30% for older patients. Prolonged hospitalization may lead to deconditioning and functional dependence. In a different population of lymphoma patients, also aged 65 and older, and treated with CHOP or CNOP, Morrison et al. [17] reported a risk of neutropenic infections around 40%. Lyman et al. [18] found that age was an independent risk factor for neutropenic infections following cytotoxic chemotherapy, and Kuderer et al. [19] demonstrated that the risk of mortality from neutropenic infections increased with the patient's age. In addition, in seven prospective studies of individuals aged 65 or 70 and older with large-cell lymphoma, the risk of neutropenia was as high as 90% and the risk of neutropenic infections as high as 50% (Table 18.2) [20–26]. Another important finding of these studies was that the risk of neutropenia and neutropenic infections, and of infection-related mortality, was highest after the first and the second course of chemotherapy [18,20–27]. In patients with acute myeloid leukemia, older age was associated with decreased tolerance of high doses of cytarabine during consolidation [6], but in this case the decreased tolerance might have been due to the effects of the disease, rather than of age, on hematopoiesis.

The influence of age on the incidence of thrombocytopenia and anemia is less clear, though both complications may be more common in older individuals.

Fortunately, hematopoietic growth factors, including filgrastim, pegfilgrastim, epoetin alpha, and darbepoetin alpha, are effective in older individuals to the same extent as they are in younger individuals. In three randomized controlled studies of patients with large-cell lymphoma, filgrastim reduced by 40% the risk of neutropenia and neutropenic infections [20,25,26]. In a recently completed study of patients aged 65 and older with a variety of solid tumors, pegfilgrastim reduced by 40% the risk of neutropenia and neutropenic infections [27].

Mucositis

Two age-related factors may conspire to increase the risk of mucositis in the older aged person. With age, proliferation of mucosal cells of the intestine increases, enhancing their susceptibility to destruction by cycle-active chemotherapy. At the same time the concentration of mucosal stem cells may be decreased, which delays the recovery after chemotherapy [4]. The drugs more likely to induce mucositis include methotrexate, the fluorinated pyrimidines, and the anthracyclines. Gelman and Taylor [9] demonstrated that adjusting the doses of methotrexate to the GFR in individuals aged 65 and older reduced the risk of myelodepression, but not that of mucositis. Jacobson *et al.* [28] reviewed the experience of the North Central Cancer Treatment Group in randomized studies involving fluorouracil or FUDR, and concluded that age was an independent risk factor for the incidence and severity of mucositis of the upper digestive tract, and for diarrhea. The prevention and management of mucositis are still unsatisfactory. A keratinocyte growth factor was recently approved by the FDA for the prevention of mucositis in patients receiving allogeneic bone-marrow transplant, but its activity in older individuals is untested [29]. A solution of glutamine, AES-14, appeared promising, but the studies so far have been inconclusive [30]. The advent of capecitabine, a prodrug of fluorouracil that is activated in the liver and in the tumor tissue, has been associated with lower risk of mucositis than fluorouracil, as the exposure of normal tissue to the active drug is reduced [31]. However, the use of capecitabine is problematic in persons with a GFR ≤30 mL/minute, as the drug is excreted from the kidneys. It needs to be emphasized that mucositis may be lethal in older individuals, who are more subject than younger people to dehydration and volume depletion due to declining body content of water with age. People who develop diarrhea and dysphagia should be offered prompt and vigorous fluid resuscitation.

Cardiotoxicity

The risk of anthracycline-induced cardiomyopathy increases with age. In two recent studies, independent risk factors for cardiomyopathy included age over 65, previous radiation therapy to the chest, total dose of doxorubicin ≥450 mg/m^2 BSA, and possibly the presence of pre-existent myocardial disease [32,33]. Of particular interest, Hequet *et al.* [32] followed 141 patients who had been treated for large-cell non-Hodgkin lymphoma with a chemotherapy combination containing doxorubicin, and demonstrated subclinical myocardial damage in approximately one-fourth of individuals over 65, several years after treatment termination. The anthracycline cardiotoxicity may be ameliorated by pharmacokinetic interventions and by antidotes. Continuous infusions of doxorubicin were found to be less cardiotoxic than pulse administration, but were associated with increased risk of mucositis [34] and required either prolonged hospitalization or the use of a home infusion pump. Except for the VAD (vincristin, adriamycin, decadron) regimen for multiple myeloma, now abandoned in most centers, this form of administration has not found widespread acceptance.

The antidotes to doxorubicin cardiotoxicity include digoxin, which prevents uptake of the drug in the myocardium [4], and dexrazoxane [35], which chelates myocardial iron, preventing the interaction of doxorubicin and iron and the formation of the free radicals that are responsible for the cardiomyopathy. In an Israeli study it was found that prophylactic use of digoxin allowed administrations of total doses of doxorubicin as high as $1400 \, mg/m^2$ BSA, without cardiac toxicity, but prophylactic use of the drug was never developed in the USA [4]. Dexrazoxane was found to reduce the risk of cardiomyopathy, but it was associated with increased risk of mucositis and myelodepression [35]. In addition, in at least one study, this drug reduced the response rate of breast cancer to doxorubicin. Currently dexrazoxane may be indicated in patients for whom total doses of doxorubicin in excess of $300 \, mg/m^2$ BSA are planned, but it is recommended that treatment with dexrazoxane be initiated after second the course of chemotherapy.

Liposomal preparations of doxorubicin, and especially pegylated liposomal doxorubicin (PLD, Doxil, Caelyx) are less cardiotoxic than doxorubicin, and may represent the ultimate solution for anthracycline cardiotoxicity [36]. Additional advantages of PLD include negligible risk of alopecia, myelosuppression, and nausea and vomiting. PLD was found as active as doxorubicin in multiple myeloma and metastatic breast cancer, and more active in ovarian cancer [36–38]. Ongoing studies explore the activity of PLD in large-cell lymphoma and in the adjuvant treatment of breast cancer.

The monoclonal antibody trastuzumab, which is active in HER2/neu-overexpressing breast cancer, may also cause a cardiomyopathy, whose mechanism is not well clarified. It appears that trastuzumab prevents the binding of neurophysins to the myocardium, and the scarcity of these substances is associated with cardiomyopathy [38]. This toxicity

is reversible with discontinuance of treatment and does not preclude further treatment at a later time [38]. According to the initial study of trastuzumab, the combination with doxorubicin was synergistic in causing cardiomyopathy [38]. However, the combination of trastuzumab with other anthracyclines, such as epirubicin and PLD, does not seem to enhance the risk of cardiotoxicity. It is not clear whether age is a risk factor for this complication.

Neurotoxicity

Peripheral neuropathy is a common complication of alkaloids, epipodophyllotoxins, taxanes, and platinum derivatives, especially cisplatin and oxaliplatin [39]. While it is not clear whether age is a risk factor for this complication, peripheral neuropathy may cause older individuals to lose their independence, by preventing fine movements of the upper extremity and jeopardizing their gait. It is possible that chronic conditions, such as diabetes, B_{12} deficiency, or ischemia, more common among the elderly, may enhance the risk of neuropathy. It is reasonable to check the circulating levels of vitamin B_{12} in older individuals developing peripheral neuropathy, as the prevalence of B_{12} deficiency may be as high as 15% after age 60, due to decreased ability to digest food-bound cyanocobalamin [40]. The widespread use of proton pump inhibitors for the management of heartburn may increase the incidence of this problem.

The clinical course of chemotherapy-related peripheral neuropathy is variable, and the symptoms may be partially reversible over the years [4]. Antiepileptic medications, especially gabapentin, may relieve neuropathic pain, but may cause somnolence and occasional gastrointestinal distress; lidocaine patches (lidoderm) are also effective, when the pain is refractory to other measures [5].

No antidotes to neuropathy are available. Preventive measures may involve trying to avoid the combination of neurotoxic agents such as cisplatin and paclitaxel. Anecdotally, simultaneous infusions of calcium and magnesium have prevented oxaliplatin-related neuropathy [40].

The possibility of *central neurotoxicity* is of special concern to older individuals, subjected as they are to degenerative and ischemic diseases of the central nervous system. The only form of central neurotoxicity that clearly increases with age is cerebellar toxicity from high doses of cytarabine [4]. This appears to be related more to age-related renal insufficiency than to increased susceptibility of the cerebellum to the drug. The toxic metabolite arauridine accumulates in the circulation when the GFR is reduced.

There are reports that chemotherapy may cause cognitive decline [41], but it is not established whether age is a risk factor for this complication. This area deserves more investigation.

A commonsense preventive measure involves the avoidance of concomitant administration of whole-brain radiation therapy and chemotherapy. Correction of anemia with erythropoietic agents may also be effective, as anemia has been associated with increased risk of dementia in dialysis patients [42], and epoetin alpha and its congeners may be neuroprotective [43].

Guidelines for the management of older individuals receiving cytotoxic chemotherapy

The National Cancer Center Network (NCCN) involves 14 NCI-designated cancer centers in the USA, whose experts every three years issue a series of consensus guidelines for the management of different clinical situations. Since 1999 the NCCN has had a panel for guidelines related to the management of cancer in the older aged person. The last edition of these guidelines, issued in 2005, are summarized in Table 18.3 [44].

Geriatric assessment

It is well established that the comprehensive geriatric assessment (CGA) allows the estimation of life expectancy and tolerance of treatment of older individuals, and the identification of reversible conditions that may interfere with the treatment. These

Table 18.3. NCCN guidelines for the management of older cancer patients with chemotherapy.

Some form of geriatric assessment is indicated in all individuals aged 70+

Adjust the doses to the individual GFR in patients aged 65+

Prophylactic use of filgrastim or pegfilgrastim in individuals aged 65+ treated with chemotherapy regimens comparable to CHOP

Maintenance of hemoglobin around 12 g/dL

When indicated, substitute fluorinated pyrimidines with capecitabine, and preferentially use pegylated liposomal doxorubicin, weekly taxanes, navelbine, or gemcitabine

include inadequate caregiving, anemia, which may increase the risk of complications, and depression, which is common among the elderly and may reduce the motivation to receive treatment (see Chapter 4). Figure 18.2 illustrates a way in which the CGA may be utilized for treatment-related decisions. Mild comorbidity may include a Cumulative Illness Rating Scale for Geriatrics (CIRS-G) score <2 or absence of comorbidity that may be life-threatening; intermediate comorbidity a CIRS-G score of 2–3, stable congestive heart failure, serum creatinine ≤3 mg/dL or presence of another malignancy that is not life-threatening; severe comorbidity a CIRS-G score of >3 or life-threatening comorbidity. It is also important to note that symptom management may involve the use of cytotoxic chemotherapy of low toxicity, including low doses of docetaxel for the management of prostate cancer metastatic to the bones, and PLD, low doses of paclitaxel, navelbine, or gemcitabine for metastatic breast cancer.

Dose adjustment to the GFR

The most practical way to determine the GFR involves a formula based on age, sex, and serum creatinine (Fig. 18.3) [4]. The formula of Wright appears more sensitive to low levels of GFR [45]. The adjustment of the dose may be calculated by the formula

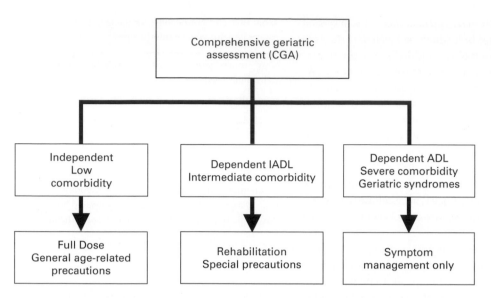

Figure 18.2 Use of the comprehensive geriatric assessment (CGA) in treatment-related decision-making.

(A) Calculation of creatinine clearance

Cockroft & Gault: CrCl = {(140 − Age) × WT × [1 − (0.15 × Sex)]}/(0.814 × SCr)

Wright: CrCl = {[98 − 0.8 × (AGE − 20)] × [1 − (0.01 × Sex)]} × (BSA/1.73)/SCr × 0.0113

(B) Calculation of the dose

Adjusted Dose = (Normal Dose) × [f(KF − 1) + 1]
f = Fraction excreted through the kidneys; KF = CrCl/120

Figure 18.3 (A) Calculation of creatinine clearance using the Cockcroft–Gault and Wright methods [45]; (B) chemotherapy dose adjustment, based on the Kintzel & Dorr formula [46].

of Kintzel and Dorr (Fig. 18.3) [46]. It is important to remember to escalate the doses if no toxicity is seen after the first course of treatment, as individual pharmacokinetics is highly variable and one wants to avoid the risk of undertreatment.

Prophylactic use of filgrastim and pegfilgrastim

A number of clinical trials have shown that both agents are active in older individuals to the same extent as in younger individuals [20,21,25–27]. It is

also clear that age 65 and older is a risk factor for myelodepression, neutropenic infection, infection-related death, and more prolonged infection-related hospitalization [14–25]. Age is also a risk factor for reduced total dose and dose-intensity of chemotherapy, and this may produce inferior outcome due to the higher incidence of therapeutic toxicity, mandating dose reduction and treatment delays. For this reason the NCCN felt that the prophylactic use of filgrastim and pegfilgrastim in patients aged 65 and over treated with a chemotherapy regimen of dose-intensity comparable to CHOP is the safest and most cost-effective course of action that may improve the overall outcome for these patients. These regimens include doxorubicin cyclophosphamide; fluorouracil doxorubicin (or epirubicin) and cyclophosphamide; docetaxel doxorubicin and cyclophosphamide; carboplatin and paclitaxel. In term of cost-effectiveness it should be remembered that older individuals are at risk of more frequent and more prolonged hospitalization for neutropenic infections than younger individuals, and of more prolonged deconditioning after hospitalization, which may result in costly rehabilitation, more frequent dose reductions, and dose delays.

Maintenance of hemoglobin around 12 g/dL

Anemia is a risk factor for chemotherapy-related toxicity, due to the fact that the majority of drugs are heavily bound to red blood cells, and in the presence of anemia the concentration of free drug in the circulation and the risk of complications increases. In addition, anemia is associated with fatigue [47], which in older individuals may lead to functional dependence [48]. The level of 12 g/dL was selected because the best improvement in fatigue was observed when the hemoglobin rose from 11 to 13 g/dL, and it is not clear whether levels >12 g/dL are safe [49].

Selection of drugs of low toxicity

The nature of this recommendation is self-evident. As already pointed out, in certain situations cytotoxic chemotherapy may represent the most effective form of symptom management. While capecitabine has a lower risk of mucositis and myelodepression than intravenous fluorinated pyrimidines, at the recommended doses it may cause substantial toxicity, especially in the presence of renal insufficiency. PLD is as effective as doxorubicin in multiple myeloma, and in metastatic cancers of the breast and ovary. Ongoing clinical trials explore the possibility of substituting this agent for doxorubicin in large-cell lymphoma and in the adjuvant setting of breast cancer.

Age and targeted cancer therapy

Targeted anti-neoplastic therapy in general is better tolerated than cytotoxic chemotherapy. As this form of treatment is relatively recent, data related to the influence of age are limited.

Bevacizumab is an antibody directed against the vascular endothelial growth factor (VEGF), and it has been associated with hypertension and bleeding, complications that appear more common with age.

Alemtuzumab is a monoclonal antibody targeted to the CD52 antigen, overxpressed on B lymphocytes, but also in normal hematopoietic precursors. This drug has an approximately 30% response rate in patients with chronic lymphocytic leukemia (CLL) refractory to chemotherapy, but is associated with significant myelotoxicity.

Tositumomab (Bexxar) and *ibritumomab tiuxetan* (Zevalin) are monoclonal antibodies targeting CD20, and they are bound respectively to radioactive iodine and yttrium. They have produced prolonged remissions in patients with low-grade lymphomas, refractory to other forms of treatment, including rituximab, but their use has been complicated by substantial myelotoxicity.

Mylotarg targets the CD33 antigen of myelopoietic cells and is active in patients with acute myeloid leukemia refractory to chemotherapy, but induces substantial myelosuppression and thrombosis of the hepatic vein.

Conclusions

This chapter deals with anti-neoplastic chemotherapy in the elderly for two reasons: first, neoplastic diseases of the hematopoietic system are among the most treatable of malignancies; second, the main toxicity of cytotoxic chemotherapy is hematopoietic.

The main conclusion of this chapter is that cancer chemotherapy may be as effective and safe in older individuals as it is in younger ones, as long as patients are properly selected in terms of life expectancy and treatment tolerance, and as long as the GFR is taken into account in the dosing of treatment, and support with hematopoietic growth factors is provided.

Other important conclusions include the fact that age is a risk factor for neutropenic infections, mucositis, neurotoxicity, and cardiotoxicity, that anemia may increase the risks of cytotoxic chemotherapy, and that targeted anti-neoplastic treatment may in the future render some forms of cytotoxic chemotherapy obsolete.

REFERENCES

1. Balducci L, Ershler WB. Cancer and ageing: a nexus at several levels. *Nat Rev Cancer* 2005; **5**: 655–62.
2. Duthie EH. Physiology of aging: relevance to symptoms, perceptions, and treatment tolerance. In Balducci L, Lyman GH, Ershler WB, Extermann M, eds, *Comprehensive Geriatric Oncology*, 2nd edn (London: Taylor and Francis, 2004), 207–22.
3. Carreca I, Balducci L, Extermann M. Cancer in the older person. *Cancer Treat Rev* 2005; **31**: 380–402.
4. Cova D, Balducci L. Cancer chemotherapy in the older patient. In Balducci L, Lyman GH, Ershler WB, Extermann M, eds, *Comprehensive Geriatric Oncology*, 2nd edn (London: Taylor and Francis, 2004), 463–88.
5. Balducci L. Management of cancer pain in geriatric patients. *J Support Oncol* 2003; **3**: 175–91.
6. Lancet JE, Willman CL, Bennett JM. Acute myelogenous leukemia and aging: clinical interactions. *Hematol Oncol Clin North Am* 2000; **16**: 251–67.
7. Rudd GN, Hartley JA, Souhani RL. Persistence of cisplatin-induced DNA interstrand crosslinking in peripheral blood mononuclear cells from elderly and younger individuals. *Cancer Chemother Pharmacol* 1995; **35**: 323–6.
8. Begg CB, Carbone P. Clinical trials and drug toxicity in the elderly: the experience of the Eastern Cooperative Oncology Group. *Cancer* 1983; **52**: 1986–92.
9. Gelman RS, Taylor SG. Cyclophosphamide, methotrexate, and 5-fluorouracil chemotherapy in women more than 65 years old with advanced breast cancer: the elimination of age trends in toxicity by using doses based on creatinine clearance. *J Clin Oncol* 1984; **2**: 1406–13.
10. Christman K, Muss HB, Case LD, Stanley V. Chemotherapy of metastatic breast cancer in the elderly. *JAMA* 1992; **268**: 57–62.
11. Giovanazzi-Bannon S, Rademaker A, Lai G, Benson AB. treatment tolerance of elderly cancer patients entered onto phase II clinical trials. An Illinois Cancer Center study. *J Clin Oncol* 1994; **12**: 2447–52.
12. Ibrahim NK, Frye DK, Buzdar AU, Walters RS, Hortobagyi GN. Doxorubicin based combination chemotherapy in elderly patients with metastatic breast cancer: tolerance and outcome. *Arch Intern Med* 1996; **156**: 882–8.
13. Ibrahim NK, Buzdar AU, Asmar L, Theriault RL, Hortobagyi GN. Doxorubicin-based adjuvant chemotherapy in elderly breast cancer patients: the M. D. Anderson experience, with long-term follow-up. *Ann Oncol* 2000; **11**: 1–5.
14. Kim YJ, Rubenstein EB, Rolston KV, *et al.* Colony-stimulating factors (CSFs) may reduce complications and death in solid tumor patients with fever and neutropenia. *Proc ASCO* 2000; **19**: 612a, abstract 2411.
15. Crivellari D, Bonetti M, Castiglione-Gertsch M, *et al.* Burdens and benefits of adjuvant cyclophosphamide, methotrexate and fluorouracil and tamoxifen for elderly patients with breast cancer: the International Breast Cancer Study Group Trial VII. *J Clin Oncol* 2000; **18**: 1412–22.
16. Chrischilles E, Delgado DJ, Stolshek BS, *et al.* Impact of age and colony stimulating factor use in hospital length of stay for febrile neutropenia in CHOP-treated non-Hodgkin's lymphoma patients. *Cancer Control* 2002; **9**: 203–11.
17. Morrison VA, Picozzi V, Scott S, *et al.* The impact of age on delivered dose-intensity and hospitalizations for febrile neutropenia in patients with intermediate-grade non-Hodgkin's lymphoma receiving initial CHOP chemotherapy: a risk factor analysis. *Clin Lymphoma* 2001; **2**: 47–56.
18. Lyman GH, Lyman CH, Agboola O. Risk models for predicting chemotherapy-induced neutropenia *Oncologist* 2005; **10**: 427–37.
19. Kuderer NM, Crawford J, Dale DC, *et al.* Meta-analysis of granulocyte colony stimulating factor (G-CSF) in cancer patients receiving chemotherapy. *Proc Am Soc Clin Oncol* 2005; **23**: 758s, abstract 8117.
20. Zinzani PL, Storti S, Zaccaria A, *et al.* Elderly aggressive-histology non-Hodgkin's lymphoma: first-line VNCOP-B regimen experience on 350 patients. *Blood* 1999; **94**: 33–8.

21. Sonneveld P, de Ridder M, van der Lelie H, *et al.* Comparison of doxorubicin and mitoxantrone in the treatment of elderly patients with advanced diffuse non-Hodgkin's lymphoma using CHOP vs CNOP chemotherapy. *J Clin Oncol* 1995; **13**: 2530–9.

22. Gomez H, Mas L, Casanova L, *et al.* Elderly patients with aggressive non-Hodgkin's lymphoma treated with CHOP chemotherapy plus granulocyte-macrophage colony-stimulating factor: identification of two age subgroups with differing hematologic toxicity. *J Clin Oncol* 1998; **16**: 2352–8.

23. Tirelli U, Errante D, Van Glabbeke M, *et al.* CHOP is the standard regimen in patients ⩾70 years of age with intermediate and high grade non-Hodgkin's lymphoma: results of a randomized study of the European organization for the Research and Treatment of Cancer Lymphoma Cooperative Study. *J Clin Oncol* 1998; **16**: 27–34.

24. Bastion Y, Blay JY, Divine M, *et al.* Elderly patients with aggressive non-Hodgkin's lymphoma: disease presentation, response to treatment and survival. A Groupe d'Etude des Lymphomes de l'Adulte Study on 453 patients older than 69 years. *J Clin Oncol* 1997; **15**: 2945–53.

25. Doorduijn JK, van der Holt B, van der Hem KG, *et al.* Randomized trial of granulocyte-colony stimulating factor (G-CSF) added to CHOP in elderly patients with aggressive non-Hodgkin's lymphoma. *Blood* 2000; **96**: 133a.

26. Osby E, Hagberg H, Kvaloy S, *et al.* CHOP is superior to CNOP in elderly patients with aggressive lymphoma while outcome is unaffected by filgrastim treatment: results of a Nordic Lymphoma Group randomized trial. *Blood* 2003; **101**: 3840–8.

27. Balducci L, Tam J, Al-Halavani H, *et al.* A large study of the older cancer patient in the community setting: initial report of a randomized controlled trial using pegfilgrastim to reduce neutropenic complications. *Proc Am Soc Clin Oncol* 2005; **23**: 756s B.

28. Jacobson SD, Cha S, Sargent DJ, *et al.* Tolerability, dose intensity and benefit of 5FU based chemotherapy for advanced colorectal cancer (CRC) in the elderly: a North Central Cancer Treatment Group study. *Proc Am Soc Clin Oncol* 2001; **20**: 384a, abstract 1534.

29. Sonis ST. Oral mucositis in cancer therapy. *J Support Oncol* 2004; **2** (6 Suppl 3): 3–8.

30. Spielberger R, Stiff P, Bensinger W, *et al.* Palifermin for oral mucositis after intensive treatment for hematologic cancer. *N Engl J Med* 2004; **351**: 2590–8.

31. Carreca I, Balducci L. Oral chemotherapy of cancer in the elderly. *Am J Cancer* 2002; **1**: 101–8.

32. Hequet O, Le OH, Moullet I, *et al.* Subclinical late cardiomyopathy after doxorubicin therapy for lymphoma in adults. *J Clin Oncol* 2004; **22**: 1864–71.

33. Swain SM, Whaley FS, Ewer MS. Congestive heart failure in patients treated with doxorubicin: a retrospective analysis of three trials. *Cancer* 2003; **97**: 2869–79.

34. Swain SM, Vici P. The current and future role of dexrazoxane as a cardioprotector in anthracycline treatment: expert panel review. *J Cancer Res Clin Oncol* 2004; **130**: 1–7.

35. Robert NJ, Vogel CL, Henderson IC, *et al.* The role of liposomal anthracyclines and other systemic therapies in the management of advanced breast cancer. *Semin Oncol* 2004; **31** (6 Suppl 13): 106–46.

36. Rifkin RM, Hussein MA, Gregory SA, *et al.* Updated results from a randomized multicenter trial of DVd vs. VAd in patients with newly diagnosed multiple myeloma. *Proc Am Soc Clin Oncol* 2004; **22**: 560s, abstract 6509.

37. Rose PG. Pegylated liposomal doxorubicin: optimizing the dosing schedule in ovarian cancer. *Oncologist* 2005; **10**: 205–14.

38. Youssef G, Links M. The prevention and management of cardiovascular complications of chemotherapy in patients with cancer. *Am J Cardiovasc Drugs* 2005; **5**: 233–43.

39. Norman EJ, Morrison JA. Screening elderly populations for cobalamin (vitamin B12) deficiency using the urinary methylmalonic acid assay by gas chromatography mass spectrometry. *Am J Med* 1993; **94**: 589–94.

40. Grothey A. Clinical management of oxaliplatin-associated neurotoxicity. *Clin Colorectal Cancer* 2005; **5** (Suppl 1): S38–S46.

41. Brezden CB, Phillips KA, Abdolell M, Bunston T, Tannock IF. Cognitive function in breast cancer patients receiving adjuvant chemotherapy. *J Clin Oncol* 2000; **18**: 2695–701.

42. Pickett JL, Theberge DC, Brown WS, Schweitzer SU, Nissenson AR. Normalizing hematocrit in dialysis patients improves brain function. *Am J Kidney Dis* 1999; **33**: 1122–30.

43. Nissenson AR. Epoetin and cognitive function. *Am J Kidney Dis* 1992; **20**: 21–4.

44. Balducci L, Cohen HJ, Engstrom PF, *et al.* The NCCN senior adult oncology practice guidelines in oncology. *J Natl Compr Canc Netw* 2005; **3**: 572–90.

45. Marx GM, Blake GM, Galani E, *et al.* Evaluation of the Cockroft–Gault, Jelliffe and Wright formulae in estimating renal function in elderly cancer patients. *Ann Oncol* 2004; **15**: 291–5.

46. Kintzel PE, Dorr RT. Anticancer drug renal toxicity and elimination: dosing guidelines for altered renal function. *Cancer Treat Rev* 1995; **21**: 33–64.

47. Respini D, Jacobsen PB, Thors C, Tralongo P, Balducci L. The prevalence and correlates of fatigue in older cancer patients. *Crit Rev Oncol Hematol* 2003; **47**: 273–9.

48. Guralnik JM, Eisenstaedt RS, Ferrucci L, Klein HG, Woodman RC. Prevalence of anemia in persons 65 years and older in the United States: evidence for a high rate of unexplained anemia. *Blood* 2004; **104**: 2263–8.

49. Curt GA, Breitbart W, Cella D, *et al.* Impact of cancer-related fatigue on the lives of patients: new findings from the Fatigue Coalition. *Oncologist* 2000; **5**: 353–60.

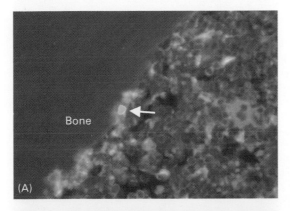

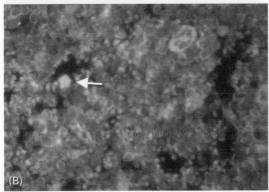

Figure 6.2 Analysis of spatial distribution following transplantation. CFSE-labeled cells (green) are designated as either endosteal (A) or central (B).

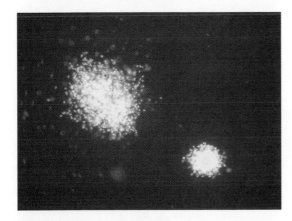

Figure 6.4 In-vitro colony-forming assay, used as a surrogate measure of hemopoietic potential.

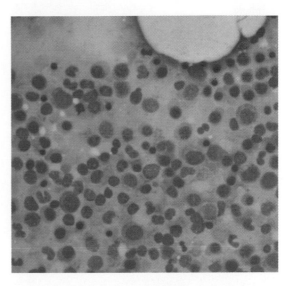

Figure 8.1 Aspirate smear showing hyperplastic and dysplastic features.

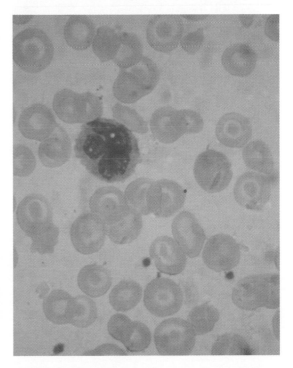

Figure 8.2 Blood smear from a patient with myelodysplastic syndrome, showing an abnormal monocyte.

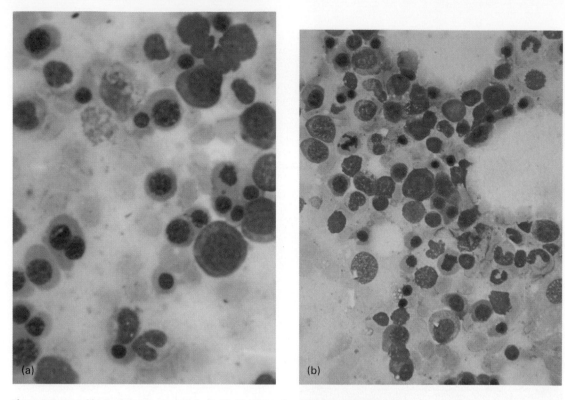

Figure 8.3 (a and b) Aspirate smear: myelodysplastic dyserythropoiesis and mitosis.

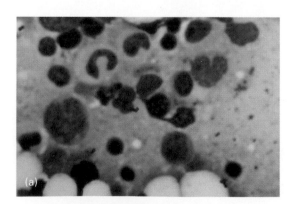

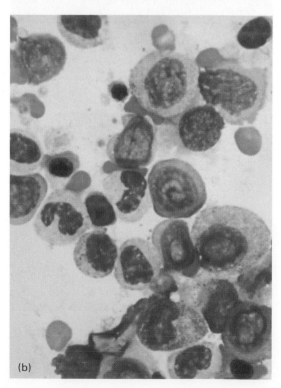

Figure 8.4 Dysgranulopoiesis. Aspirate smears from (a) a 48-year-old man with granule deficiency; (b) a 79-year-old man with bicytopenia and maturation defect in the granulopoiesis.

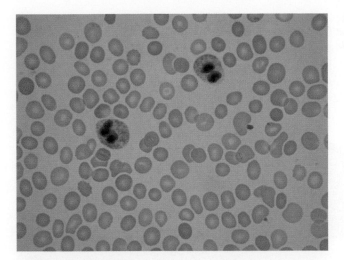

Figure 8.5 Blood smear from a patient with refractory cytopenia, showing two neutrophils with bilobed nuclei.

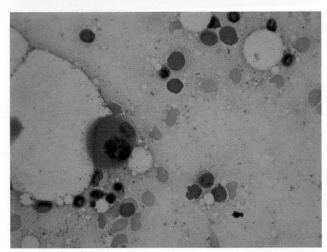

Figure 8.6 Dysplastic megakaryocyte: aspirate smear from a 77-year-old female with bicytopenia and thrombocytosis (5q–syndrome).

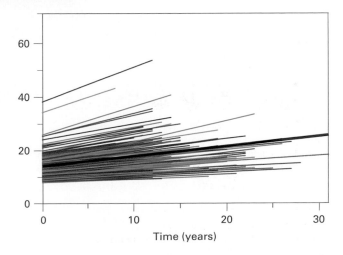

Figure 12.2 Predicted erythropoietin levels over time. Baltimore Longitudinal Study in Aging [58].

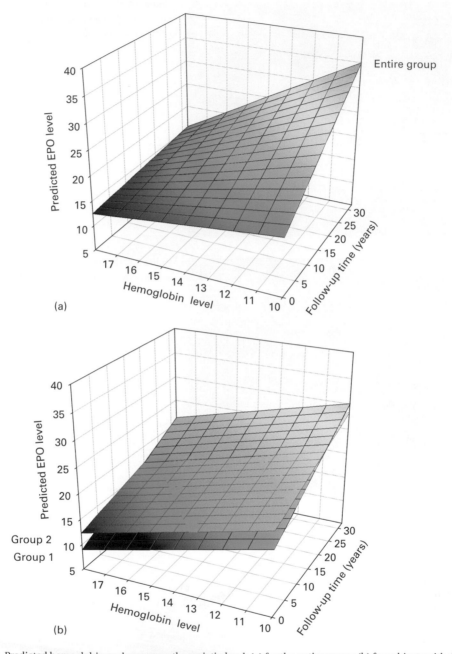

Figure 12.3 Predicted hemoglobin and serum erythropoietin level: (a) for the entire group; (b) for subjects with diabetes or hypertension (group 2) compared to subjects with these conditions (group 1). Baltimore Longitudinal Study in Aging [58].

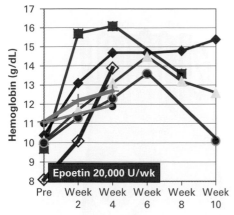

Figure 12.4 Hemoglobin response for epoetin alpha treatment of elderly with unexplained anemia [50].

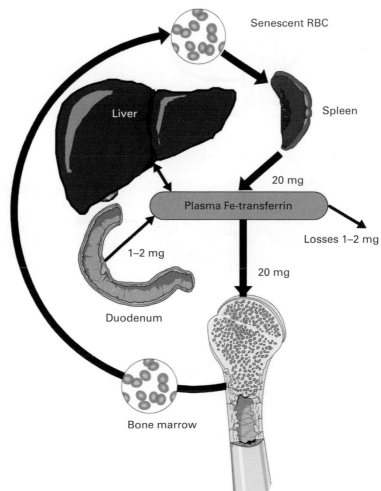

Figure 13.1 Major iron flows during normal iron homeostasis. Most iron enters plasma from macrophages that recycle senescent erythrocytes, with smaller amounts coming from hepatocyte stores and dietary absorption in the duodenum. Most plasma iron is destined for the hemoglobin in developing erythrocytes in the bone marrow. In the absence of bleeding, iron losses from desquamation of intestinal epithelia and skin are relatively minor.

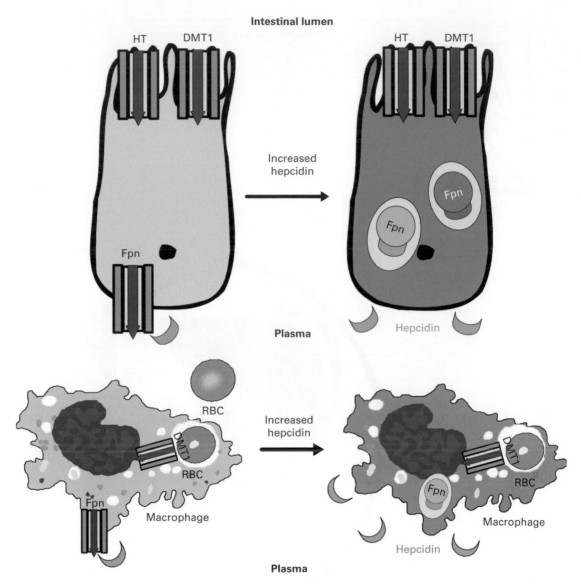

Figure 13.2 Hepcidin–ferroportin interaction regulates the flow of iron into plasma. Absorptive enterocytes acquire iron from the diet through the DMT1 iron transporter, and as heme, using apical heme transporters (HT) (top panel). DMT1 is also involved in the translocation of iron across the phagosomal membrane of macrophages (bottom panel). The red arrows indicate iron flows through channels. Cytoplasmic iron from duodenal enterocytes and macrophages is exported into plasma through the iron channel ferroportin (Fpn). Hepcidin binds to ferroportin, and induces its internalization and degradation. The loss of ferroportin results in decreased efflux of iron from cells into plasma and accumulation of iron in cytoplasmic ferritin (blue color).

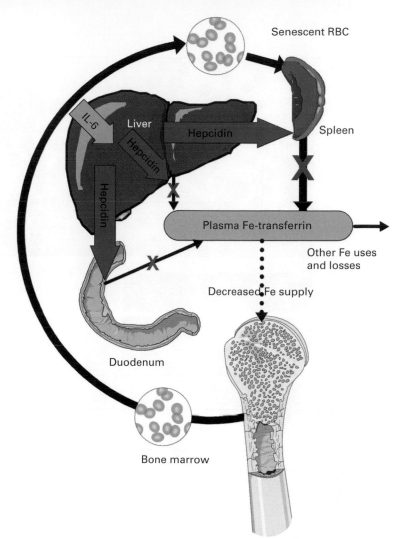

Figure 13.3 Changes of iron flows during inflammation. IL-6 and other cytokines induce hepcidin production and increased concentrations of hepcidin inhibit iron efflux from erythrocyte-recycling macrophages (predominantly in the spleen), from hepatic storage, and from the duodenum into plasma. Hypoferremia develops, and erythropoiesis becomes iron-limited.

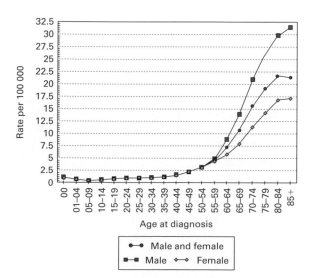

Figure 19.1 Incidence of AML in the US population by age and sex, 1969–2002 [7].

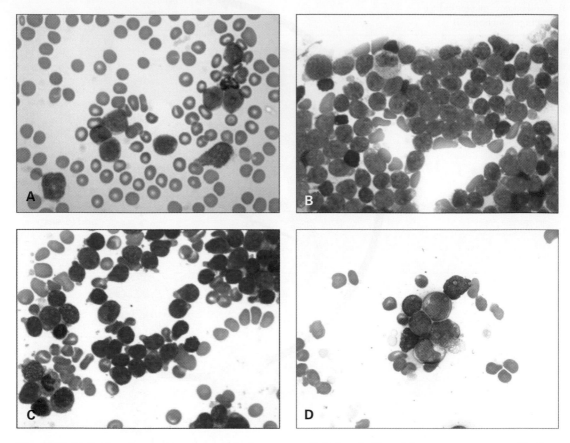

Figure 20.1 (A) ALL lymphocytes in peripheral blood smear; (B) ALL L3 lymphoblasts in bone-marrow aspirate; (C) ALL hand-mirror variant; (D) ALL granular variant.

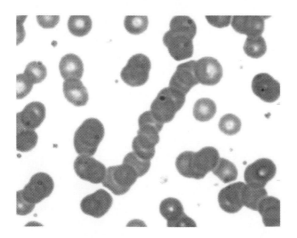

Figure 21.1 Peripheral smear showing rouleaux formation. Lazarchick, J., ASH Image Bank 2001: 101085. Copyright American Society of Hematology. All rights reserved.

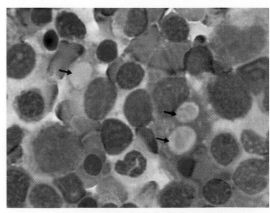

Figure 21.2 High-power view of plasma cells with large cytoplasmic inclusions known as Russell bodies (arrows). Maslak, P., ASH Image Bank 2001: 100211. Copyright American Society of Hematology. All rights reserved.

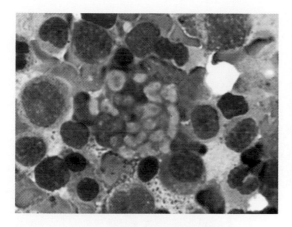

Figure 21.3 Mott cells have a cytoplasm filled with Russell bodies. Maslak, P., ASH Image Bank 2001: 100211. Copyright American Society of Hematology. All rights reserved.

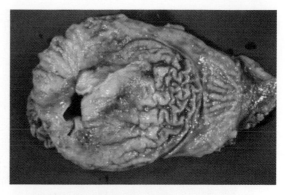

Figure 22.2 Gastric MALT lymphoma: gross pathology. Normal gastric mucosa disrupted by MALT lymphoma. Kadin, M., ASH Image Bank 2003: 100693. Copyright American Society of Hematology. All rights reserved.

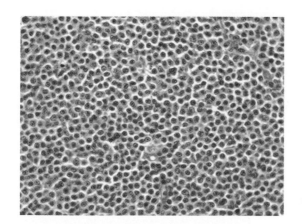

Figure 22.1 Marginal zone lymphoma: neoplastic marginal zone cells with moderately abundant cytoplasm have plasmacytoid appearance. Kadin, M., ASH Image Bank 2004: 101238. Copyright American Society of Hematology. All rights reserved.

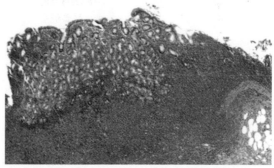

Figure 22.3 Gastric MALT lymphoma: marginal zone cells colonize and obliterate germinal centers of reactive B-cell follicles. Kadin, M., ASH Image Bank 2003: 100693. Copyright American Society of Hematology. All rights reserved.

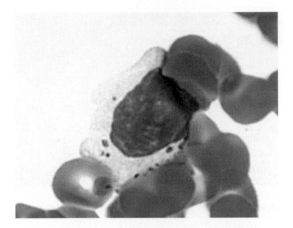

Figure 23.1 Large granular lymphocyte may appear as an atypical lymphocyte with scattered prominent granules in the cytoplasm. Maslak, P., ASH Image Bank 2004: 101068. Copyright American Society of Hematology. All rights reserved.

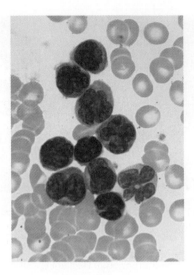

Figure 23.3 ATLL: peripheral blood smear showing abnormal lymphocytes with nuclear indentation or lobulation (Wright's stain). Myoshi, I. *et al.*, ASH Image Bank 2003: 100715. Copyright American Society of Hematology. All rights reserved.

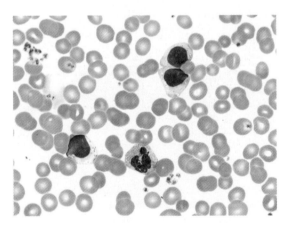

Figure 23.2 LGL leukemia: atypical lymphocytes are noted in the peripheral smear. Jurcic, J. & Maslak, P., ASH Image Bank 2004: 101229. Copyright American Society of Hematology. All rights reserved.

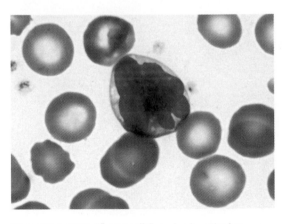

Figure 23.4 ATLL: "flower cells" can be described as having pleomorphic nuclei with deeply basophilic cytoplasm. Maslak, P., ASH Image Bank 2006: 6-00002. Copyright American Society of Hematology. All rights reserved.

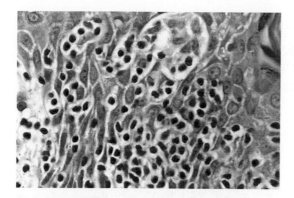

Figure 23.5 Mycosis fungoides: epidermotropism of atypical lymphocytes with cerebriform nuclei. Kadin, M., ASH Image Bank 2005: 101309. Copyright American Society of Hematology. All rights reserved.

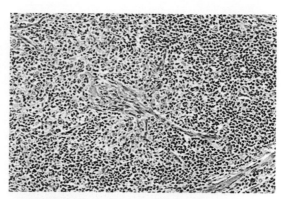

Figure 23.7 AITL: arborizing blood vessel(s) (1996). Kadin, M., ASH Image Bank 2003: 100652. Copyright American Society of Hematology. All rights reserved.

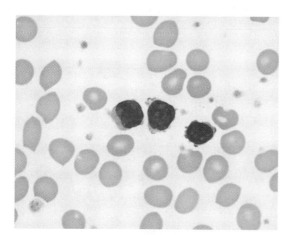

Figure 23.6 Sézary cells: the nuclear convolutions are most apparent in the cell in the center in this view. Lazarchick, J., ASH Image Bank 2004: 101081. Copyright American Society of Hematology. All rights reserved.

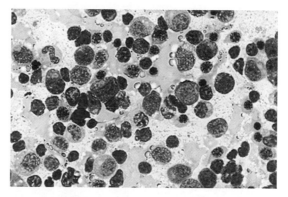

Figure 23.8 AITL: immunoblasts in bone marrow aspirate stained with Giemsa (1995). Kadin, M., ASH Image Bank 2003: 100652. Copyright American Society of Hematology. All rights reserved.

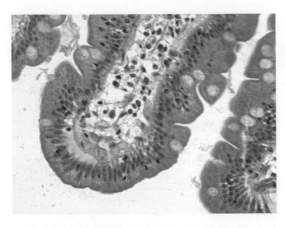

Figure 23.9 High magnification of normal duodenal mucosa for comparison to abnormal mucosa in enteropathy type T cell lymphoma. Kadin, M., ASH Image Bank 2003: 100846. Copyright American Society of Hematology. All rights reserved.

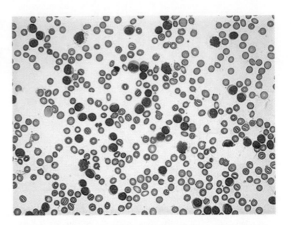

Figure 24.2 This mixed-cell variant of CLL contains a dimorphic population of cells. Kadin, M., ASH Image Bank 2003: 100935. Copyright American Society of Hematology. All rights reserved.

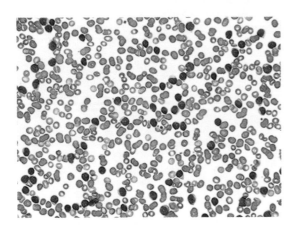

Figure 24.1 This peripheral smear shows that there can be heterogeneity in the appearance of the abnormal lymphocytes in CLL. Kadin, M., ASH Image Bank 2003: 100690. Copyright American Society of Hematology. All rights reserved.

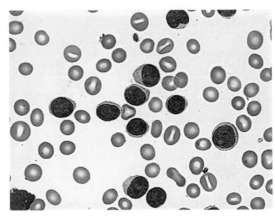

Figure 24.3 PLL variant of CLL: prominent nuclei characterize the prolymphocytes. Kadin, M., ASH Image Bank 2003: 100935. Copyright American Society of Hematology. All rights reserved.

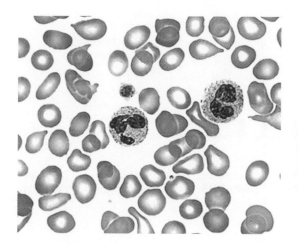

Figure 25.1 Idiopathic myelofibrosis: a typical picture in the peripheral blood may include dacrocytes, dysplastic granulocytes and large platelets. Maslak, P., ASH Image Bank 2004: 101216. Copyright American Society of Hematology. All rights reserved.

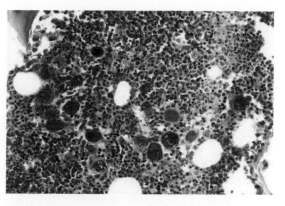

Figure 25.2 Bone marrow biopsy showing clustering of megakaryocytes with mature cytoplasm, and variable nuclear lobulations. Lazarchick, J., ASH Image Bank 2001: 100172. Copyright American Society of Hematology. All rights reserved.

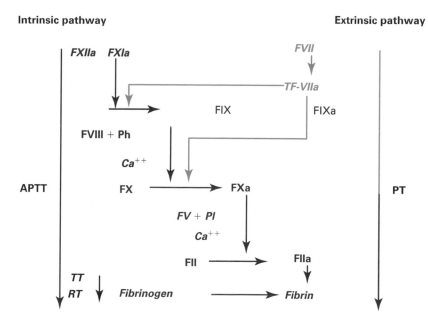

Figure 26.1 Simplified scheme of the coagulation cascade and laboratory tests; intrinsic (in blue), extrinsic (in green), and common (in red) pathway. TF, tissue factor; PH, phospholipid; APTT, activated partial thromboplastin time; PT, prothrombin time; RT, reptilase time.

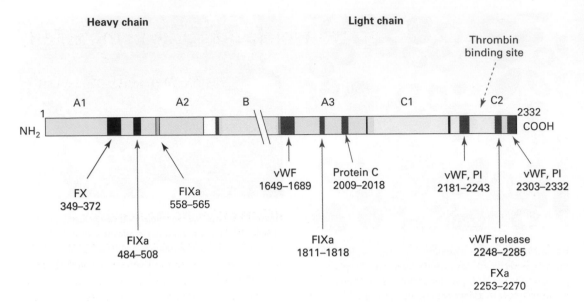

Figure 26.2 FVIII structure (simplified as relevant to the present discussion). Heavy chain (A1, A2, B domains) and light chain (A3, C1, C2 domains). Arrows indicate the binding sites of the major FVIII ligands as mapped by the use of alloantibodies: FIXa, FX, FXa, vWF, phospholipids (Pl), and protein C. Blue indicates target of FVIII inhibitors. Dotted arrow indicates that the inhibitor target is not mapped to date. From Saenko *et al*. 2002 [48], reproduced with permission of the author.

19

Acute myeloid leukemia in the elderly

Magda Melchert, Jeffrey Lancet

Introduction

Acute myeloid leukemia (AML) is a clonal hematologic malignancy characterized by proliferation and accumulation of myeloid progenitors within the bone marrow, leading ultimately to hematopoietic failure. In the peripheral blood, there is often profound pancytopenia, with the attendant complications of infection and bleeding. In some patients, the white blood count may become markedly elevated, resulting in leukostatic complications such as cerebrovascular or cardiovascular insufficiency. AML may occur *de novo* or arise secondarily from pre-existing clonal hematologic diseases such as myelodysplastic syndrome (MDS) or myeloproliferative syndromes. In rare cases, AML may develop as a consequence of exposure to previously administered chemotherapeutic agents such as alkylators or epipodophyllotoxins.

Recent years have witnessed an expanded understanding of AML, in terms of both pathophysiology and classification. Several new oncogenes and molecular targets have been discovered, therapies directed at these targets have been developed, and notable advances in supportive care through antibiotics and blood-product support are undisputed. Despite these advances, however, AML remains incurable in the majority of patients. In the case of older patients, outcomes are especially dismal. This chapter will examine the epidemiologic, biologic, and therapeutic aspects of AML that are unique to older individuals, highlighting the challenges associated with treating such patients.

Unique challenges to treating AML in the elderly

Major obstacles to defining optimal therapy in older adults with AML, and many other cancers for that matter, may result both from under-representation of the elderly in clinical trials and from a high degree of selection for patients treated with "curative" intent. To illustrate this point, the Southwest Oncology Group (SWOG) analyzed the proportion of patients enrolled onto clinical trials compared with the corresponding rates in the USA of patients with cancer, and found that patients over age 65 were under-represented [1]. In AML specifically, there are lower rates of enrollment onto clinical trials for older patients than for younger ones [2,3]. An important reason for exclusion of elderly patients from clinical cancer trials is the presence and severity of comorbidities. In fact, over 25% of cancer patients above age 75 have six or more comorbidities [4]. While the presence and severity of medical comorbidities appear to adversely affect survival of cancer patients, including those with AML [2,5], it remains unclear whether the comorbidities themselves are responsible for the poor outcomes, as patients may be denied intensive therapy on this basis. In support of this assertion is the fact that several retrospective studies have demonstrated that a majority of elderly AML patients are often treated with supportive or palliative measures only [2,3,6]. Hence, great caution must be exercised in interpreting and extrapolating results of therapeutic trials in elderly AML patients, given not only the heterogeneity of the disease, but also

Blood Disorders in the Elderly, ed. Lodovico Balducci, William Ershler, Giovanni de Gaetano.
Published by Cambridge University Press. © Cambridge University Press 2008.

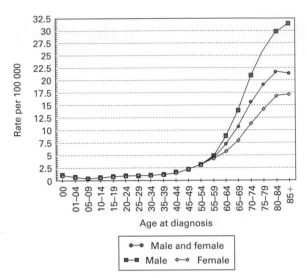

Figure 19.1 Incidence of AML in the US population by age and sex, 1969–2002 [7]. *See color plate section.*

the selection of patients upon whom these results are based.

Epidemiology

Incidence

It is clear that AML is a disease that primarily affects older individuals. In the USA, the incidence peaks at a rate of 20–25 per 100 000 in people over age 75, compared with less than 2.5 per 100 000 in people under age 55 (Fig. 19.1). Unfortunately, the mortality rate closely parallels the incidence in older individuals, speaking to the high degree of lethality of the disease, despite its relatively low incidence compared with other malignancies.

Environmental exposures

There are few known causative environmental factors in AML, though exposure to certain toxins has been associated with an increased risk of disease. Chronic benzene exposure is one of the best-described environmental risk factors for the development of AML [8–10]. Another environmental exposure to which the development of AML has been implicated is external radiation, which may result

in a two- to six fold increase in relative risk [10–12]. Systemic exposure to a multitude of chemotherapeutic agents, including alkylating agents, epipodophyllotoxins, and topoisomerase II inhibitors have been clearly associated with an increased risk for AML [13–15]. Such treatment-related AML is characterized by cytogenetic anomalies in chromosomes 5, 7, and 11, and is nearly invariably associated with a very poor prognosis [15–17]. Hydroxyurea, a commonly used agent for several myeloproliferative diseases, may also impart an increased risk for the development of AML with the deletion of the short arm of chromosome 17 [18]. Several reports have also clearly indicated an increased risk of secondary AML and MDS following high-dose therapy and autologous transplantation for diseases such as non-Hodgkin lymphoma and multiple myeloma [13,19]. Finally, cigarette smoking appears to impart a modestly increased risk for AML, and this risk appears to be exacerbated in adults over age 60 [10,20].

Diagnosis and classification

AML is a disease in which diagnosis and classification are made upon morphologic, and more recently cytogenetic, criteria. A comparison of the

Table 19.1. Comparison of French–American–British (FAB) and World Health Organization (WHO) classification of AML [21].

FAB classification	WHO classification
M0 AML, minimally differentiated ≥30% blasts bone marrow	AML with recurrent cytogenetic abnormalities ≥20% blasts bone marrow t(8;21)(q22;q22) (AML1/ETO) inv(16)(p13q22) or t(16;16)(p13;q22) (CBFβ/MYH 11) t(15;17)(q22;q12) (PML/RARα), APL 11q23 (MLL)
M1 AML, without maturation ≥30% blasts bone marrow	AML with multilineage dysplasia ≥20% blasts bone marrow Following MDS or MDS/MPD Without MDS or MDS/MPD, but with dysplasia involving >50% cells in 2 or more lineages
M2 AML, with maturation ≥30% blasts bone marrow	AML and MDS, therapy-related Alkylating agent/radiation-related type Topoisomerase II inhibitor-related type Others
M3 acute promyclocytic leukemia (APL) ≥30% blasts bone marrow M4 acute myelomonocytic leukemia ≥30% blasts bone marrow M5 acute monoblastic leukemia ≥30% blasts bone marrow M6 acute erythroleukemia ≥30% blasts bone marrow M7 acute megakaryoblastic leukemia ≥30% blasts bone marrow	AML, not otherwise categorized ≥20% blasts bone marrow

French–American–British (FAB) classification system and the more recent World Health Organization (WHO) system is shown in Table 19.1. One important difference in the WHO system is the lowering of the threshold for diagnosis of AML from 30% to 20% blasts in the bone-marrow aspirate or peripheral blood. This change subsequently eliminated the former FAB-delineated MDS category of refractory anemia with excess blasts in transformation (RAEB-T). One category in the WHO classification system also specifies AML with multilineage dysplasia. Since a significant proportion of AML in the elderly is thought to arise from MDS, the WHO system may be particularly relevant for older patients.

Another category, AML with recurrent cytogenetic abnormalities, refers to those cases with translocations involving chromosome 11q23, between 15 and 17 (acute promyelocytic leukemia), 8 and 21, 16 and 16, and chromosome 16 inversion. This category of AML occurs primarily in younger individuals [22].

Biologic characteristics of AML in elderly patients

Cytogenetic abnormalities

A clonal disorder, AML is characterized by molecular lesions that are often recognized as chromosomal

Table 19.2. Prognostic classification of karyotype analysis [30,31].

Favorable	Intermediate	Unfavorable
Inv(16), t(16;16), del(16q)	Normal karyotype	Monosomy 5, 5q–
t(8;21)	Trisomy 6	Monosomy 7, 7q–
t(15;17)	–Y	Trisomy 8
	Del(12p)	Abn 3q
	Other non-complex	Abn 9q
	karyotype	11q23 (MLL)
		t(9;22)
		20q–
		21q–
		17p
		t(6;9)
		Complex karyotype (involving 4 or more unrelated mutations)

aneuploidy or translocations. The specific leukemic karyotype can then be prognostically categorized further into favorable, intermediate, or unfavorable subtypes (Table 19.2). The frequency of specific leukemic karyotypes as well as the prognostic category differs between older adults and younger ones [23,24]. Specifically, cytogenetic abnormalities involving t(15;17), t(8;21), and inversion 16 [t(16;16)] are rarely encountered in older adults with AML [23,25–27]. Conversely, the frequency of specific karyotypes that fall within the unfavorable subgroup, such as full or partial deletions of chromosomes 5 and 7, trisomy 8, or 11q23, are higher in the elderly AML setting [23–27]. Additionally, AML secondary to previous exposure to cytotoxic chemotherapy or environmental carcinogens appears to be more frequently associated with abnormalities of chromosomes 5 and 7. Topoisomerase II inhibitors such as etoposide, mitoxantrone, and doxorubicin have shown a strong association with the mixed-lineage leukemia (*MLL*) gene at 11q23 [28]. Complex karyotype is also more frequently seen in older adults, and consistently confers an inferior complete remission rate and long-term survival [23,29].

Molecular anomalies

In the last decade, several other molecular abnormalities have been found to be associated with AML. These markers have been identified in both older and younger AML patients, and have been identified as prognostically important only in younger patients with normal karyotype. FMS-like tyrosine kinase (FLT3) is expressed on early hematopoietic and lymphoid progenitors, and appears to play an important role in myeloid differentiation and stem-cell survival [32]. Internal tandem duplications of the *FLT3* gene (FLT3-ITD) involving the juxtamembrane region have now been described to be present in 17–34% of patients with AML [32–34]. A point mutation in codon 835 of the *FLT3* gene has also been discovered and involves the activating loop of the tyrosine kinase domain (TKD), although it is detected with considerable lower frequency [35]. Using mouse models, transfection of the FLT3-ITD mutation into myeloid cell lines induces leukemia-type disease in syngeneic mice [36]. Further in-vitro studies have shown that FLT3-ITD causes a ligand-independent receptor dimerization with subsequent constitutive activation of Ras, MAP kinase, and Stat5 pathways, and thus unregulated cell proliferation [36,37]. AML patients with FLT3-ITD and TKD mutations often present at diagnosis with higher white blood cell counts, a higher percentage of blasts, higher LDH, and more commonly with *de novo* AML [37]. While complete remission rates are generally unaffected by the presence of *FLT3* abnormalities, a significantly inferior disease-free survival and overall survival have been described by most authors [32,37–39].

Also of considerable importance in cytogenetically normal AML is the presence of nucleophosmin member 1 gene (*NPM1*) mutations. Heterozygous mutations involving exon 12 of the *NPM1* gene result in translocation of the nucleophosmin gene product from the nucleus to the cytoplasm [40]. Concurrent FLT3-ITD mutations can be identified in up to 40% of patients with mutated *NPM1*. Increased bone-marrow blast percentage, female sex, increased lactate dehydrogenase levels, higher white blood cell count, lower platelet count, and low or absent CD34+ expression have all been associated with *NPM1* mutations [40,41]. Also functionally important to normal myeloid maturation is the gene CCAAT/enhancer-binding protein α (CEBPA). Mutations of this gene are also present in increased frequency in patients with normal cytogenetics, in approximately 15–20% of cases. Mutated CEBPA has been associated with lower platelet counts, higher percentages of peripheral blood blasts, less extramedullary involvement and less lymphadenopathy [40,42].

Another molecular abnormality that has been described with considerable frequency in AML is the *Ras* proto-oncogene. The majority of *Ras* mutations involve point mutations at codons 12, 13, and 61, leading to constitutive activation of Ras protein. Mutations at one of the three functional *Ras* genes leads to decreased GTPase activity of the Ha-, Ki-, or N-ras proteins, which in turn causes leukemic transformation [43,44]. N-ras has been detected in 15–30% of AML samples, and multiple groups have attempted to stratify prognostically according to the presence of one of these mutations. Despite evidence that the presence of the N-*ras* proto-oncogene in patients with MDS confers a higher risk

of progression to AML and inferior overall survival [45], the majority of clinical correlates have failed to show an unfavorable outcome in patients with AML [38,43,46,47].

Of considerable interest in recent years is the multi-drug resistance phenotype, with the associated gene (*MDR1*) located on the long arm of chromosome 7. *MDR1* encodes a 170 kD glycoprotein, or P-glycoprotein (Pgp), that functions as an ATP-dependent efflux pump. In-vitro models have shown that over-expression of Pgp has led to increased cellular export of anti-neoplastic drugs, including anthracyclines, vinca alkaloids, epipodophyllotoxins, and taxol [48]. The MDR1 phenotype in elderly patients with AML confers a resistance to anthracycline chemotherapy with a significantly inferior complete remission rate, disease-free survival, and overall survival [27,49]. In the SWOG 9031 trial, 71% of patients greater than age 55 exhibited the MDR1 phenotype, while in the SWOG 8600 trial, with patients younger than 55, the incidence of MDR1 overexpression was approximately 30% [27]. The increased incidence of Pgp overexpression in the elderly supports the finding that conventional induction therapy in the elderly is less efficacious than in younger adults. Therapeutic strategies to inhibit Pgp cellular export of anthracyclines have been investigated, with compounds such as cyclosporine, quinine, and PSC-833, with variable success [49,50]. These will be discussed in further detail later in the chapter.

Treatment

While the majority of patients with AML are considered to be elderly, their response to standard chemotherapy has been historically poor, with lower response rates and increased treatment-related mortality. Complete remission (CR) rates for patients younger than age 55–60 generally range 60–80%, while CR rates in elderly patients are reported in most studies as 30–50% (Table 19.3). Tolerability of intensive induction therapy has also been sub-optimal, due in part to the high risk of infection with prolonged cytopenias and also to the prevalence of

Table 19.3. Comparison of outcomes for induction therapy for AML in younger (<55–60) and older (>55–60) patients.

Trial	Year	Age >55–60		Age <55–60	
		CR (%)	ED (%)	CR (%)	ED (%)
AMLCG [52]	1985	51	33	68	25
CALGB [53]	1987	41	31/45	65	21
CALGB [54]	1991	41	43	69	15
SECSG [55]	1992	53/63	NA	63/79	NA
CALGB [56]	1994	47	31	71	13
BMRC [57]	1996	46	30	73	12
IAMLSG [58]	1997	64[a]	NA	74[a]	NA
SWOG [27]	1997	45	32	NA	NA
SWOG [59]	1998	NA	NA	70	7
MRC: AML10, 11 [23,60]	2001	43	20	59	8
SWOG [61]	2002	34/43	17	NA	NA
ECOG [62]	2004	42	17	NA	NA

CR, complete remission; ED, early death; NA, not available; [a] stratified by age <50 or ≥50 years

significant comorbidities in the elderly [51]. The frequency of early death in younger patients exposed to standard induction chemotherapy has been as high as 10–20%, but it is 20–40% in the elderly. However, treatment-related mortality rates continue to decline as supportive care measures improve with time. In order to increase remission rates and minimize toxicities, various strategies to optimize induction therapy for the elderly have been explored. Some of the studies aimed at improving chemotherapy have utilized less intensive regimens, alternative dosing or choice of anthracyclines, addition of alternative chemotherapies, and use of hematopoietic growth factors both as priming and as supportive care. Finally, several new targeted agents have been explored for the treatment of patients unable to tolerate standard intensive therapy, or in the salvage chemotherapy setting.

Supportive care versus induction chemotherapy

Given the high treatment-related mortality and suboptimal response to chemotherapy, several groups in the 1980s evaluated the benefit of induction chemotherapy in elderly patients with AML [63–65]. However, only one study by the EORTC was designed prospectively and provided a basis for further studies of intensive chemotherapy in elderly patients [65]. In this trial, elderly AML patients who were randomized to supportive care achieved a median overall survival of 11 weeks, versus a 22-week median survival for those receiving intensive chemotherapy. This study confirmed that elderly patients have an improved survival with intensive chemotherapy when compared to supportive care alone.

Induction chemotherapy

A standard regimen for induction chemotherapy in elderly AML patients is cytarabine 100 mg/m^2 by continuous intravenous infusion (CIVI) over seven days with daunorubicin 45–60 mg/m^2 daily for three days (7 + 3 regimen). In order to identify a more effective induction regimen with additional agents, the Medical Research Council (MRC) AML11 trial randomized over 1000 elderly patients to two cycles of one of three regimens: daunorubicin, cytarabine, thioguanine (DAT) vs. cytarabine, daunorubicin, etoposide (ADE) vs. mitoxantrone and cytarabine (MAC) [25]. Patients receiving DAT experienced a statistically significant improvement in CR when compared to ADE or MAC, although five-year overall survival rates were similar in all three induction groups. Given these results, it is reasonable to conclude that the addition of thioguanine can improve CR rates in the elderly, although no benefits are seen with respect to survival.

The anthracycline idarubicin has been shown in studies with younger patients to have modestly superior CR rates, although also without clear benefits in overall survival [55,66].

Multiple groups have investigated the benefits of mitoxantrone or idarubicin in older patients, with variable improvements in remission rates. A large randomized controlled trial by ECOG was recently reported evaluating the optimal choice of anthracycline [62]. Over 350 AML patients older than 55 years received cytarabine in addition to one of three anthracyclines: idarubicin $12\,mg/m^2$ (IA) vs. daunorubicin $45\,mg/m^2$ (DA) vs. mitoxantrone $12\,mg/m^2$ (MA). In the subset of patients aged 55–70, there was a significant improvement in CR with idarubicin, but this benefit diminished in patients over the age of 70. Furthermore, there was no significant difference between the three regimens with respect to disease-free survival (DFS) or overall survival (OS). Given the lack of clear benefit in survival with other anthracyclines, daunorubicin remains the standard anthracycline of choice in elderly patients when given with cytarabine.

The optimal dose of daunorubicin in elderly patients has been heavily investigated, with most doses ranging from $30\,mg/m^2$ to $60\,mg/m^2$ for 1–4 days. While it is difficult to make direct comparisons among various studies, a large metanalysis of over 2000 patients found a clear benefit in terms of CR rates and five-year DFS for patients who received at least $90\,mg/m^2$ total dose of anthracycline [67]. The incidence of early death in these two groups was essentially identical. Hence there is no clear benefit to reducing the daunorubicin dose in the elderly.

With a goal of minimizing treatment-related morbidity and mortality, less intensive chemotherapy regimens have also been explored [61,68,69]. In a large phase III SWOG study comparing the standard therapy of daunorubicin and cytarabine with mitoxantrone and etoposide, the non-cytarabine arm was inferior with lower CR rates and lower two-year OS [61]. Furthermore, a less intensive regimen of oral idarubicin and etoposide resulted in a 36% CR rate in elderly patients who would not otherwise receive standard therapy [70]. Another minimally toxic regimen consists of low-dose cytarabine $10\,mg/m^2$ subcutaneously, twice a day for 7–14 days, in addition to etoposide $100\,mg$ daily for 3 days and either low-dose mitoxantrone or 6-thioguanine. A 50% CR rate was reported with this well-tolerated protocol [71]. Cytarabine as a single agent has also been used in the treatment of elderly AML patients unable to receive standard chemotherapy. When compared to hydroxyurea (Hydrea), there was a significant improvement in CR rates and OS [72]. For patients with comorbidities precluding the use of intensive chemotherapy, a low-dose therapy regimen may be a reasonable alternative to offer patients. However, given the data supporting the use of intensive chemotherapy in "fit" elderly patients, they should not be recommended universally to patients older than age 60.

Growth factors

Leukemic blasts of elderly patients with AML are more commonly resistant to standard chemotherapy, as evidenced by inferior remission rates. Priming of the leukemia with growth factors, such as granulocyte colony-stimulating factor (G-CSF) or granulocyte-monocyte colony-stimulating factor (GM-CSF), has been of interest to several groups [62,73]. Both G-CSF and GM-CSF have been shown to alter the cell-cycle kinetics of the leukemia blasts, rendering them more susceptible to agents such as cytarabine, which has cell-cycle-dependent cytotoxicity [74]. In younger patients, the addition of G-CSF to induction chemotherapy with idarubicin and cytarabine, followed by amascrine and cytarabine, resulted in significant improvements in DFS and OS [73]. However, a large ECOG study revealed no CR or survival benefit from GM-CSF priming in elderly AML patients given just prior to induction chemotherapy [62]. It appears unlikely that growth-factor priming has any benefit in leukemia outcomes, but delays in the initiation of induction chemotherapy may adversely affect CR rates.

A more common use of growth factors, both in clinical trials and in standard practice, has been in the post-chemotherapy stage of treatment. There is generally a two- to three-week delay in the recovery of neutrophil number following the completion of chemotherapy, and elderly patients in particular are at high risk for severe infection and early death. One complicating factor has been the theoretical concern that growth-factor use would stimulate residual leukemia cells to proliferate, thus limiting the effectiveness of induction therapy. Preclinical studies have supported this theory with the finding that G-CSF and GM-CSF can upregulate procaspase protein levels in leukemia cell lines, further promoting cell survival and proliferation [74]. Several groups have investigated the use of growth factors on various days following the completion of chemotherapy, and there has been no evidence of inferior clinical outcome [25,60,67,75,76]. With the use of G-CSF or GM-CSF following induction, there have been reports of a two- to six-day improvement in neutrophil recovery time. In some studies, this has resulted in fewer hospitalization days and reduced incidence of severe infections. However, only one study to date has reported an improved overall survival with the use of GM-CSF [76]. Given the current evidence, the use of growth-factor support after induction chemotherapy is unlikely to be harmful and may reduce the number of days the patient remains neutropenic and thus susceptible to severe infections.

Multi-drug resistance gene

Leukemia cells that overexpress Pgp have clearly been shown via in-vitro model systems to demonstrate resistance to cytotoxic chemotherapy [48].

The ability to effectively block Pgp export of anthracyclines might be of considerable benefit to elderly AML patients, who frequently express this phenotype [27]. SWOG conducted a trial using placebo vs. cyclosporine A (CsA), a potent competitive Pgp inhibitor, in conjunction with sequential cytarabine and infusional daunorubicin [49]. The results from over 200 adult AML patients indicated that there was a significant reduction in the amount of resistant disease in the patients who received CsA with chemotherapy in comparison to placebo (31% vs. 47%). Although there was no difference in CR rate between the two arms, CsA-treated patients had modestly improved DFS and OS. Unfortunately, other trials utilizing Pgp inhibitors have not yielded positive results [50,77,78], so this strategy remains investigational. However, because of the high prevalence of the MDR1 phenotype in the elderly population, there is continued investigation into the use of more potent and specific inhibitors of Pgp function.

Consolidation

The majority of older adult patients with AML will experience relapse of their disease, with only 0–20% of elderly patients achieving long-term survival (Fig. 19.2) [24]. Given this dismal prognosis, attempts to reduce the risk of relapse with consolidation chemotherapy, maintenance therapy, and transplant have been explored. Younger patients with good or intermediate prognosis have shown clear benefit with one to four cycles of high-dose cytarabine, although the optimal number of cycles has not yet been defined [56]. Unfortunately, no standard consolidation regimen has been identified in elderly patients, owing in part to the resistant nature of their disease and also to relative intolerance of high-dose chemotherapy. The majority of studies have utilized one or two courses of the same regimen that was used in induction, or an intermediate dose of cytarabine, with resultant long-term survival rates in the range of 10–15% [61,62,68,75]. There has been no clear evidence to date that a more prolonged consolidation phase will improve clinical outcome.

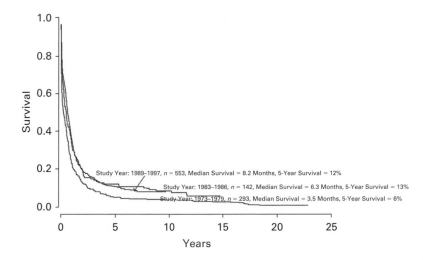

Figure 19.2 Patients >55 years with newly diagnosed AML treated on Eastern Cooperative Oncology Group (ECOG) protocols since 1973. From Appelbaum *et al.*, *Hematology Am Soc Hematol Educ Program* 2001; 62–86 [80].

In the MRC AML11 trial, elderly patients were randomized to shorter (3) or longer (6) courses of combination chemotherapy as consolidation [25]. No improvements were seen with respect to DFS or OS in patients treated on the longer chemotherapy regimen. Furthermore, there have been no randomized studies indicating that there is a benefit of additional chemotherapy beyond cytarabine alone. When single-agent cytarabine (100 mg/m^2 CIVI for 7 days) was compared to cytarabine (500 mg/m^2 every 12 hours for 6 doses) and mitoxantrone (5 mg/m^2 every 12 hours for 6 doses) in elderly AML patients in complete remission, there was no improvement with respect to leukemic relapse or overall survival with the addition of anthracycline [79].

The optimal regimen of consolidation cytarabine for adult patients with AML was investigated by the Cancer and Leukemia Group B (CALGB). Over 1000 patients received standard induction chemotherapy with daunorubicin and cytarabine, and were randomized upon confirmation of remission to one of three chemotherapy arms: cytarabine 100 mg/m^2 CIVI for 5 days (low dose) vs. cytarabine 400 mg/m^2 CIVI for 5 days (intermediate dose) vs. cytarabine 3 g/m^2 given every 12 hours on days 1, 3, and 5 (high dose) [56]. For patients younger than 60, DFS was superior in the high-dose arm. However, in the elderly patients, there was no significant difference

between arms. This finding was related in part to the poor tolerability of the high-dose cytarabine in the elderly cohort, with the main adverse event being neurotoxicity. As a result, high-dose cytarabine cannot be routinely recommended as consolidation therapy for patients older than 60. Strategies utilizing an intermediate dose of cytarabine have shown acceptable tolerability, but still with disappointingly low DFS rates [62,81]. Thus there is no established standard consolidation regimen for elderly patients. Post-remission therapy must be tailored to the individual patient, taking into consideration associated comorbidities and demonstrated tolerance to induction chemotherapy. One to two cycles of intermediate-dose cytarabine or repeated cycles of combination chemotherapy represent reasonable options.

Maintenance chemotherapy

Over the last few decades, various maintenance therapies have been investigated as post-remission therapy in elderly patients with AML. Interferon, interleukin 2 (IL-2), low-dose cytarabine, and combination chemotherapy are some of the treatments that have been administered for various lengths of time post-consolidation [25,56,60,62,82]. Unfortunately, in studies that have compared maintenance therapy to placebo in the elderly, they have been unsuccessful in reducing the risk of relapse or improving OS [25,60]. It is clear that post-remission therapy in elderly patients needs to be optimized, as the majority of those that achieve CR will ultimately relapse.

Transplant

Older adults are under-represented in transplantation trials in AML, making it difficult to predict survival and treatment-related mortality (TRM) rates. Historically, patients older than 55 or 60 were not considered to be eligible for transplant, because of concerns of early death or debilitating morbidity. However, there have been substantial changes in transplantation protocols over the last decade, with the use of more tolerable conditioning regimens, substitution of peripheral-blood progenitor cells (PBPC) for bone-marrow cells in transplant, and improved supportive care measures.

Autologous transplant in the elderly has been studied in a small feasibility study including 19 patients between the ages of 60 and 70 after induction chemotherapy and one cycle of consolidation [83]. While only two toxic deaths were reported as a result of transplantation, 14 of the 19 patients experienced early relapse following autologous transplant. Conversely, a large retrospective review of 193 patients between the ages of 60 and 75 who underwent autologous transplantation between 1984 and 1998 in first complete remission (CR1) did demonstrate a 47% three-year overall survival, suggesting a possible benefit to aggressive post-remission therapy [84]. However, TRM was significant at 15%. The European Bone Marrow Transplant group published a similar experience in 111 patients between the ages of 50 and 60 who underwent allografting in CR1 [85]. The four-year leukemia-free survival was also promising at 34%, but the TRM remained substantial at 28%. Hence it appears that while autografting for AML in older adults potentially promotes extended survival, severe regimen-related toxicity remains a barrier to optimal outcomes.

While outcomes have been generally poor for ablative allogeneic transplants in the elderly [86], somewhat more promising outcomes may be seen with non-myeloablative and reduced-intensity allogeneic regimens [87–89]. Reduced-intensity strategies have been employed to take advantage of the T-cell-mediated graft versus leukemia (GVL) effect without the added toxicity of high-dose chemotherapy. In a small study of 19 elderly patients with active leukemia, reduced-intensity conditioning regimen followed by allogeneic stem-cell transplant resulted in an overall one-year survival of 68% and one-year non-relapse mortality of 22% [88]. Non-myeloablative regimens have produced similarly promising outcomes, with relatively low TRM and favorable one-year survival rates [87,90]. However, reduced-intensity and non-myeloablative regimens have significant relapse rates. Larger, prospective multicenter trials are needed to further elucidate the benefit of allogeneic transplant in the elderly [91]. While transplant cannot be routinely recommended for elderly patients with AML, further investigation of reduced-intensity allogeneic regimens or autologous transplant is warranted.

Salvage chemotherapy

The majority of elderly patients with AML who achieve CR will eventually relapse, and salvage therapy thus becomes an option for many of these patients. Unfortunately, response rates with subsequent chemotherapy drop precipitously, with the remission rates in most studies ranging from 10% to 80% [92–94]. The large variability in response is essentially due to various prognostic factors, such as the length of first remission and cytogenetics. The most important predictor of response to salvage therapy is the length of the patient's CR1. For remissions lasting at least one year, CR rates of 40–60% can be expected, in contrast to a 10–20% CR rate for those patients who have refractory disease or shorter remission durations [92,93,95,96]. Because of the unfavorable outcomes, salvage chemotherapy is often used as a bridge to allogeneic transplant once a second or third CR is achieved. This is usually not a viable option for the vast majority of patients over the age of 60. There is, however, a small portion of patients (approximately 10–15%) who can survive long term following a second remission induction, thus making salvage therapy alone a reasonable option for elderly patients [93]. Multiple chemotherapy regimens have been used in this setting, but there is no clear optimal choice for second-line treatment.

Cytarabine-based regimens remain the most commonly administered of the salvage protocols. For patients with an initial remission duration greater than one year, cytarabine alone or in combination with other drugs can significantly improve OS when compared to those who received investigational agents [93]. The same is not true for patients with short CR1 or refractory disease. The addition of an anthracycline to high-dose cytarabine can improve rates of second CR and length of disease-free survival, especially in patients who exhibit resistance to cytarabine alone [97]. When etoposide is used concurrently with cytarabine and an anthracycline (idarubicin) as salvage therapy in refractory/relapsed AML, comparable remission rates are seen (40%) with reasonable toxicity profiles [98]. A randomized phase III trial that explored the benefit of adding etoposide to high-dose cytarabine did reveal an improvement in remission duration (11.9 months vs. 25 months); however, there was no difference in OS, and the effect was diminished in patients over the age of 50 [99]. The combination of mitoxantrone, etoposide, and cytarabine is a commonly used treatment strategy, generally producing CR rates of 40–80% with a favorable toxicity profile [94,100]. The addition of purine analogs to cytarabine has also produced promising results in relapsed or refractory patients. Cytarabine and G-CSF with 2-chlorodeoxyadenosine (2-CdA), or the CLAG regimen, has produced CR rates of approximately 50% for patients initially unsuccessful with standard induction therapy [101,102]. The FLAG regimen, which is composed of fludarabine, cytarabine, and G-CSF, similarly has resulted in CR rates of 50–70% for the treatment of AML and high-risk MDS in the first-line setting [103,104]. Fludarabine with cytarabine in the relapsed/refractory setting has a reported CR rate of 36% [105].

Non-cytarabine regimens have also been investigated in the salvage setting. This is of particular interest to the elderly population, given the higher incidence of neurotoxicity associated with this drug in patients over age 60. For example, continuous infusion of carboplatin has modest activity as salvage therapy in AML, with complete response rates of 7–16% being reported [106].

The only new agent to gain FDA approval in the past several years for the treatment of AML is gemtuzumab ozogamicin (GO; Mylotarg). GO is a humanized monoclonal antibody directed against CD33, which is present on myeloid blast cells in over 80% of patients with AML, and is conjugated to an anti-tumor antibiotic, calicheamicin. Approved for the treatment of older adults with AML in first relapse, this drug has a reported CR rate of 26%, but carries the risks of prolonged myelosuppression and hepatic veno-occlusive disease [107].

Novel therapies

Acute leukemia in the elderly has a distinct disease biology, more commonly arising from myelodysplasia or secondary to cytotoxic chemotherapy. As a result, cytogenetic and other molecular abnormalities are frequently associated, leading to an inherent resistance to our standard drugs. As specific molecular abnormalities are identified in leukemic blast cells, i.e., FLT3-ITD, *Ras* proto-oncogene, and MDR1, novel therapies are developed to target these abnormalities. For example, multiple small-molecule tyrosine kinase inhibitors of FLT3 are currently under investigation. Phase I and II trials with agents such as CEP-70, PKC, and SU11248 have shown promise, with hematologic and bone-marrow responses in patients with refractory or recurrent AML and documented activating mutations [108–110]. These drugs are generally well tolerated, and may eventually prove to be especially useful in AML, when combined with standard chemotherapeutic agents.

Another promising class of drugs for the treatment of AML are the farnesyl transferase inhibitors (FTIs). Farnesyl transferase is an enzyme that catalyzes a 15-carbon farnesyl group to Ras, which is a process that is required for Ras to attach to the cell membrane. Ras, in its membrane-bound form, will then initiate phosphorylation of several downstream proteins, such as Raf, Mek1, and ERKs, leading to the promotion of cell proliferation and survival [44]. Tipifarnib, an orally bioavailable inhibitor of farnesyl transferase, is currently under active investigation in several settings. Significant activity was confirmed in a multi-center phase II trial involving elderly patients with untreated poor-risk AML or high-risk MDS who were not otherwise candidates for standard induction therapy [111]. A complete response rate of 17% was seen, with additional patients achieving partial response, hematologic improvement, or stable disease. Interestingly, CRs were maintained for more than six months, and achievement of CR appeared to correlate with extended survival. Such responses were observed even in the 75-plus age group, a population that often receives supportive care or low-dose chemotherapy as sole treatment. New strategies currently under development include the use of FTIs as maintenance therapy as well as in combination with cytotoxic chemotherapy.

Hypomethylating agents have acquired new interest in recent years, although initial studies with these drugs in leukemia began three decades ago [112]. Hypermethylation of DNA is an important event in carcinogenesis and leads to epigenetic silencing of tumor suppressor genes [113]. 5-Azacitidine is a DNA methyltransferase inhibitor that can cause direct tumor cell cytotoxicty through inhibition of thymidylate synthase, and it causes hypomethylation of DNA with resultant inhibition of DNA, RNA, and protein synthesis [113]. It was recently approved for the treatment of MDS, notably with an ability to delay the transformation to AML by a median of eight months [114]. Small phase I/II studies in AML or MDS/AML have shown overall response rates in the range of 50%, with reasonable toxicity profiles [115,116]. In the same family of agents is 5-aza-2′-deoxycytidine, or decitabine, which forms an irreversible bond with DNA methyltransferase leading to gene hypomethylation and subsequent reactivation of silenced genes [113]. Decitabine was investigated in a recent phase I trial of refractory AML or MDS, revealing a 65% overall response rate with acceptable toxicity [117]. Larger studies are needed to confirm these results, but hypomethylating agents show considerable promise in the treatment of poor-risk AML or AML/MDS.

Monoclonal antibodies have been studied in various hematologic malignancies, with gemtuzumab being the only FDA-approved agent for the treatment of AML in this class. Bevacizumab is a monoclonal antibody to vascular endothelial growth factor (VEGF), which has demonstrated activity in a number of solid tumors. Furthermore, this agent has shown activity when combined with chemotherapy in a variety of hematologic malignancies, including early studies in AML. Studies of bone-marrow stroma from acute leukemia show that there is increased evidence of angiogenesis when compared to normal marrows, and that the vessel density actually decreases when clinical response to chemotherapy is seen [118,119]. A phase I/II clinical trial using bevacuzimab in combination with mitoxantrone and 1-β-D-arabinofuranosylcytosine (AraC) has been reported in patients with relapsed or refractory AML. A single 10 mg/kg dose of bevacuzimab was administered on day 8 following a 72-hour infusion of AraC and mitoxantrone 40 mg/m^2 on day 4. Over half of the patients were refractory to one or more previous chemotherapies and the majority of patients presented with adverse cytogenetic features. Despite these poor-risk features, the overall response rate was 48%, with 33% of patients achieving a CR. However, significant toxicities were noted and were primarily cardiovascular, with reports of diminished ejection fraction and cerebrovascular bleeding. Future studies in AML with this drug or others that target VEGF and other angiogenic markers will likely further define the benefit of this therapeutic approach.

Treatment of the 70-plus age group

Largely under-represented in the majority of leukemia trials, patients over the age of 70 make up approximately one-third of the adult leukemia population [82]. The most commonly cited reason for clinical-trial exclusion in leukemia was age and comorbidity [2]. Thus it is difficult to extrapolate outcomes from the few elderly AML trials that exist to those patients who have significant comorbidities or who are beyond the age of 70. Additionally, this cohort of patients rarely receive standard induction chemotherapy due to age alone, functional status, comorbid conditions, or the perceived benefits of therapy [82,120]. In a review of Medicare claims between 1991 and 1996 of patients with AML over the age of 65, only 30% received induction chemotherapy [121]. For those patients who did receive intensive chemotherapy, there was a six-month improvement in median survival and a 21% improvement in one-year OS. A retrospective analysis from France compared the outcomes of patients over the age of 75 who received standard induction chemotherapy, low-dose palliative chemotherapy, or supportive care alone to patients between the ages of 65 and 74 who were treated during the same period [122]. For those over 75 receiving an anthracycline-based regimen, CR and OS rates were not significantly different from those achieved by the under-75 age group, and they are also comparable to those obtained in previous studies of intensive chemotherapy in an elderly population over the age of 60 years [23,55,61,62,73,123].

Nonetheless, treatment-related mortality remains high for elderly patients, and as patients become older than 70 they are much less likely to tolerate intensive chemotherapy. There are no strict guidelines for an age "cutoff," and treatment decisions should be based on the individual patient. However, the M. D. Anderson experience suggests that patients older than 80 should not receive standard induction chemotherapy [124]. This is based on a single institutional experience with 30 patients over age 80 treated between 1980 and 1994 with induction chemotherapy consisting of an anthracycline alone, anthracycline plus cytarabine, or fludarabine with cytarabine. The median survival of these treated patients was a mere 3–4 weeks, with only two patients surviving beyond one year. For the nine patients who achieved CR, eight died in remission or from relapse at a median of 11 weeks. This is in comparison to a 10-week median survival of age-matched controls older than 80 years who did not receive induction therapy. As a result, it is reasonable to consider palliative chemotherapy, supportive care, or clinical trial as an option for all patients over the age of 80 [124,125].

Prognosis

Elderly patients with AML demonstrate consistently inferior outcomes when compared to their younger counterparts. Five-year OS rates for patients greater than age 60 range from less than 5% to as high as 30%, with median survival reported between 6 and 12 months [24,25,29,121,126]. This is due, in large part, to a higher prevalence of adverse cytogenetic features, which remains the most powerful prognostic indicator of response to standard therapeutic strategies. A review of elderly patients treated on CALGB protocols between 1984 and 1999 reported a five-year OS for patients with complex karyotype, rare chromosomal aberrations, and core binding factor leukemias of 0%, 0%, and 19.4% respectively [29]. Similarly, Appelbaum *et al.* reported outcomes on elderly patients treated on SWOG protocols, and within each prognostic category of favorable, intermediate, or poor cytogenetic features, long-term survival continued to deteriorate with increasing age [24]. Aside from karyotype, functional status, lactate dehydrogenase level, leukocyte count, MDR1 expression, and secondary AML have also been identified as independent factors that can negatively impact prognosis and are more frequently encountered in older adults [24,25,27,126]. Early death with standard induction, in particular, is highly dependent on poor performance status at leukemia diagnosis in elderly patients [24]. While the molecular phenotype of NPM1-mutated/FLT3-ITD wild-type has been associated with a favorable prognosis in younger patients with cytogenetically normal AML, the significance of these and other molecular abnormalities in older adults has yet to be defined. Thus, elderly patients with adverse prognostic factors such as complex karyotype or poor performance status should be strongly considered for investigational strategies in order to improve long-term outcomes and minimize toxicity.

Conclusion

AML remains an incurable disease for the vast majority of patients diagnosed with this hematologic malignancy. Standard chemotherapy regimens offer inferior rates of CR and long-term survival in elderly patients as compared to their younger counterparts. A higher prevalence of adverse prognostic features is largely responsible for these unfavorable rates of survival. The decision to offer standard induction or post-remission chemotherapies should be based on patient preference, karyotype, performance status, and other prognostic factors. Further investigation of the molecular abnormalities such as FLT-3, NPM1, and MDR1 in older patients, may eventually help stratify patients regarding therapeutic decisions, and provide molecular targets for novel agents. Strong consideration should be given to clinical trial participation for elderly patients, in order to improve outcomes for this population.

REFERENCES

1. Hutchins LF, Unger JM, Crowley JJ, Coltman CA Jr, Albain KS. Underrepresentation of patients 65 years of age or older in cancer-treatment trials. *N Engl J Med* 1999; **341**: 2061–7.

2. Mengis C, Aebi S, Tobler A, Dahler W, Fey MF. Assessment of differences in patient populations selected for excluded from participation in clinical phase III acute myelogenous leukemia trials. *J Clin Oncol* 2003; **21**: 3933–9.

3. Baudard M, Marie JP, Cadiou M, Viguie F, Zittoun R. Acute myelogenous leukaemia in the elderly: retrospective study of 235 consecutive patients. *Br J Haematol* 1994; **86**: 82–91.

4. Yancik R. Cancer burden in the aged: an epidemiologic and demographic overview. *Cancer* 1997; **80**: 1273–83.

5. Piccirillo JF, Tierney RM, Costas I, Grove L, Spitznagel EL Jr. Prognostic importance of comorbidity in a hospital-based cancer registry. *JAMA* 2004; **291**: 2441–7.

6. Taylor PR, Reid MM, Stark AN, Bown N, Hamilton PJ, Proctor SJ. De novo acute myeloid leukaemia in patients over 55-years-old: a population-based study of incidence, treatment and outcome. Northern Region Haematology Group. *Leukemia* 1995; **9**: 231–7.

7. AML Incidence 1969–2002, T.U.S. National Cancer Institute, DCCPS, Surveillance Research Program, Cancer Statistics Branch. Surveillance, Epidemiology, and End Results (SEER), April 2005. www.seer.cancer.gov. Accessed August 1, 2006.

8. Schnatter AR, Nicolich MJ, Bird MG. Determination of leukemogenic benzene exposure concentrations: refined analyses of the Pliofilm cohort. *Risk Anal* 1996; **16**: 833–40.

9. Smith MT, Zhang L, Wang Y, *et al*. Increased translocations and aneusomy in chromosomes 8 and 21 among workers exposed to benzene. *Cancer Res* 1998; **58**: 2176–81.

10. Groves FD, Linet MS, Devesa SS. Epidemiology of leukemia: overview and patterns of occurrence. In Henderson ES, Lister TA, Greaves MF, eds, *Leukemia*, 6th edn (Cambridge, MA: Saunders, 1996), 145–59.

11. Moloney WC. Radiogenic leukemia revisited. *Blood* 1987; **70**: 905–8.

12. Sandler D. Epidemiology of acute myelogenous leukemia. *Semin Oncol* 1987; **14**: 359–64.

13. Pedersen-Bjergaard J, Andersen MK, Christiansen DH. Therapy-related acute myeloid leukemia and myelodysplasia after high-dose chemotherapy and autologous stem cell transplantation. *Blood* 2000; **95**: 3273–9.

14. Pedersen-Bjergaard J, Philip P. Balanced translocations involving chromosome bands 11q23 and 21q22 are highly characteristic of myelodysplasia and leukemia following therapy with cytostatic agents targeting at DNA-topoisomerase II. *Blood* 1991; **78**: 1147–8.

15. Pedersen-Bjergaard J, Philip P, Larsen SO, Jensen G, Byrsting K. Chromosome aberrations and prognostic factors in therapy-related myelodysplasia and acute nonlymphocytic leukemia. *Blood* 1990; **76**: 1083–91.

16. Smith SM, Le Beau MM, Huo D, *et al*. Clinical-cytogenetic associations in 306 patients with therapy-related myelodysplasia and myeloid leukemia: the University of Chicago series. *Blood* 2003; **102**: 43–52.

17. van Leeuwen FE, Chorus AM, van den Belt-Dusebout AW, *et al*. Leukemia risk following Hodgkin's disease: relation to cumulative dose of alkylating agents,

treatment with teniposide combinations, number of episodes of chemotherapy, and bone marrow damage. *J Clin Oncol* 1994; **12**: 1063–73.

18. Sterkers Y, Preudhomme C, Lai JL, *et al.* Acute myeloid leukemia and myelodysplastic syndromes following essential thrombocythemia treated with hydroxyurea: high proportion of cases with 17p deletion. *Blood* 1998; **91**: 616–22.

19. Friedberg JW, Neuberg D, Stone RM, *et al.* Outcome in patients with myelodysplastic syndrome after autologous bone marrow transplantation for non-Hodgkin's lymphoma. *J Clin Oncol* 1999; **17**: 3128–35.

20. Sandler DP, Shore DL, Anderson JR, *et al.* Cigarette smoking and risk of acute leukemia: associations with morphology and cytogenetic abnormalities in bone marrow. *J Natl Cancer Inst* 1993; **85**: 1994–2003.

21. Vardiman JW, Harris NL, Brunning RD. The World Health Organization (WHO) classification of the myeloid neoplasms. *Blood* 2002; **100**: 2292–302.

22. Brunning RD, Matutes E, Harris NL, *et al.* Acute myeloid leukaemia. In Jaffe ES, Harris NL, Stein H, Vardiman JW, eds, *World Health Organization Classification of Tumours* (Lyon: IARC Press, 2001), 75–107.

23. Grimwade D, Walker H, Harrison G, *et al.* The predictive value of hierarchical cytogenetic classification in older adults with acute myeloid leukemia (AML): analysis of 1065 patients entered into the United Kingdom Medical Research Council AML11 trial. *Blood* 2001; **98**: 1312–20.

24. Appelbaum F, Gundacker H, Head D, *et al.* Age and acute myeloid leukemia. *Blood* 2006; **107**: 3481–5.

25. Goldstone AH, Burnett AK, Wheatley K, *et al.* Attempts to improve treatment outcomes in acute myeloid leukemia (AML) in older patients: the results of the United Kingdom Medical Research Council AML11 trial. *Blood* 2001; **98**: 1302–11.

26. Lowenberg B. Post-remission treatment of acute myelogenous leukemia. *N Engl J Med* 1995; **332**: 260–2.

27. Leith CP, Kopecky KJ, Godwin J, *et al.* Acute myeloid leukemia in the elderly: assessment of multidrug resistance (MDR1) and cytogenetics distinguishes biologic subgroups with remarkably distinct responses to standard chemotherapy: a Southwest Oncology Group study. *Blood* 1997; **89**: 3323–9.

28. Libura J, Slater DJ, Felix CA, Richardson C. Therapy-related acute myeloid leukemia-like MLL rearrangements are induced by etoposide in primary human CD34+ cells and remain stable after clonal expansion. *Blood* 2005; **105**: 2124–31.

29. Farag S, Archer K, Mrozek K, *et al.* Pretreatment cytogenetics add to other prognostic factors predicting complete remission and long-term outcome in patients 60 years of age or older with acute myeloid leukemia: results from Cancer and Leukemia Group B 8461. *Blood* 2006; **108**: 63–73.

30. Slovak ML, Kopecky KJ, Cassileth PA, *et al.* Karyotypic analysis predicts outcome of preremission and post-remission therapy in adult acute myeloid leukemia: a Southwest Oncology Group/Eastern Cooperative Oncology Group study. *Blood* 2000; **96**: 4075–83.

31. Wolman SR, Gundacker H, Appelbaum FR, *et al.* Impact of trisomy 8 (+8) on clinical presentation, treatment response, and survival in acute myeloid leukemia: a Southwest Oncology Group study. *Blood* 2002; **100**: 29–35.

32. Thiede C, Steudel C, Mohr B, *et al.* Analysis of FLT3-activating mutations in 979 patients with acute myelogenous leukemia: association with FAB subtypes and identification of subgroups with poor prognosis. *Blood* 2002; **99**: 4326–35.

33. Schnittger S, Schoch C, Dugas M, *et al.* Analysis of FLT3 length mutations in 1003 patients with acute myeloid leukemia: correlation to cytogenetics, FAB subtype, and prognosis in the AMLCG study and usefulness as a marker for the detection of minimal residual disease. *Blood* 2002; **100**: 59–66.

34. Nakao M, Yokota S, Iwai T, *et al.* Internal tandem duplication of the flt3 gene found in acute myeloid leukemia. *Leukemia* 1996; **10**: 1911–18.

35. Yamamoto Y, Kiyoi H, Nakano Y, *et al.* Activating mutation of D835 within the activation loop of FLT3 in human hematologic malignancies. *Blood* 2001; **97**: 2434–9.

36. Mizuki M, Fenski R, Halfter H, *et al.* Flt3 mutations from patients with acute myeloid leukemia induce transformation of 32D cells mediated by the Ras and STAT5 pathways. *Blood* 2000; **96**: 3907–14.

37. Frohling S, Schlenk RF, Breitruck J, *et al.* Prognostic significance of activating FLT3 mutations in younger adults (16 to 60 years) with acute myeloid leukemia and normal cytogenetics: a study of the AML Study Group Ulm. *Blood* 2002; **100**: 4372–80.

38. Kiyoi H, Naoe T, Nakano Y, *et al.* Prognostic implication of FLT3 and N-RAS gene mutations in acute myeloid leukemia. *Blood* 1999; **93**: 3074–80.

39. Yanada M, Matsuo K, Suzuki T, Kiyoi H, Naoe T. Prognostic significance of FLT3 internal tandem duplication and tyrosine kinase domain mutations for acute

myeloid leukemia: a meta-analysis. *Leukemia* 2005; **19**: 1345–9.

40. Mrozek K, Bloomfield C. Chromosome aberrations, gene mutations and expression changes, and prognosis in adult acute myeloid leukemia. *Hematology Am Soc Hematol Educ Program* 2006; 169–77.

41. Thiede C, Koch S, Creutzig E, *et al*. Prevalence and prognostic impact of NPM1 mutations in 1485 adult patients with acute myeloid leukemia (AML). *Blood* 2006; **107**: 4011–20.

42. Frohling S, Schlenk RF, Stolze I, *et al*. CEBPA mutations in younger adults with acute myeloid leukemia and normal cytogenetics: prognostic relevance and analysis of cooperating mutations. *J Clin Oncol* 2004; **22**: 624–33.

43. Radich JP, Kopecky KJ, Willman CL, *et al*. N-ras mutations in adult de novo acute myelogenous leukemia: prevalence and clinical significance. *Blood* 1990; **76**: 801–7.

44. Karp JE, Lancet JE, Kaufmann SH, *et al*. Clinical and biologic activity of the farnesyltransferase inhibitor R115777 in adults with refractory and relapsed acute leukemias: a phase 1 clinical-laboratory correlative trial. *Blood* 2001; **97**: 3361–9.

45. Paquette RL, Landaw EM, Pierre RV, *et al*. N-ras mutations are associated with poor prognosis and increased risk of leukemia in myelodysplastic syndrome. *Blood* 1993; **82**: 590–9.

46. Stirewalt DL, Kopecky KJ, Meshinchi S, *et al*. FLT3, RAS, and TP53 mutations in elderly patients with acute myeloid leukemia. *Blood* 2001; **97**: 3589–95.

47. Bowen DT, Frew ME, Hills R, *et al*. RAS mutation in acute myeloid leukemia is associated with distinct cytogenetic subgroups but does not influence outcome in patients <60 yrs. *Blood* 2005; **106**: 2113–19.

48. Chin KV, Pastan I, Gottesman MM, Function and regulation of the human multidrug resistance gene. *Adv Cancer Res* 1993; **60**: 157–80.

49. List AF, Kopecky KJ, Willman CL, *et al*. Benefit of cyclosporine modulation of drug resistance in patients with poor-risk acute myeloid leukemia: a Southwest Oncology Group study. *Blood* 2001; **98**: 3212–20.

50. Baer MR, George SL, Dodge RK, *et al*. Phase 3 study of the multidrug resistance modulator PSC-833 in previously untreated patients 60 years of age and older with acute myeloid leukemia: Cancer and Leukemia Group B Study 9720. *Blood* 2002; **100**: 1224–32.

51. Extermann M, Overcash J, Lyman GH, Parr J, Balducci L. Comorbidity and functional status are independent in older cancer patients. *J Clin Oncol* 1998; **16**: 1582–7.

52. Buchner T, Urbanitz D, Hiddemann W, *et al*. Intensified induction and consolidation with or without maintenance chemotherapy for acute myeloid leukemia (AML): two multicenter studies of the German AML Cooperative Group. *J Clin Oncol* 1985; **3**: 1583–9.

53. Preisler H, Davis R, Kirshner J, *et al*. Comparison of three remission induction regimens and two postinduction strategies for the treatment of acute nonlymphocytic leukemia: a Cancer and Leukemia Group B study. *Blood* 1987; **69**: 1441–9.

54. Dillman R, Davis R, Green M, *et al*. A comparative study of two different doses of cytarabine for acute myeloid leukemia: a phase III trial of the Cancer and Leukemia Group B. *Blood* 1991; **78**: 2520–6.

55. Vogler WR, Velez-Garcia E, Weiner RS, *et al*. A phase III trial comparing idarubicin and daunorubicin in combination with cytarabine in acute myelogenous leukemia: a Southeastern Cancer Study Group study. *J Clin Oncol* 1992; **10**: 1103–11.

56. Mayer RJ, Davis RB, Schiffer CA, *et al*. Intensive postremission chemotherapy in adults with acute myeloid leukemia. *N Engl J Med* 1994; **331**: 896–903.

57. Rees J, Gray R, Wheatley K. Dose intensification in acute myeloid leukaemia: greater effectiveness at lower cost. Principal report of the Medical Research Council's AML9 study. MRC Leukaemia in Adults Working Party. *Br J Haematol* 1996; **94**: 89–98.

58. Heil G, Hoelzer D, Sanz M, *et al*. A randomized, double-blind, placebo-controlled, phase III study of filgrastim in remission induction and consolidation therapy for adults with de novo acute myeloid leukemia. *Blood* 1997; **90**: 4710–18.

59. Cassileth P, Harrington D, Appelbaum F, *et al*. Chemotherapy compared with autologous or allogeneic bone marrow transplantation in the management of acute myeloid leukemia in first remission. *N Engl J Med* 1998; **339**:1649–56.

60. Lowenberg B, Suciu S, Archimbaud E, *et al*. Use of recombinant granulocyte-macrophage colony-stimulating factor during and after remission induction chemotherapy in patients aged 61 years and older with acute myeloid leukemia (AML): Final Report of AML-11, a phase III randomized study of the Leukemia Cooperative Group of European Organization for the Research and Treatment of Cancer (EORTC-LCG) and the Dutch Belgian Hemato-Oncology Cooperative Group (HOVON). *Blood* 1997; **90**: 2952–61.

61. Anderson JE, Kopecky KJ, Willman CL, *et al*. Outcome after induction chemotherapy for older patients with

acute myeloid leukemia is not improved with mitoxantrone and etoposide compared to cytarabine and daunorubicin: a Southwest Oncology Group study. *Blood* 2002; **100**: 3869–76.

62. Rowe JM, Neuberg D, Friedenberg W, *et al*. A phase 3 study of three induction regimens and of priming with GM-CSF in older adults with acute myeloid leukemia: a trial by the Eastern Cooperative Oncology Group. *Blood* 2004; **103**: 479–85.

63. Sebban C, Archimbaud E, Coiffier B, *et al*. Treatment of acute myeloid leukemia in elderly patients. *Cancer* 1981; **61**: 227–31.

64. Keating MJ, McCredie KB, Benjamin RS, *et al*, Treatment of patients over 50 years of age with acute myelogenous leukemia with a combination of rubidazone and cytosine arabinoside, vincristine, and prednisone (ROAP). *Blood* 1981; **58**: 584–91.

65. Lowenberg B, Zittoun R, Kerkhofs H, *et al*. On the value of intensive remission-induction chemotherapy in elderly patients of 65+ years with acute myeloid leukemia: a randomized phase III study of the European Organization for Research and Treatment of Cancer Leukemia Group. *J Clin Oncol* 1989; **7**: 1268–74.

66. Berman E, Heller G, Santorsa J, *et al*. Results of a randomized trial comparing idarubicin and cytosine arabinoside with daunorubicin and cytosine arabinoside in adult patients with newly diagnosed acute myelogenous leukemia. *Blood* 1991; **77**: 1666–74.

67. Hiddemann W, Kern W, Schoch C, *et al*. Management of acute myeloid leukemia in elderly patients. *J Clin Oncol* 1999; **17**: 3569–76.

68. Liu Yin JA, Johnson PR, Davies JM, Flanagan NG, Gorst DW, Lewis MJ. Mitozantrone and cytosine arabinoside as first-line therapy in elderly patients with acute myeloid leukaemia. *Br J Haematol* 1991; **79**: 415–20.

69. Leoni F, Ciolli S, Giuliani G, *et al*. Attenuated-dose idarubicin in acute myeloid leukaemia of the elderly: pharmacokinetic study and clinical results. Br J Haematol 1995; **90**: 169–74.

70. Jackson GH, Taylor PR, Iqbal A, *et al*. The use of an all oral chemotherapy (idarubicin and etoposide) in the treatment of acute myeloid leukemia in the elderly: A report of toxicity and efficacy. *Leukemia* 1997; **11**: 1193–6.

71. Manoharan A, Baker RI, Kyle PW. Low-dose combination chemotherapy for acute myeloid leukemia in elderly patients: A novel approach. *Am J Hematol* 1997; **55**: 115–17.

72. Burnett AK, Milligan DW, Prentice AG *et al*. Low dose ara-C versus hydroxyurea with or without retinoid in older patients not considered fit for intensive chemotherapy: the UK NCRI AML14 trial. ASH Annual Meeting Abstracts. *Blood* 2004; **104**: abstract 872.

73. Lowenberg B, van Putten W, Theobald M, *et al*. Effect of priming with granulocyte colony-stimulating factor on the outcome of chemotherapy for acute myeloid leukemia. *N Engl J Med* 2003; **349**: 743–52.

74. Faderl S, Harris D, Van Q, Kantarjian HM, Talpaz M, Estrov Z. Granulocyte-macrophage colony-stimulating factor (GM-CSF) induces antiapoptotic and proapoptotic signals in acute myeloid leukemia. *Blood* 2003; **102**: 630–7.

75. Stone RM, Berg DT, George SL, *et al*. Granulocyte-macrophage colony-stimulating factor after initial chemotherapy for elderly patients with primary acute myelogenous leukemia. *N Engl J Med* 1995; **332**: 1671–7.

76. Rowe JM, Andersen JW, Mazza JJ, *et al*. A randomized placebo-controlled phase III study of granulocyte-macrophage colony-stimulating factor in adult patients (>55 to 70 years of age) with acute myelogenous leukemia: a study of the Eastern Cooperative Oncology Group (E1490). *Blood* 1995; **86**: 457–62.

77. Ross DD, Joneckis CC, Schiffer CA. Effects of verapamil on in vitro intracellular accumulation and retention of daunorubicin in blast cells from patients with acute nonlymphocytic leukemia. *Blood* 1986; **68**: 83–8.

78. Solary E, Drenou B, Campos L, *et al*. Quinine as a multidrug resistance inhibitor: a phase 3 multicentric randomized study in adult de novo acute myelogenous leukemia. *Blood* 2003; **102**: 1202–10.

79. Stone RM, Berg DT, George SL, *et al*. Postremission therapy in older patients with de novo acute myeloid leukemia: a randomized trial comparing mitoxantrone and intermediate-dose cytarabine with standard-dose cytarabine. *Blood* 2001; **98**: 548–53.

80. Appelbaum FR, Rowe JM, Radich J, Dick JE. Acute myeloid leukemia. *Hematology Am Soc Hematol Educ Program* 2001; 62–86.

81. Sperr WR, Piribauer M, Wimazal F, *et al*. A novel effective and safe consolidation for patients over 60 years with acute myeloid leukemia: Intermediate dose cytarabine (2×1 g/m^2 on days 1, 3, and 5). *Clin Cancer Res* 2004; **10**: 3965–71.

82. Ferrara F, Annunziata M, Copia C, Magrin S, Mele G, Mirto S. Therapeutic options and treatment results for patients over 75 years of age with acute myeloid leukemia. *Haematologica* 1998; **83**: 126–31.

83. Archimbaud E, Jehn U, Thomas X, *et al*. Multicenter randomized phase II trial of idarubicin vs. mitoxantrone,

combined with VP-16 and cytarabine for induction/consolidation therapy, followed by a feasibility study of autologous peripheral blood stem cell transplantation in elderly patients with acute myeloid leukemia. *Leukemia* 1999; **13**(6): 843–9.

84. Gorin NC, Labopin M, Pichard P, *et al.* Feasibility and recent improvement of autologous stem cell transplantation for acute myelocytic leukaemia in patients over 60 years of age: importance of the source of stem cells. *Br J Haematol* 2000; **110**: 887–93.

85. Cahn JY, Labopin M, Mandelli F, *et al.* Autologous bone marrow transplantation for first remission acute myeloblastic leukemia in patients older than 50 years: a retrospective analysis of the European Bone Marrow Transplant Group. *Blood* 1995; **85**: 575–9.

86. Wallen H, Gooley TA, Deeg HJ, *et al.* Ablative allogeneic hematopoietic cell transplantation in adults 60 years of age and older. *J Clin Oncol* 2005; **23**: 3439–46.

87. McSweeney PA, Niederwieser D, Shizuru JA, *et al.* Hematopoietic cell transplantation in older patients with hematologic malignancies: replacing high-dose cytotoxic therapy with graft-versus-tumor effects. *Blood* 2001; **97**: 3390–400.

88. Bertz H, Potthoff K, Finke J. Allogeneic stem-cell transplantation from related and unrelated donors in older patients with myeloid leukemia. *J Clin Oncol* 2003; **21**: 1480–4.

89. Claxton DF, Ehmann C, Rybka W. Control of advanced and refractory acute myelogenous leukaemia with sirolimus-based non-myeloablative allogeneic stem cell transplantation. *Br J Haematol* 2005; **130**: 256–64.

90. Mohty M, de Lavallade H, Ladaique P, *et al.* The role of reduced intensity conditioning allogeneic transplantation in patients with acute myeloid leukemia: a donor vs. no-donor comparison. *Leukemia* 2005; **19**: 916–20.

91. Kassim AA, Chinratanalab W, Ferrara JL, Mineishi S. Reduced-intensity allogeneic hematopoitic stem cell transplantation for acute leukemias: "what is the best recipe?" *Bone Marrow Transplant* 2005; **36**: 565–74.

92. Keating MJ, Kantarjian H, Smith TL, *et al.* Response to salvage therapy and survival after relapse in acute myelogenous leukemia. *J Clin Oncol* 1989; **7**: 1071–80.

93. Estey E. Treatment of relapsed and refractory acute myelogenous leukemia. *Leukemia* 2000; **14**: 476–9.

94. Archimbaud E, Leblond V, Michallet M, *et al.* Intensive sequential chemotherapy with mitoxantrone and continuous infusion etoposide and cytarabine for previously treated acute myelogenous leukemia. *Blood* 1991; **77**: 1894–900.

95. Hiddemann W, Martin WR, Sauerland CM, Heinecke A, Buchner T. Definition of refractoriness against conventional chemotherapy in acute myeloid leukemia: a proposal based on the results of retreatment by thioguanine, cytosine arabinoside, and daunorubicin (TAD 9) in 150 patients with relapse after standardized first line therapy. *Leukemia* 1990; **4**: 184–8.

96. Estey E, Kornblau S, Pierce S, Kantarjian H, Beran M, Keating M. A stratification system for evaluating and selecting therapies in patients with relapsed or primary refractory acute myelogenous leukemia. *Blood* 1996; **88**: 756.

97. Herzig RH, Lazarus HM, Wolff SN, Phillips GL, Herzig GP. High-dose cytosine arabinoside therapy with and without anthracycline antibiotics for remission reinduction of acute nonlymphoblastic leukemia. *J Clin Oncol* 1985; **3**: 992–7.

98. Carella AM, Carlier P, Pungolino E, *et al.* Idarubicin in combination with intermediate-dose cytarabine and VP-16 in the treatment of refractory or rapidly relapsed patients with acute myeloid leukemia. The GIMEMA Cooperative Group. *Leukemia* 1993; **7**: 196–9.

99. Vogler WR, McCarley DL, Stagg M, *et al.* A phase III trial of high-dose cytosine arabinoside with or without etoposide in relapsed and refractory acute myelogenous leukemia: a Southeastern Cancer Study Group trial. *Leukemia* 1994; **8**: 1847–53.

100. Thomas X, Fenaux P, Dombret H, *et al.* Granulocyte-machrophage colony-stimulating factor (GM-CSF) to increase efficacy of intensive sequential chemotherapy with etoposide, mitoxantrone and cytarabine (EMA) in previously treated acute myeloid leukemia: a multicenter randomized placebo-controlled trial (EMA91 Trial). *Leukemia* 1999; **13**: 1214–20.

101. Robak T, Wrzesien-Kus A, Lech-Maranda E, Kowal M, Dmoszynska A. Combination regimen of cladribine (2-chlorodeoxyadenosine), cytarabine and G-CSF (CLAG) as induction therapy for patients with relapsed or refractory acute myeloid leukemia. *Leuk Lymphoma* 2000; **39**: 121–9.

102. Wrzesien-Kus A, Robak T, Lech-Maranda E, *et al.* A multicenter, open, non-comparative, phase II study of the combination of cladribine (2-chlorodeoxyadenosine), cytarabine, and G-CSF as induction therapy in refractory acute myeloid leukemia: a report of the Polish Adult Leukemia Group (PALG). *Eur J Haematol* 2003; **71**: 155–62.

103. Estey E, Thall P, Andreeff M, *et al.* Use of granulocyte colony-stimulating factor before, during, and after

fluadarabine plus cytarabine induction therapy of newly diagnosed acute myelogenous leukemia or myelodysplastic syndromes: comparison with fludarabine plus cytarabine without granulocyte colony-stimulating factor. *J Clin Oncol* 1994; **12**: 671–8.

104. Ossenkoppele GJ, Graveland WJ, Sonneveld P, *et al.* The value of fludarabine in addition to ARA-C and G-CSF in the treatment of patients with high-risk myelodysplastic syndromes and AML in elderly patients. *Blood* 2004; **103**: 2908–13.

105. Estey E, Plunkett W, Gandhi V, Rios MB, Kantarjian H, Keating MJ. Fludarabine and arabinosylcytosine therapy of refractory and relapsed acute myelogenous leukemia. *Leuk Lymphoma* 1993; **9**: 343–50.

106. Welborn JL, Kopecky KJ, Meyers FJ, *et al.* Carboplatin infusion in relapsed and refractory acute myeloid leukemia: a Southwest Oncology Group trial. *Leukemia* 1995; **9**: 1126–9.

107. Sievers EL, Larson RA, Stadtmauer EA, *et al.* Efficacy and safety of gemtuzumab ozogamicin in patients with CD33-positive acute myeloid leukemia in first relapse. *J Clin Oncol* 2001; **19**: 3244–54.

108. Stone RM, DeAngelo DJ, Klimek V, *et al.* Patients with acute myeloid leukemia and an activating mutation in FLT3 respond to a small-molecule FLT3 tyrosine kinase inhibitor, PKC412. *Blood* 2005; **105**: 54–60.

109. Smith BD, Levis M, Beran M, *et al.* Single-agent CEP-701, a novel FLT3 inhibitor, shows biologic and clinical activity in patients with relapsed or refractory acute myeloid leukemia. *Blood* 2004; **103**: 3669–76.

110. Fiedler W, Serve H, Dohner II, *et al.* A phase 1 study of SU11248 in the treatment of patients with refractory or resistant acute myeloid leukemia (AML) or not amenable to conventional therapy for the disease. *Blood* 2005; **105**: 986–93.

111. Lancet JE, Gotlib J, Gojo I, *et al.* Tipifarnib (ZARNESTRA™) in previously untreated poor-risk AML of the elderly: updated results of a multicenter phase 2 trial. ASH Annual Meeting Abstracts. *Blood* 2004; **104**: abstract 874.

112. Vogler WR, Miller DS, Keller JW. 5-Azacytidine (NSC 102816): a new drug for the treatment of myeloblastic leukemia. *Blood* 1976; **48**: 331–7.

113. Christman J. 5-Azacytidine and 5-aza-2'-deoxycytidine as inhibitors of DNA methylation: mechanistic studies and their implications for cancer therapy. *Oncogene* 2002; **21**: 5483–95.

114. Silverman LR, Demakos EP, Peterson BL, *et al.* Randomized controlled trial of azacitidine in patients with the myelodysplastic syndrome: a study of the cancer and leukemia group B. *J Clin Oncol* 2002; **20**: 2429–40.

115. Gore SD, Baylin SB, Dauses T, *et al.* Changes in promoter methylation and gene expression in patients with MDS and MDS-AML treated with 5-azacitidine and sodium phenylbutyrate. ASH Annual Meeting Abstracts. *Blood* 2004; **104**: abstract 469.

116. Shadduck RK, Rossetti JM, Faroun Y, *et al.* AML induction therapy with outpatient azacitidine. ASH Annual Meeting Abstracts. *Blood* 2004; **104**: abstract 1800.

117. Issa JP, Garcia-Manero G, Giles FJ, *et al.* Phase 1 study of low-dose prolonged exposure schedules of the hypomethylating agent 5-aza-2'-deoxycytidine (decitabine) in hematopoietic malignancies. *Blood* 2004; **103**: 1635–40.

118. Karp JE, Gojo I, Pili R, *et al.* Targeting vascular endothelial growth factor for relapsed and refractory adult acute myelogenous leukemias: therapy with sequential 1-beta-d-arabinofuranosylcytosine, mitoxantrone, and bevacizumab. *Clin Cancer Res* 2004; **10**: 3577–85.

119. Gerber HP, Malik AK, Solar GP, *et al.* VEGF regulates haematopoietic stem cell survival by an internal autocrine loop mechanism. *Nature* 2002; **417**: 954–8.

120. Sekeres MA, Stone RM, Zahrieh D, *et al.* Decision-making and quality of life in older adults with acute myeloid leukemia or advance myelodysplastic syndrome. *Leukemia* 2004; **18**: 809–16.

121. Menzin J, Lang K, Earle C, Derney D, Mallick R. The outcomes and costs of acute myeloid leukemia among the elderly. *Arch Intern Med* 2002; **162**: 1597–603.

122. Vey N, Coso D, Bardou VJ, *et al.* The benefit of induction chemotherapy in patients age > or = 75 years. *Cancer* 2004; **101**: 325–31.

123. Lowenberg B, Downing JR, Burnett A. Acute myeloid leukemia. *N Engl J Med* 1999; **341**: 1051–62.

124. DeLima M, Ghaddar H, Pierce S, Estey E. Treatment of newly-diagnosed acute myelogenous leukaemia in patients aged 80 years and above. *Br J Haematol* 1996; **93**: 89–95.

125. Estey EH. How I treat older patients with AML. *Blood* 2000; **96**: 1670–3.

126. Gupta V, Chun K, Yi QL, *et al.* Disease biology rather than age is the most important determinant of survival of patients > or = 60 years with acute myeloid leukemia treated with uniform intensive therapy. *Cancer* 2005; **103**: 2082–90.

20

Acute lymphoblastic leukemia in the elderly patient: diagnosis and therapy

Salvador Bruno, Fermina Mazzella, Oscar Ballester

Epidemiology

In adults, acute lymphoblastic leukemia (ALL) is a rare disease with a poor prognosis. An estimated 3970 new cases of ALL (all ages) were diagnosed in the USA during 2005. The incidence of the disease peaks in the age group 1 to 4 years, with 7.2 cases per 100 000. From ages 20 to 60 years the incidence decreases to less than 1 per 100 000. A secondary increase is noted after age 60, peaking at age 85+ with 1.6 cases expected per 100 000 [1]. Among adults, approximately 30% of ALL cases arise in patients aged 60 years or older.

Similar findings have been reported from other countries, such as the population-based study by Taylor and coworkers from the Northern Health Region of England (approximately 3 million people). Over the 8.5-year study period, 157 cases of ALL in adults (age >15) were identified. Of these cases, 31% were individuals aged over 60 (annual incidence 0.9 per 100 000) [2]. In the Western Swedish Health Care Region, the incidence of ALL was 0.72 per 100 000 in patients over the age of 65 (1982–96). In this study, the three-year overall survival (OS) rate for elderly ALL patients was 14.2% [3]. These data are similar to those reported by SEER in the USA: a five-year OS rate of 7.9% for individuals age 65 or older.

Table 20.1 shows the five-year relative survival rates for ALL by age group in the USA and Europe [1,4]. Comparative data on acute myeloid leukemia (AML) are also given.

The poor outcomes in elderly patients have been attributed to low complete remission (CR) rates,

Table 20.1. Five-year relative survival rates by age for acute lymphoblastic leukemia (ALL) acute myeloid leukemia (AML) (SEER and Eurocare data).

Age	ALL		AML	
	USA	Europe	USA	Europe
<45	74.4	67	45.5	56
45–54	27.9	49	26.0	37
55–64	19.8	43	17.4	31
65–74	8.6	38	5.3	17
75+	7.3	19	1.9	11

which in turn is the result of (1) high induction-related mortality, (2) use of attenuated "age-adjusted" chemotherapy protocols or low-dose "palliative chemotherapy," and (3) high prevalence of drug resistance. Further, it seems that even for those patients who achieve a CR, disease-free survival (DFS) and OS are very short.

The clustering of ALL cases in time and space has supported the hypothesis of a link with an infectious etiology [5]. However, this clustering effect is seen only in children, suggesting that perhaps adult ALL results from a different etiologic mechanism. After accounting for phenotype and cytogenetics, gene mapping studies have not demonstrated significant differences in gene expression patterns between adult and pediatric cases [6]. This is surprising in view of the epidemiologic data, and considering also the different outcomes of children and adults with ALL.

Blood Disorders in the Elderly, ed. Lodovico Balducci, William Ershler, Giovanni de Gaetano.
Published by Cambridge University Press. © Cambridge University Press 2008.

The lack of randomized clinical trials that define the best approach for the management of elderly patients with ALL is of utmost importance. When faced with treatment decisions in elderly ALL patients, physicians often need to extrapolate data from studies done in young adults or to pool data from small non-randomized trials. In either case, this might be a risky undertaking.

Clinical presentation of ALL in the elderly patient

The clinical features of ALL in elderly patients differ from those of younger adults and children. Thomas *et al.* [7] compared the characteristics of 69 ALL patients older than 60 years (median age 68) to those of 309 younger adults (median age 29). Significant differences included a history of prior malignant disorder (14% vs. 3%) and a lower incidence of peripheral lymphadenopathy (21% vs. 51%). Elderly patients presented with lower peripheral-blood leukocyte counts (median 8.4×10^9/L vs. 13.2×10^9/L), a lower incidence of FAB L1 morphology (41% vs. 59%) and T-cell lineage phenotype, and a higher rate of B-cell lineage phenotype (89% vs. 66%). These differences were also noted in Philadelphia-chromosome-positive (Ph+) cases, the most important subset of elderly ALL patients. Elderly Ph+ ALL patients also presented with lower leukocyte counts, and lower rates of FAB L1 morphology and peripheral lymphadenopathy than their younger counterparts [8].

These differences can, at least in part, explain the poor prognosis of older patients. Indicators of poor prognosis such as Ph+ and B-cell phenotype are seen more often in older patients, while good risk indicators such as T-cell phenotype are seen less frequently.

Pathology: diagnosis and differential diagnosis

ALL typically involves bone marrow and blood, but may occasionally involve nodal or extranodal sites. The diagnosis of ALL is usually not difficult. However, some conditions may be confused with ALL in certain instances. These include hyperplasia of hematogones, chronic lymphocytic leukemia, acute myeloid leukemia without maturation, acute bilineage leukemia, acute biphenotypic leukemia, neuroblastoma, infectious mononucleosis, prolymphocytic leukemia, Sézary syndrome (especially the blastic type), and sometimes even hairy-cell leukemia. These can typically be distinguished on the basis of clinical setting, morphology, immunophenotyping, and immunohistochemistry.

Morphology of lymphoblasts

The French–American–British (FAB) classification separated the ALLs into three groups based upon morphology (Table 20.2). The most important discerning criteria are amount and color of cytoplasm, nuclear features, and the presence or absence of cytoplasmic vacuoles. Lymphoblasts are somewhat homogeneous in appearance, with round to oval nuclei which may manifest varying degrees of convolution of the nuclear membrane. The chromatin is fine and nucleoli are generally inconspicuous. The cytoplasm is pale and scant to moderate in amount for L1 and L2 type blasts, but dark blue and abundant in L3. Cytoplasmic vacuoles are a characteristic feature of L3, but may also be seen in other types of B and T ALL. The morphologic features of B and T lymphoblastic proliferations are similar and cannot be used as a distinguishing feature of immunophenotype [9,10]. Typically, the identification of L3 (Burkitt) cells is clear-cut. However, distinction between L1 and L2 may be difficult. L1 accounts for over 80% of ALL cases in childhood and 30% in adults. The majority of ALL cases in adults are L2. L3 (Burkitt) makes up 3–5% of ALL cases in children and adults. Burkitt lymphoma (tissue counterpart of L3) is being seen with more frequency with the AIDS epidemic (Fig. 20.1b).

Hand-mirror cell variant

Hand-mirror cells are lymphocytes or blasts with a uropod. The hand-mirror cell configuration is

Table 20.2. FAB classification of acute lymphoblastic leukemia.

	FAB L1	FAB L2	FAB L3
Morphology			
Size	Small & homogeneous	Large & pleomorphic	Medium & homogeneous
N/C ratio	Higher in >95%	Lower in >25%	Variable
Nucleoli	Inconspicuous	Prominent	Prominent, multiple
Vacuolization	No	No	Sharply defined
Basophilia	Moderate	Moderate	Deep
Cytochemistry			
MPO	−	−	−
NSE	+/−	+/−	−
PAS	+	+	−
AP	+	+	−

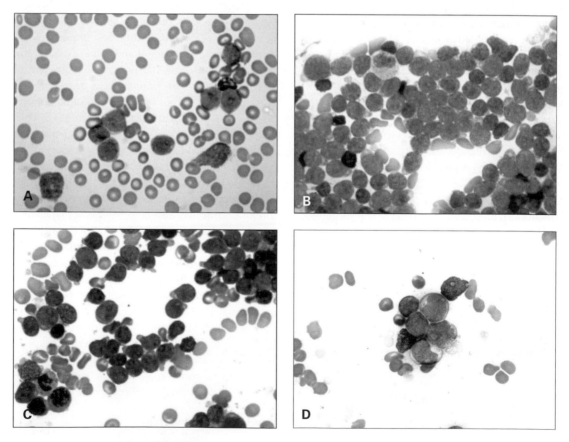

Figure 20.1 (A) ALL lymphocytes in peripheral blood smear; (B) ALL L3 lymphoblasts in bone-marrow aspirate; (C) ALL hand-mirror variant; (D) ALL granular variant. *See color plate section.*

believed to occur when adhesion molecules are triggered by their corresponding ligands. Most reports are of T-cell or mixed T-cell/myeloid lineage (Fig. 20.1c) [11,12].

Granular variant

This is a rare variant of ALL in the pediatric population, and even rarer in adults. It is characterized by myeloid-appearing blasts, with at least 5% of the blasts demonstrating coarse azurophilic granules, but no Auer rods (Fig. 20.1d). The blasts are of early B-precursor or common B phenotype, with no myeloid differentiation. This malignancy has been associated with a single or double Philadelphia chromosome, poor response to induction chemotherapy, and poor prognosis [13].

Classification

The World Health Organization has recently consolidated and reclassified the acute lymphoblastic leukemias as either "precursor B-ALL" and "precursor T-ALL." [14]. These diseases are then subclassified into high-, intermediate-, or low-risk ALL according to the cytogenetics.

Laboratory findings

The white cell count may be elevated, normal, or even low. Hyperleukocytosis at diagnosis is a characteristic feature of early B-precursor ALL, and is also an independent poor prognostic indicator.

Bone-marrow examination almost always reveals replacement of normal marrow elements by sheets of lymphoblasts. These blasts should exceed 30% of all nucleated cells in the bone marrow and are commonly more than 50%. Marrow biopsies are most often hypercellular, but on occasion may be hypocellular or necrotic. The number of mitotic figures usually varies, and are typically more numerous in T-cell than in B-cell ALL. A "starry sky" appearance is characteristic of L3, but may be seen in the other types of ALL as well [15].

Extramedullary involvement is frequent, with a particular predilection for the central nervous system. Lymph nodes, spleen, liver, and gonads may be involved in B-cell ALL, and the mediastinum for T-cell ALL.

Cytochemistry

ALL cells are characteristically negative for MPO and CAE. The lymphoblasts are usually negative with Sudan black B and non-specific esterase, but may on occasion stain less intensely than myeloblasts. PAS stain often demonstrates coarse red granules or blocks of positive material in some or many of the lymphoblasts. The granules and blocks are found in a clear background, in contrast to the acute myeloid leukemias, where there is a finely granular or diffusely positive background. Acid phosphatase will usually stain the lymphoblasts of T-ALL as a strong, red dot-like Golgi zone pattern. ALL L3 blasts often stain with oil red O due to the presence of neutral lipids within the cytoplasmic vacuoles.

Terminal deoxynucleotidyl transferase (TdT) is a deoxynucleotide polymerizing enzyme. It can be detected by cytochemical or immunohistochemical staining, or by flow cytometry. The majority of blasts in ALL are TdT-positive. However, T-cell ALLs may be negative. Occasionally, myeloblasts will express TdT, but usually < 50% of the blasts will be positive. ALL L3 is characteristically negative [15].

Immunophenotyping

The lymphoblasts in B-ALL are TdT-positive, HLA-DR-positive, and are almost always positive for CD19. The lymphoblasts are positive for CD10 and CD24 in most cases; however, the lymphoblasts in early B-precursor ALL are usually CD10-negative and frequently CD24-negative. There is variable expression of CD22 and CD20. CD45 may be absent. Cytoplasmic CD22 is considered lineage-specific. Surface immunoglobulin is characteristically absent, although if present does not exclude a diagnosis of B-ALL [16].

Table 20.3. Immunophenotyping of acute lymphoblastic leukemia.

Stage of maturation	CD19	CD20	CD10	CD34	cCD22	sCD22	sIg	TdT
Early B precursor	+	–	–	+	+	–	–	+
Common B	+	–	+/–	–/+	+	–/+	–	+
Pre B cell	+	–/+	+	–	+	–/+	–/+	+
B cell	+	+	+	–	+	+	+	–

	CD2	CD7	CD5	cCD3	sCD3	CD1	TdT	
Early thymocyte	+	+	+	+	–	–	+/–	
Common thymocyte	+	+	+	+	–	+	+/–	
Mature thymocyte	+	+	+	+	+	–	+/–	

The lymphoblasts in T-ALL are usually but not always positive for TdT, and may or may not express CD1a, CD2, CD3, CD4, CD5, CD7, and CD8. Of these, CD7 and cytoplasmic CD3 are most often positive. Only CD3 is considered lineage-specific. CD4 and CD8 may be coexpressed or both absent on the blasts. CD10 may be positive.

One or both of the myeloid-associated antigens CD13 and CD33 may be expressed, but the presence of these markers does not exclude a diagnosis of ALL. However, when present, a diagnosis of acute bilineage leukemia or acute biphenotypic leukemia must be excluded. CD34 may be positive in any of the subtypes, but is most frequently present in early B-precursor ALL. It is considered a good prognostic indicator, in contrast to AML, where CD34 expression is considered a poor prognostic indicator.

An immunophenotypic classification of ALL has been established (Table 20.3). Over 50% of all ALL cases have common B phenotype. About 20% are pre-B ALL, 5% B-ALL (Burkitt), and 1–2% are early B-precursor ALL. Approximately 20% have a T-cell phenotype. In the older adult population, pre-B and common B-ALL are most frequently encountered, while T-cell ALL is under-represented when compared to the younger age groups. Interestingly, T-cell ALLs also show age-related differences in phenotype, with a shift from predominantly TCR-expressing type in younger patients to an immature stage of maturation arrest in adults [17].

Early B-precursor ALL and common ALL can have FAB L1 or L2 morphology. Pre-B ALL usually has L1 morphology; and B-ALL has L3 morphology. T-ALL usually has L2 morphology.

Expression of P-glycoprotein and Bcl-2 have been reported to be independent prognostic factors, which may contribute to a worse outcome in adult ALL [18].

Cytogenetics and molecular pathology

The cytogenetic abnormalities in B-ALL are traditionally classified into hypodiploid, hyperdiploid <50, hyperdiploid >50, pseudodiploid, and translocations. These findings are prognostically important [19,20].

Good prognostic groups are hyperdiploid >50 and the t(12;21)(p13;q22). The t(12;21)(p13;q22) is the result of fusion of the *TEL* gene at 12p13 with the transcription factor-encoding *AML1* gene at 21q22. As this translocation cannot be detected by routine karyotyping, molecular techniques are required for its recognition.

Abnormalities such as del(6q), del(9p), del(12p), hyperdiploidy <50, near-triploidy, and near-tetraploidy are associated with an intermediate prognosis.

Poor-prognosis cytogenetic findings include the t(9;22)(q34;q11), hypodiploidy, the t(1;19)(q23; p13.3), and the t(4;11)(q21;q23), which is usually found in early B-precursor ALL. Other transloca-tions at the 11q23 locus may be found, and result in fusion of the *MLL* locus with various partner genes. ALL with 11q23 abnormalities may also occur as a therapy-related leukemia.

The most common structural chromosomal abnormality in adult B-ALL is the Philadelphia chro-mosome, t(9;22)(q34;q11) [21]. This translocation is seen in over 30% of adult patients but in only 3–5% of pediatric patients. Morphologically the Ph chro-mosome in ALL appears to be the same as the trans-location in chronic myelogenous leukemia (CML); but at the molecular level the break in the *BCR* gene is at the minor *bcr* region. This translocation is associated with the L1 and L2 morphology and the phenotypes of early B-precursor, common, and pre-B ALL. Coexpression of myeloid markers is seen in approximately 20% of cases. Secondary cytoge-netic aberrations are seen in 68% of patients at the time of diagnosis. These most frequently include +der(22)t(9;22), +21, 9p abnormalities, high hyper-diploidy (>50 chromosomes), +8, −7, and +X. Relapse-free survival is significantly shorter in cases with double Ph+, trisomy 8, and del(9p21).

The detection of Ph+ has a significant adverse effect on survival. In fact, in a prospective study including 478 patients, univariate and multivariate analysis revealed BCR-ABL (present in 37% of the cases) as the leading factor for poor prognosis, and the DFS at three years was 13% vs. 47% ($p < 0.0001$) [22]. The prognosis of the Ph+ ALL does not seems to be affected by the presence of any additional chromosomal abnormality, except for the presence of −7 as the sole secondary abnormality, associated with a significantly lower CR rate [23].

The chromosomal aberration t(4;11)(q21;q23) is seen in about 5% of all B-ALL cases, and is equal in frequency among adults and infants younger than 1 year. This translocation is associated with the L1 and L2 morphology and the early B-precursor phenotype. The blasts often express the myeloid antigen CD15. These patients tend to have a high white cell count and splenomegaly at diagnosis, and a poor prognosis.

The t(1;19)(q23;p13) is associated with the L1 morphology and pre-B ALL phenotype. Patients with this abnormality also have a poor prognosis.

The t(8;14)(q24;q32) is seen in the majority of cases with L3 B-ALL (Burkitt). This translocation involves the translocation of the *c-myc* proto-oncogene on chromosome 8 and the immunoglob-ulin heavy chain gene on chromosome 14. Patients with this abnormality have a high rate of central nervous system involvement and a poor prognosis.

Some genetically defined entities have character-istic immunophenotypes [23,24]. These include the *MLL*-rearranged leukemias, which are characteristi-cally CD10-negative, and frequently CD24-negative and CD15-positive, and t(12;21), which typically demonstrates a high density expression of CD10 and HLA-DR, but negativity for CD19 and CD20.

About one-third of T-ALL cases have translocations involving the alpha and delta T-cell receptor loci at 14q11.2, the beta locus at 7q35, and the gamma locus at 7p14–15. These genes are involved with a vari-ety of partner genes, including transcription factors *MYC* (8q24.1), *TAL1* (1p32), *RBTN1* (11p15), *RBTN2* (11p13), and *HOX11* (10q24), and the cytoplasmic tyrosine kinase *LCK* (1p34.3–35). In most cases, these translocations lead to a dysregulation of transcription of the partner gene by juxtaposition with the regula-tory region of one of the T-cell receptor loci.

Treatment of ALL

Treatment outcome in children with ALL has stead-ily improved in the last four decades, with current ten-year cure rates of 80% [23]. Although consider-able progress has also occurred in the treatment of adults aged 16–60 years, the results lag behind those of children, with overall long-term survival of only 40–45%. Moreover, in the elderly ALL population aged 60 or older results remain dismal, with long-term OS of barely 10% [25,26].

Treatment response and outcomes have been universally found to be a function of age. In 197 adult ALL patients, including 18 older than 60 years, the CALGB study 8811 demonstrated a 94% CR in patients less than 30 years, 85% for those aged 30–59, and only 39% for those aged 60 or older. Induction mortality in the older group of patients accounted for 50% of deaths, mostly related to infections, compared to 1% for the those under 30, and 8% for those aged 30–59 years [27]. Moreover, among the older patients, those aged 70 and older responded less well than those aged 60–69 years, with a marked drop in CR rate (27% vs. 67%) and a very high death rate during induction (38% vs. 4%) [25].

Prognostic factors

Numerous risk factors have been assessed in the search for an explanation of the poor outcome of elderly patients with ALL.

Patients may be divided into two risk groups: those with favorable, standard, or good-risk ALL, encompassing 25% of the cases, and those with unfavorable or poor-risk ALL, accounting for an overwhelming majority of 75% of elderly ALL cases.

Favorable pretreatment characteristics, as assessed by subsequent DFS and OS, have included: younger age (<60 years); achievement of CR; high white blood cell count; presence of mediastinal mass or lymphadenopathy; L1 morphology; T immunophenotype; performance status (ECOG < than 2); *MLL*-rearrangement-negative and the absence of Ph chromosome or other karyotype or molecular abnormalities like t(4;11)/MLL-AFA4, t(1;19)/E2A-PBX1, 9p/p15-p16 deletions, and 6q deletions; minimal-residual-disease- (MRD)-negative status; absence of bleeding; time to leukemia cell clearance; preserved organ function; selection of favorable genes by gene expression profiling; negative MDR1 protein expression; elevated VEGF; and BCL2 expression among others [27–36]. Certainly, age and cytogenetic abnormalities are the most important and the best defined risk factors for treatment outcome [37].

In a recent report of the ECOG/MRC trial, which included over 1500 patients, a simplified prognostic score was proposed based on age (under or over 35 years), white blood count at diagnosis (>30 000 × 10^9/L for B-cell phenotype, >100 000 × 10^9/L for T-cell phenotype), and presence of the Ph chromosome. Four prognostic groups are defined, with expected five-year OS decreasing from 55% to 5% (Table 20.4). Interestingly, individuals over the age

Table 20.4. Prognostic risk groups for adult ALL (MRC UKALL XII/ECOG E2993).

Risk group	Ph chromosome	Age	WBC	OS at 5 years
Low	Negative	<35	Low	55%
Intermediate	Negative	<35	High	34%
		>35	Low	
High	Positive	Any	Any	25%
Very high	Negative	>35	High	5%

WBC, white blood cell count at diagnosis; Low, <30 000 for B-cell phenotypes, <100 000 for T-cell phenotypes; High, >30 000 for B-cell phenotype, >100 000 for T-cell phenotype.

of 35 with an initial elevated white blood cell count had the worst prognosis, even worse than those with Ph-positive disease [26].

Standard treatment of adult ALL

Adult ALL protocols were originally based on previous pediatric protocols, with an induction phase combining an anthracycline (daunorubicin or doxorubicin), vincristine, prednisone or dexamethasone, and L-asparaginase. Induction was followed by a consolidation phase (with or without intensification) with the use of repeated courses of high doses of alternating non-cross-resistant agents, and a final consolidation and maintenance phase, generally shorter than in the pediatric protocols. The subsequent introduction in the induction or consolidation phases of drugs aimed at lineage-specific ALL subsets included cyclophosphamide (mature B-cell ALL), high-dose methotrexate (MTX) (B-cell lineage, protection of CNS relapse), and high-dose Ara-C (T-lineage ALL). These may have contributed to the overall therapy results, but the particular influence of each drug is difficult to assess. Patients with CNS leukemia at diagnosis have been treated with MTX intrathecally, alone or associated with Ara-C, with the addition of high-dose intravenous MTX and/or radiotherapy. Post-remission consolidation with allogeneic transplant in patients aged over 50 years with a compatible sibling donor

Table 20.5. Results of selected studies on adult ALL patients.

Study group	No. patients	Age*	CR%	OS
MRC/ECOG	1521	<60	91	45% at 5 years for CR patients
CALGB 8811	197	10% >60	85	Median 36 m; patients >60: 1 m
U of CA	60	<60	93	47% at 5 years
GIMEMA	778	<60	82	Median 2.2 years
GMALL	432	<65	78	47% for Ph (−), 13% for Ph (+) at 3 years
PETHEMA	108	25% >50	86	47% at 5 years
MDA	288	20% >60	92	38% for <60, 17% for >60 at 5 years
GALGB 9111	198	10% >60	82	43% at 3 years
GET-LALA	92	<55	84	19% at 3 years

* Age limit for inclusion, % of patients over stated age.

have been generally advocated for poor prognosis (such as Ph+) patients [38,39].

With this or similar approaches, consistent induction results with CR rates of over 85% have been achieved by most study groups, even with exclusion of L-asparaginase and vincristine from the treatment protocols. But the long-term survival continues to be lower (40–55%) than in the pediatric population, whether single-institution or cooperative group studies are analyzed (Table 20.5). Achieving a CR with induction therapy is a *sine qua non* for a long-term survival in adult ALL, with only 5% OS in those patients not achieving a CR with the initial therapy [2,27,39–43].

The M. D. Anderson Center piloted a novel dose-intense schedule, built on the treatment for Burkitt lymphoma with high-dose fractionated cyclophosphamide (favorable bioactivity and metabolic autoinduction) and high doses of MTX and cytarabine, with the addition of vincristine, doxorubicin, and dexamethasone (hyper-CVAD). The hyper-CVAD regimen administered to 288 ALL patients (59 older than 60 years, 20%) resulted in a 92% CR rate (99% for those age < 60 vs. 80% for those ≥ 60 years, mostly related to higher mortality). Induction mortality rate was 5% (2% if patient age was <60 years and 15% if ≥ 60 years). With a median follow-up time of 63 months, five-year DFS and OS rates were 38%. For patients ≥ 60 years the five-year OS rate was

only 17%, compared to 30% for those aged 40–59 and 50% for those under 40. Among the 14 patients who experienced induction death, 9 (64%) were aged over 60 years.

Historical comparison with the previous VAD study revealed that the induction mortality rates were similar for both regimens (5%) but with a better CR rate (92% vs. 75%) and a better five-year OS (38% vs. 21%), favoring the most intensive hyper-CVAD regimen [44].

Other investigators have explored the possibility of achieving remission with a short induction regimen with high doses of cytarabine 3 g/m^2 per day for five days and mitoxantrone 80 mg/m^2 as a single course, producing a CR rate of 84% in a seemingly shorter time than in the previous standard regimen experience at the Sloan-Kettering Institute [45]. Furthermore, in an expanded randomized study including 161 ALL patients, the cytarabine/mitoxantrone combination appeared superior to the standard regimen in frequency of CR, failure due to resistant disease, activity in Ph+ cases, and in five-year OS (35%) [46].

Treatment of the elderly ALL patient

The treatment of ALL in the elderly (aged 60 years and older) remains a challenge, with little progress

Table 20.6. Results of selected studies in older ALL patients.

Ref	Age group	No. patients	CR (No. treated with curative intent)	OS (median, in months)	Long-term survivors
2	>60	49	45% (22)	1–3	4% at 5 years
50	>55	40	77.5% (40)	14	20% at 2 years
54	>60	69	62% (64)	7	7% at 3 years
47	>60	87	45% (75)	5	4.5% at 3 years

Ref, reference; CR, complete remission; OS, overall survival.

made in the last decades. The published studies are few, mostly single-institution reports, with limited numbers of patients, treated with various protocols, and performed over lengthy periods, precluding a fair comparison with the studies in younger adult patients (Table 20.6) [47–51].

Pagano *et al.* reviewed 12 studies encompassing 514 patients aged over 55 years from 1990 to 2001. The CR rate for those over 60 years was below 70%, and the median OS was only 7 months, compared to more than 90% and 2 years for patients younger than 60 years [48].

In view of comorbidities, poor organ function, and poor performance status, many trials have an age-adapted design, with generally less aggressive chemotherapy in the elderly [44,49–53]. Indeed, a number of non-randomized sequential trials have found age-adapted therapy to be superior to young-adult-like therapy in terms of CR rate (96% vs. 60%). However, no significant benefit in DFS or OS was noted [7]. Others have reported a standard chemotherapy induction regimen (daunorubicin, vincristine, prednisone, and L-asparaginase) with comparable results to the milder combination of vincristine and prednisone [53]. Further, M.D. Anderson investigators and others have suggested the opposite: more intensive chemotherapy regimens significantly improved survival in the elderly compared to historical data from gentler treatment protocols (hyper-CVAD vs. VAD regimens) [44].

New approaches for the treatment of ALL in the elderly patient

Hematopoietic growth factors

The high failure rate of elderly ALL patients is related, at least in part, to a high treatment-related mortality, particularly from infections. In an effort to ameliorate these complications, the CALGB 9111 study was designed as a randomized, controlled, double-blind trial of filgrastim (G-CSF) versus placebo during remission induction and consolidation chemotherapy [54]. A total of 198 patients (41 older than 60 years) were accrued. For patients aged over 60, the induction chemotherapy doses of cyclophosphamide, daunorubicin, and prednisone were reduced and vincristine and L-asparaginase were excluded. For the 21 patients over 60 years old assigned to G-CSF treatment, the CR rate was 81%, and 10% died during induction. For the 20 patients over 60 years old assigned to placebo, the CR rate was 55%, and 25% died during induction. These differences, however, did not reach statistical significance. Unfortunately, the ultimate outcome was not markedly modified by the G-CSF treatment. After median follow-up of 4.7 years, there were no significant differences in either DFS or OS for the patients assigned to G-CSF compared to those assigned to placebo [54].

Similar conclusion were drawn by the multi-center French GET-LALA Group study, which included 236 adult ALL patients randomized to receive G-CSF, GM-CSF, or no growth factor. Overall, growth factors showed a trend for a reduced incidence of severe infections, days with antibiotics, and duration of hospitalization. CR rate was higher in the GM-CSF group compared to the control group, but there were no significant differences between the three groups in terms of DFS [55].

Monoclonal antibodies

ALL cells express a number of well-characterized antigens in their cell surface which could be the target of monoclonal antibodies. Preliminary reports in refractory patients indicate that rituximab (anti-CD20), gentuzumab ozogamicin (anti-CD33), and alemtuzumab (anti-CD52) have in-vitro and in-vivo anti-tumor activity against ALL [56–60]. These monoclonal antibodies are currently approved for clinical use, and a number of others are in various stages of development (anti-CD19, anti-CD22). Monoclonal antibodies could potentially enhance the activity of induction, consolidation, or maintenance chemotherapy regimens without significantly increasing their toxicity profiles. This could be particularly attractive for the elderly ALL population.

Targeted therapies: role of imatinib

The t(9;22) translocation leads to constitutive expression of an abnormal ABL tyrosine kinase, which is implicated in the pathogenesis of Ph+ leukemias. Imatinib, a selective inhibitor of the abnormal tyrosine kinase, has demonstrated substantial activity against CML, but also in acute leukemias characterized by the BCR-ABL fusion protein [61].

The role of imatinib as salvage therapy, as well as the addition of imatinib to standard chemotherapy during induction and during consolidation or as maintenance, has been explored in several trials. Single-agent imatinib has shown significant activity in refractory/relapsed Ph+ ALL. The landmark dose-seeking study of imatinib included 20 patients with CML in lymphoblastic transformation or with previously treated Ph+ ALL. Hematologic responses

were seen in ten patients including four CR, with two of these patients achieving a major cytogenetic response. Nevertheless, all patients who had a response relapsed within four months [61,62]. Scheuring and others reported on 56 patients with refractory or relapsed Ph+ ALL treated with imatinib [63]. All patients were previously treated with chemotherapy and some had received an allogeneic (n = 18) or autologous transplant (n = 4). Forty of the 56 patients (71%) achieved a response, with a median time to progression of 8.7 months. Other studies have reported similar results [62,64,65].

The Japan Adult Leukemia Study Group treated 24 newly diagnosed patients with Ph+ ALL (15–64 years of age) with induction chemotherapy plus imatinib. Twenty-three of 24 (96%) achieved a CR after a single course of induction therapy, and 78% achieved PCR-negativity. Fifteen patients received allogeneic transplants. The DFS and OS rates at one year were estimated at 68% and 89%, respectively. No increased toxicity appeared evident with the addition of imatinib [66].

The M. D. Anderson Center reported on the addition of imatinib on days 1 to 14 of each course of the induction hyper-CVAD regimen. Twenty patients, aged 17 to 75, (11 with *de novo* disease, 4 refractory, 5 in CR) entered the study. CR rates were achieved in 100% of the 15 patients with active disease. With a median follow-up of 20 months, 15 of 20 patients treated with imatinib remained in CR [67]. Anecdotally, the successful use of imatinib combined with second-line chemotherapy in relapsed ALL patients has been reported [68].

The GIMEMA LAL0201 study A was designed for Philadelphia-positive adults aged 18–60 years who, after standard induction and consolidation, received daily imatinib for six months as maintenance. After a median follow-up of 20 months, 18 of 22 patients remained in hematological CR with the probability of DFS at two years of 79%. Study B was designed for patients age 60 and older. Induction therapy consisted of imatinib 800 mg/day and prednisone 40 mg/day, for 30 days. Ten of the 12 patients enrolled achieved a CR [69]. Other investigators have reported similar results [70].

The French Group for Research on Adult Acute Lymphocytic Leukemia designed a trial with imatinib for patients 55 years and older. Following a pre-induction with steroids for a week, Ph-positive ALL patients received an induction with chemotherapy followed by imatinib combined with intermittent doses of steroids for two months. Patients in CR were then treated with alternating chemotherapy courses, including two with imatinib, for a total of two years. Fifteen of 19 patients achieved CR [71].

In another study, patients who achieved a CR after induction with hyper-CVAD were assigned to imatinib alternating with consolidation chemotherapy. Twenty-two of the 23 patients who achieved a CR remained in sustained first CR until the time of transplant. For patients not in CR after hyper-CVAD, imatinib was administered for salvage as single agent. In this group of six patients with refractory disease three achieved CR [72].

A trial with imatinib to prevent relapse was designed for patients in molecular positive BRC-ABL status after transplant. Imatinib was given to 27 patients (16–63 years) who had undergone allogeneic ($n = 24$) or autologous transplants ($n = 3$). Fourteen of 27 patients (52%) achieved a molecular remission as defined by the decrease of BCR-ABL transcripts below the detection threshold. Eleven of 14 patients remained in molecular remission after a median follow-up of 15.6 months. Three patients experienced bone-marrow relapse (2) or CNS relapse (1), all after discontinuation of imatinib. The probability of DFS and OS after two years was 54% and 80% in the molecular CR group. The molecular response rate did not differ significantly between patients with and without graft-versus-host disease (GVHD) [73].

While many of these trials have few patients and short follow-ups, as a whole the preliminary results are quite encouraging.

Hematopoietic stem-cell transplantation in ALL: role of autologous and allogeneic transplants

A comprehensive discussion of the role of hematopoietic stem-cell transplantation (HSCT) for ALL is beyond the scope of this chapter. The reader is referred to two excellent reviews [72,73].

The role of autologous HSCT remains controversial. Autologous transplantation has not shown clearly and consistently superior outcomes to those of standard chemotherapy [74]. On the other hand, outcomes of autologous HSCT have been consistently inferior to those of allogeneic HSCT [75,76]. Autologous HSCT may improve the outcomes of good-risk patients. This issue should be further explored in the elderly patient, since autologous HSCT can be performed in individuals well into their seventies. However, good-risk patients represent only a small subset of the elderly ALL population.

In general terms, allogeneic HSCT can improve the DFS and OS of adult patients with high-risk ALL, such as those who are PH-positive. While in selected cases allogeneic HSCT can be attempted in individuals over the age of 60, it is probably not an option for most patients, primarily due to the high transplant-related mortality associated with allogeneic HSCT in older individuals. The recent development of non-myeloablative and reduced-intensity conditioning (NMA/RIC) regimens, with their decreased transplant-related morbidity and mortality, could make allogeneic HSCT more suitable for the elderly population. Allogeneic transplantation with NMA/RIC relies on a graft-versus-leukemia (GVL) effect for its anti-leukemic activity, since no intensive chemotherapy is administered. A GVL effect can be indirectly inferred by the association of the occurrence of GVHD with a reduced relapse rate. Directly, it can be demonstrated by the induction of tumor responses with donor lymphocyte infusions in patients who relapsed after allogeneic HSCT.

Early reports appeared to indicate that ALL was relatively insensitive to a GVL effect. More recent studies, however, clearly demonstrate a significantly reduced risk of relapse in patients who develop GHVD, particularly with chronic GVHD. In some studies the reduced relapse risk is offset by a higher transplant-related mortality, resulting in no significantly improved overall survival.

In a study of 170 adults with high-risk ALL, of whom two-thirds were beyond first CR, the

Table 20.7. Results of selected trials of NMA/RIC transplants for adult ALL patients.

Ref	No. patients	Median age	Disease status	aGVHD	cGVHD	Outcome
83	27	50	41% Ph+ 85% >1st CR	48%	72%	DFS 51%, OS 31% at 2 years
84	22	46	11 no prior SCT	8/11	5/9	3/11 alive at 5–30 m5
		11 prior SCT	7/10	2/6	1/11 alive at 19 m	
85	33	55	33% Ph+ 66% >1st CR	45%	64%	DFS 30%, OS 39% at 1 year

Ref, reference number; aGVHD, acute graft-versus-host disease; cGVHD, chronic graft-versus-host disease; DFS, disease-free survival; OS, overall survival; m, months.

occurrence of chronic GVHD was the most important factor predicting survival [77]. Similar results were found in a review of IBMTR data including 1132 patients of all ages with ALL in first or second CR. The relative risk of relapse for patients transplanted in first CR who developed acute or chronic GVHD was 0.34 for T-cell lineage ALL and 0.44 for B-cell lineage ALL, and 0.54 and 0.61 respectively for those patients transplanted in second CR [78].

A GVL effect is also demonstrated in the subset of patients with Ph+ ALL. In a study of 121 patients, first CR status and occurrence of acute GVHD were the most relevant prognostic factors for relapse [79]. This study and others have also reported the successful use of donor lymphocyte infusions (DLI) to treat post-transplant relapse [80,81].

The presence of a GVL effect even in the absence of GVHD has been suggested by an analysis of EBMT data including 1785 ALL patients who received autologous, syngeneic or allogeneic HSCT. Allografted patients who did not develop GHVD had a lower relapse risk than patients receiving autografts [82].

The confirmation of a GVL effect in ALL opened the way to explore NMA/RIC allogeneic HSCT in this disease. Some early reports are summarized in Table 20.7 [83–85]. These studies have included older patients with median ages in the 46–55 range. A majority of patients had high-risk disease: 33–41% were Ph+, 66–85% were beyond first CR, and in one of the studies half of the patients had a prior HSCT. These studies are difficult to interpret because of the small number of patients and their short follow-up. However, it is encouraging that some patients have remained free of relapse for periods of up to 2–3

years. These preliminary results, if confirmed, would indicate that NMA/RIC could be an effective and safe approach to harness a GVL effect in elderly patients.

Summary

ALL is a rare but lethal disease in the elderly patient. Results of conventional chemotherapy programs are disappointing in this age group. In part, this is due to increased treatment-related morbidity and mortality; and in part, due to adverse biological features which renders the disease more resistant to chemotherapy. The introduction in treatment protocols of targeted drugs, such as imatinib and perhaps monoclonal antibodies, holds the promise of improving outcomes of selected subsets of patients. The possibility of harnessing a GVL effect safely, such as NMA/RIC approaches, may further improve the outcomes of ALL patients.

REFERENCES

1. Ries LAG, Eisner MP, Kosary CL, *et al.*, eds, *SEER Cancer Statistics Review, 1975–2002* (Bethesda, MD: National Cancer Institute). http: //seer.cancer.gov/csr/1975_2002, based on November 2004 SEER data submission, posted to the SEER web site 2005.
2. Taylor PR, Reid MM, Bown N, Hamilton PJ, Proctor SJ. Acute lymphoblastic leukemia in patients aged 60 years and over: a population-based study of incidence and outcome. *Blood* 1992; **80**: 1813–17.
3. Luik E, Palk K, Everaus H, *et al.* The incidence and survival of acute de novo leukaemias in Estonia and in a

well-defined region of western Sweden during 1982–1996: a survey of patients aged > or = 65. *J Intern Med* 2004; **256**: 79–85.

4. Carli PM, Coebergh JWW, Verdecchia A. Variation in survival of adult patients with haematological malignancies in Europe since 1978. *Eur J Cancer* 1998; **34**: 2253–63.

5. McNally RJQ, Alexander FE, Birch JM. Space-time clustering analyses of childhood acute lymphoblastic leukemia by immunophenotype. *Br J Cancer* 2002; **87**: 513–15.

6. Kuchinskaya E, Heyman M, Grander D, *et al.* Children and adults with acute lymphoblastic leukemia have similar gene expression profiles. *Eur J Haematol* 2005; **74**: 466–80.

7. Thomas X, Olteanu N, Charrin C, Lheritier V, Magaud JP, Fiere D. Acute lymphoblastic leukemia in the elderly: the Edouard Herriot Hospital experience. *Am J Hematol* 2001; **67**: 73–83.

8. Houot R, Tavernier E, Le QH, Lheritier V, Thiebaut A, Thomas X. Philadelphia chromosome-positive acute lymphoblastic leukemia in the elderly: prognostic factors and treatment outcome. *Hematology* 2004; **9**: 369–76.

9. Bennett JM, Catovsky D, Daniel MT, *et al.* Proposals for the classification of the acute leukaemias. French–American–British (FAB) co-operative group. *Br J Haematol* 1976; **33**: 451–8.

10. Bennett JM, Catovsky D, Daniel MT, *et al.* The morphological classification of acute lymphoblastic leukaemia: concordance among observers and clinical correlations. *Br J Haematol* 1981; **47**: 553–61.

11. Wibowo A, Pankowsky D, Mikhael A, Wright T, Steele PE, Schumacher H. Adult acute leukemia: hand mirror variant. *Hematopath Mol Hematol* 1996; **10**: 85–98.

12. Kovarik P, Shrit MA, Yuen B, Radvany R, Schumacher HR. Hand mirror variant of adult acute lymphoblastic leukemia. Evidence for a mixed leukemia. *Am J Clin Pathol* 1992; **98**: 526–30.

13. Hay CR, Barnett D, James V, Woodcock BW, Brown MG, Lawrence AC. Granular common acute lymphoblastic leukaemia in adults: a morphological study. *Eur J Haematol* 1987; **39**: 299–305.

14. Brunning RD, Borowitz M, Head D, *et al.* Precursor B-cell and T-cell neoplasms. In *World Health Organization Classification of Tumours: Tumours of Haematopoietic and Lymphoid Tissues* (Washington, DC: IARC Press, 2001), 110–17.

15. Brissette MD, Cotelingam JD. Acute leukemia and myelodysplastic syndrome. In Schumacher HR, Rock WA, Stass SA, eds, *Handbook of Hematologic Pathology* (New York, NY: Marcel Dekker, 2000), 195–201.

16. Thalhammer-Scherrer R, Mitterbauer G, Simonitsch I, *et al.* The immunophenotype of 325 adult acute leukemias: relationship to morphologic and molecular classification and proposal for a minimal screening program highly predictive for lineage discrimination. *Am J Clin Pathol* 2002; **117**: 380–9.

17. Asnafi V, Beldjord K, Libura M, *et al.* Age-related phenotypic and oncogenic differences in T-cell acute lymphoblastic leukemias may reflect thymic atrophy. *Blood* 2004; **104**: 4173–80.

18. Del Principe MI, Del Poeta G, Maurillo L, *et al.* P-glycoprotein and BCL-2 levels predict outcome in adult acute lymphoblastic leukaemia. *Br J Haematol* 2003; **121**: 730–8.

19. Brunning RD. Classification of acute leukaemias. *Semin Diagn Pathol* 2003; **20**: 142–53.

20. Khalidi HS, Chang KL, Medieros LJ, *et al.* Acute lymphoblastic leukemia. Survey of immunophenotype, French–American–British classification, frequency of myeloid antigen expression, and karyotypic abnormalities in 210 paediatric and adult cases. *Am J Clin Pathol* 1999; **111**: 467–76.

21. Primo D, Tabernero MD, Perez JJ, *et al.* Genetic heterogeneity of BCR/ABL+ adult B-cell precursor acute lymphoblastic leukemia: impact on the clinical, biological and immunophenotypical disease characteristics. *Leukemia* 2005; **19**: 713–20.

22. Wetzler M, Dodge RK, Mrozek K, *et al.* Additional cytogenetic abnormalities in adults with Philadelphia chromosome-positive acute lymphoblastic leukaemia: a study of the Cancer and Leukaemia Group B. *Br J Haematol* 2004; **124**: 275–88.

23. Pui CH, Relling MV, Downing JR. Mechanisms of disease: acute lymphoblastic leukemia. *N Engl J Med* 2004; **350**: 1535–48.

24. Westbrook CA. Molecular subsets and prognostic factors in acute lymphoblastic leukemia. *Leukemia* 1997, **11** (Suppl 4): S8–S10.

25. Legrand O, Marie JP, Marjanovic Z, *et al.* Prognostic factors in elderly acute lymphoblastic leukemia. *Br J Haematol* 1997; **97**: 596–602.

26. Rowe JM, Buck G, Burnett AK, *et al.* Induction therapy for adult with acute lymphoblastic leukemia: results of more than 1500 patients from the international ALL trial: MRC UKALL XII/ECOG E2993. *Blood* 2005; **106**: 3760–7.

27. Larson RA, Dodge RK, Burns CP, *et al.* A five-drug remission induction regimen with intensive consolidation for

adults with acute lymphoblastic leukemia; a Cancer and Leukemia Group B Study 8811. *Blood* 1995; **65**: 2025–37.

28. Schuer P, Arlin ZA, Mertelsmann R, *et al*. Treatment of acute lymphoblastic leukemia in adults: result of the L-10 and L-10M protocols. *J Clin Oncol* 1983; **1**: 462–70.

29. Hoelzer D, Thiel H, Loffler H, *et al*. Prognostic factors in a multicenter study for treatment of acute lymphoblastic leukemia in adults. *Blood* 1988; **71**: 123–31.

30. Tafuri A, Chiara G, Petrucci M, *et al*. MDR1 protein expression is an independent predictor of complete remission in newly diagnosed adult acute lymphoblastic leukemia. *Blood* 2002; **100**: 974–81.

31. Chiaretti S, Li X, Gentleman R, *et al*. Gene expression profile of adult T-cell acute lymphocytic leukemia identifies distinct subsets of patients with different response to therapy and survival. *Blood* 2004; **103**: 2771–8.

32. Mortuza FY, Papaioannou M, Moreira IM, *et al*. Minimal residual disease tests provide an independent predictor of clinical outcome in adult acute lymphoblastic leukemia. *J Clin Oncol* 2002; **20**: 1094–104.

33. Foa R, Vitale A, Mancini M, *et al*. E2A-PBX1 fusion in adult acute lymphoblastic leukemia: biological and clinical features. *Br J Haematol* 2003; **120**: 484–7.

34. Mancini M, Scappaticci D, Cimino G, *et al*. A comprehensive genetic classification of adult acute lymphoblastic leukemia (ALL): analysis of the GIMEMA 0496 protocol. *Blood* 2005; **105**: 3434–41.

35. Faderl S, Do KA, Johnson MM, *et al*. Angiogenic factors may have a different prognostic role in adult acute lymphoblastic leukemia (ALL). *Blood* 2005; **106**: 4303–7.

36. Gleissner B, Goekbuget N, Rieder H, *et al*. CD-10-negative pre-B acute lymphoblastic leukemia (ALL): a distinct high-risk group of adult ALL associated with a high frequency of MLL aberrations. Result of the German Multicenter Trials for Adult ALL (GMALL). *Blood* 2005; **106**: 4054–6.

37. Secker-Walker LM, Craig JM, Hawkins JM, *et al*. Philadelphia positive acute lymphoblastic leukemia in adults: age distribution, BCR breakpoint and prognostic significance. *Leukemia* 1991; **5**: 196–9.

38. Dombret H, Gabert J, Boiron JM, *et al*. Outcome of treatment in adults with Philadelphia chromosome-positive acute lymphoblastic leukemia—results of the prospective multicenter LALA-94 trial. *Blood* 2002; **100**: 2357–66.

39. Thomas X, Boiron JM, Huguet F, *et al*. Outcome of treatment in adults with acute lymphoblastic leukemia: analysis of the LALA-94 trial. *J Clin Oncol* 2004; **22**: 4075–86.

40. Annino L, Vegna ML, Camer A, *et al*. Treatment of adult acute lymphoblastic leukemia (ALL): long term follow up of the GIMEMA ALL 0288 randomized study. *Blood* 2002; **99**: 863–71.

41. Linker C, Damon L, Ries C, Navarro W. Intensified and shortened cyclical chemotherapy for adult acute lymphoblastic leukemia. *J Clin Oncol* 2002; **20**: 2464–71.

42. Castagnola C, Lunghi M, Caberlon S, *et al*. Long-term outcome of Ph-negative acute lymphoblastic leukemia in adults: a single centre experience. *Acta Haematol* 2005; **113**: 234–40.

43. Ribera JM, Ortega JJ, Oriol A, *et al*. Late intensification chemotherapy has not improved the results of intensive chemotherapy in acute lymphoblastic leukemia. Results of prospective multicenter randomized trial (PETHEMA ALL-89). *Haematologica* 1998; **83**: 222–30.

44. Kantarjian H, Thomas D, O'Brien S, *et al*. Long-term follow-up results of hyperfractionated cyclophosphamide, vincristine, doxorubicin, and dexamethasone (hyper-CVAD), a dose-intensive regimen, in acute lymphocytic leukemia. *Cancer* 2004; **101**: 2788–801.

45. Weiss M, Maslak P, Feldman E, *et al*. Cytarabine with high-dose mitoxantrone induces rapid complete remission in adult acute lymphoblastic leukemia without the use of vincristine or prednisone. *J Clin Oncol* 1996; **14**: 2480–5.

46. Weiss MA, Heffner L, Lamanna N, *et al*. A randomized trial of cytarabine with high-dose mitoxantrone compared to a standard vincristine/prednisone-based regimen as induction therapy for adult patients with ALL. *J Clin Oncol* 2005; **23**: abstract 6516.

47. Robak T, Szmigielska A, Wrzesien A. Acute lymphoblastic leukemia in the elderly: the Polish Adult Leukemia Group (PALG) experience. *Ann Hematol* 2003; **83**: 225–31.

48. Pagano L, Mele L, Trape G, Leone G. The treatment of acute lymphoblastic leukemia in the elderly. *Leuk Lymphoma* 2004; **45**: 117–23.

49. Offidani M, Corvatta L, Malerba L, *et al*. Comparison of two regimens for the treatment of elderly patients with acute lymphoblastic leukemia (ALL). *Leuk Lymphoma* 2005; **46**: 233–8.

50. Delannoy A, Ferrant A, Bosly A, *et al*. Acute lymphoblastic leukemia in the elderly. *Eur J Haematol* 1990; **45**: 90–3.

51. Kantarjian HM, O'Brien S, Smith T, *et al*. Acute lymphoblastic leukemia in the elderly: characteristics and

outcome with the vincristine-adriamycin-dexamethasone (VAD) regimen. *Br J Haematol* 1994; **88**: 94–100.

52. Spath-Schalbe E, Heil G, Heimpel H. Acute lymphoblastic leukemia in patients over 59 years of age: experience in a single center over a 10-year period. *Ann Hematol* 1994; **69**: 291–6.

53. Ferrari A, Annino L, Crescenzi S, *et al*. Acute lymphoblastic leukemia in the elderly: results of two different treatment approaches in 49 patients during a 25-year period. *Leukemia* 1995; **10**: 1643–7.

54. Larson RA, Dodge RK, Linker CA, *et al*. A randomized trial of filgrastim during remission induction and consolidation chemotherapy for adults with acute lymphoblastic leukemia: CALGB 9111. *Blood* 1998; **92**: 1556–64.

55. Thomas X, Boiron JM, Huguet F, *et al*. Efficacy of granulocyte and granulocyte-macrophage colony-stimulating factors in the induction treatment of adult acute lymphoblastic leukemia: a multicenter randomized study. *Hematol J* 2004; **5**: 384–94.

56. Gokbuget N, Hoelzer D. Treatment with monoclonal antibodies in acute lymphoblastic leukemia: current knowledge and future prospects. *Ann Hematol* 2004; **83**: 201–5.

57. de Vries MJ, Veerman AJ, Zwaan CM. Rituximab in three children with relapsed/refractory B-cell acute lymphoblastic leukemia/Burkitt non-Hodgkin's lymphoma. *Br J Haematol* 2002; **125**: 414–15.

58. Pfeiffer M, Stanojevic S, Feuchtinger T, *et al*. Rituximab mediates in vitro antileukemia activity in pediatric patients after allogeneic transplantation. *Bone Marrow Transplant* 2005; **36**: 91–7.

59. Golay J, Di Gaetano N, Amico D, *et al*. Gentuzumab ozogamicin (Mylotarg) has therapeutic activity against CD33 acute lymphoblastic leukemias in vitro and in vivo. *Br J Haematol* 2005; **128**: 310–17.

60. Piccaluga PP, Martinelli G, Malagola M, *et al*. Anti-leukemic and anti-GVHD effects on campath-1H in acute lymphoblastic leukemia relapsed after stem cell transplantation. *Leuk Lymphoma* 2004; **45**: 731–3.

61. Druker BJ, Sawyers CL, Kantarjian A, *et al*. Activity of a specific inhibitor of the BCR-ABL tyrosine kinase in the blast crisis of chronic myeloid leukemia and acute lymphoblastic leukemia with the Philadelphia chromosome. *N Engl J Med* 2001; **344**: 1038–42.

62. Lahaye T, Riehm B, Berger U, *et al*. Response and resistance in 300 patients with BCR-ABL-positive leukemias treated with imatinib in a single center: a 4.5 year follow up. *Cancer* 2005; **103**: 1559–69.

63. Ottmann OG, Druker BJ, Sawyers CL, *et al*. A phase II study of imatinib in patients with relapsed or refractory Philadelphia chromosome-positive acute lymphoid leukemias. *Blood* 2002; **100**: 1965–71.

64. Wassmann B, Pfeifer H, Scheuring UJ, *et al*. Early prediction of response in patients with relapsed or refractory Philadelphia chromosome-positive acute lymphoblastic leukemia (Ph+ ALL) treated with imatinib. *Blood* 2004; **103**: 1495–8.

65. Lee KH, Choi SJ, Lee JH, *et al*. Clinical effect of imatinib added to intensive combination chemotherapy for newly diagnosed Philadelphia chromosome-positive acute lymphoblastic leukemia. *Leukemia* 2005; **19**: 1509–16.

66. Towatari M, Yanada M, Usui N, *et al*. Combination of intensive chemotherapy and imatinib can rapidly induce high-quality complete remission in the majority of patients with newly diagnosed BCR-ABL acute lymphoblastic leukemia. *Blood* 2004; **14**: 3507–12.

67. Thomas DA, Faderl S, Cortes J, *et al*. Treatment of Philadelphia chromosome-positive acute lymphoblastic leukemia with hyper-CVAD and imatinib mesylate. *Blood* 2004; **103**: 4396–407.

68. Lee S, Kim DW, Kim YJ, *et al*. Minimal residual disease-based role of imatinib as first-line interim therapy prior to allogeneic stem cell transplantation in Philadelphia chromosome-positive acute lymphoblastic leukemia. *Blood* 2003; **102**: 3068–70.

69. Fruehauf S, Topaly J, Buss E, *et al*. Combination of imatinib and established treatment modalities for otherwise refractory BCRAL positive lymphoblastic leukemia. *Haematologica* 2002; **87**: ECR38.

70. Potenza L, Luppi M, Riva G, *et al*. Efficacy of imatinib mesylate as maintenance therapy in adults with acute lymphoblastic leukemia in first complete remission. *Haematologica* 2005; **90**: 1275–7.

71. Delannoy A, Lheritier V, Thomas X, *et al*. Treatment of Philadelphia-positive acute lymphocytic leukemia (Ph+ ALL) in the elderly with imatinib mesylate (STI571) and chemotherapy, an interim analysis of the (GRAALL) AFR09 trial. *Blood* 2004; **104**: abstract 2735.

72. Popat U, Carrum G, Heslop HE. Haematopoietic stem cell transplantation for acute lymphoblastic leukaemia. *Cancer Treat Rev* 2003; **29**: 3–10.

73. Gorin NC. Autologous stem cell transplantation in acute lymphocytic leukemia. *Stem Cells* 2002; **20**: 3–10.

74. Abdallah A, Egerer G, Goldschmidt H, Wannenmacher M, Korbling M, Ho A. Continuous complete remission in adult patients with acute lymphocytic leukemia at a

median observation of 12 years after autologous bone marrow transplantation. *Br J Haematol* 2001; **112**: 1012–15.

75. Attal M, Blaise D, Marit G, *et al*. Consolidation treatment of adult acute lymphoblastic leukemia: a prospective, randomized trial comparing allogeneic versus autologous bone marrow transplantation and testing the impact of recombinant interleukin-2 after autologous bone marrow transplantation. *Blood* 1995; **86**: 1619–28.

76. Hunault M, Harousseau JL, Delai M, *et al*. Better outcome of adult acute lymphoblastic leukemia after early genoidentical allogeneic bone marrow transplant (BMT) than after late high-dose therapy and autologous BMT: a GOELAMS trial. *Blood* 2004; **104**: 3028–37.

77. Zikos P, Van Lint MT, Lamparelli T, *et al*. Allogeneic hematopoietic stem cell transplantation for patients with high-risk acute lymphoblastic leukemia: favorable impact of chronic graft-versus-host disease on survival and relapse. *Haematologica* 1998; **83**: 896–903.

78. Passweg JR, Tiberghien P, Cahn JY, *et al*. Graft-versus-leukemia effects in T lineage and B lineage acute lymphoblastic leukemia. *Bone Marrow Transplant* 1998; **21**: 153–8.

79. Esperou H, Boiron JM, Cayuela JM, *et al*. A potential graft-versus-leukemia effect after hematopoietic stem cell transplantation for patients with Philadelphia chromosome positive acute lymphoblastic leukemia: results from the French Bone Marrow Transplantation Society. *Bone Marrow Transplant* 2003; **31**: 909–18.

80. Choi SJ, Lee JH, Kim S, *et al*. Treatment of relapsed acute lymphoblastic leukemia after allogeneic bone marrow transplantation with chemotherapy followed by G-CSF-primed donor lymphocyte infusion: a prospective study. *Bone Marrow Transplant* 2005; **36**: 163–9.

81. Patriarca F, Sperotto A, Skert C, Damiani D, Prosdocimo S, Fanin R. Successful treatment of hematological and extramedullary relapse of MLL-positive acute lymphoblastic leukemia after bone marrow transplantation using donor lymphocyte infusion. *Ann Hematol* 2004; **83**: 667–9.

82. Rigden O, Labopin M, Gorin NC, *et al*. Is there a graft-versus-leukemia effect in the absence of graft-versus-host disease in patients undergoing bone marrow transplantation for acute leukaemia? *Br J Haematol* 2000; **111**: 1130–7.

83. Martino R, Giralt S, Caballero MD, *et al*. Allogeneic hematopoietic stem cell transplantation with reduced-intensity conditioning in acute lymphoblastic leukemia: a feasibility study. *Haematologica* 2003; **88**: 555–60.

84. Arnold R, Massenkeil G, Bornhauser M, *et al*. Nonmyeloablative stem cell transplantation in adults with high-risk ALL may be effective in early but not in advanced disease. *Leukemia* 2002; **16**: 2423–8.

85. Hamaki T, Kami M, Kanda Y, *et al*. Reduced-intensity stem-cell transplantation for adult acute lymphoblastic leukemia: a retrospective study of 33 patients. *Bone Marrow Transplant* 2005; **35**: 549–56.

21

Multiple myeloma

Todd J. Alekshun, Melissa Alsina

Introduction

Multiple myeloma represents approximately 10% of all hematologic malignancies, and accounts for 1% of all cancers in the USA [1]. It is the second most common hematologic malignancy, and mortality rates from multiple myeloma have increased over the previous three decades. An estimated 15 980 new cases with 11 300 deaths resulting from this disease were expected in 2005 [1]. Incidence and prevalence rates are highest among the elderly, men (male : female ratio of 1.1 : 1), African-Americans, and Pacific Islanders. Mortality rates are highest among the elderly and blacks. The median age at diagnosis is 66 years, and the median survival with treatment is approximately three years [2]. Even with conventional treatment using melphalan plus prednisone (MP) or vincristine, doxorubicin plus dexamethasone (VAD) chemotherapy, or high-dose chemotherapy (HDT) followed by stem-cell transplantation, multiple myeloma still remains an incurable disease.

HDT followed by autologous peripheral-blood stem-cell transplants (ASCT) has shown disease-free and overall survival advantages when compared to standard-dose chemotherapy, but has failed to induce long-term responses in the majority of these patients. Presently, HDT followed by ASCT remains the most effective therapy for treating multiple myeloma with respect to improving disease-free intervals and overall survival, when compared with traditional therapies. Even for the geriatric population, HDT and ASCT are feasible and offer disease-free interval and survival advantages. However, for those who cannot tolerate HDT and ASCT there have been novel therapeutic developments within the past five years that have increased treatment options for induction, as well as for relapsed disease. The advent of these novel entities has broadened the therapeutic armamentarium and remains quite effective in inducing disease stabilization and affording acceptable qualities of life. Still, the challenge remains to develop more effective therapies that will prolong survival and induce long-term remissions while minimizing toxicities in elderly patients with multiple myeloma.

Pathogenesis

The exact etiology responsible for multiple myeloma has eluded the scientific community for many years, but particular associations do remain firm. Monoclonal gammopathy of undetermined significance (MGUS) is an hematologic entity that occurs in approximately 3% of those who are older than 70 years of age, and in approximately 1% of those who are older than 50 years [3]. This condition is characterized by the presence of an M-protein <3 g/dL, <10% plasma cells in the bone marrow, trace or absence of a urinary M-protein, along with an absence of anemia, hypercalcemia, renal insufficiency, and lytic bone lesions [3]. As derived from population-based studies, the risk for progression of MGUS to multiple myeloma is approximately 1% per year, although the mechanisms inducing this transformation are poorly understood [4,5]. Likely, these mechanisms involve a

Blood Disorders in the Elderly, ed. Lodovico Balducci, William Ershler, Giovanni de Gaetano.
Published by Cambridge University Press. © Cambridge University Press 2008.

complex interplay between processes unique to aberrant plasma cells such as chromosomal alterations and expression of soluble chemokines that alter the bone-marrow microenvironment, influence angiogenesis, and support the proliferation of this abnormal cell population. Among the more well-described chemokines that are involved in the pathophysiology of multiple myeloma are tumor necrosis factor α, interleukin 6 (IL-6), interleukin 1β, receptor activator of nuclear factor κB ligand (RANKL), and macrophage inflammatory protein 1α [3,6]. Exposures to pesticides, heavy metals, and ionizing radiation are among the described environmental factors associated with multiple myeloma [7,8]. However, the mechanisms by which these exposures cause multiple myeloma are speculative. Although conclusive evidence for an etiology that induces multiple myeloma does not exist, the understanding of pathobiologic mechanisms is rapidly evolving.

The transformed plasma cells or plasmablasts, the malignant cell population constituting multiple myeloma, arise from post-germinal center B cells [5]. Under normal physiologic circumstances, the plasma cell represents a terminally differentiated B cell that functions to produce immunoglobulin. The evolution and differentiation of a B cell is rather complex, and involves a relationship between the bone-marrow microenvironment, extramedullary lymphatic tissues, and soluble chemokines. B-cell development first occurs within the bone marrow, and extramedullary lymphatic tissues are critical for supporting further B-cell maturation. Upon exposure of B cells to antigens within a primary lymphatic organ (i.e., lymph-node follicle), these B cells are activated and undergo subsequent clonal proliferation. Centroblasts, which are clonally proliferating B cells, undergo somatic hypermutation of previously fully assembled V/J and V/D/J chains. Through the process of somatic hypermutation immunoglobulin affinity to encountered antigens is increased. During somatic hypermutation, B cells undergo random but specific point mutations within their V/J and V/D/J exons at an extremely high velocity. B cells completing this process are then selected for further immune responses. Upon leaving the

Table 21.1. IgH translocations. Adapted from Bergsagel PL, Kuehl WM. Chromosome translocations in multiple myeloma. *Oncogene* 2001; **20**: 5611–22 [10].

Translocations involving 14q32	Pathogenic mechanism
11q13 t(11;14) (q13;q32)	Dysregulated cyclin D1
4p16 t(4;14) (p16;q32)	Dysregulated FGFR3 (fibroblast growth factor receptor 3)
	Dysregulated MMSET (multiple myeloma SET domain)
16q23 t(14;16) (q32;q23)	Dysregulated c-maf
	Possible overexpression of c-maf
6p21 t(6;14) (p21;q32)	Overexpression of cyclin D3
20q11	Dysregulated mafB

lymphoid organ, and prior to migration back to the bone marrow, where further plasma cell differentiation occurs, these somatically mutated B cells undergo immunoglobulin heavy chain class (IgH) switching resulting in clonal selection. B cells, or centrocytes, surviving this selection process emerge from the germinal center as either plasma cells or memory B cells [9]. Early pathogenesis of MGUS and multiple myeloma involves non-random chromosomal translocation errors, or non-hyperdiploid lesions, involving this process of IgH class switching. Five recurrent translocations, all involving the IgH gene locus found on chromosome 14q32, have been described to occur in MGUS, multiple myeloma, and plasma cell leukemias (Table 21.1). Hyperdiploid lesions involving trisomies constitute other myeloma oncogenic events [5]. IgH translocations are the most frequent structural abnormalities involved in the pathogenesis of multiple myeloma. Through aberrant mechanisms and errors in switch recombination, the juxtaposition of IgH gene sequences with non-immunoglobulin sequences results in illegitimate switch rearrangements. These oncogenes are influenced by enhancer regions at the IgH locus, and therefore result in the activation of oncogenes and in many cases promote cell immortalization.

MGUS represents a low-burden clone of M-protein-producing plasma cells that do not result in the clinical or pathologic sequelae seen with multiple myeloma. Rather, MGUS most likely represents a harbinger of disease transformation, yet may remain indefinitely silent. Translocations involving immunoglobulin heavy chain genes (IgH) are among the unique biologic observations similar to both MGUS and multiple myeloma [11,12]. Primary IgH translocations are early and potentially initiating events in myelomagenesis, whereas secondary translocations occur throughout disease evolution [5]. It is estimated that approximately 50% of MGUS patients, 60–75% of multiple myeloma patients, and 85% of those with plasma cell leukemias harbor translocations involving the immunoglobulin heavy-chain gene locus located on chromosome 14q32 [13,14]. Five recurrent partner translocations have been described, including the following: 11q13, 4p16.3, 6p21, 16q23, and 20q11 [5,13,14]. One of these aforementioned loci becomes erroneously translocated as a result of an error in IgH switch recombination, which occurs in normal B-cell development in the germinal centers of primary lymphatic organs.

Presently, there are no discriminating factors that will reliably predict the progression of MGUS to multiple myeloma, although particular observations have been reported from retrospective analyses. Kyle and Rajkumar have reported higher risks of progression proportional to the magnitude of the serum M-protein at diagnosis [15]. Twenty years after the diagnosis of MGUS, the risk of progression to multiple myeloma was 14% for those who presented with an initial M-protein of ≤0.5 g/dL, while the risk was 49% for an initial M-protein of 2.5 g/dL. Cesana *et al.*, and others, found that the total burden of bone-marrow plasma cells was an independent predictor of disease transformation, whereby the risk of transformation was proportional to the total number of bone-marrow plasma cells [3,16,17]. Other postulated factors that may predict a higher risk of transformation of MGUS to multiple myeloma includes the presence of an IgA M-protein and the presence of an abnormal kappa to lambda serum free light chain ratio [3,18,19]. A risk-stratification model has been proposed by Rajkumar *et al.* for predicting progression of MGUS [20]. The risk stratification is based upon three factors: presence of an abnormal serum free light chain ratio, serum M-protein level ≥1.5 g/dL, and the presence of a non-IgG paraprotein. The absolute risk of progression at 20 years for patients demonstrating all three factors is 58%, while the absolute risks of progression at 20 years for those demonstrating one factor and those lacking any factors are 21% and 5%, respectively [20].

Diagnosis/staging/prognostic factors

By virtue of age, the elderly are prone to developing various neoplasms. Often the primary origin of a neoplasm is obscured at presentation by non-specific symptoms of back pain and fatigue, or the detection of biochemical or radiographic abnormalities such as anemia, hypercalcemia, and lytic skeletal lesions. Multiple myeloma is a heterogeneous disease manifesting at various stages with a spectrum of complications. As the manifestations of the disease are heterogeneous, non-specific abnormalities can make the diagnosis of multiple myeloma much more challenging; therefore, the clinician must have a high index of suspicion and be familiar with these heterogeneous manifestations. The presence of lytic bone lesions, found either incidentally or upon evaluating particular symptoms, should lead to a differential diagnosis whereby multiple myeloma must be considered. The most frequent manifestations of multiple myeloma are fatigue, back pain, and recurrent infections usually resulting from encapsulated bacterial organisms, *Streptococcus pneumoniae* and *Haemophilus influenzae*, as well as enteric Gram-negative bacilli. Oral candidiasis can also be a recurrent complication. Patients may be prone to bleeding due to platelet dysfunction, or from the development of an acquired coagulopathy. Kyle *et al.* reviewed the presenting features of 1027 patients with newly diagnosed multiple myeloma and found that bone pain was experienced by 58% of patients, fatigue was described by approximately 30% of patients, and weight loss occurred in 24% of newly diagnosed patients [21]. Furthermore, hypercalcemia was documented in 13%, serum creatinine level >2 mg/dL in 19%, and a neuropathy in 5% of patients.

Often, multiple myeloma is suspected upon incidentally detecting an elevated total protein, anemia, or proteinuria on routine laboratory analyses. Once suspected, the evaluation should include the following: a thorough history and physical examination, serum protein electrophoresis with immunofixation, urine protein electrophoresis with immunofixation obtained from a 24-hour urinary collection to also evaluate both total proteinuria and creatinine clearance, quantitative immunoglobulins, unilateral bone-marrow biopsy with aspirate, cytogenetic analysis, skeletal survey, serum and urine quantitative free light chains, serum calcium, CBC with differential, β2-microglobulin, LDH, and a comprehensive metabolic panel. Serum protein electrophoresis will detect an M-protein in approximately 82% of patients with multiple myeloma, while immunofixation will detect an M-protein in 93% of those with multiple myeloma [22]. Under particular clinical circumstances further diagnostic evaluation with MRI, non-contrasted CT scans, and serum viscosity can be helpful. Fluorescence in-situ hybridization (FISH) testing may also be helpful in detecting particular chromosomal aberrations that standard karyotypic analysis fails to detect, and it may add useful prognostic information. Presently, the role for positron emission tomography (PET) in evaluating patients with multiple myeloma is unclear.

The diagnosis of multiple myeloma can be established by the presence of each of the following: ≥10% abnormal plasma cells in a bone-marrow specimen or the presence of a biopsy-proven plasmacytoma, presence of a monoclonal protein in the serum (usually >3 g/dL) and/or urine (usually >1 g/dL), and either elevated serum calcium levels (>10.5 mg/ L or upper limit of normal), renal insufficiency (serum creatinine >2 mg/dL), anemia (hemoglobin <10 g/dL or at least 2 g/dL below normal), or the presence of lytic bone lesions or osteoporosis [23]. The characteristic serologic pattern seen in multiple myeloma is an elevation in the level of the monoclonal immunoglobulin and a decrease in all other, uninvolved, immunoglobulins. Patients with

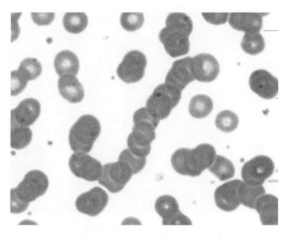

Figure 21.1 Peripheral smear showing rouleaux formation. Lazarchick, J., ASH Image Bank 2001: 101085. Copyright American Society of Hematology. All rights reserved. *See color plate section.*

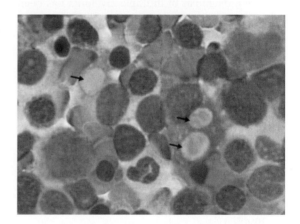

Figure 21.2 High-power view of plasma cells with large cytoplasmic inclusions known as Russell bodies (arrows). Maslak, P., ASH Image Bank 2001: 100211. Copyright American Society of Hematology. All rights reserved. *See color plate section.*

non-secretory myeloma are those with no demonstrable monoclonal protein and must have ≥30% abnormal monoclonal plasma cells within the bone marrow or a biopsy-proven plasmacytoma to fulfill the criteria for multiple myeloma. Salient hematologic findings of multiple myeloma are shown in Figs. 21.1 to 21.3.

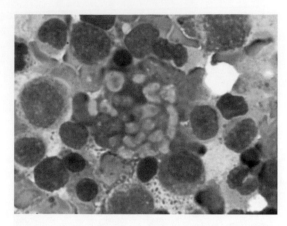

Figure 21.3 Mott cells have a cytoplasm filled with Russell bodies. Maslak, P., ASH Image Bank 2001: 100211. Copyright American Society of Hematology. All rights reserved. *See color plate section.*

Once a diagnosis of multiple myeloma has been established, there are two major systems that define staging, as well as guide treatment strategies and provide estimates of prognosis [24,25]. The International Staging System for Myeloma (ISS) [24] utilizes two variables, β2-microglobulin and serum albumin, and stratifies patients into three stages with associated survival (measured in months) as follows:

(1) Stage I – β2-microglobulin <3.5, albumin ≥3.5, survival 62 months
(2) Stage II – not meeting Stage I or Stage II criteria, survival 44 months
(3) Stage III – β2-microglobulin >5.5, survival 29 months

The more commonly used staging system was developed by Durie and Salmon [25]. The Durie–Salmon system employs the total burden of myeloma through various radiographic and biochemical factors such as presence or absence of lytic lesions, anemia, serum calcium levels, and serum and urine immunoglobulin levels, together with the presence or absence of renal insufficiency. As in the ISS, three stages have been designated, either with the absence (designated A) or presence (designated B) of renal insufficiency (renal insufficiency defined as a serum creatinine of ≥2 mg/dL).

Apart from factors specific to either the Durie–Salmon Staging System or the ISS, other independent factors that are used to prognosticate outcomes in multiple myeloma are performance status, deletion of chromosome 13, hypodiploidy, translocations involving chromosomes 4;14 or 14;16 by FISH, deletion of the short arm of chromosome 17, elevated LDH, plasmablastic morphology, and a high plasma cell labeling index [26–29]. As demonstrated by Facon *et al.*, patients with an elevated β2-microglobulin and deletion of chromosome 13 by FISH who undergo a stem-cell transplantation will have a median survival of 25 months. Similar patients with the presence of only one of these factors will have a median survival of 47 months, and patients without an elevated β2-microglobulin or deletion of chromosome 13 have median survival of 111 months [22,26]. The most frequent recurrent chromosomal deletion in multiple myeloma, deletion of chromosome 13q, is strongly associated with an unfavorable prognosis. This deletion occurs in approximately 40–55% of newly diagnosed patients with multiple myeloma, while approximately 50% of patients with MGUS will harbor deletion of 13q. Deletions involving chromosome 13q14, the site of a putative tumor suppressor gene, occur through interstitial breaks, deletions of large segmental proportions, or loss of the entire chromosomal arm [10].

Smoldering or indolent multiple myeloma, which is also synonymous to Stage IA myeloma by the Durie–Salmon staging system, is also defined by the same criteria for multiple myeloma, but with the absence of myeloma-related organ involvement or patient symptoms. This distinction is important, because treating this population of patients with smoldering/indolent or asymptomatic multiple myeloma with systemic therapies has no proven benefit with respect to improving overall survival [30,31].

Treatment

Much of the focus in the development of new therapeutic strategies for multiple myeloma has shifted away from primarily targeting the aberrant plasma cell with cytotoxic agents. The focus of drug development in treating multiple myeloma has shifted toward altering one, or many, of the complex interactions between myeloma cells and the bone-marrow microenvironment. The understanding of the mechanisms by which the bone-marrow microenvironment influences myeloma cell growth, and imparts selective drug resistance to cytotoxic agents, has gained momentum. As a result of this understanding, interest has emerged in the development and utilization of novel and rational agents, such as bortezomib, thalidomide, and lenalidomide.

On multiple levels, the bone-marrow microenvironment is uniquely influential in imparting selective tumor survival advantages among many varying hematologic malignancies, one of which includes multiple myeloma. Numerous in-vitro models have demonstrated the major impact of bone-marrow stromal cells in regulating malignant cell growth and inducing drug resistance [32–37]. Regulation of myeloma cell growth occurs via the effects of soluble mediators such as IL-6, oncostatin M, leukemia inhibitory factor, IL-10, and insulin-like growth factor 1, which are all elaborated by the bone-marrow microenvironment.

Induction

Therapeutic induction strategies for multiple myeloma focus upon achieving optimal responses, as the magnitude of response correlates with improved survival [38–40]. The approach to establishing therapy for multiple myeloma is based upon symptoms, disease stage, and most importantly the eligibility of these patients to undergo high-dose chemotherapy followed by autologous stem-cell rescue. Age no longer remains a criterion for determining transplant eligibility, rather organ function and performance status are better predictors of clinical outcome [23,41]. The use of alkylating agents as induction therapy for patients who are eligible for high-dose chemotherapy and stem-cell rescue should be avoided.

For those who are deemed to be ineligible autologous stem-cell transplantation candidates, standard induction therapies that are used to treat multiple myeloma include MP, high-dose dexamethasone, thalidomide plus dexamethasone, or VAD. Since the initial reports of the use of melphalan to treat multiple myeloma in 1958, this agent still remains the most commonly used therapy for this patient population. However, prednisone in combination with melphalan is preferred due to the enhanced efficacy provided by the addition of prednisone, as compared to single-agent melphalan [42]. However, few clinical data support this finding. Although complete response (CR) rates from MP are typically <5%, improvements in overall survival have been demonstrated when compared with supportive care. Overall response rates from MP range from 50% to 55%, and meaningful disease stabilization is achieved. In a randomized study, Facon *et al.* evaluated outcomes of standard MP compared to melphalan plus dexamethasone, single-agent dexamethasone, and dexamethasone plus recombinant interferon alpha in 489 newly diagnosed patients aged 65–75 years [43]. Overall survival from all four therapies was similar. However, those patients who did not receive melphalan had significantly shorter event-free survival (EFS) rates, as follows: MP 21.1 months, melphalan plus dexamethasone 23.1 months, versus dexamethasone 12.4 months and dexamethasone plus recombinant interferon alpha 15.2 months ($p < 0.0001$). The authors concluded that outcomes from these dexamethasone-containing regimens were equivalent to MP.

The largest meta-analysis to date, performed by the Myeloma Trialists' Collaborative Group, has compared outcomes from combination chemotherapy versus MP in 6633 evaluable patients derived from 27 randomized trials [44]. The median overall survival for patients who received MP and combination chemotherapy was 29 months. Both groups had similar overall survival rates. This publication suggested that patients who received combination chemotherapy achieved a 60% median overall response rate, compared to the 53.2% overall response rates achieved from MP ($p < 0.00001$). However, caution should be used when interpreting response data, as the authors mention that certain clinical information was incomplete and data could not be reliably interpreted.

Differences do exist between therapies with respect to how quickly responses can be achieved. MP is tolerable in the elderly and is capable of producing responses and improving overall survival, but the time to response can often be delayed when compared to other induction regimens.

The combination of vincristine, doxorubicin, and dexamethasone (VAD) is expected to produce overall response rates of 55–65% when used as induction therapy [45–47]. Although this regimen remains a well-studied and acceptable first-line therapy, there are certain disadvantages. Doxorubicin and vincristine do potentially cause alopecia, neuropathies, mucositis, neutropenia, and cardiomyopathy. Furthermore, this regimen requires central venous access, which can also be potentially problematic with respect to infections, thrombosis, and expense. This regimen can be inconvenient to many patients because of the four-day doxorubicin continuous infusion. VAD is dosed as follows: vincristine 0.4 mg/day IV and doxorubicin 9 mg/m^2/day as continuous IV infusion, both given for four consecutive days, along with dexamethasone 40 mg on days 1–4, 9–12, and 17–20. Each cycle is repeated every 28 days [45]. Approximately 85% of the efficacy of the VAD regimen is derived from dexamethasone, while doxorubicin is expected to provide a 10–15% benefit with respect to the probability of inducing a response [23,47]. As vincristine produces toxicities and adds very little to the overall efficacy of VAD, novel VAD modifications such as the substitution of pegylated liposomal doxorubicin have been tested [48].

Further understanding of multiple myeloma biology and the influence of the bone-marrow microenvironment on myeloma pathogenesis has led to the employment of immunomodulatory agents such as thalidomide and lenalidomide (CC-5013). The data generated from a number of phase II clinical studies utilizing thalidomide in combination with dexamethasone have led to the use of this therapeutic combination as induction for newly diagnosed multiple myeloma patients [49–51]. The USA Food and Drug Administration (FDA) has approved the use of thalidomide for the treatment of newly diagnosed patients with multiple myeloma. The following studies support its efficacy as induction therapy [52]. Rajkumar *et al.* demonstrated an overall response rate of 64% in 50 patients who received induction therapy with thalidomide (200 mg/day) plus monthly dexamethasone 40 mg/day given on days 1–4, 9–12, and 17–20 (on odd cycles) and on days 1–4 (even cycles) [49]. An additional 28% developed a minor reduction in paraprotein levels or stabilization of disease. The use of thalidomide and dexamethasone as induction therapy did not compromise stem-cell collection for those who proceeded to transplantation or stem-cell cryopreservation. Twelve percent of patients treated with the thalidomide plus dexamethasone combination developed deep venous thromboses, and one patient died from a fatal pulmonary embolism. The development of thromboses, which appears to be related to this combination, has led to the recommendation of concurrent administration of low-molecular-weight heparin (40 mg once daily of enoxaparin or its equivalent), warfarin to achieve a target INR of 2–3, or full-dose aspirin when patients receive this combination [50,52,53].

Similar results were demonstrated by Weber *et al.* in a phase II trial with 28 patients who were treated with thalidomide alone, and 40 patients who were treated with thalidomide combined with dexamethasone [50]. Both populations of patients were newly diagnosed and chemonaive; patients treated with thalidomide alone were asymptomatic, whereas the patients treated with thalidomide plus dexamethasone were symptomatic from their myeloma. These asymptomatic patients who were treated were felt to be at high risk for disease progression based upon the presence of selected risk factors. The median maximum tolerated thalidomide dose was 400 mg in those patients treated with thalidomide alone, and 200 mg in those treated with combination thalidomide and dexamethasone. The overall response rates, defined as partial responses or better, were 36% in those receiving thalidomide alone and 72% in those receiving combination therapy. Sixteen percent of those treated with thalidomide and dexamethasone achieved a complete response. Furthermore, the median time to response was 4.2 months and 0.7 months for those treated with thalidomide and thalidomide with dexamethasone, respectively. A 25% incidence of thromboembolic events was noted in the first 24 patients treated with combination thalidomide and dexamethasone (these patients did not receive concurrent or pre treatment anticoagulation). The incidence of thromboembolic events in patients treated with full-dose anticoagulation is rare.

The Eastern Cooperative Oncology Group (E1A00) has concluded its phase III trial comparing the combination of thalidomide plus dexamethasone with dexamethasone as a single agent as induction therapy for patients with newly diagnosed multiple myeloma [54]. The dosing schema for the combination arm is thalidomide 200 mg orally once daily with dexamethasone 40 mg orally on days 1–4, 9–12, and 17–20, repeated monthly. Overall response rates, the primary endpoint, are defined as a decrease in serum and urine monoclonal protein by 50% and greater. Among the 207 randomly assigned patients, responses were observed in 63% of those receiving the combination therapy and in 41% who received dexamethasone alone ($p = 0.0017$). Median time to response was 1.1 months in both treatment groups. Importantly, 17% of those receiving thalidomide plus dexamethasone developed a deep venous thrombosis, compared to 3% of those receiving dexamethasone.

Although not without toxicities, induction treatment with single-agent pulse dexamethasone can also be employed for those not willing to receive thalidomide or vincristine plus doxorubicin, or in cases where these treatments are contraindicated. Response rates for single-agent dexamethasone can be as high as 40–50%, and a standard dosing regimen would be 40 mg/day (20 mg/m²/day) given on days 1–4, 9–12, and 17–20, repeated monthly [23,55].

Lenalidomide is a thalidomide analog that possesses a 200- to 1000-fold more potent immunomodulatory activity. Among the mechanisms by which lenalidomide induces a pharmacologic effect is by inhibiting the release of IL-6, vascular endothelial growth factor, and tumor necrosis factor α. Through its effects on modulating various cytokines, lenalidomide disrupts angiogenesis, alters adhesion of myeloma cells to bone-marrow stroma, and facilitates apoptosis [56–58]. Furthermore, lenalidomide appears to have better tolerability and a more favorable side-effect profile than thalidomide. Rajkumar et al. have reported an overall response rate of 91% in 34 symptomatic patients treated with lenalidomide (25 mg orally given consecutively for 21 days of a 28-day cycle) plus dexamethasone (40 mg orally on days 1–4, 9–12, 17–20) as induction therapy for newly diagnosed multiple myeloma [59]. These responses included: 6% complete response, 32% very good partial response, and 53% partial response. The median time to response was four weeks.

Two phase II studies have evaluated the role of bortezomib as first-line treatment for multiple myeloma [60,61]. Oakervee et al. reported overall response rates of 95% in 21 symptomatic, newly diagnosed multiple myeloma patients who received bortezomib together with doxorubicin, and dexamethasone (PAD) as induction therapy prior to ASCT [61]. This treatment consisted of four cycles of bortezomib 1.3 mg/m² administered on days 1, 4, 8, and 11 along with dexamethasone 40 mg on days 1–4, 8–11, 15–18 during cycle 1, and days 1–4 of cycles 2–4. Furthermore, patients received escalating doses of doxorubicin until 9 mg/m² was achieved on days 1–4 of each cycle. There were no reported dose-limiting toxicities, and 90% of patients received all four planned cycles of therapy. Following induction with PAD, 24% achieved a complete response, and 20 of 21 had undergone stem-cell mobilization, with 18 of 20 patients proceeding to receive HDT plus ASCT.

High-dose chemotherapy and autologous stem-cell transplantation

High-dose chemotherapy (HDT) followed by autologous peripheral-blood stem-cell rescue is the standard and preferred primary treatment approach for patients with multiple myeloma who are less than 70 years old and who have adequate organ function [2,39,40]. Although advanced age is not an absolute

Table 21.2. Prospective randomized autologous stem-cell transplant trials.

Trial	No. of patients	Median age (years)	CR or VGPR (HDT+ASCT vs. CC)	Overall survival (months) (HDT+ASCT vs. CC)
IFM 90 [39]	200	57.4	38% vs. 14% ($p < 0.001$)	57 vs. 44 ($p = 0.03$)
MRC VII [40]	401	55	44% vs. 8% ($p < 0.001$)	54.1 vs. 42.3 ($p = 0.04$)
Trial	No. of patients	Median age (years)	CR or VGPR (IDT + ASCT vs. CC)	Overall survival (months) (IDT + ASCT vs. CC)
Palumbo *et al.* [62]	194	65	25% vs. 6% ($p = 0.0002$)	58+ vs. 42.5 ($p = 0.005$)

CR, complete response; VGPR, very good partial response; HDT, high-dose chemotherapy; IDT, intermediate-dose chemotherapy; ASCT, autologous stem-cell transplant; CC, conventional chemotherapy.

contraindication for treatment with HDT and ASCT, the two randomized prospective trials confirming a survival benefit using this approach were conducted in patients aged less than 65 years [39,40]. A third randomized trial confirmed a survival benefit among newly diagnosed patients with multiple myeloma who were older than 65 years (range 51–70), but these patients received intermediate-dose melphalan (IDT) followed by ASCT (Table 21.2) [62]. Palumbo *et al.* randomized 194 newly diagnosed patients to receive either two cycles of intermediate-dose melphalan (100 mg/m^2) followed by ASCT or conventional MP. Unique among these patients' characteristics were the median ages of those randomized to both treatment arms, 65 years for those receiving IDT plus ASCT and 63 years for those receiving conventional MP. Forty-six percent of patients randomized to the IDT treatment arm were ≥65 years. Superior overall survival, event-free survival, and response rates were demonstrated in those receiving IDT followed by ASCT. Furthermore, patients older than 65 years also derived superior overall survival, event-free survival, and overall response rates from this approach.

In general, estimated overall response rates and CR rates following HDT and ASCT, when used as part of induction therapeutic programs, are 75–90% and 20–40%, respectively, and estimated median survival is 4–5 years [2,39,63–65]. Compared with conventional chemotherapy, HDT followed by ASCT affords a 13-month longer median duration of overall survival and higher rates of EFS in some studies [39,63]. In the large MRC VII trial, Child *et al.* reported CR rates of 44% in patients treated with HDT and ASCT, while those treated with conventional chemotherapy achieved CR rates of 8% ($p < 0.001$) [40]. The median overall survival was 54.1 months in those patients receiving HDT and ASCT, compared to 42.3 months in patients who received conventional chemotherapy. Higher rates of progression-free survival, 32 months versus 20 months ($p < 0.001$), were also seen in the HDT group. The results of this trial were recently updated and reflect a median follow-up of 68 months [66]. Overall survival was 14.1 months longer in those receiving HDT and ASCT (median overall survival of 56.3 months in the HDT and ASCT group versus 42.2 months in the conventional therapy arm, $p = 0.004$), while a significant improvement in the median progression-free survival was seen in the HDT and ASCT arm compared with the conventional therapy arm, 31.2 months and 19.5 months ($p = 0.0001$), respectively. Further evidence supporting the benefits of HDT followed by ASCT over conventional chemotherapy were reported by Attal *et al.* from the IFM-90 trial [39]. Complete response or very good partial response was achieved by 38% of the patients receiving HDT and ASCT, as compared with 14% randomized to the conventional chemotherapy arm ($p < 0.001$). After a median follow-up of 108 months, EFS was superior in the HDT arm (28 months versus 18 months, $p = 0.01$), and a seven-year probability of overall survival of 35% versus 20% ($p = 0.03$) was demonstrated favoring the HDT arm. Based upon these data and others [67–71], HDT followed by ASCT significantly enhances CR and EFS rates, and, in the case of the IFM-90 and MRC VII trials, it also improves overall survival. Achievement and maintenance of durable disease control in multiple myeloma strongly correlates with early development of CR, which is considerably enhanced by HDT followed by ASCT.

Still, very few people have been cured to date. Although less toxic and more available than allogeneic transplantation, autologous peripheral-blood stem-cell transplantation is problematic for two reasons: lack of a graft-versus-myeloma effect, and contamination of the graft with myeloma cells. Efforts to further reduce tumor cell contamination through tandem autologous transplantations have occurred, and results have been reported [71–76]. In a landmark trial, the French Myeloma Intergroup reported an overall survival benefit among patients undergoing tandem autologous stem-cell transplantation [76]. Patients who failed to achieve a very good partial response after a single autologous transplant seemed to benefit the most from tandem autologous transplantation. Both the seven-year EFS, 20% versus 10% ($p < 0.03$), and seven-year overall survival, 42% versus 21% ($p = 0.01$), were double among those in the tandem transplant cohort. Among patients failing to achieve a very good partial response within three months after a single autologous transplantation, the estimated overall seven-year survival advantage was nearly fourfold in those receiving a tandem transplant [76].

In a randomized trial, Vesole et al. were among the first to apply tandem ASCT to a large number of multiple myeloma patients, and subsequently demonstrated the safety and benefits of extensions in EFS and overall survival resulting from this treatment. Furthermore, they demonstrated CR rates increased from 24% to 43% following the first ASCT and second ASCT, respectively [73]. Barlogie et al. also demonstrated the safety and feasibility of tandem ASCT, as well as improved outcomes resulting from its use. In Total Therapy I, Barlogie et al. demonstrated improved response rates and overall survival among patients who received tandem

autologous transplants as compared with matched controls (receiving standard therapy) or those receiving single autologous transplants. At ten years of follow-up, the median overall survival and EFS of the 152 patients who received a tandem autologous transplant were 79 months (33%) ($p < 0.001$) and 37 months (15%) ($p < 0.001$), respectively. The median overall survival and EFS, among the comparative 152 matched controls who received standard therapy, were 43 months (15%) and 16 months (5%), respectively [71].

Other randomized trials comparing single autologous transplants to tandem autologous transplants have been published with mixed results [77–81]. These studies, however, differ in design and have shorter intervals of median follow-up. Therefore, overall conclusions are challenging and require cautious interpretation [2].

The optimal conditioning regimen for autologous stem-cell transplantation in multiple myeloma has not yet been determined. Therefore, new effective regimens and approaches are warranted.

Relapsed disease

The behavior of multiple myeloma is such that almost every patient will experience a disease relapse at some point during the disease course. The development of novel therapeutic compounds to treat multiple myeloma has resulted from our continued understanding of multiple myeloma biology, and has expanded the therapeutic armamentarium for treating patients with relapsed disease. The novel agent bortezomib is one example. Bortezomib gained FDA approval in May 2003 for the treatment of patients with relapsed multiple myeloma after treatment with at least two prior regimens. The FDA has now approved its use for the treatment of relapsed disease following treatment with one prior regimen. In a non-randomized, multi-center, phase II trial evaluating the efficacy of bortezomib in patients with relapsed, refractory multiple myeloma, 193 patients were evaluated after having received bortezomib 1.3 mg/m^2 on days 1, 4, 8, and 11 every 21 days for a median duration of treatment of 3.8 months [82].

Ninety-two percent of these patients had received three or more prior therapies, and most were refractory to their most recent therapy. Follow-up after 24 weeks of treatment revealed an overall response rate (including minor responses) of 35%, and 27% of patients who received bortezomib achieved either a complete or partial response. Of these responses, 4% developed a CR and 6% developed a near-CR (myeloma protein only demonstrable by immunofixation). The median overall survival and duration of response were 16 months and 12 months, respectively. Grade 4 toxicities included thrombocytopenia (3%), diarrhea, and neutropenia (3%), while grade 3 toxicities included (but were not limited to) thrombocytopenia (28%), neutropenia (11%), and peripheral neuropathy (12%).

One other phase II study, by Jagannath *et al.*, evaluated 54 multiple myeloma patients who failed or relapsed after first-line therapy [83]. Two doses of bortezomib ($1.0 \, \text{mg/m}^2$ and $1.3 \, \text{mg/m}^2$) were given twice weekly, in a three-week cycle, for eight cycles. The complete and partial response rates among those who received bortezomib $1.3 \, \text{mg/m}^2$ were 38%, while the complete and partial response rates among those who received bortezomib $1.0 \, \text{mg/m}^2$ were 30%.

Many alternate strategies exist for treating patients with relapsed disease. Some of these include re-treatment with the induction regimen if relapse occurs more than six months after initial treatment, HDT followed by ASCT, thalidomide-based regimen, or treatment under the guidance of a clinical trial. At the time of disease relapse, treatment with HDT followed by ASCT offers the same survival advantage compared to employing this treatment modality immediately after induction therapy [22]. This has been demonstrated through prospective studies [67].

Thalidomide-based therapies, either as a single agent or in combination with glucocorticoids or cytotoxic agents, have activity in treating relapsed disease. When single-agent thalidomide is used to treat patients with relapsed disease, expected response rate, defined as ≥50% reduction in M-protein, is 25–35%, with median duration and time to response of 12 months and 1–2 months, respectively [84–88]. Combining thalidomide with dexamethasone in this treatment setting can enhance response rates to approximately 50% [22,89,90].

Primary refractory disease

Approximately 20–30% of patients with newly diagnosed multiple myeloma fail to respond to induction treatment regimens such as VAD or thalidomide and dexamethasone [91]. As a result, these patients have primary refractory disease. Even though these patients still benefit from high-dose chemotherapy, their progression-free survival ranges from four to eight months, while overall survival is approximately 12 months [92]. This is significantly lower than for patients with responsive disease at diagnosis.

The pathogenesis of primary resistance to chemotherapy is poorly understood, but likely involves factors intrinsic to the myeloma cells, as well as those posed by the bone-marrow microenvironment. Regarding the latter, it is well known that adhesion of myeloma cells to stroma renders these cells resistant to chemotherapy [93]. This is a form of *de novo* drug resistance, and these phenotypes have been described for multiple chemotherapeutic agents [33,94,95]. Protection against drug-induced cytotoxicity occurs via direct contact with stromal elements, and this most probably accounts for poor response rates to chemotherapy in those patients with primary refractory multiple myeloma. Several mechanisms involving this phenomenon, in both hematologic and non-hematologic cell lines, have been proposed. NF-κB is one important, and perhaps the major, regulatory pathway that mediates resistance of myeloma cells when adhered to fibronectin. Increases of NF-κB activity in multiple myeloma correlates with an increase in tumor cell survival [96–99]. Interestingly, when myeloma cells are adherent to fibronectin this resistance is overcome by the proteasome inhibitor bortezomib. This suggests a role for bortezomib to overcome *de novo* drug resistance and sensitize multiple myeloma cells to chemotherapy. Several investigators have shown that bortezomib sensitizes myeloma cells to chemotherapy, in particular melphalan [37].

Regulation of anti-apoptotic products via NF-κB activation is one example of cell-adhesion-mediated drug resistance (CAM-DR). Anti-apoptotic signal transduction pathways are activated and gene products, which are regulated by the NF-κB superfamily, are altered through myeloma cell interactions with elements of their bone-marrow microenvironment – most specifically, fibronectin [93]. Landowski et al. have described a signal transduction pathway that contributes to an important anti-apoptotic phenotype in myeloma cells [100]. Resulting from interactions between myeloma cells and fibronectin, they demonstrated increased expression of 53 gene products. Eleven of these gene products are regulated by a pathway involving the NF-κB superfamily. Among these eleven NF-κB-regulated genes are apoptosis inhibitor-2, tumor necrosis factor-α-induced protein 2, MAX protein, IL-6, nuclear factor of kappa light polypeptide gene enhancer in B-cell inhibitor alpha, IL-8, and CD83 antigen. In this study, it was found that the RPMI 8226, ARH 77, H 929, and MM.1S myeloma cell lines all undergo a significant time-dependent induction of NF-κB DNA binding activity upon adhesion to fibronectin. A specific member of the NF-κB family, RelB, was preferentially activated, thereby adding another molecular dimension to myeloma cell resistance against drug-induced apoptosis. Hideshima et al. have proposed another mechanism explaining de novo myeloma cell drug resistance imparted by the bone-marrow microenvironment [32]. This pathway involves TNF-α-mediated expression of NF-κB by the stromal elements. Bortezomib has been shown to reduce binding interactions between myeloma cells and bone-marrow stromal cells [32]. Bortezomib has also been shown to sensitize highly resistant myeloma cell lines to chemotherapy [37]. Ma et al. demonstrated that bortezomib sensitized resistant myeloma cell lines to melphalan and other chemotherapeutic agents, thereby overcoming drug resistance by enhancing apoptosis [37]. It has been established that levels of phosphorylated IκBα, a cytoplasmic NF-κB inhibitory protein, increase in myeloma cells following exposure to

chemotherapy [37]. Phosphorylated IκBα becomes a selective target for ubiquitination and subsequent cytoplasmic degradation by the proteosome, a process that is inhibited by bortezomib.

Other mechanisms of intrinsic or acquired drug resistance include both quantitative and qualitative changes in intracellular drug targets, increases in p27^{kip1} levels, overexpression of multidrug resistance-associated protein (MRP), P-glycoprotein (Pgp), and lung-resistance protein (LRP) [100–104].

HDT followed by ASCT has recently been shown to benefit patients with primary refractory multiple myeloma [91]. Overall response rates were demonstrated in 46 of the 50 (92%) evaluable patients who received high-dose melphalan followed by ASCT. Ten of the 50 patients (20%) achieved a CR ($p = 0.06$). The one-year estimated progression-free survival for this group of patients was 70% ($p = 0.65$). Alexanian et al. evaluated the outcomes of early (within one year of diagnosis) intensive therapy followed by ASCT in 113 patients with primary refractory disease [105]. These patients were compared to 81 matched controls who continued to receive standard therapy. The overall response rate in the intensive-therapy group was 58%. Of these patients, 17% achieved a CR, while 88% achieved a partial response within two months. The median survival was 4 years in the intensive therapy group compared to 2.8 years in the matched control group ($p = 0.02$). Furthermore, the median survival was 6.9 years for those achieving a CR, 4.3 years for those achieving a PR, and 3.1 years for non-responders ($p < 0.02$). In another study performed by the Royal Marsden Group, 40% of 43 patients with primary refractory disease achieved a CR following high-dose melphalan and autologous transplantation [106]. The event-free and overall survival rates at five years for patients with primary refractory disease who achieved a CR were similar to those who achieved a response to initial induction therapy. Vesole et al. reported improved EFS (23 versus 14 months) and overall survival (39 versus 25 months) in patients with primary refractory multiple myeloma who received HDT followed by tandem ASCT when compared to patients with resistant relapse [107]. Overall, data support that patients with primary refractory multiple myeloma benefit from HDT and both single and tandem ASCT [73,91,105,106,108–113].

Plasma cell leukemia

There are only anecdotal data relating to patients with plasma cell leukemia who have undergone HDT followed by ASCT. To date, no optimal regimen exists for treating patients with plasma cell leukemia. For eligible patients with plasma cell leukemia, the preferred treatment approach is HDT followed by ASCT [114–123].

Conclusions

Multiple myeloma is a common hematologic malignancy, primarily affecting the aged population. This disease presents with heterogeneous manifestations and is complicated by significant degrees of morbidity. No defined etiology has been identified, but much progress has been made in multiple myeloma therapeutics, with positive impacts on quality of life and survival. Within the arena of all hematologic malignancies, multiple myeloma has been unequivocally influenced by the development and employment of multiple, novel therapies that have influenced our management of this disorder. Among these novel breakthroughs are a greater understanding of proteosome biology and the development of bortezomib, an understanding of angiogenesis biology and the role of the bone-marrow microenvironment in myeloma, which has led to the use of thalidomide and lenalidomide, the role for tandem ASCT, and the use of kyphoplasty and bisphosphonates for treating skeletal complications resulting from multiple myeloma. Unfortunately, none of these novel interventions has cured this hematologic malignancy. Therefore, a considerable amount of knowledge and understanding, with respect to myeloma biology and the mechanisms responsible for drug resistance, still remains to be conquered.

The magnitude of responses translates into better overall survival rates [38–40]. In addition, overall response rates, CR rates, and overall survival rates resulting from HDT followed by autologous peripheral-blood stem-cell transplantation exceed those obtained from conventional chemotherapy [39,40,63].

REFERENCES

1. Jemal A, Clegg LX, Ward E, *et al.* Annual report to the nation on the status of cancer, 1975–2001, with a special feature regarding survival. *Cancer* 2004; **101**: 3–27.
2. Barlogie B, Shaughnessy J, Tricot G, *et al.* Treatment of multiple myeloma. *Blood* 2004; **103**: 20–32.
3. Kyle RA, Rajkumar SV. Monoclonal gammopathy of undetermined significance. *Clin Lymphoma Myeloma* 2005; **6**: 102–14.
4. Kyle RA, Therneau TM, Rajkumar SV, *et al.* A long-term study of prognosis in monoclonal gammopathy of undetermined significance. *N Engl J Med* 2002; **346**: 564–9.
5. Hideshima T, Bergsagel PL, Kuehl WM, Anderson KC. Advances in biology of multiple myeloma: clinical applications. *Blood* 2004; **104**: 607–18.
6. Lust JA, Donovan KA. The role of interleukin-1 beta in the pathogenesis of multiple myeloma. *Hematol Oncol Clin North Am* 1999; **13**: 1117–25.
7. Bertazzi PA, Pesatori AC, Bernucci I, Landi MT, Consonni D. Dioxin exposure and human leukemias and lymphomas: lessons from the Seveso accident and studies on industrial workers. *Leukemia* 1999; **13** (Suppl 1): S72–S74.
8. Schwartz GG. Multiple myeloma: clusters, clues, and dioxins. *Cancer Epidemiol Biomarkers Prev* 1997; **6**: 49–56.
9. DeFranco. B-cell development and the humoral immune response. In Parslow T, Stites D, Terr A, Imboden J, eds, *Medical Immunology* (San Francisco, CA: McGraw-Hill, 2001).
10. Bergsagel PL, Kuehl WM. Chromosome translocations in multiple myeloma. *Oncogene* 2001; **20**: 5611–22.
11. Avet-Loiseau H, Li JY, Facon T, *et al.* High incidence of translocations t(11;14)(q13;q32) and t(4;14)(p16;q32) in patients with plasma cell malignancies. *Cancer Res* 1998; **58**: 5640–5.
12. Fonseca R, Bailey RJ, Ahmann GJ, *et al.* Genomic abnormalities in monoclonal gammopathy of undetermined significance. *Blood* 2002; **100**: 1417–24.

13. Kuehl WM, Bergsagel PL. Multiple myeloma: evolving genetic events and host interactions. *Nat Rev Cancer* 2002; **2**: 175–87.

14. Seidl S, Kaufmann H, Drach J. New insights into the pathophysiology of multiple myeloma. *Lancet Oncol* 2003; **4**: 557–64.

15. Kyle RA, Rajkumar SV. Monoclonal gammopathies of undetermined significance: a review. *Immunol Rev* 2003; **194**: 112–39.

16. Baldini L, Guffanti A, Cesana BM, *et al*. Role of different hematologic variables in defining the risk of malignant transformation in monoclonal gammopathy. *Blood* 1996; **87**: 912–18.

17. Cesana C, Klersy C, Barbarano L, *et al*. Prognostic factors for malignant transformation in monoclonal gammopathy of undetermined significance and smoldering multiple myeloma. *J Clin Oncol* 2002; **20**: 1625–34.

18. Blade J, Lopez-Guillermo A, Rozman C, *et al*. Malignant transformation and life expectancy in monoclonal gammopathy of undetermined significance. *Br J Haematol* 1992; **81**: 391–4.

19. Rajkumar SV, Kyle RA, Therneau TM, *et al*. Presence of monoclonal free light chains in the serum predicts risk of progression in monoclonal gammopathy of undetermined significance. *Br J Haematol* 2004; **127**: 308–10.

20. Rajkumar SV, Kyle RA, Therneau TM, *et al*. Serum free light chain ratio is an independent risk factor for progression in monoclonal gammopathy of undetermined significance. *Blood* 2005; **106**: 812–17.

21. Kyle RA, Gertz MA, Witzig TE, *et al*. Review of 1027 patients with newly diagnosed multiple myeloma. *Mayo Clin Proc* 2003; **78**: 21–33.

22. Rajkumar SV, Kyle RA. Multiple myeloma: diagnosis and treatment. *Mayo Clin Proc* 2005; **80**: 1371–82.

23. Durie BG, Kyle RA, Belch A, *et al*. Myeloma management guidelines: a consensus report from the Scientific Advisors of the International Myeloma Foundation. *Hematol J* 2003; **4**: 379–98.

24. Greipp PR, Miguel JS, Durie BGM, *et al*. International staging system for multiple myeloma. *J Clin Oncol* 2005; **23**: 3412–20.

25. Durie BG, Salmon SE. A clinical staging system for multiple myeloma. Correlation of measured myeloma cell mass with presenting clinical features, response to treatment, and survival. *Cancer* 1975; **36**: 842–54.

26. Facon T, Avet-Loiseau H, Guillerm G, *et al*. Chromosome 13 abnormalities identified by FISH analysis and serum beta2-microglobulin produce a powerful myeloma staging system for patients receiving high-dose therapy. *Blood* 2001; **97**: 1566–71.

27. Rajkumar SV, Fonseca R, Lacy MQ, *et al*. Plasmablastic morphology is an independent predictor of poor survival after autologous stem-cell transplantation for multiple myeloma. *J Clin Oncol* 1999; **17**: 1551–7.

28. Kyle RA. Prognostic factors in multiple myeloma. *Stem Cells* 1995; **13** (Suppl 2): 56–63.

29. Rajkumar SV, Greipp PR. Prognostic factors in multiple myeloma. *Hematol Oncol Clin North Am* 1999; **13**: 1295–314.

30. Hjorth M, Hellquist L, Holmberg E, Magnusson B, Rodjer S, Westin J. Initial versus deferred melphalan-prednisone therapy for asymptomatic multiple myeloma stage I: a randomized study. Myeloma Group of Western Sweden. *Eur J Haematol* 1993; **50**: 95–102.

31. Riccardi A, Mora O, Tinelli C, *et al*. Long-term survival of stage I multiple myeloma given chemotherapy just after diagnosis or at progression of the disease: a multicentre randomized study. Cooperative Group of Study and Treatment of Multiple Myeloma. *Br J Cancer* 2000; **82**: 1254–60.

32. Hideshima T, Richardson P, Chauhan D, *et al*. The proteasome inhibitor PS-341 inhibits growth, induces apoptosis, and overcomes drug resistance in human multiple myeloma cells. *Cancer Res* 2001; **61**: 3071–6.

33. Damiano JS, Cress AE, Hazlehurst LA, Shtil AA, Dalton WS. Cell adhesion mediated drug resistance (CAM-DR): role of integrins and resistance to apoptosis in human myeloma cell lines. *Blood* 1999; **93**: 1658–67.

34. Garrido SM, Appelbaum FR, Willman CL, Banker DE. Acute myeloid leukemia cells are protected from spontaneous and drug-induced apoptosis by direct contact with a human bone marrow stromal cell line (HS-5). *Exp Hematol* 2001; **29**: 448–57.

35. Hazlehurst LA, Dalton WS. Mechanisms associated with cell adhesion mediated drug resistance (CAM-DR) in hematopoietic malignancies. *Cancer Metastasis Rev* 2001; **20**: 43–50.

36. Hazlehurst LA, Valkov N, Wisner L, *et al*. Reduction in drug-induced DNA double-strand breaks associated with beta1 integrin-mediated adhesion correlates with drug resistance in U937 cells. *Blood* 2001; **98**: 1897–903.

37. Ma MH, Yang HH, Parker K, *et al*. The proteasome inhibitor PS-341 markedly enhances sensitivity of multiple myeloma tumor cells to chemotherapeutic agents. *Clin Cancer Res* 2003; **9**: 1136–44.

38. Harousseau JL, Moreau P. Evolving role of stem cell transplantation in multiple myeloma. *Clin Lymphoma Myeloma* 2005; **6**: 89–95.

39. Attal M, Harousseau JL, Stoppa AM, *et al*. A prospective, randomized trial of autologous bone marrow transplantation and chemotherapy in multiple myeloma. Intergroupe Francais du Myelome. *N Engl J Med* 1996; **335**: 91–7.

40. Child JA, Morgan GJ, Davies FE, *et al*. High-dose chemotherapy with hematopoietic stem-cell rescue for multiple myeloma. *N Engl J Med* 2003; **348**: 1875–83.

41. Sirohi B, Powles R, Treleaven J, *et al*. The role of autologous transplantation in patients with multiple myeloma aged 65 years and over. *Bone Marrow Transplant* 2000; **25**: 533–9.

42. Alexanian R, Haut A, Khan AU, *et al*. Treatment for multiple myeloma. Combination chemotherapy with different melphalan dose regimens. *JAMA* 1969; **208**: 1680–5.

43. Facon T, Mary J, Attal M, *et al*. Melphalan-prednisone versus dexamethasone-based regimens for newly diagnosed myeloma patients aged 65–75 years. Final analysis of the IFM 95-01 trial on 489 patients. *Blood* 2003; **102** (11): abstract 507.

44. Combination chemotherapy versus melphalan plus prednisone as treatment for multiple myeloma: an overview of 6,633 patients from 27 randomized trials. Myeloma Trialists' Collaborative Group. *J Clin Oncol* 1998; **16**: 3832–42.

45. Barlogie B, Smith L, Alexanian R. Effective treatment of advanced multiple myeloma refractory to alkylating agents. *N Engl J Med* 1984; **310**: 1353–6.

46. Alexanian R, Barlogie B, Tucker S. VAD-based regimens as primary treatment for multiple myeloma. *Am J Hematol* 1990; **33**: 86–9.

47. Kyle RA, Rajkumar SV. Multiple myeloma. *N Engl J Med* 2004; **351**: 1860–73.

48. Hussein MA, Anderson KC. Role of liposomal anthracyclines in the treatment of multiple myeloma. *Semin Oncol* 2004; **31** (6 Suppl 13): 147–60.

49. Rajkumar SV, Hayman S, Gertz MA, *et al*. Combination therapy with thalidomide plus dexamethasone for newly diagnosed myeloma. *J Clin Oncol* 2002; **20**: 4319–23.

50. Weber D, Rankin K, Gavino M, Delasalle K, Alexanian R. Thalidomide alone or with dexamethasone for previously untreated multiple myeloma. *J Clin Oncol* 2003; **21**: 16–19.

51. Cavo M, Zamagni E, Tosi P, *et al*. First-line therapy with thalidomide and dexamethasone in preparation for autologous stem cell transplantation for multiple myeloma. *Haematologica* 2004; **89**: 826–31.

52. Dimopoulos MA, Anagnostopoulos A, Weber D. Treatment of plasma cell dyscrasias with thalidomide and its derivatives. *J Clin Oncol* 2003; **21**: 4444–54.

53. Rajkumar SV. Thalidomide therapy and deep venous thrombosis in multiple myeloma. *Mayo Clin Proc* 2005; **80**: 1549–51.

54. Rajkumar SV, Blood E, Vesole D, Fonseca R, Greipp PR. Phase III clinical trial of thalidomide plus dexamethasone compared with dexamethasone alone in newly diagnosed multiple myeloma: a clinical trial coordinated by the Eastern Cooperative Oncology Group. *J Clin Oncol* 2006; **24**: 431–6.

55. Alexanian R, Dimopoulos MA, Delasalle K, Barlogie B. Primary dexamethasone treatment of multiple myeloma. *Blood* 1992; **80**: 887–90.

56. Dredge K, Marriott JB, Macdonald CD, *et al*. Novel thalidomide analogues display anti-angiogenic activity independently of immunomodulatory effects. *Br J Cancer* 2002; **87**: 1166–72.

57. Hideshima T, Chauhan D, Podar K, Schlossman RL, Richardson P, Anderson KC. Novel therapies targeting the myeloma cell and its bone marrow microenvironment. *Semin Oncol* 2001; **28**: 607–12.

58. Mitsiades N, Mitsiades CS, Poulaki V, *et al*. Apoptotic signaling induced by immunomodulatory thalidomide analogs in human multiple myeloma cells: therapeutic implications. *Blood* 2002; **99**: 4525–30.

59. Rajkumar SV, Hayman SR, Lacy MQ, *et al*. Combination therapy with lenalidomide plus dexamethasone (Rev/Dex) for newly diagnosed myeloma. *Blood* 2005; **106**: 4050–3.

60. Jagannath S, Durie BG, Wolf J, *et al*. Bortezomib therapy alone and in combination with dexamethasone for previously untreated symptomatic multiple myeloma. *Br J Haematol* 2005; **129**: 776–83.

61. Oakervee HE, Popat R, Curry N, *et al*. PAD combination therapy (PS-341/bortezomib, doxorubicin and dexamethasone) for previously untreated patients with multiple myeloma. *Br J Haematol* 2005; **129**: 755–62.

62. Palumbo A, Bringhen S, Petrucci MT, *et al*. Intermediate-dose melphalan improves survival of myeloma patients aged 50 to 70: results of a randomized controlled trial. *Blood* 2004; **104**: 3052–7.

63. Attal M, Harousseau JL. Randomized trial experience of the Intergroupe Francophone du Myelome. *Semin Hematol* 2001; **38**: 226–30.

64. Barlogie B, Jagannath S, Epstein J, *et al.* Biology and therapy of multiple myeloma in 1996. *Semin Hematol* 1997; **34** (1 Suppl 1): 67–72.

65. Rajkumar SV, Fonseca R, Dispenzieri A, *et al.* Effect of complete response on outcome following autologous stem cell transplantation for myeloma. *Bone Marrow Transplant* 2000; **26**: 979–83.

66. Child JA. Update on high dose therapy: MRC studies. *Haematologica* 2005; **90** (S1): 40–1.

67. Fermand JP, Ravaud P, Chevret S, *et al.* High-dose therapy and autologous peripheral blood stem cell transplantation in multiple myeloma: up-front or rescue treatment? Results of a multicenter sequential randomized clinical trial. *Blood* 1998; **92**: 3131–6.

68. Fermand P, Ravaud P, Katsahian S. *Blood* 2004; **94**: abstract 396.

69. Palumbo A, Bringhen S, Rus C, *et al. Blood* 2001; **98**: abstract 849.

70. Blade J, Sureda A, Ribera J, *et al.* High-dose therapy autotransplantation/intensification vs. continued conventional chemotherapy in multiple myeloma patients responding to initial treatment chemotherapy. Results of a prospective randomized trial from the Spanish Cooperative Group. *Blood* 2001; **98**: abstract 815.

71. Barlogie B, Jagannath S, Vesole DH, *et al.* Superiority of tandem autologous transplantation over standard therapy for previously untreated multiple myeloma. *Blood* 1997; **89**: 789–93.

72. Harousseau JL, Milpied N, Laporte JP, *et al.* Double-intensive therapy in high-risk multiple myeloma. *Blood* 1992; **79**: 2827–33.

73. Vesole DH, Barlogie B, Jagannath S, *et al.* High-dose therapy for refractory multiple myeloma: improved prognosis with better supportive care and double transplants. *Blood* 1994; **84**: 950–6.

74. Barlogie B, Jagannath S, Desikan KR, *et al.* Total therapy with tandem transplants for newly diagnosed multiple myeloma. *Blood* 1999; **93**: 55–65.

75. Bjorkstrand B. European Group for Blood and Marrow Transplantation Registry studies in multiple myeloma. *Semin Hematol* 2001; **38**: 219–25.

76. Attal M, Harousseau JL, Facon T, *et al.* Single versus double autologous stem-cell transplantation for multiple myeloma. *N Engl J Med* 2003; **349**: 2495–502.

77. Segeren CN, Sonneveld P, van der Holt B, *et al.* Intensive versus double intensive therapy in previously untreated multiple myeloma: a prospective randomized phase III study in 450 patients. Banff, Canada: *VIII International Myeloma Workshop Book*, 2001: 31.

78. Segeren CM, Sonneveld P, van der Holt B, *et al.* Overall and event-free survival are not improved by the use of myeloablative therapy following intensified chemotherapy in previously untreated patients with multiple myeloma: a prospective randomized phase 3 study. *Blood* 2003; **101**: 2144–51.

79. Fermand JP, Marolleau JP, Alberti C. Single versus tandem high-dose therapy (HDT) supported with autologous blood stem cell (ABSC) transplantation using unselected or CD-34 enriched ABSC: preliminary results of a two by two design randomized trial in 230 young patients with multiple myeloma. Banff, Canada: *VIII International Myeloma Workshop Book*, 2001: 147.

80. Cavo M, Tosi P, Zamagni E, *et al.* The Bologna 96 clinical trial of single versus double PBSC transplantation for previously untreated MM: results of an interim analysis. Banff, Canada: *VIII International Myeloma Workshop Book*, 2001: 29.

81. Barlogie B, Jacobson J, Sawyer J, *et al.* Increasing CR frequency as a strategy toward extending event-free survival (EFS) and overall survival (OS) in multiple myeloma (MM): 4-year results of Total Therapy II (TT II) versus Total Therapy I (TT I). *Blood* 2003; **102** (11): abstract 136.

82. Richardson PG, Barlogie B, Berenson J, *et al.* A phase 2 study of bortezomib in relapsed, refractory myeloma. *N Engl J Med* 2003; **348**: 2609–17.

83. Jagannath S, Barlogie B, Berenson J, *et al.* A phase 2 study of two doses of bortezomib in relapsed or refractory myeloma. *Br J Haematol* 2004; **127**: 165–72.

84. Singhal S, Mehta J, Desikan R, *et al.* Antitumor activity of thalidomide in refractory multiple myeloma. *N Engl J Med* 1999; **341**: 1565–71.

85. Juliusson G, Celsing F, Turesson I, Lenhoff S, Adriansson M, Malm C. Frequent good partial remissions from thalidomide including best response ever in patients with advanced refractory and relapsed myeloma. *Br J Haematol* 2000; **109**: 89–96.

86. Rajkumar SV, Fonseca R, Dispenzieri A, *et al.* Thalidomide in the treatment of relapsed multiple myeloma. *Mayo Clin Proc* 2000; **75**: 897–901.

87. Barlogie B, Desikan R, Eddlemon P, *et al.* Extended survival in advanced and refractory multiple myeloma

after single-agent thalidomide: identification of prognostic factors in a phase 2 study of 169 patients. *Blood* 2001; **98**: 492–4.

88. Yakoub-Agha I, Attal M, Dumontet C, *et al.* Thalidomide in patients with advanced multiple myeloma: a study of 83 patients–report of the Intergroupe Francophone du Myelome (IFM). *Hematol J* 2002; **3**: 185–92.

89. Palumbo A, Giaccone L, Bertola A, *et al.* Low-dose thalidomide plus dexamethasone is an effective salvage therapy for advanced myeloma. *Haematologica* 2001; **86**: 399–403.

90. Anagnostopoulos A, Weber D, Rankin K, Delasalle K, Alexanian R. Thalidomide and dexamethasone for resistant multiple myeloma. *Br J Haematol* 2003; **121**: 768–71.

91. Kumar S, Lacy MQ, Dispenzieri A, *et al.* High-dose therapy and autologous stem cell transplantation for multiple myeloma poorly responsive to initial therapy. *Bone Marrow Transplant* 2004; **34**: 161–7.

92. Alexanian R, Dimopoulos M. The treatment of multiple myeloma. *N Engl J Med* 1994; **330**: 484–9.

93. Dalton WS, Hazlehurst L, Shain K, Landowski T, Alsina M. Targeting the bone marrow microenvironment in hematologic malignancies. *Semin Hematol* 2004; **41** (2 Suppl 4): 1–5.

94. Damiano JS, Hazlehurst LA, Dalton WS. Cell adhesion-mediated drug resistance (CAM-DR) protects the K562 chronic myelogenous leukemia cell line from apoptosis induced by BCR/ABL inhibition, cytotoxic drugs, and gamma-irradiation. *Leukemia* 2001; **15**: 1232–9.

95. Mudry RE, Fortney JE, York T, Hall BM, Gibson LF. Stromal cells regulate survival of B-lineage leukemic cells during chemotherapy. *Blood* 2000; **96**: 1926–32.

96. Andela VB, Schwarz EM, Puzas JE, O'Keefe RJ, Rosier RN. Tumor metastasis and the reciprocal regulation of prometastatic and antimetastatic factors by nuclear factor kappaB. *Cancer Res* 2000; **60**: 6557–62.

97. Huang Y, Johnson KR, Norris JS, Fan W. Nuclear factor-kappaB/IkappaB signaling pathway may contribute to the mediation of paclitaxel-induced apoptosis in solid tumor cells. *Cancer Res* 2000; **60**: 4426–32.

98. Kim JY, Lee S, Hwangbo B, *et al.* NF-kappaB activation is related to the resistance of lung cancer cells to TNF-alpha-induced apoptosis. *Biochem Biophys Res Commun* 2000; **273**: 140–6.

99. Palombella VJ, Rando OJ, Goldberg AL, Maniatis T. The ubiquitin–proteasome pathway is required for processing the NF-kappa B1 precursor protein and the activation of NF-kappa B. *Cell* 1994; **78**: 773–85.

100. Landowski TH, Olashaw NE, Agrawal D, Dalton WS. Cell adhesion-mediated drug resistance (CAM-DR) is associated with activation of NF-kappa B (RelB/p50) in myeloma cells. *Oncogene* 2003; **22**: 2417–21.

101. Dalton WS, Salmon SE. Drug resistance in myeloma: mechanisms and approaches to circumvention. *Hematol Oncol Clin North Am* 1992; **6**: 383–93.

102. Abbaszadegan MR, Futscher BW, Klimecki WT, List A, Dalton WS. Analysis of multidrug resistance-associated protein (MRP) messenger RNA in normal and malignant hematopoietic cells. *Cancer Res* 1994; **54**: 4676–9.

103. Grogan TM, Spier CM, Salmon SE, *et al.* P-glycoprotein expression in human plasma cell myeloma: correlation with prior chemotherapy. *Blood* 1993; **81**: 490–5.

104. Nooter K, Burger H, Stoter G. Multidrug resistance-associated protein (MRP) in haematological malignancies. *Leuk Lymphoma* 1996; **20**: 381–7.

105. Alexanian R, Weber D, Delasalle K, Giralt S, Champlin R. Value of intensive therapy supported by autologous stem cells (IT+ASCT) for primary resistant multiple myeloma. *Blood* 2002; **100** (11): abstract 672.

106. Singhal S, Powles R, Sirohi B, Treleaven J, Kulkarni S, Mehta J. Response to induction chemotherapy is not essential to obtain survival benefit from high-dose melphalan and autotransplantation in myeloma. *Bone Marrow Transplant* 2002; **30**: 673–9.

107. Vesole DH, Tricot G, Jagannath S, *et al.* Autotransplants in multiple myeloma: what have we learned? *Blood* 1996; **88**: 838–47.

108. Alexanian R, Dimopoulos MA, Hester J, Delasalle K, Champlin R. Early myeloablative therapy for multiple myeloma. *Blood* 1994; **84**: 4278–82.

109. Blade J, Esteve J. Treatment approaches for relapsing and refractory multiple myeloma. *Acta Oncol* 2000; **39**: 843–7.

110. Dimopoulos MA, Hester J, Huh Y, Champlin R, Alexanian R. Intensive chemotherapy with blood progenitor transplantation for primary resistant multiple myeloma. *Br J Haematol* 1994; **87**: 730–4.

111. Jagannath S, Barlogie B, Dicke K, *et al.* Autologous bone marrow transplantation in multiple myeloma: identification of prognostic factors. *Blood* 1990; **76**: 1860–6.

112. Schenkein DP, Koc Y, Alcindor T, *et al.* Treatment of primary resistant or relapsed multiple myeloma with high-dose chemoradiotherapy, hematopoietic stem cell rescue, and granulocyte-macrophage

colony-stimulating factor. Biol *Blood Marrow Transplant* 2000; **6**: 448–55.

113. Alexanian R, Dimopoulos MA, Delasalle KB, Hester J, Champlin R. Myeloablative therapy for primary resistant multiple myeloma. *Stem Cells* 1995; **13** (Suppl 2): 118–21.

114. Ghosh K, Gosavi S, Pathare A, Madkaikar M, Rao VB, Mohanty D. Low cost autologous peripheral blood stem cell transplantation performed in a municipal hospital for a patient with plasma cell leukaemia. *Clin Lab Haematol* 2002; **24**: 187–90.

115. Hayman SR, Fonseca R. Plasma cell leukemia. *Curr Treat Options Oncol* 2001; **2**: 205–16.

116. Hovenga S, de Wolf JT, Klip H, Vellenga E. Consolidation therapy with autologous stem cell transplantation in plasma cell leukemia after VAD, high-dose cyclophosphamide and EDAP courses: a report of three cases and a review of the literature. *Bone Marrow Transplant* 1997; **20**: 901–4.

117. Kosmo MA, Gale RP. Plasma cell leukemia. *Semin Hematol* 1987; **24**: 202–8.

118. Mak YK, Chan CH, Chen YT, Lau SM, So CC, Wong KF. Consolidation therapy with autologous blood stem cell transplantation in a patient with primary plasma cell leukaemia. *Clin Lab Haematol* 2003; **25**: 55–8.

119. McElwain TJ, Powles RL. High-dose intravenous melphalan for plasma-cell leukaemia and myeloma. *Lancet* 1983; **2**: 822–4.

120. Panizo C, Rifon J, Rodriguez-Wilhelmi P, Cuesta B, Rocha E. Long-term survival in primary plasma cell leukemia after therapy with VAD, autologous blood stem cell transplantation and interferon-alpha. *Acta Haematol* 1999; **101**: 193–6.

121. Sica S, Chiusolo P, Salutari P, *et al.* Long-lasting complete remission in plasma cell leukemia after aggressive chemotherapy and CD34-selected autologous peripheral blood progenitor cell transplant: molecular follow-up of minimal residual disease. *Bone Marrow Transplant* 1998; **22**: 823–5.

122. Yang CH, Lin MT, Tsay W, Liu LT, Wang CH, Chen YC. Autologous bone marrow transplantation for plasma cell leukemia: report of a case. *Transplant Proc* 1992; **24**: 1531–2.

123. Yeh KH, Lin MT, Tang JL, Yang CH, Tsay W, Chen YC. Long-term disease-free survival after autologous bone marrow transplantation in a primary plasma cell leukaemia: detection of minimal residual disease in the transplant marrow by third-complementarity-determining region-specific probes. *Br J Haematol* 1995; **89**: 914–16.

22

Non-Hodgkin lymphoma

Nicole Jacobi, Bruce A. Peterson

Introduction

Non-Hodgkin lymphoma (NHL) is a topic of increasing significance in an aging population. According to the National Cancer Institute's SEER program, the overall incidence of NHL increased by 75% between 1973 and 1994, or approximately 3% each year [1]. However, not only is the incidence rising, but one-half of all lymphomas are diagnosed in patients over 65 years of age, and the incidence by age keeps increasing at least until age 85 [2]. In the context of an aging population, the absolute number of patients over 65 years with lymphoma is expected to double within the next 25 years [3]. Fortunately, our understanding of lymphoma biology is also steadily growing, leading to innovative treatments that capitalize upon this new understanding.

Lymphomas are biologically heterogeneous, and for most subtypes the etiology is unknown. Although epidemiologic factors, often incompletely understood, such as geography, environmental exposure, immunodeficiency, and specific preconditions, play a role, there is a strong relationship between aging and the development of NHL [4–10]. To some extent this may relate to exposure and opportunity, but with aging also come aberrations in immune function and response. The heterogeneity of lymphomas extends to their clinical behavior. Although the behavior of specific subtypes of NHL tends to be similar regardless of age, the impact of the disease and the individual's ability to tolerate the necessary interventions may vary. Thus, it is important to have an appreciation of the varieties of NHL and their management in an older population.

Classification and clinical evaluation

In order to make appropriate clinical decisions it is vital to appreciate the differences in various subtypes of NHL. This chapter focuses on the largest group, mature B-cell lymphomas. In the past, an imperfect understanding of lymphoma biology and multiple systems of classification contributed to complexity and confusion. In 1982, the International Working Formulation began to address these problems by providing a common language that bridged different nomenclatures in use throughout the world [11]. The Revised European–American Classification of Lymphoid Neoplasms (REAL) [12] then integrated distinctive biological with morphological features as the forerunner of the current World Health Organization (WHO) classification of Tumors of Hematopoietic and Lymphoid Tissue (Table 22.1) [13]. The WHO Classification utilizes relevant morphologic, immunologic and genetic features to distinguish entities that are biologically and clinically relevant.

Upon discerning the diagnostic subtype, clinical behavior can be anticipated, an appropriate evaluation initiated, and management options identified. The anticipated clinical behavior of each subtype can be characterized as indolent or aggressive. Indolent lymphomas, usually disseminated, may be associated with a life expectancy of several years, but often without prospect of cure. Aggressive lymphomas, on the other hand, present no middle ground with the choice between cure-directed treatment, or palliation and an unrelenting course to death.

Blood Disorders in the Elderly, ed. Lodovico Balducci, William Ershler, Giovanni de Gaetano.
Published by Cambridge University Press. © Cambridge University Press 2008.

Table 22.1. WHO classification of mature
B-cell neoplasms [13].

Chronic lymphocytic leukemia/small lymphocytic
  lymphoma
Lymphoplasmacytic lymphoma
Splenic marginal zone lymphoma
Extranodal marginal zone B-cell lymphoma of mucosa-
  associated lymphoid tissue (MALT lymphoma)
Nodal marginal zone B-cell lymphoma
Follicular lymphoma
Mantle cell lymphoma
Diffuse large B-cell lymphoma
Mediastinal (thymic) large B-cell lymphoma
Intravascular large B-cell lymphoma
Primary effusion lymphoma
Burkitt lymphoma

Table 22.2. Ann Arbor staging system for non-Hodgkin
lymphoma.

Stage I	Involvement of a single lymph-node region or a single extralymphatic site
Stage II	Involvement of two or more lymph-node regions on the same side of the diaphragm with or without localized involvement of an extralymphatic site
Stage III	Involvement of lymph-node regions on both sides of the diaphragm with or without localized involvement of an extralymphatic site
Stage IV	Diffuse or disseminated involvement of one or more extralymphatic sites

Presence or absence of symptoms noted with each stage
designation:
A, asymptomatic
B, fever, night sweats, weight loss

The Ann Arbor staging system, originally developed
for Hodgkin lymphoma, is an important adjunct to
the WHO classification in the initial evaluation of the
patient with NHL (Table 22.2). There are some draw-
backs to its use in NHL, but rigorous staging according
to a predetermined schedule of tests has numerous
advantages. Staging (1) facilitates the identification
of inapparent disease that might constitute a clinical

threat; (2) provides assistance in deciding among
therapeutic options; (3) allows an estimate of prognosis; (4) allows the baseline identification of disease
sites that can be used to assess response; and (5)
establishes uniformity for patients included in clinical trials. Studies routinely recommended for staging
and prognostic evaluation include adequate biopsies,
including bone-marrow aspirates and cores, and laboratory and radiologic tests. Multiple bone-marrow
core biopsies will more likely identify involvement
because it is often focal. FDG-PET/CT fusion scans can
delineate involved sites not otherwise identified and
clarify questionable radiographic findings. However,
metabolic activity may not be sufficient in indolent
lymphomas to routinely provide useful PET imaging.
Laboratory studies (e.g., hemoglobin and serum LDH)
aid in establishing prognosis and assess potential
problems, such as organ dysfunction, hypercalemia,
hyperuricemia, and spontaneous tumor lysis.

In addition to histopathologic subtype and stage,
there are other important factors that also contribute to an estimation of prognosis. Age almost always
emerges as important in prognosis and is most likely
a surrogate for aggregate factors, such as comorbidity and functional capability [14–17]. Comorbidity
is a significant risk factor for shorter survival [18],
and a poor performance status can largely replace
advanced chronologic age as an adverse factor
for the risk of treatment-related death [19]. The
Comprehensive Geriatric Assessment (CGA) score
may help to even better identify frail patients, but
still has to be evaluated in a prospective trial [20–23].

Standard multifactorial prognostic indices that
consider both host and tumor characteristics
are important. The most commonly used are the
International Prognostic Index (IPI) [15] and the
Follicular Lymphoma International Prognostic Index
(FLIPI) (Table 22.3) [17]. In 1993, the IPI was developed for diffuse aggressive lymphomas, based an on
analysis of patients treated with curative intent. Five
easily established clinical factors provide an important tool to assess prognosis. The number of factors
present (0–5) predicts complete response rates that
range from 91% to 36% and five-year survival between
56% and 21% (Table 22.4) [15]. Although the IPI was

Table 22.3. Prognostic indices for non-Hodgkin lymphoma.

	International Prognostic Index (IPI) [15]	Follicular Lymphoma International Prognostic Index (FLIPI) [17]
Factor		
Age >60 years	+	+
Serum LDH > normal	+*	+*
Ann Arbor Stage III–IV	+*	+*
Extranodal sites >1	+	—
Performance status ≥2	+*	—
Hemoglobin <12 gm/L	—	+*
Nodal sites >4	—	+*
Risk group	**Number of factors**^{a}	**Number of factors**^{a}
Low	0–1 (0)	0–1 (1)
Low/intermediate	2 (1)	—
Intermediate	—	2 (2)
High/intermediate	3 (2)	—
High	4–5 (3)	≥3 (≥3)

* Only those factors identified by asterisk should be used if index restricted to patients over 60 years.

^{a} Number of factors in parentheses is used if index restricted to patients over 60 years.

not specifically developed for elderly patients, it discriminates well those at highest risk. In the indolent follicular lymphomas, it has proven more difficult to meaningfully identify patients at substantial risk. Although the IPI has been applied with modest success, the FLIPI may be more pertinent [17]. On the basis of five factors, three groups of patients with follicular lymphoma can be identified that have ten-year survival rates ranging from 70% to 30% (Table 22.4).

Genetic features of NHL can serve as distinguishing diagnostic or prognostic characteristics and can, in some cases, be used in the detection of inapparent disease. In follicular lymphomas the t(14;18)(q32;q21) juxtaposes *BCL-2* with the immunoglobulin heavy chain gene, and is pathogenetic [24–28]. Its presence may assist in the diagnosis or in the detection of residual disease. Additional genetic changes in follicular lymphoma, such as those involving *BCL-6* [29] or altered expression of *C-MYC* [30], predict a higher risk of transformation.

Patterns of multiple gene expression may suggest responsiveness to individual agents, such as rituximab [31], or overall prognosis [32]. In diffuse large B-cell lymphoma (DLBCL) at least three major subtypes can be distinguished by microarray analysis [33–36]. It can have the molecular signature of activated B cells, germinal-center B cells, or a less common subtype, type 3. Those with the activated B-cell pattern have a relatively unfavorable outcome with chemotherapy [37], but this may be abrogated by the inclusion of rituximab with chemotherapy [38]. Precise molecular findings may not have the same significance in patients of different ages. For example, the overexpression of *BCL-2* and *p53* in DLBCL does not appear to have the same adverse prognostic significance in older as in younger patients [39]. Undoubtedly, new biological features will continue to emerge, and will permit even greater refinements in classification, prognosis, and treatment selection.

Table 22.4. Outcome by risk group in prognostic indices.

	Distribution of patients (%)	Survival		
		2 year (%)	5 year (%)	10 year (%)
International Prognostic Index [15]				
All patients				
Risk group				
Low	35	84	73	—
Low/intermediate	27	66	51	—
High/intermediate	22	54	43	—
High	16	34	26	—
Age-adjusted >60 years				
Risk group				
Low	18	80	56	—
Low/intermediate	31	68	44	—
High/intermediate	35	48	37	—
High	16	31	21	—
Follicular Lymphoma International Prognostic Index [17]				
All patients				
Risk group				
Low	36	—	91	71
Intermediate	37	—	78	51
High	27	—	52	36
Age-adjusted >60 years				
Risk group				
Low	20	—	85	70
Intermediate	32	—	70	45
High	48	—	45	30

Clinical management of indolent B-cell lymphomas

Indolent lymphomas, despite important differences between subtypes, are characterized by slow progression and, often, the absence of any symptoms for prolonged periods of time. These lymphomas account for 30% of adult NHL, but one subgroup, follicular lymphoma, makes up the great majority and is second in frequency only to DLBCL [11,13,40,41]. The other subtypes, including small lymphocytic, lymphoplasmacytic, and marginal zone lymphomas, are far less common. Small lymphocytic lymphoma is related to chronic lymphocytic leukemia, which is discussed in Chapter 24.

Follicular lymphoma

Follicular lymphomas have been extensively studied, and often serve as the prototype for management of other indolent lymphomas. Lymphadenopathy that may be modest and long-standing is most often the presenting finding. Patients are typically in their sixth or seventh decade. Most patients are asymptomatic, and less than a third will have B symptoms. Involvement of the bone marrow can be detected morphologically in up to 65%, but even more patients may have disseminated disease demonstrated by sensitive molecular tests. Fortunately, the finding of lymphoma in the bone marrow has little impact on prognosis. Nearly 85% will be stage III–IV. The architecture of the lymph node shows a follicular or nodular pattern, and based on the proportion of large cells in the malignant nodules, follicular lymphomas can be graded 1 through 3 [13,41]. Grade 3 generally has more rapid clinical growth [42]. The t(14;18)(q32;q21) can be detected in 90% of the cases by either classical banded cytogenetics or molecular techniques [24,43].

The general approach to patients with follicular lymphoma does not need to vary because of age. Since the disease is often indolent, patients asymptomatic, and treatments generally not curative, therapy can often be deferred until clinically necessary without jeopardizing the patient's prognosis while enhancing quality of life [44–50]. Median survival is eight to ten years. However, the rare patient with localized disease may have prolonged disease-free survival following irradiation [51,52]. In view of this possibility, whether patients with localized disease should be observed or treated should be individualized [44,49,51].

When treatment is necessary in the patient with advanced disease, a wide range of possibilities exists, extending from the use of single drugs (e.g., alkylating agents [53–56], nucleoside analogs [57–62], rituximab [63–67]) to modest combinations, such as CVP (cyclophosphamide, vincristine, prednisone) [54,56,68] or combinations based on fludarabine [62,69–73], to those combinations commonly reserved for patients with aggressive lymphomas, such as CHOP (cyclophosphamide, doxorubicin, vincristine, prednisone) [55,74–76].

Clinical trials in follicular lymphomas largely have not focused special attention on the elderly. Fortunately, this has not been a major issue because even the most innocuous therapies are likely to be initially as effective as more aggressive treatments. The use of a single alkylator, either chlorambucil or cyclophosphamide, is as effective for most patients as combinations such as CVP [54,56,68] or CHOP

[55,76], and may induce a significant response in 90% of patients. As single agents, these drugs are generally very well tolerated in old and young alike, but have toxicities (e.g., hemorrhagic cystitis and myelosuppression) that must be considered. Fludarabine is the most commonly used nucleoside analog and is also generally well tolerated [60,77,78]. It may not be as active as alkylating agents and may induce a more lasting impairment of the immune system. The use of fludarabine also has been associated with a heightened risk of earlier transformation [79,80], and both alkylating agents and nucleoside analogs have been associated with secondary leukemias [81–84]. Any of these approaches can yield a meaningful response, but relapse is almost inevitable. When the disease returns and treatment is again necessary, depending on the quality of the original response, re-treatment with the original therapy may be appropriate.

Rituximab, initially introduced for the relapsed patient, can also be useful as initial therapy. Although response rates appear to be lower than with commonly used chemotherapies, an objective response can be obtained in approximately 50–60% of patients, with little toxicity [64–67]. The median time to progression is about 18–20 months. A strategy of maintenance therapy, repeating rituximab at specified intervals, leads to longer remissions, but whether this is the best overall strategy is still not settled [64,65].

Success with rituximab in various settings has led to studies of its inclusion as a component of drug combinations. However, since controlled clinical trials are essential to clarify the benefits of new therapies, the role of rituximab in combination is not established. In a randomized study, the addition of rituximab to CVP (R-CVP) as initial treatment resulted in an improved response rate and prolonged time to progression [85]. However, there was not a significant increase in survival. In relapsed patients, a small phase III study assessed fludarabine, cyclophosphamide, and mitoxantrone with (R-FCM) or without rituximab (FCM) [70]. An improved response rate (94% vs. 70%, $p = 0.011$) and progression-free survival (median >36 months vs. 21 months, $p = 0.0139$) were seen with R-FCM, but survival was not significantly affected by the addition of rituximab. In a study of fludarabine plus mitoxantrone (FM) versus CHOP, each with or without rituximab, the complete response rate was higher with FM. However, again this did not translate into an improvement in progression-free or overall survival [86]. Radiolabelled monoclonal antibodies, I-131 tositumomab and ibritumomab tiuxetan, have also become available for use in follicular lymphomas, and hold promise. Their role in the overall scheme of management of follicular lymphomas remains to be determined [87–90].

For the older patient with follicular lymphoma who requires treatment, the choice is myriad. Certain interventions may offer higher rates of initial response, sometimes with increased toxicity, cost, or inconvenience. Occasionally, this translates into an improvement in time to failure, but almost never to an extension of survival. Thus, a strategy for patients needing treatment begins with the least burdensome therapy associated with an acceptable response rate, providing meaningful intervention while limiting unnecessary side effects, inconvenience, and risk. This does not eliminate future options, and more toxic or risky treatments are reserved for when necessary.

Lymphoplasmacytic lymphoma

Lymphoplasmacytic lymphoma, accounting for less than 2% of all adult lymphomas, presents most commonly in males and almost always after 50 years of age [13,40,91,92]. Although a monoclonal IgG or IgA protein may be present, classically, this subtype is accompanied by monoclonal IgM and called Waldenström macroglobulinemia. Frequent sites of involvement include nodes, spleen, and the gastrointestinal tract. The marrow is usually involved and up to 80% of patients will be stage IV. With extensive marrow infiltration, anemia and pancytopenia are common. Lymphoplasmacytic lymphoma may be associated with amyloidosis. Prior infection with hepatitis C may play a role in pathogenesis.

The systemic symptoms of fevers, night sweats, and weight loss are infrequent. Fatigue, often related to anemia, is a common symptom. Hypercalcemia, as a result of lytic bone disease, cryoglobulinemia, and cold agglutinins can each lead to manifestations. Most notably, IgM forms large pentameric aggregates that can increase the serum viscosity to the extent that clinical hyperviscosity, mucosal bleeding, fatigue, mental status changes, and blurred vision are seen in 15% of patients. Increased viscosity can lead to strokes, cardiac ischemia, and high-output cardiac failure. Unfortunately, measured serum viscosity does not correlate very well with clinically significant hyperviscosity [93,94].

The median life expectancy of an individual with Waldenström macroglobulinemia is 5–7 years. However, extensive marrow replacement is adverse and predicts a median survival of a year or less [95]. Other correlates of a poorer prognosis are hemoglobin less than 10 gm/dL, very high monoclonal peak, weight loss, and age over 60 years. The t(9;14)(p13;q32) is a frequent cytogenetic finding, but does not seem to carry prognostic significance [24,91,96].

As with other indolent B-cell lymphomas, asymptomatic patients with lymphoplasmacytic lymphoma who are not anemic or experiencing significant problems may be observed without initial therapy [91,93,94]. Close monitoring for disease progression, renal and metabolic derangements, and potential manifestations of hyperviscosity is required. Once the necessity of treatment is established, many of the same options appropriate for follicular lymphoma can be considered. An alkylating agent, chlorambucil, is a standard first choice and results in partial responses for 50–75% of patients. The addition of prednisone is not beneficial unless needed for an immunologic problem. Combinations such as CHOP are also not more useful than single agents in the initial phase of treatment. Although the nucleoside analogs, fludarabine [77,97] and 2-chlorodeoxyadenosine [95,98], produce response rates similar to chlorambucil, 2′-chlorodeoxyadenosine has been reported to more rapidly reduce the monoclonal protein, dropping the level by more than half within two months. Newer treatments [93,94,98,99] include rituximab, interferon alpha, thalidomide, bortezomib, and in highly selected cases with problematic disease, high-dose therapy with stem-cell transplant [100,101]. The use of rituximab, active in 30–40% of patients, may be associated with a rapid rise in serum IgM precipitating manifestations of hyperviscosity [102,103]. For those patients presenting with hyperviscosity syndrome, plasmapheresis can almost immediately reduce the monoclonal protein and rapidly improve the clinical situation. In this setting chemotherapy should be instituted soon after plasmapheresis to control the disease over the longer term.

Marginal zone lymphomas

There are three varieties of marginal zone lymphoma (Fig. 22.1) identified in the WHO classification: splenic, nodal, and extranodal [13]. Each has unique characteristics that may influence the clinical approach.

Splenic marginal zone lymphoma

Splenic marginal zone lymphoma is rare [40,104–108]. It occurs most frequently in women and at a median age of 68 years. In some cases it has been associated

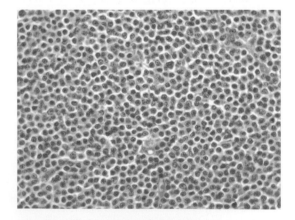

Figure 22.1 Marginal zone lymphoma: neoplastic marginal zone cells with moderately abundant cytoplasm have plasmacytoid appearance. Kadin, M., ASH Image Bank 2004: 101238. Copyright American Society of Hematology. All rights reserved. *See color plate section.*

with chronic hepatitis C infection, and treatment for hepatitis C with interferon has been reported to result in improvement [109]. Splenomegaly is the unifying finding and accounts for most of the problems. Fatigue from a moderate anemia caused by splenic sequestration is common. Substantial lymphadenopathy is unusual, and B symptoms are very rare. Peripheral blood involvement, sometimes with cells that have small cytoplasmic villous projections, is frequent, but usually modest. A monoclonal gammopathy is seen in half of the patients. The t(11;14)(q13;q32), a translocation more commonly associated with mantle cell lymphoma, and allelic loss of 7(q21–32) have been reported, but a characteristic cytogenetic abnormality has not been described.

Although modest chemotherapy may be helpful [110–112], most patients in need of treatment are best served by splenectomy [105,107,109,112]. This approach corrects symptoms in the great majority of patients and the benefits can be quite durable. Median survival is approximately nine years.

Nodal marginal zone lymphoma

Nodal marginal zone lymphoma is only slightly more common than the splenic variety, accounting for less than 2% of adult NHL [13,40,113,114]. It also affects more women than men, and patients at diagnosis have a median age of 64 years. Lymphadenopathy, especially of peripheral nodes, is common, and the spleen is enlarged in most patients. When nodes are involved in a setting of extranodal disease, the nodes should be considered an extension of the extranodal process. Nearly three-quarters will have advanced-stage disease, two-thirds will have splenomegaly, and one-third bone-marrow involvement. There are no unique diagnostic cytogenetic or molecular abnormalities.

The prognosis is slightly worse than that of other indolent B-cell lymphomas; the median survival is approximately five years. However, the approaches used in follicular lymphomas, observation without initial therapy in asymptomatic patients and interventions tied to particular situations, are still most appropriate [115,116]. In the uncommon setting of localized disease, involved-field irradiation may be considered.

Extranodal marginal zone lymphoma of mucosa-associated lymphoid tissue (MALT)

The MALT lymphomas (Figs. 22.2, 22.3) are especially interesting because an etiology or predisposition can often be identified [13,117–119]. Many occur

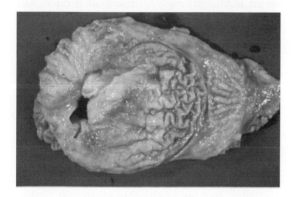

Figure 22.2 Gastric MALT lymphoma: gross pathology. Normal gastric mucosa disrupted by MALT lymphoma. Kadin, M., ASH Image Bank 2003: 100693. Copyright American Society of Hematology. All rights reserved. *See color plate section.*

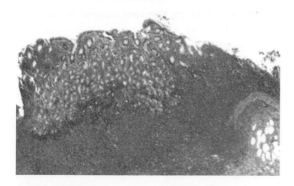

Figure 22.3 Gastric MALT lymphoma: marginal zone cells colonize and obliterate germinal centers of reactive B-cell follicles. Kadin, M., ASH Image Bank 2003: 100693. Copyright American Society of Hematology. All rights reserved. *See color plate section.*

in sites where chronic infectious, autoimmune, or inflammatory stimuli pre-exist. The relationship between gastrointestinal infection with *Helicobacter pylori* and some cases of gastric MALT lymphoma is well established [120–122]. More recently, evidence of a role for *Borrelia burgdorferi* and *Chlamydophila psittaci* has been reported in the evolution of cutaneous [122–124] and ocular adnexal [117] MALT lymphomas, respectively. As first demonstrated for *H. pylori*, and now for both *B. burgdorferi* and *C. psittaci*, treatment directed at the bacteria may cause tumor regression.

MALT lymphomas affect a wide range of primary sites in addition to those noted above, including thyroid, salivary gland, breast, and lung [13,40,125–128]. Together, they make up about 8% of all lymphomas. In keeping with the potential etiologic role of chronic inflammation, Hashimoto's thyroiditis often precedes MALT lymphomas of the thyroid, and Sjögren's syndrome may precede MALT lymphomas of the salivary glands. Most patients are over 60 years of age, and presenting symptoms are non-specific but relate directly to the tissue involved. Thus, in gastric MALT lymphomas, symptoms associated with gastritis or ulcers may be present. Ocular adnexal involvement may lead to mild eye discomfort, visual blurring, conjunctival thickening, or small tumor nodules. Chronic respiratory symptoms may be seen with pulmonary disease. MALT lymphomas arising at other sites usually present with slowly growing masses.

One-half of MALT lymphomas are gastric, and evidence for *H. pylori* should be sought, because, if present, appropriate antibiotics plus proton pump inhibitors can usually eradicate the organism, and if *H. pylori* is eliminated, about 80% of patients will have subsequent tumor regression and may not need other therapy [120–122]. Since 80–90% of gastric MALT lymphomas are isolated, if antibiotics fail or the tumor is not associated with *H. pylori*, gastric irradiation can still be curative [129,130].

The best approach to localized extranodal lymphomas at other sites may involve the use of irradiation, since there is not yet sufficient data to recommend antibiotics as first-line therapy [131,132]. However, in selected cases, observation also may be appropriate. For patients in need of systemic treatment, single alkylating agents, nucleoside analogs, and rituximab are effective [127,133–135]. Combination chemotherapy is reserved for those with resistant or transformed disease.

Clinical management of aggressive B-cell lymphomas

The topic of aggressive B-cell lymphomas is dominated by a focus on the treatment of DLBCL, which accounts for 35% of adult NHL [13,40]. In this subtype of NHL there are multiple clinical trials of treatment in older patients. Less common subtypes of aggressive B-cell lymphomas include mantle cell and Burkitt lymphoma.

Diffuse large B-cell lymphoma

Diffuse large B-cell lymphoma presents as nodal disease in the majority of patients, but also can involve extranodal sites [13,40]. Approximately 50% of patients will be stage III or IV. The bone marrow is involved in 15–20% and indicates a higher risk of central nervous system involvement. The IPI applies directly to patients with DLBCL, and age is a prominent component of this index [15]. Approximately 60% of patients are over 60 years. Within DLBCL there are subtypes that can be identified by different biological characteristics, such as by cytogenetic or molecular profiling. There also are uncommon but clinically distinct subtypes [40], including primary mediastinal (thymic) B-cell lymphoma, which usually occurs in young patients, and intravascular large B-cell lymphoma, which is extremely rare and typically involves small vessels, often of the skin and central nervous system.

Prior to the introduction of effective drug combinations, complete remissions in DCBCL were rare and median survival was less than a year. It was not until the combinations C-MOPP (cyclophosphamide, vincristine, procarbazine, prednisone) and CHOP were introduced that durable remissions were reported with regularity. Soon after its introduction in 1976, CHOP became the standard treatment for advanced DLBCL [136].

There have been multiple attempts to improve upon CHOP for patients of all ages. Second- and third-generation regimens derived from the addition of several other chemotherapeutic agents to the four drugs in CHOP were initially promising. However, large phase III studies did not substantiate an advantage for any of these more complex and toxic treatments compared to CHOP [137,138]. A trial involving 899 patients, 40% of whom were over 60 years old and 25% over 65 years, compared three of these more promising new regimens to CHOP [137]. Although some were substantially more toxic, none was more effective than CHOP either in younger or in older patients. CHOP yielded an overall complete response rate of about 55% and long-term disease-free survival of 35%.

Despite the widespread adoption of CHOP, there remains concern about its use in the elderly. Toxicities, such as myelosuppression and cardiotoxicity, may be more pronounced in older patients, especially if there are comorbidities [139]. Also, CHOP may not be as effective in older patients. When the age-adjusted IPI is applied to patients above or below the age of 60 years, five-year survival for the lowest- and highest-risk groups under 60 years is 83% and 32%, respectively. For the same risk groups over 60 years, five-year survival is only 56% and 21% [15].

The inclusion of doxorubicin in CHOP raises the concern of cardiomyopathy in an elderly population that frequently harbors covert heart disease. In an attempt to retain the efficacy of CHOP but reduce cardiotoxicity, doxorubicin has been replaced with other, potentially less cardiotoxic, agents. Alternative anthracyclines, such as THP-doxorubicin (pirarubicin) [140–142], epirubicin [143,144], and idarubicin [143], have been investigated. Unfortunately, in these studies, the control arm was not CHOP, did not include an anthracycline, or was not concurrent – and thus it becomes difficult to assess the true utility of these drugs. However, none appears to eliminate the risk of cardiomyopathy.

Table 22.5. Selected clinical trials in elderly patients with diffuse aggressive non-Hodgkin lymphoma.

Reference	Regimen	No. of patients	Median age (range in years)	Complete response rate	Overall survival rate
Sonneveld et al. [145]	CHOP	72	70 (60–82)	49%	42% @ 3 years
	CNOP	76	71 (60–84)	31%	26% @ 3 years
				($p = 0.03$)	($p = 0.029$)
Tirelli et al. [146]	CHOP	60	74 (70–93)	45%	65% @ 2 years
	VMP	60	76 (70–93)	27%	30% @ 2 years
				($p = 0.06$)	($p = 0.004$)
Doorduijn et al. [148]	CHOP	192	73 (65–90)	55%	22% @ 5 years
	CHOP+G-CSF	197	72 (65–90)	52%	24% @ 5 years
				($p = 0.63$)	($p = 0.76$)
Tilly et al. [149]	CHOP	312	65 (61–69)	56%	38% @ 5 years
	ACVBP	323	65 (61–69)	58%	46% @ 5 years
				($p = 0.5$)	($p = 0.036$)
Pfreundschuh et al. [150]	CHOP-21	178	(61–75)	60%	41% @ 5 years
	CHOP-14	172	(61–75)	76%	53% @ 5 years ($p < 0.001$)*
	CHOEP-21	170	(61–75)	70%	45% @ 5 years ($p = 0.109$)*
	CHOEP-14	169	(61–75)	72%	50% @ 5 years ($p = 0.035$)*
					*versus CHOP-21
Coiffier et al. [151]	CHOP-R	202	69 (60–80)	76%	58% @ 5 years
				($p = 0.005$)	($p < 0.0073$)
Habermann et al. [152]	CHOP	279	70 (60–80+)	NA	57% @ 3 years
	CHOP-R	267	69 (60–80+)	NA	67% @ 3 years
					($p = 0.05$)

NA, not available; CHOP, cyclophosphamide, doxorubicin, vincristine, and prednisone; CNOP, cyclophosphamide, mitoxantrone, vincristine, and prednisone; VMP, etoposide, mitoxantrone, and prednimustine; G-CSF, recombinant granulocyte colony-stimulating factor; ACVBP, doxorubicin, cyclophosphamide, vindesine, bleomycin, and prednisone induction followed by multiple consolidations; CHOP-21, CHOP every 21 days; CHOP-14, CHOP every 14 days; CHOEP-21, cyclophosphamide, doxorubicin, vincristine, etoposide, prednisone every 21 days; CHOEP-14, CHOEP every 14 days; CHOP-R, CHOP plus rituximab.

Studies in which CHOP was used as a control (Table 22.5) have not demonstrated the superiority of alternatives to doxorubicin. Mitoxantrone, an anthracenedione considered effective yet less cardiotoxic than doxorubicin, has been extensively studied [18,145–147]. Tirelli et al. tested the combination of etoposide, mitoxantrone, and prednimustine (VMP) [147]. When VMP was compared to CHOP in a phase III trial, complete response rates were comparable, but CHOP showed superior progression-free and overall survival, and toxicity, including cardiotoxicity, was not significantly changed [146]. Mitoxantrone has been directly substituted for the doxorubicin in CHOP, yielding CNOP (cyclophosphamide, mitoxantrone, vincristine, prednisone). CNOP has been compared to the original CHOP in a prospective multicenter phase III trial of patients over 60 years [145]. Mitoxantrone did not significantly reduce cardiomyopathy or other toxicities, and the use of doxorubicin resulted in both a significantly better response rate and survival. Thus, substitution for doxorubicin may jeopardize outcome without reducing toxicity.

Although dose reductions minimize the myelosuppression of CHOP, they are also associated with adverse outcomes [153–155]. The introduction of recombinant growth factors permits a strategy to maintain or increase dose in CHOP and still afford protection from severe myelosuppression [156]. The routine initiation of G-CSF in support of chemotherapy permits a high proportion of elderly patients to receive full-dose therapy [157,158]. Whether this translates into an improved outcome when compared to the traditional approach of standardized dose reductions is unclear. In a randomized study, of CHOP alone versus CHOP with G-CSF [148], G-CSF support resulted in higher relative dose intensities of myelosuppressive drugs, but this did not translate into reductions in severe infections. Others, however, have demonstrated a reduction in both severe neutropenia and severe infection, but improved control of the NHL has not been seen [158–160]. Although it may be possible to identify older individuals who should receive empiric growth factor support with standard chemotherapy, it is most reasonable to apply American Society of Clinical Oncology Guidelines [161].

The use of growth factor support to substantially increase dose intensity has been evaluated in the elderly patient with DLBCL [149,150]. Of particular interest is a German study conducted in patients between 61 and 75 years of age [150]. Patients were randomized to receive either CHOP or CHOP plus etoposide (CHOEP) administered at standard three-week intervals or at two-week intervals with G-CSF support. This shortening of the treatment interval increases the amount of drug delivered by 50%. The shortened schedule for CHOP raised the complete response rate (76% vs. 60%) and prolonged overall survival at five years (53% vs. 41%, $p < 0.001$) without significantly affecting toxicity. The addition of etoposide primarily added toxicity.

Rituximab is active in relapsed aggressive B-cell lymphomas [162] and can be combined with near impunity with standard CHOP because it adds little to toxicity [163]. Two large phase III studies of CHOP compared to combinations of rituximab plus CHOP have been completed in older patients [151,152,164]. In both studies, patients who experienced significant neutropenia were given recombinant growth factors. In Europe, 398 patients, 60–80 years of age, with

stage II–IV DLBCL and a fair to good performance status were randomized to receive either eight cycles of CHOP or CHOP plus rituximab (R-CHOP) on day 1 of each cycle [151,173]. Both the complete response rate, 76% versus 63%, and event-free survival were superior with R-CHOP. At five years, 58% treated with R-CHOP and 45% treated with CHOP were alive ($p = 0.0073$) and there were no differences in serious adverse effects [164]. Grade 3–4 infection occurred in approximately 16%, and 4% of patients died of infection. The incidence of grade 3 or 4 congestive heart failure or ventricular dysfunction was 9%. A subsequent report suggests a slight excess of late cardiac deaths associated with the use of rituximab [165].

In North America, 632 patients over 60 years were randomized to initial therapy with either CHOP or R-CHOP. In this study, rituximab was administered on a different schedule [152]. Responders were subsequently randomized to either observation or four courses of maintenance rituximab given every six months for two years. The use of rituximab either during induction or as maintenance prolonged failure-free survival. Lethal toxicities occurred in 4% of the patients, including 2% due to infection and nearly 2% due to cardiac factors. Together, these two studies have established R-CHOP as the new standard of therapy for older adults with DLBCL and, in view of the apparent benefits of a two-week schedule [150], underscore the rationale for a prospective study of R-CHOP administered at two-week intervals.

In suitable patients who have stage I or II DLBCL, combined-modality treatment with CHOP-based therapy plus involved irradiation is preferable to either chemotherapy or radiation used alone [166,167]. The number of chemotherapy cycles given before the irradiation may be as few as three, but the specific question of optimal chemotherapy has not been adequately studied.

The treatment of the older patient with relapsed or refractory DLBCL remains problematic. Although there are many available treatments, none is likely to provide significant long-term benefits in the patient who has already failed CHOP. In younger patients the use of autologous stem-cell transplant is established in the relapsed setting. However, fear of excessive toxicity has limited research on autologous PBSCT in the elderly. Small studies demonstrate that PBSCT is a feasible option for older patients, but they must be carefully selected and the long-term benefits have not been established [168,169].

Mantle cell lymphoma

Patients of all ages with mantle cell lymphoma present a difficult challenge. Despite the use of intensive therapies the patient is usually neither cured outright nor compensated with the expectation of a long life expectancy. Median survival times range from three to four years [13,40,170,171]. Mantle cell lymphoma is seen predominantly in the elderly, especially men; the median age at diagnosis in a population-based cohort was 68 years [172]. It accounts for 6–10% of lymphomas. Mantle cell lymphoma has a characteristic translocation, t(11;14)(q13;q32), with the resultant overexpression of the protein cyclin D1 [13,40].

Over two-thirds of patients present with stage IV disease. Nodes, spleen, bone marrow, blood, and the gastrointestinal tract are common sites. The bone marrow is positive in more than half of patients. Involvement of the gastrointestinal tract often takes the form of small polyps, which can lead to a variety of symptoms, including gastrointestinal bleeding.

Although a rare patient may have localized disease and benefit from irradiation, most patients with mantle cell lymphoma require systemic treatment. Since most therapies are likely to provide only temporary benefit, single-agent therapy or CVP is often utilized as initial treatment. Response rates for chlorambucil or fludarabine range from 40% to 60% [172–176]. Rituximab has an objective response rate of about 30% [177,178]. Unfortunately, evidence that more intensive therapies such as CHOP are particularly beneficial when used as initial treatment is weak [170,173,174], and the importance of doxorubicin, unlike in DLBCL, has not been established. The addition of rituximab to CHOP may increase the response rate in mantle cell lymphoma but, also unlike in DLBCL, it has little impact on survival [179,180]. Thus, since neither CHOP nor

R-CHOP provides a greater advantage, except perhaps in response rate, they have been used as a bridge to autologous transplantation in suitable young patients [181]. Some young patients do well with allogeneic [182] or autologous [181,183] stem-cell transplantation, but these are options rarely applicable to the older individual. Attempts to improve the outcome in older patients through the administration of intensified cyclical therapy, such as Hyper-CVAD, a regimen that includes moderately high doses of cyclophosphamide and dexamethasone, plus doxorubicin and vincristine followed by methotrexate and cytarabine, have produced response rates of over 90% in patients 65 years and older, similar to R-CHOP [184]. Unfortunately, also similar to R-CHOP, these responses are not durable.

In previously treated patients with mantle cell lymphoma, the addition of rituximab to the combination of fludarabine, cyclophosphamide, and mitoxantrone (R-FCM) has slightly improved overall survival ($p = 0.002$) [70]. The question of how R-FCM would compare to R-CHOP in relapsed patients remains unaddressed. In patients with relapsed disease there is also growing experience with new agents [176]. Perhaps of greatest interest is the proteasome inhibitor bortezomib, which has shown responses in 40–50% of patients, some of which have lasted over one year [185,186].

Burkitt lymphoma

Burkitt lymphoma is a highly aggressive malignancy with the potential for extremely rapid growth. Although an endemic variety exists in equatorial Africa, most cases in North America and Europe are either sporadic or occur in the setting of severe immunodeficiency, such as HIV. Burkitt lymphoma is rare, making up only about 1–2% of NHL, and is thought of as a disease of children and young adults [13,40,187]. In adult series, the median age is often around 30 years. However, when it occurs in an elderly or infirm patient, dramatic deterioration may happen from rapid tumor progression.

The Epstein–Barr virus plays an etiologic role in some cases, especially in the endemic type of Burkitt lymphoma [188]. Most cases of Burkitt lymphoma will have a genetic abnormality involving *C-MYC* [13], with the exception of the Burkitt-like lymphomas [189]. Approximately 80% of cases demonstrate the presence of t(8;14) in which the immunoglobulin heavy chain gene on chromosome 14 is juxtaposed with *C-MYC* on chromosome 8. The remaining cases may have translocations involving the kappa or lambda light chain loci on chromosomes 2 or 22, and chromosome 8.

The clinical presentation of Burkitt lymphoma is rarely subtle. Bulky disease, often involving abdominal or pelvic sites, may lead to major symptoms. Typically, the disease is not localized; bone marrow is positive in 30–40%, and all patients are at risk of central nervous system involvement. If a complete remission is not obtained with systemic therapy, death usually follows in weeks to months.

Successful treatment of Burkitt lymphoma requires high doses of drugs repeated frequently over the space of a few months [190–193]. Such high-intensity programs often include cyclophosphamide, vincristine, methotrexate, cytarabine, doxorubicin, and other drugs along with central nervous system prophylaxis. The doses are substantial and growth-factor support is generally required. In patients with bulky disease, the initiation of therapy often precipitates the metabolic sequelae of tumor lysis syndrome. Expectant attention to fluids, electrolytes, uric acid, and the coagulation status is mandatory. Prospective comparative studies in Burkitt lymphoma have not been conducted, but it appears that CHOP and related programs are primarily palliative, and that the intensive regimens are truly necessary. Most current regimens appear to produce high complete response rates, 80–90%, with nearly one-half of the patients cured. Although age is an important factor, specific treatments for the elderly have not been evaluated.

REFERENCES

1. *Surveillance, Epidemiology and End Results (SEER) Review 1973–1997*. Bethesda, MD: National Cancer Institute, 2000.

2. Glass A, Karnell L, Menck H. The National Cancer Data Base Report on non-Hodgkin's lymphoma. *Cancer* 1997; **80**: 2311–20.

3. McNeil C. Non-Hodgkin's lymphoma trials in elderly look beyond CHOP. *J Natl Cancer Inst* 1998; **90**: 266–7.

4. Biggar R, Rabkin C. The epidemiology of acquired immunodeficiency syndrome-related lymphomas. *Curr Opin Oncol* 1992; **4**: 883–93.

5. Brandt L, Kristoffersson U, Olsson H, Mittelman F. Relation between occupational exposure to organic solvents and chromosome aberrations in non-Hodgkin's lymphoma. *Eur J Haematol* 1989; **42**: 298–302.

6. Isaacson PG. Mucosa-associated lymphoid tissue lymphoma. *Semin Hematol* 1999; **36**: 139–47.

7. Muller A, Ihorst G, Mertelsmann R, Engelhardt M. Epidemiology of non-Hodgkin's lymphoma (NHL): trends, geographic distribution, and etiology. *Ann Hematol* 2005; **84**: 1–12.

8. Wick G, Grubeck-Loebenstein B. The aging immune system: primary and secondary alterations of immune reactivity in the elderly. *Exp Gerontol* 1997; **32**: 401–13.

9. Zahm S, Weisenburger D, Babbitt P, *et al.* A case-control study of non-Hodgkin's lymphoma and the herbicide 2,4-dichlorophenoxyacetic acid (2,4-d) in eastern Nebraska. *Epidemiology* 1990; **1**: 349–56.

10. Zintzaras E, Voulgarelis M, Moutsopoulos H. The risk of lymphoma development in autoimmune diseases. *Arch Intern Med* 2005; **165**: 2337–44.

11. Non-Hodgkin's Lymphoma Pathologic Classification Project. National Cancer Institute sponsored study of classifications of non-Hodgkin's lymphomas. Summary and description of a working formulation for clinical usage. *Cancer* 1982; **49**: 2112–35.

12. Harris NL, Jaffe ES, Stein H, *et al.* A revised European-American Classification of lymphoid neoplasms: a proposal from the International Lymphoma Study Group. *Blood* 1994; **84**: 1361–92.

13. Jaffe ES, Harris NL, Stein H, Vardiman JW. *World Health Organization Classification of Tumours: Pathology and Genetics of Tumours of Haematopoietic and Lymphoid Tissues* (Lyon: IARC Press; 2001).

14. Frederico M, Vitolo U, Zinzani P, *et al.* Prognosis of follicular lymphoma: a predictive model based on a retrospective analysis of 987 cases. Intergruppo Italiano Linfoni. *Blood* 2000; **95**: 783–9.

15. International Non-Hodgkin's Lymphoma Prognostic Factors Project: a predictive model for aggressive non-Hodgkin's lymphoma. *N Engl J Med* 1993; **329**: 987–94.

16. Maartense E, le Cessie S, Kluin-Nelemans H, *et al.* Age-related differences among patients with follicular lymphoma and the importance of prognostic scoring systems: analysis from a population-based non-Hodgkin's lymphoma registry. *Ann Oncol* 2002; **13**: 1275–84.

17. Solal-Celigny P, Roy P, Colombat P, *et al.* Follicular Lymphoma International Prognostic Index. *Blood* 2004; **104**: 1258–65.

18. Jelic S, Milanovic N, Tomasevic Z, Matovic S, Gavrilovic D. Comparison of two non-anthracycline-containing regimens for elderly patients with diffuse large-cell non Hodgkin's lymphoma: possible pitfalls in results reporting and interpretation. *Neoplasma* 1999; **46**: 394–9.

19. Gomez H, Hidalgo M, Casanova L, *et al.* Risk factors for treatment-related death in elderly patients with aggressive non-Hodgkin's lymphoma: results of a multivariate analysis. *J Clin Oncol* 1998; **16**: 2065–9.

20. Balducci L, Extermann M. A practical approach to the older patient with cancer. *Cancer* 2001; **25**: 6–76.

21. McCorkle R, Strumpf N, Nuamah I, *et al.* A specialized home care intervention improves survival among older post-surgical cancer patients. *J Am Geriatr Soc* 2000; **48**: 1707–13.

22. Monfardini S, Balducci L. A comprehensive geriatric assessment (CGA) is necessary for the study and the management of cancer in the elderly. *Eur J Cancer* 1999; **35**: 1771–2.

23. Repetto L, Frantino L, Audisio R, *et al.* Comprehensive geriatric assessment adds information to Eastern Cooperative Oncology Group performance status in elderly cancer patients: an Italian Group for Geriatric Oncology Study. *J Clin Oncol* 2002; **20**: 494–502.

24. Capello D, Gaidano G. Molecular pathophysiology of indolent lymphoma. *Haematologica* 2000; **85**: 105–201.

25. Korsemeyer S. Bcl-2 initiates a new category of oncogenes: regulators of cell death. *Blood* 1992; **80**: 879–86.

26. Tsujimoto Y, Cossman J, Jaffe E, Croce C. Involvement of the bcl-2 gene in human follicular lymphoma. *Science* 1985; **228**: 1440–3.

27. Vaux D, Cory S, Adams M. bcl-2 gene promotes haemopoietic cell survival and cooperates with c-myc to immortalize pre-B cells. *Nature* 1988; **335**: 440–2.

28. Weiss L, Warnke R, Sklar J, Cleary M. Molecular analysis of the t(14; 18) chromosomal translocation in malignant lymphomas. *N Engl J Med* 1987; **317**: 1185–9.

29. Akasaka T, Lossos I, Levy R. BCL6 gene translocation in follicular lymphoma: a harbinger of eventual transformation to diffuse aggressive lymphoma. *Blood* 2003; **102**: 1443–8.

30. Lossos I, Alizadeh A, Diehn M, *et al.* Transformation of follicular lymphoma to diffuse large-cell lymphoma: alternative patterns with increased or decreased expression of c-myc and its regulated genes. *Proc Natl Acad Sci USA* 2002; **99**: 8886–91.

31. Bohen S, Troyanskaya O, Alter O, *et al.* Variation in gene expression patterns in follicular lymphoma and the response to rituximab. *Proc Natl Acad Sci USA* 2003; **100**: 1926–30.

32. Dave S, Wright G, Tan B, *et al.* Prediction of survival in follicular lymphoma based on molecular features of tumor-infiltrating immune cells. *N Engl J Med* 2004; **351**: 2159–69.

33. Abramson J, Shipp MA. Advances in the biology and therapy of diffuse large B-cell lymphoma: moving toward a molecularly targeted approach. *Blood* 2005; **106**: 1164–74.

34. Lossos I, Czerwinski D, Alizadeh A, *et al.* Prediction of survival in diffuse large-B-cell lymphoma based on the expression of six genes. *N Engl J Med* 2004; **350**: 1828–37.

35. Monti S, Savage K, Kutok J, *et al.* Molecular profiling of diffuse large B-cell lymphoma identifies robust subtypes including one characterized by host inflammatory response. *Blood* 2005; **105**: 1851–61.

36. Shipp M, Ross K, Tamayo P, *et al.* Diffuse large B-cell lymphoma outcome prediction by gene-expression profiling and supervised machine learning. *Nature Med* 2002; **8**: 68–74.

37. Rosenwald A, Wright G, Chan W, *et al.* The use of molecular profiling to predict survival after chemotherapy for diffuse large-B-cell lymphoma. *N Engl J Med* 2002; **346**: 1937–47.

38. Mounier N, Briere J, Gisselbrecht C, *et al.* Rituximab plus CHOP (R-CHOP) overcomes bcl-2-associated resistance to chemotherapy in elderly patients with diffuse large B-cell lymphoma (DLBCL). *Blood* 2003; **101**: 4279–84.

39. Maartense E, Kramer M, le Cessie S, *et al.* Lack of prognostic significance of BCL2 and p53 protein overexpression in elderly patients with diffuse large B-cell non-Hodgkin's lymphoma: results for a population-based non-Hodgkin's lymphoma registry. *Leuk Lymphoma* 2004; **45**: 101–7.

40. A clinical evaluation of the International Lymphoma Study Group classification of non-Hodgkin's lymphoma. The Non-Hodgkin's Lymphoma Classification Project. *Blood* 1997; **89**: 3909–18.

41. Harris NL, Jaffe ES, Diebold J, *et al.* World Health Organization Classification of neoplastic diseases of

the hematopoietic and lymphoid tissues: report of the Clinical Advisory Committee Meeting, Airlie House, Virginia, November 1997. *J Clin Oncol* 1999; **17**: 3835–49.

42. Martin AR, Weisenburger DD, Chan WC, *et al.* Prognostic value of cellular proliferation and histologic grade in follicular lymphoma. *Blood* 1995; **85**: 3671–8.

43. Lopez-Guillermo A, Cabanillas F, McDonnell TI, *et al.* Correlation of Bcl-2 rearrangement with clinical characteristics and outcome in indolent follicular lymphoma. *Blood* 1999; **93**: 3081–7.

44. Advani R, Rosenberg S, Horning SJ. Stage I and II follicular non-Hodgkin's lymphoma: long-term follow-up of no initial therapy. *J Clin Oncol* 2004; **22**: 1454–9.

45. Ardeshna K, Smith P, Norton A, *et al.* Long-term effect of a watch and wait policy versus immediate systemic treatment for asymptomatic advanced-stage non-Hodgkin's lymphoma: a randomized controlled trial. *Lancet* 2003; **362**: 516–22.

46. Brice P, Bastion Y, Lepage E, *et al.* Comparison in low-tumor-burden follicular lymphomas between an initial no-treatment policy, prednimustine, or interferon alfa: a randomized study from the Group D'Etude des Lymphomes Folliculaires. *J Clin Oncol* 1997; **15**: 1110–17.

47. Horning SJ, Rosenberg SA. The natural history of initially untreated low-grade non-Hodgkin's lymphomas. *N Engl J Med* 1984; **311**: 1471–5.

48. Portlock CS, Rosenberg SA. No initial therapy for stage III and IV non-Hodgkin's lymphomas of favorable histologic types. *Ann Intern Med* 1979; **90**: 10–13.

49. Soubeyran P, Eghbali H, Trojani M, Bonichon F, Richaud P, Hoerni B. Is there any place for a wait-and-see policy in stage I_0 follicular lymphoma? A study of 43 consecutive patients in a single center. *Ann Oncol* 1996; **7**: 713–18.

50. Young RC, Longo DL, Glatstein E, Inde DC, Jaffe ES, DeVita VT Jr. The treatment of indolent lymphomas. Watchful waiting *v* aggressive combined modality treatment. *Semin Hematol* 1988; **25**: 11–26.

51. MacManus M, Hoppe R. Is radiotherapy curative for stage I and II low-grade follicular lymphoma? Results of a long-term follow-up study of patients treated at Stanford University. *J Clin Oncol* 1996; **14**: 1282–90.

52. Wilder R, Jones D, Tucker S, *et al.* Long-term results with radiotherapy for stage I-II follicular lymphomas. *Int J Radiat Oncol Biol Phys* 2001; **51**: 1219–27.

53. Kennedy BJ, Bloomfield CD, Kiang DT, Vosika G, Peterson BA, Theologides A. Combination versus successive single agent chemotherapy in lymphocytic lymphoma. *Cancer* 1978; **41**: 23–8.

54. Lister TA, Cullen MH, Beard MEJ, *et al.* Comparison of combined and single-agent chemotherapy in non-Hodgkin's lymphomas of favourable histologic type. *Br Med J* 1978; **1**: 533–7.

55. Peterson B, Petroni G, Frizzera G, *et al.* Prolonged single-agent versus combination chemotherapy in indolent follicular lymphomas: a study of the Cancer and Leukemia Group B. *J Clin Oncol* 2003; **21**: 5–15.

56. Portlock CS, Rosenberg SA, Glatstein E, Kaplan HS. Treatment of advanced non-Hodgkin's lymphomas with favorable histologies: preliminary results of a prospective trial. *Blood* 1976; **47**: 747–56.

57. Cheson BD. New prospects in the treatment of indolent lymphomas with purine analogues. *Cancer J Sci Am* 1998; **4** (Suppl 2): S27–S36.

58. Hoffman M, Tallman MS, Hakimian D, *et al.* 2-chlorodeoxyadenosine is an active salvage therapy in advanced indolent non-Hodgkin's lymphoma. *J Clin Oncol* 1994; **12**: 788–92.

59. Kay AC, Saven A, Carrera CJ, *et al.* 2-Chlorodeoxyadenosine treatment of low-grade lymphomas. *J Clin Oncol* 1992; **10**: 371–7.

60. Solal-Celigny P, Brice P, Brousse H, *et al.* Phase II trial of fludarabine monophosphate as first-line treatment in patients with advanced follicular lymphoma: A multicenter study by the Group d-Etude des Lymphomes de l'Adulte. *J Clin Oncol* 1996; **14**: 514–19.

61. Tallman MS, Hakimian D. Purine nucleoside analogs: emerging roles in indolent lymphoproliferative disorders. *Blood* 1995; **86**: 2463–74.

62. Zinzani PL, Magagnoli M, Moretti L, *et al.* Randomized trial of fludarabine versus fludarabine and idarubicin as frontline treatment in patients with indolent or mantle-cell lymphoma. *J Clin Oncol* 2000; **18**: 773–9.

63. Cohen Y, Solal-Celigny P, Polliack A. Rituximab therapy for follicular lymphoma: a comprehensive review of its efficacy as primary treatment, treatment for relapsed disease, re-treatment and maintenance. *Haematologica* 2003; **88**: 811–23.

64. Ghielmini M, Schmitz SF, Cogliatti S, *et al.* Prolonged treatment with rituximab in patients with follicular lymphoma significantly increases event-free survival and response duration compared with the standard weekly x 4 schedule. *Blood* 2004; **103**: 4416–23.

65. Hainsworth J, Litchy S, Shaffer D, Lackey V, Grimaldi M, Greco F. Maximizing therapeutic benefit of

rituximab: maintenance therapy versus re-treatment at progression in patients with indolent non-Hodgkin's lymphoma. A randomized phase II trial of the Minnie Pearl Cancer Research Network. *J Clin Oncol* 2005; **23**: 1088–95.

66. Hainsworth JD, Burris HA, Morrissey LH, *et al.* Rituximab monoclonal antibody as initial systemic therapy for patients with low-grade non-Hodgkin lymphoma. *Blood* 2000; **95**: 3052–6.

67. Witzig T, Vukov A, Habermann TM, *et al.* Rituximab therapy for patients with newly diagnosed, advanced-stage, follicular grade I non-Hodgkin's lymphoma: a phase II trial in the North Central Cancer Treatment Group. *J Clin Oncol* 2005; **23**: 1103–8.

68. Hoppe RT, Kushain P, Kaplan HS, Rosenberg SA, Brown BW. The treatment of advanced stage favorable histology non-Hodgkin's lymphoma: a preliminary report of a randomized trial comparing single agent chemotherapy, combination chemotherapy, and whole body irradiation. *Blood* 1981; **58**: 592–8.

69. Flinn IW, Byrd JC, Morrison C, *et al.* Fludarabine and cyclophosphamide with filgrastim support in patients with previously untreated indolent lymphoid malignancies. *Blood* 2000; **96**: 71–5.

70. Forstpointner R, Dreyling M, Repp R, *et al.* The addition of rituximab to a combination of fludarabine, cyclophosphamide, mitoxantrone (FCM) significantly increases the response rate and prolongs survival as compared with FCM alone in patients with relapsed and refractory follicular and mantle cell lymphomas: results of a prospective randomized study of the German Low-Grade Lymphoma Study Group. *Blood* 2004; **104**: 3064–71.

71. Foussard C, Deconinck E, Desablens B, *et al.* A randomized trial of fludarabine, mitoxantrone (FM) versus doxorubicin, cyclophosphamide, vindesine, prednisone (CHVP), as first line treatment in patients with advanced low-grade non-Hodgkin lymphoma (LG-NHL): a multicenter study by GOELAMS Group. *Blood* 1998; **92** (Suppl 10): 316e.

72. Hochster HS, Oken MM, Winter JN, *et al.* Phase I study of fludarabine plus cyclophosphamide in patients with previously untreated low-grade lymphoma: results and long-term follow-up: a report from the Eastern Cooperative Oncology Group. *J Clin Oncol* 2000; **18**: 987–94.

73. Kimby E, Cavallin-Stahl E, Haapaniemi E, *et al.* Fludarabine in combination with idarubicin as treatment of untreated and relapsed low-grade lymphoma.

Preliminary results of a multicenter phase II study. *Blood* 1999; **94** (Suppl 1): 95a.

74. Czuczman MS, Grillo-Lopez AJ, White CA, *et al.* Treatment of patients with low-grade B-cell lymphoma with the combination of chimeric anti-CD20 monoclonal antibody and CHOP chemotherapy. *J Clin Oncol* 1999; **17**: 268–76.

75. Dana B, Dahlberg S, Bharat N, *et al.* Long term follow up of patients with low grade malignant lymphomas treated with doxorubicin-based chemotherapy or chemoimmunotherapy. *J Clin Oncol* 1993; **11**: 644–51.

76. Kimby E, Bjorkholm M, Gahrton G, *et al.* Chlorambucil/prednisone vs. CHOP in symptomatic low-grade non-Hodgkin's lymphomas: a randomized trial from the Lymphoma Group of Central Sweden. *Ann Oncol* 1994; **5** (Suppl 2): 67–71.

77. Foran JM, Rohatiner AZ, Coiffier B, *et al.* Multicenter phase II study of fludarabine phosphate for patients with newly diagnosed lymphoplasmacytoid lymphoma, Waldenstrom's macroglobulinemia, and mantle-cell lymphoma. *J Clin Oncol* 1999; **17**: 546–53.

78. Zinzani PL, Bendandi M, Magagnoli M, *et al.* Results of a fludarabine induction and alpha-interferon maintenance protocol in pretreated patients with chronic lymphocytic leukemia and low-grade non-Hodgkin's lymphoma. *Eur J Haematol* 1997; **59**: 82–8.

79. Cohen Y, Da'as N, Libster D, Amir G, Berrebi A, Polliack A. Large-cell transformation of chronic lymphocytic leukemia and follicular lymphoma during or soon after treatment with fludarabine-rituximab-containing regimens: natural history or therapy-related complication? *Eur J Haematol* 2002; **68**: 80–3.

80. Thornton P, Bellas C, Santori A, *et al.* Richter's transformation of chronic lymphocytic leukemia. The possible role of fludarabine and the Epstein–Barr virus in its pathogenesis. *Leuk Res* 2005; **29**: 389–95.

81. Armitage J, Carbone P, Connors J, Levine A, Bennett J, Kroll S. Treatment-related myelodysplasia and acute leukemia in non-Hodgkin's lymphoma patients. *J Clin Oncol* 2003; **21**: 897–906.

82. Cheson BD, Vena DA, Barrett J, Freidlin B. Second malignancies as a consequence of nucleoside analog therapy for chronic lymphoid leukemia. *J Clin Oncol* 1999; **17**: 2454–60.

83. Pedersen-Bjergaard J, Ersboll J, Sorensen H, *et al.* Risk of acute nonlymphocytic leukemia and preleukemia in patients treated with cyclophosphamide for non-Hodgkin's lymphomas: comparison with results obtained in patients treated for Hodgkin's

disease and ovarian carcinoma with other alkylating agents. *Ann Intern Med* 1985; **103**: 195–200.

84. Van Den Neste E, Louviaux I, Michaux JL, *et al.* Myelodysplastic syndrome with monosomy 5 and/or 7 following therapy with 2-chloro-2'-deoxyadenosine. *Br J Haematol* 1999; **105**: 268–70.

85. Marcus R, Imrie K, Belch A, *et al.* CVP chemotherapy plus rituximab compared with CVP as first-line treatment for advanced follicular lymphoma. *Blood* 2005; **105**: 1417–23.

86. Zinzani P, Pulsoni A, Perrotti A, *et al.* Fludarabine plus mitoxantrone with and without rituximab versus CHOP with and without rituximab as front-line treatment for patients with follicular lymphoma. *J Clin Oncol* 2004; **22**: 2654–61.

87. Kaminski M, Estes J, Zasadny K, *et al.* Radioimmunotherapy with iodine 131I tositumomab for relapsed or refractory B-cell non-Hodgkin lymphoma: updated results and long-term follow-up of the University of Michigan experience. *Blood* 2000; **96**: 1259–66.

88. Kaminski M, Tuck M, Estes J, *et al.* 131I-tositumomab therapy as initial treatment for follicular lymphoma. *N Engl J Med* 2005; **352**: 441–9.

89. Witzig T, Flinn I, Gordon L, *et al.* Treatment with ibritumomab tiuxetan radioimmunotherapy in patients with rituximab refractory follicular non-Hodgkin's lymphoma. *J Clin Oncol* 2002; **20**: 3262–9.

90. Witzig T, Gordon LI, Cabanillas F, *et al.* Randomized controlled trial of yttrium-90-labeled ibritumomab tiuxetan radioimmunotherapy verus rituximab immunotherapy for patients with relapsed or refractory low-grade, follicular, or transformed B-cell non-Hodgkin's lymphoma. *J Clin Oncol* 2002; **20**: 2453–63.

91. Dimopoulos M, Kyle R, Anagnostopoulos A, Treon S. Diagnosis and management of Waldenstrom's macroglobulinemia. *J Clin Oncol* 2005; **23**: 1564–77.

92. Owen R, Treon S, Al-Katib A, *et al.* Clinicopathological definition of Waldenstrom's macroglobulinemia: consensus panel recommendations from the Second International Workshop on Waldensrom's Macroglobulinemia. *Semin Oncol* 2003; **30**: 110–15.

93. Chen C. Treatment for Waldenstrom's macroglobulinemia. *Ann Oncol* 2004; **15**: 550–8.

94. Gertz M. Waldenstrom macroglobulinemia: a review of therapy. *Am J Hematol* 2005; **79**: 147–57.

95. Gertz MA, Fonseca R, Rajkumar SV. Waldenstrom's macroglobulinemia. *Oncologist* 2000; **5**: 63–7.

96. Sarris A, Ford R. Recent advances in the molecular pathogenesis of lymphomas. *Curr Opin Oncol* 1999; **11**: 351–63.

97. Zinzani PL, Gherlinzoni F, Bendandi M, *et al.* Fludarabine treatment in resistant Waldenstrom's macroglobulinemia. *Eur J Haematol* 1995; **54**: 120–3.

98. Gertz M, Anagnostopoulos A, Anderson K, *et al.* Treatment recommendations in Waldenstrom's macroglobulinemia: consensus panel recommendations from the Second International Workshop on Waldenstrom's Macroglobulinemia. *Semin Oncol* 2003; **30**: 121–6.

99. Zeldis J, Schafer P, Bennett B, Mercurio F, Stirling D. Potential new therapeutics for Waldenstrom's macroglobulinemia. *Semin Oncol* 2003 **30**: 275–81.

100. Martino R, Shah A, Romero P, *et al.* Allogeneic bone marrow transplantation for advanced Waldenstrom's macroglobulinemia. *Bone Marrow Transplant* 1999; **23**: 747–9.

101. Munshi N, Barlogie B. Role for high-dose therapy with autologous hematopoietic stem cell support in Waldenstrom's macroglobulinemia. *Semin Oncol* 2003; **30**: 282–5.

102. Dimopoulos M, Alexandian R, Gika D, *et al.* Treatment of Waldenstrom's macroglobulinemia with rituximab: prognostic factors for response and progression. *Leuk Lymphoma* 2004; **45**: 2057–61.

103. Gertz M, Rue M, Blood E, Kaminer L, Vesole D, Greipp P. Multicenter phase 2 trial of rituximab for Waldenstrom macroglobulinemia (WM): an Eastern Cooperative Oncology Group Study (E3A98). *Leuk Lymphoma* 2004; **45**: 2047–55.

104. Catovsky D, Matutes E. Splenic lymphoma with circulating villous lymphocytes/splenic marginal-zone lymphoma. *Semin Hematol* 1999; **36**: 148–54.

105. Franco V, Florena A, Iannitto E. Splenic marginal zone lymphoma. *Blood* 2003; **101**: 2464–72.

106. Hammer RD, Glick AD, Greer JP, Collins RD, Cousar JB. Splenic marginal zone lymphoma. A distinct B-cell neoplasm. *Am J Surg Pathol* 1996; **20**: 613–26.

107. Thieblemont C, Felman P, Callet-Bauchu E, *et al.* Splenic marginal-zone lymphoma: a distinct clinical and pathological entity. *Lancet Oncol* 2003; **4**: 95–103.

108. Troussard X, Valensi F, Duchayne E, *et al.* Splenic lymphoma with villous lymphocytes: clinical presentation, biology and prognostic factors in a series of 100 patients. Groupe Francais d'Hematologie Cellulaire (GFHC). *Br J Haematol* 1996; **93**: 731–6.

109. Hermine O, Lefrere F, Bronowicki JP, *et al.* Regression of splenic lymphoma with villous lymphocytes after treatment of hepatitis C virus infection. *N Engl J Med* 2002; **347**: 89–94.

110. Bolam S, Orchard J, Oscier D. Fludarabine is effective in the treatment of splenic lymphoma with villous lymphocytes. *Br J Haematol* 1997; **99**: 158–61.

111. Lefrere F, Hermine O, Belanger C, *et al.* Fludarabine: an effective treatment in patients with splenic lymphoma with villous lymphocytes. *Leukemia* 2000; **14**: 573–5.

112. Mulligan SP, Matutes E, Dearden C, Catovsky D. Splenic lymphoma with villous lymphocytes: natural history and response to therapy in 50 cases. *Br J Haematol* 1991; **78**: 206–9.

113. Campo E, Miquel R, Krenacs L, Sorbara L, Raffeld M, Jaffe ES. Primary nodal marginal zone lymphomas of splenic and MALT type. *Am J Surg Pathol* 1999; **23**: 59–68.

114. Nathwani BM, Drachenberg MR, Hernandez AM, Levine AM, Sheibani K. Nodal monocytoid B-cell lymphoma (nodal marginal-zone B-cell lymphoma). *Semin Hematol* 1999; **36**: 128–38.

115. Berger R, Felman P, Thieblemont C, *et al.* Non-MALT marginal zone B-cell lymphomas: a description of clinical presentation and outcome in 124 patients. *Blood* 2000; **95**: 1950–6.

116. Bertoni F, Zucca E. State-of-the-art therapeutics: marginal-zone lymphoma. *J Clin Oncol* 2005; **23**: 6415–20.

117. Ferreri A, Ponzoni M, Guidoboni M, *et al.* Regression of ocular adnexal lymphoma after Chlamydia psittaci-eradicating antibiotic therapy. *J Clin Oncol* 2005; **23**: 5067–73.

118. Greiner A, Knorr C, Seeberger H, Schultz A, Muller-Hermelink HK. Tumor biology of mucosa-associated lymphoid tissue lymphomas. *Recent Results Cancer Res* 2000; **156**: 19–27.

119. Van Kriken JHJM, Hoeve MA. Epidemiological and prognostic aspects of gastric MALT-lymphoma. *Recent Results Cancer Res* 2000; **156**: 3–8.

120. Bayerdorffer E, Neubauer A, Rudolph B, *et al.* Regression of primary gastric lymphoma of mucosa-associated lymphoid tissue type after cure of Helicobacter pylori infection. *Lancet* 1995; **345**: 1591–4.

121. Fischbach W, Goebeler-Kolve M-E, Dragnosics B, Greiner A, Stolte M. Long term outcome of patients with gastric marginal zone B cell lymphoma of mucosa associated lymphoic tissue (MALT) following exclusive Helicobacter pylori eradication therapy: experience from a large prospective series. *Gut* 2004; **53**: 34–7.

122. Ruggero E, Zucca E, Pinotti G, *et al.* Eradication of Helicobacter pylori infection in primary low-grade gastric lymphoma of mucosa-associated lymphoid tissue. *Ann Intern Med* 1995; **122**: 767–9.

123. Cerroni L, Zochling N, Putz B, Kerl H. Infection by Borrelia burgdorferi and cutaneous B-cell lymphoma. *J Cutan Pathol* 1997; **24**: 457–61.

124. Kodama K, Massone C, Chott A, Mertze D, Kerl H, Cerroni L. Primary cutaneous large B-cell lymphomas: clinicopathologic features, classification, and prognostic factors in a large series of patients. *Blood* 2005; **106**: 2491–7.

125. Bhattacharyya N, Frankenthaler RA, Gomolin HI, Kadin ME, Lauretano AM. Clinical and pathologic characterizations of mucosa-associated lymphoid tissue lymphoma of the head and neck. *Ann Otol Rhinol Laryngol* 1998; **107**: 801–6.

126. Hoefnagel J, Vermeer M, Jansen P, *et al.* Primary cutaneous marginal zone B-cell lymphoma. Clinical and therapeutic features in 50 cases. *Arch Dermatol* 2005; **141**: 1139–45.

127. Thieblemont C, Berger F, Dumontet C, *et al.* Mucosa-associated lymphoid tissue lymphoma is a disseminated disease in one third of 158 patients analyzed. *Blood* 2000; **95**: 802–6.

128. Zinzani PL, Magagnoli M, Ascani S, *et al.* Nongastrointestinal mucosa-associated lymphoid tissue (MALT) lymphomas: clinical and therapeutic features of 24 localized patients. *Ann Oncol* 1997; **8**: 883–6.

129. Gospodarowicz MK, Pintilie M, Tsang R, Patterson B, Bezjak A, Wells W. Primary gastric lymphoma: brief overview of the recent Princess Margaret Hospital experience. *Recent Results Cancer Res* 2000; **156**: 108–15.

130. Schechter NR, Portlock CS, Yahalom J. Treatment of mucosa-associated lymphoid tissue lymphoma of the stomach with radiation alone. *J Clin Oncol* 1998; **16**: 1916–21.

131. Matsuo T, Yoshino T. Long-term follow-up results of observation or radiation for conjunctival malignant lymphoma. *Ophthalmology* 2004; **111**: 1233–7.

132. Tsang R, Gospodarowicz M, Pintilie M, *et al.* Localized mucosa-associated lymphoid tissue lymphoma treated with radiation therapy has excellent clinical outcome. *J Clin Oncol* 2003; **21**: 4157–64.

133. Conconi A, Martinelli G, Thieblemont C, *et al.* Clinical activity of rituximab in extranodal marginal zone B-cell lymphoma of MALT type. *Blood* 2003; **102**: 2741–5.

134. Hammel P, Haioun C, Chaumette MT, *et al.* Efficacy of single-agent chemotherapy in low-grade B-cell mucosa-associated lymphoid tissue lymphoma with prominent gastric expression. *J Clin Oncol* 1995; **13**: 2524–9.

135. Martinelli G, Laszlo D, Ferreri A, *et al.* Clinical activity of rituximab in gastric marginal zone non-Hodgkin's lymphoma resistant to or not eligible for anti-Helicobacter pylori therapy. *J Clin Oncol* 2005; **23**: 1979–83.

136. McKelvey EM, Gottlieb JA, Wilson HE, *et al.* Hydroxydaunomycin (Adriamycin) combination chemotherapy in malignant lymphoma. *Cancer* 1976; **38**: 1484–93.

137. Fisher R, Gaynor E, Dahlberg S, *et al.* Comparison of a standard regimen (CHOP) with three intensive chemotherapy regimens for advanced non-Hodgkin's lymphoma. *N Engl J Med* 1993; **328**: 1002–6.

138. Gordon LI, Harrington D, Andersen J, *et al.* Comparison of a second-generation chemotherapeutic regimen (m-BACOD) with a standard regimen (CHOP) for advanced diffuse non-Hodgkin's lymphoma. *N Engl J Med* 1992; **327**: 1342–9.

139. Armitage J, Potter J. Aggressive chemotherapy for diffuse histiocytic lymphoma in the elderly: increased complications with advancing age. *J Am Geriatr Soc* 1984; **32**: 269–73.

140. Bastion Y, Blay J, Divine M, *et al.* Elderly patients with aggressive non-Hodgkin's lymphoma: disease presentation, response to treatment, and survival: A Groupe d'Etude des Lymphomes de l'Adulte study on 453 patients older than 69 years. *J Clin Oncol* 1997; **15**: 2945–53.

141. Niitsu N, Umeda M. THP-COPBLM (pirarubicin, cyclophosphamide, vincristine, prednisone, bleomycin and procarbazine) regimen combined with granulocyte colony-stimulating factor (G-CSF) for non-Hodgkin's lymphoma in elderly patients: a prospective study. *Leukemia* 1997; **11**: 1817–20.

142. Niitsu N, Umeda M. Response and adverse drug reactions to combination chemotherapy in elderly patients with aggressive non-Hodgkin's lymphoma: comparison of CHOP, COP-BLAM, COP-BLAM III, and THP-COPBLM. *Eur J Haematol* 1999; **63**: 337–44.

143. Aviles A, Nambo M, Talavera A, *et al.* Epirubicin (CEOP-Bleo) versus idarubicin (CIOP-Bleo) in the treatment of elderly patients with aggressive non-Hodgkin's lymphoma: dose escalation studies. *Anticancer Drugs* 1997; **8**: 937–42.

144. Veneri D, Zanetti F, Franchini M, Krampera M, Pizzolo G. Low-dose epirubicin in combination with cyclophosphamide, vinblastine and prednisone (mini-CEOP) for the treatment of aggressive non-Hodgkin's lymphoma in elderly patients. *Haematologica* 2002; **87**: ELT43.

145. Sonneveld P, de Ridder M, Van der Lelie H, *et al.* Comparison of doxorubicin and mitoxantrone in the treatment of elderly patients with advanced diffuse non-Hodgkin's lymphoma using CHOP versus CNOP chemotherapy. *J Clin Oncol* 1995; **13**: 2530–9.

146. Tirelli U, Errante D, van Glabbeke M, *et al.* CHOP is the standard regimen in patients > or = 70 years of age with intermediate-grade and high-grade non-Hodgkin's lymphoma: results of a randomized study of the European Organization for Research and the Treatment of Cancer Lymphoma Cooperative Study Group. *J Clin Oncol* 1998; **16**: 27–34.

147. Tirelli U, Zagonel V, Errante D, *et al.* A prospective study of a new combination chemotherapy regimen in patients older than 70 years with unfavorable non-Hodgkin's lymphoma. *J Clin Oncol* 1992; **10**: 228–36.

148. Doorduijn J, van der Holt B, van Imhoff G, *et al.* CHOP compared with CHOP plus granulocyte colony-stimulating factor in elderly patients with aggressive non-Hodgkin's lymphomas. *J Clin Oncol* 2003; **21**: 3041–50.

149. Tilly H, Lepage E, Coiffier B, *et al.* Intensive conventional chemotherapy (ACVBP regimen) compared with standard CHOP for poor-prognosis aggressive non-Hodgkin lymphoma. *Blood* 2003; **102**: 4284–9.

150. Pfreundschuh M, Trumper L, Kloess M, *et al.* Two-weekly or 3-weekly CHOP chemotherapy with or without etoposide for the treatment of elderly patients with aggressive lymphomas: results of the NHL-B2 trial of the DSHNHL. *Blood* 2004; **104**: 634–41.

151. Coiffier B, Lepage E, Briere J, *et al.* CHOP chemotherapy plus rituximab compared with CHOP alone in elderly patients with diffuse large-B-cell lymphomas. *N Engl J Med* 2002; **346**: 235–42.

152. Habermann TM, Morrison VA, Cassileth PA, *et al.* Phase III trial of rituximab-CHOP (R-CHOP) vs. CHOP with a second randomization to maintenance rituximab (MR) or observation in patients 60 years

of age and older with diffuse large B-cell lymphoma (DLBCL). *Proc Am Soc Hematol* 2003; **102**: abstract 8.

153. Dixon D, Neilan B, Jones S, *et al*. Effect of age on the therapeutic outcome in advanced diffuse histiocytic lymphoma: the Southwest Oncology Group experience. *J Clin Oncol* 1986; **4**: 295–305.

154. Gottlieb A, Anderson J, Ginsberg S, *et al*. A randomized comparison of methotrexate dose and the addition of bleomycin to CHOP therapy for diffuse large cell lymphoma and other non-Hodgkin's lymphomas: Cancer and Leukemia Group B study 7851. *Cancer* 1990; **66**: 1888–96.

155. Vose J, Armitage J, Weisenburger D, *et al*. The importance of age in survival of patients treated with chemotherapy for aggressive non-Hodgkin's lymphoma. *J Clin Oncol* 1988; **6**: 1838–44.

156. Meyer R, Gyger M, Langley R, Lesperance B, Caplan S. A phase I trial of standard and cyclophosphamide dose-escalated CHOP with granulocyte colony stimulating factor in elderly patients with non-Hodgkin's lymphoma. *Leuk Lymphoma* 1998; **30**: 591–600.

157. Niitsu N, Tijima K. Full-dose CHOP chemotherapy combined with granulocyte colony-stimulating factor for aggressive non-Hodgkin's lymphoma in elderly patients: a prospective study. *Ann Hematol* 2001; **80**: 602–6.

158. Zinzani P, Pavone E, Storti S, *et al*. Randomized trial with or without granulocyte colony-stimulating factor as adjunct to induction VNCOP-B treatment of elderly high-grade non-Hodgkin's lymphoma. *Blood* 1997; **89**: 3974–9.

159. Gerhartz H, Engelhard M, Meusers P, *et al*. Randomized, double-blind, placebo-controlled, phase III study of recombinant human granulocyte-macrophage colony-stimulating factor as adjunct to induction treatment of high-grade malignant non-Hodgkin's lymphoma. *Blood* 1993; **82**: 2329–39.

160. Pettengell R, Gurney H, Radford J, *et al*. Granulocyte colony-stimulating factor to prevent dose-limiting neutropenia in non-Hodgkin's lymphoma: a randomized controlled trial. *Blood* 1992; **80**: 1430–6.

161. Ozer H, Armitage J, Bennett C, *et al*. 2000 update of recommendations for the use of hematopoietic colony-stimulating factors: evidence-based, clinical practice guidelines. *J Clin Oncol* 2000; **18**: 3558–85.

162. Coiffier B, Haioun C, Ketterer N, *et al*. Rituximab (anti-CD20 monoclonal antibody) for the treatment of patients with relapsing or refractory aggressive lymphoma: a multicenter phase II study. *Blood* 1998; **92**: 1927–32.

163. Vose J, Link B, Grossbard M, *et al*. Phase II study of rituximab in combination with CHOP chemotherapy in patients with previously untreated, aggressive non-Hodgkin's lymphoma. *J Clin Oncol* 2001; **19**: 389–97.

164. Feugier P, Van Hoof A, Sebban C, *et al*. Long-term results of the R-CHOP study in the treatment of elderly patients with diffuse large B-cell lymphoma: a study by the Groupe d'Etude des Lymphomes de l'Adulte. *J Clin Oncol* 2005; **23**: 4117–26.

165. Hequet O, Le G, Moullet I, *et al*. Subclinical late cardiomyopathy after doxorubicin therapy for lymphoma in adults. *Ann Oncol* 2004; **22**: 1864–71.

166. Horning SJ, Weller E, Kim K, *et al*. Chemotherapy with or without radiotherapy in limited-stage diffuse aggressive non-Hodgkin's lymphoma: Eastern Cooperative Oncology Group Study 1482. *J Clin Oncol* 2004; **22**: 3032–8.

167. Miller T, Dahlberg S, Cassady J, *et al*. Chemotherapy alone compared with chemotherapy plus radiotherapy for localized intermediate- and high-grade non-Hodgkin's lymphoma. *N Engl J Med* 1998; **339**: 21–6.

168. Jantunen E, Mahlamaki E, Nousiainen T. Feasibility and toxicity of high-dose chemotherapy supported by peripheral blood stem cell transplantation in elderly patients (>/-60 years) with non-Hodgkin's lymphoma: comparison with patients <60 years treated within the same protocol. *Bone Marrow Transplant* 2000; **26**: 737–41.

169. Magagnoli M, Castagna L, Balzarotti M, *et al*. Feasibility and toxicity of high-dose therapy (HDT) supported by peripheral blood stem cells in elderly patients with multiple myeloma and non-Hodgkin's lymphoma: survey from a single institution. *Am J Hematol* 2003; **73**: 267–72.

170. Fisher RI, Dahlberg S, Nathwani B, Banks P, Miller TP, Grogan T. A clinical analysis of two indolent lymphoma entities: mantle cell lymphoma and marginal zone lymphoma (including the mucosa-associated lymphoid tissue and monocytoid B-cell subcategories). A Southwest Oncology Group Study. *Blood* 1995; **85**: 1075–82.

171. Hiddemann W, Unterhalt M, Herrmann R, *et al*. Mantle-cell lymphomas have more widespread disease and a slower response to chemotherapy compared with follicle-center lymphomas: results of a prospective comparative analysis of German Low-Grade Lymphoma Study Group. *J Clin Oncol* 1998; **16**: 1922–30.

172. Velders G, Kluin-Nelemans J, De Boer C, *et al.* Mantle-cell lymphoma: a population-based clinical study. *J Clin Oncol* 1996; **14**: 1269–74.

173. Meusers P, Engelhard M, Bartels H, *et al.* Multicentre randomized therapeutic trial for advanced centro-cytic lymphoma: anthracycline does not improve the prognosis. *Hematol Oncol* 1989; **7**: 365–80.

174. Meusers P, Hense J. Management of mantle cell lymphoma. *Ann Hematol* 1999; **78**: 485–94.

175. Teodorovic I, Pittaluga S, Kluin-Nelemans J, *et al.* Efficacy of four different regimens in 64 mantle-cell lymphoma cases: clinico-pathologic comparison with 498 other non-Hodgkin's lymphoma subtypes. *J Clin Oncol* 1995; **13**: 2819–26.

176. Williams M, Densmore J. Biology and therapy of mantle cell lymphoma. *Curr Opin Oncol* 2005; **17**: 425–31.

177. Foran J, Cunningham D, Coiffier B, *et al.* Treatment of mantle-cell lymphoma with rituximab (chimeric monoclonal anti-CD20 antibody): analysis of factors associated with response. *Ann Oncol* 2000; **11**: 117–21.

178. Ghielmini M, Schmitz SF, Cogliatti S, *et al.* Effect of single-agent rituximab given at the standard schedule or as prolonged treatment in patients with mantle cell lymphoma: a study of the Swiss Group for Clinical Cancer Research (SAKK). *J Clin Oncol* 2005; **23**: 705–11.

179. Howard O, Gribben J, Neuberg D, *et al.* Rituximab and CHOP induction therapy for newly diagnosed mantle-cell lymphoma: molecular complete responses are not predictive of progression-free survival. *J Clin Oncol* 2002; **20**: 1288–94.

180. Lenz G, Dreyling M, Hoster E, *et al.* Immuno-chemotherapy with rituximab and cyclophosphamide, doxorubicin, vincristine, and prednisone significantly improves response and time to treatment failure, but not long-term outcome in patients with previously untreated mantle cell lymphoma: results of a prospective randomized trial of the German Low Grade Lymphoma Study Group (GLCS). *J Clin Oncol* 2005; **23**: 1984–92.

181. Dreyling M, Lenz G, Hoster E, *et al.* Early consolidation by myeloablative radiochemotherapy followed by autologous stem cell transplantation in first remission significantly prolongs progression-free survival in mantle cell lymphoma – results of a Prospective Randomized Trial of the European MDL Network. *Blood* 2005; **105**: 2677–84.

182. Maris M, Sandmaier B, Storer B, *et al.* Allogeneic hematopoietic cell transplantation after fludarabine and 2 GY total body irradiation for relapsed and refractory mantle cell lymphoma. *Blood* 2004; **104**: 3535–42.

183. Gianni A, Magni M, Martelli M, *et al.* Long-term remission in mantle cell lymphoma following high-dose sequential chemotherapy and in vivo rituximab-purged stem cell autografting (R-HDS regimen). *Blood* 2003; **102**: 749–55.

184. Romaguera JE, Khouri I, Kantarjian H, *et al.* Untreated aggressive mantle cell lymphoma: results with intensive chemotherapy without stem cell transplant in elderly patients. *Leuk Lymphoma* 2000; **39**: 77–85.

185. Goy A, Younes A, McLaughlin P, *et al.* Phase II study of proteasome inhibitor bortezomib in relapsed or refractory B-cell non-Hodgkin's lymphoma. *J Clin Oncol* 2005; **23**: 667–75.

186. O'Connor O, Wright J, Moskowitz C, *et al.* Phase II clinical experience with the novel proteasome inhibitor bortezomib in patients with indolent non-Hodgkin's lymphoma and mantle cell lymphoma. *J Clin Oncol* 2005; **23**: 676–84.

187. Blum K, Lozanski G, Byrd J. Adult Burkitt leukemia and lymphoma. *Blood* 2004; **104**: 3009–20.

188. Thorley-Lawson D, Gross A. Persistence of the Epstein-Barr virus and the origins of associated lymphomas. *N Engl J Med* 2004; **350**: 1328–37.

189. Braziel R, Arber D, Slovak M, *et al.* The Burkitt-like lymphomas: a Southwest Oncology Group study delineating phenotypic, genotypic, and clinical features. *Blood* 2001; **97**: 3713–20.

190. Cortes J, Thomas D, Rios A, *et al.* Hyperfractionated cyclophosphamide, vincristine, doxorubicin, and dexamethasone and highly active antiretrovial therapy for patients with acquired immunodeficiency syndrome-related Burkitt lymphoma/leukemia. *Cancer* 2002; **94**: 1492–9.

191. Lee E, Petroni GR, Schiffer C, *et al.* Brief-duration high-intensity chemotherapy for patients with small noncleaved-cell lymphoma or FAB L3 acute lymphocytic leukemia: results of Cancer and Leukemia Group B study 9251. *J Clin Oncol* 2001; **19**: 4014–22.

192. Rizzieri D, Johnson J, Niedzwiecki D, *et al.* Intensive chemotherapy with and without cranial radiation for Burkitt leukemia and lymphoma. Final results of Cancer and Leukemia Group B study 9251. *Cancer* 2004; **100**: 1438–48.

193. Thomas D, Cortes J, O'Brien S, *et al.* Hyper-CVAD program in Burkitt's-type adult acute lymphoblastic leukemia. *J Clin Oncol* 1999; **17**: 2461–70.

23

Unusual lymphomas in the elderly

Youssef Gamal, Samuel Kerr, Thomas P. Loughran

Introduction

This chapter discusses hematologic malignancies of T-cell and NK-cell origin, as classified by the World Health Organization (WHO). These malignancies are unusual in that they generally occur at low frequency. The discussion is fairly complete although some entities in WHO classification are not included because they occur primarily in younger individuals, e.g., hepatosplenic gamma/delta T-cell lymphoma.

Large granular lymphocyte and natural killer cell disorders

Large granular lymphocytes (LGL) are a distinct morphologic lymphoid subpopulation involved in cell cytotoxicity (Fig. 23.1). They comprise 10–15% of peripheral blood mononuclear cells and belong to one of two major lineages: CD3-positive in-vivo-activated cytotoxic T cells and CD3-negative natural killer (NK) cells. LGL and NK-cell lymphomas are relatively rare. T-cell and NK-cell disorders as a whole account for only 12% of all non-Hodgkin lymphomas, with the individual incidence of LGL and NK-cell neoplasms estimated to be less than 2% [1]. In general they are diseases of the older population, with a median presentation in the sixth and seventh decade. The exception is the aggressive NK-cell leukemia, which affects younger patients with a median age of 39 years. The current WHO classification of hematolymphoid malignancies considers these tumors under the subtype of mature peripheral T-cell

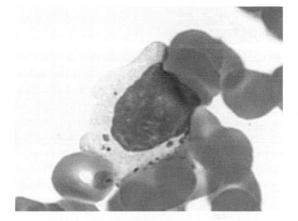

Figure 23.1 Large granular lymphocyte may appear as an atypical lymphocyte with scattered prominent granules in the cytoplasm. Maslak, P., ASH Image Bank 2004: 101068. Copyright American Society of Hematology. All rights reserved. *See color plate section.*

neoplasms [2]. These disorders will be discussed first in this chapter; they include T-cell LGL leukemia, aggressive NK-cell leukemia, extranodal NK/T-cell lymphoma nasal type, and blastic NK-cell lymphoma.

T-cell LGL leukemia

Overview

LGL leukemia was first defined in 1985 based on identification of clonal cytogenetic abnormalities and demonstration of tissue infiltration of marrow, liver, and spleen [3]. Classification into two phenotypically and clinically distinct subtypes of LGL leukemia was proposed in 1993 [4]. The most common type, occurring in 85% of cases, arises from a CD3+ T-cell lineage and displays a relatively indolent behavior manifested by chronic neutropenia and/or anemia [5]. The less common form, occurring in 15% of cases, arises from a CD3− NK-cell lineage and has been characterized by a very aggressive clinical course. This form has been classified by the current WHO classification system as a separate subtype of the mature peripheral T-cell neoplasms, and has been termed aggressive NK-cell leukemia.

Clinical features

T-LGL leukemia is primarily a disorder of the elderly, with a median age of 60 years at presentation (range 4–88 years) [5,6]. The disease is uncommon in patients under 40 years old (less than 10% of cases), and pediatric presentations are rare. There is no gender predominance. Approximately one-third of patients are asymptomatic at the time of diagnosis. The most common manifestations are recurrent bacterial infections (20–40%) and fever related to neutropenia [4,6]. Infections most commonly involve the skin, oropharynx, sinuses, and perirectal areas, but more serious infections such as sepsis and pneumonia can occur. Opportunistic infections are rare. Typical B symptoms of fever, night sweats, and weight loss are present in 20–30% of patients. Fatigue may be the presenting symptom, especially in patients with LGL leukemia that manifests as pure red-cell aplasia (PRCA). The most common physical finding is organomegaly, with splenomegaly present in 20–50% of patients and hepatomegaly present in 10–20% [7]. Lymphadenopathy is an uncommon finding (<5%). Lung involvement, presenting as pulmonary hypertension [8], and neuropathy are other rare occurrences in T-LGL leukemia.

Associated disorders

T-LGL leukemia is frequently associated with other diseases, especially autoimmune diseases. Rheumatoid arthritis (RA) is the most frequent associated syndrome, occurring in approximately 25% of patients with T-LGL leukemia [4,9]. Felty's syndrome, defined by the clinical triad of RA, neutropenia, and variable splenomegaly, has a clinical presentation similar to that of T-LGL leukemia with RA. There is no significant difference in age, sex, frequency of infections, or articular manifestations between the two disease entities. The presence of T-cell clonality is indicative of T-LGL leukemia with RA, and has been the distinguishing characteristic between the two syndromes [10]. However, there are data to suggest that Felty's syndrome and T-LGL leukemia share a common pathogenetic link and may be part of a disease continuum rather than separate disorders. The HLA-DR4 allele is found with high frequency in T-LGL leukemia with RA and in Felty's syndrome, occurring in 90% and 86% of patients respectively. Conversely, only 33% of patients with T-LGL without RA have the HLA-DR4 allele [11,12]. Furthermore, increased numbers of cells with a T-LGL phenotype have been found in blood and synovial fluid of patients with RA [13]. T-LGL leukemia has also occasionally been reported in association with several other autoimmune disorders including systemic lupus erythematosis, Sjögren's syndrome, recurrent uveitis, myasthenia gravis, and systemic sclerosis [6,14,15].

T-LGL leukemia can occur with other myeloid and lymphoid diseases. Particularly interesting is the association of T-LGL leukemia with other bone-marrow failure syndromes including aplastic anemia [16], paroxysmal nocturnal hemoglobinuria [17,18], and myelodysplastic syndrome [6,19]. Common characteristics that link these disorders together are cytopenias related to antigen-driven T-cell expansions and a response to immunosuppressive therapy. Clonal T-LGL proliferations have also been described in B-lymphoproliferative disorder [20]. Sporadic cases of concurrent T-LGL leukemia with B-cell chronic lymphocytic leukemia [21] and multiple myeloma [22] have been reported.

Expansion of T-LGL cells following allogeneic hematopoietic stem-cell transplant is commonly observed [23,24]. This could represent graft-versus-host disease, immune reconstitution, or viral (CMV) infection. T-LGL expansion in these patients may play a role in a disease control through an anti-leukemic effect, suggested by a low relapse rate [25]. Clonal T-LGL proliferations have also been reported in solid organ transplants, including liver [26] and kidney [27] transplants.

Hematologic features

T-LGL leukemia typically presents with lymphocytosis, neutropenia, and/or anemia. A lymphocyte count greater than 5.0×10^9/L is present in 60% of patients. Examination of the peripheral blood smear reveals lymphocytes that are large (15–18 µm) with abundant pale blue cytoplasm containing azurophilic granules and a reniform or round nucleus (Fig. 23.2). Careful review of the peripheral blood smear is imperative for diagnosis since up to 20% of patients will present with a normal lymphocyte count. Also, cytoplasmic granules can be absent in up to 5% of cases with a typical LGL phenotype, indicating a need for immunophenotyping of lymphocytes in patients with unexplained cytopenias or other characteristics suggestive of T-LGL leukemia. The LGL count range in normal individuals is 0.20×10^9/L $\pm$ 0.1 by morphology and 0.22×10^9/L $\pm$ 0.1 by cell flow cytometry. Proliferation of LGL cells of more than 0.5×10^9/L

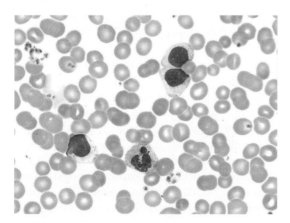

Figure 23.2 LGL leukemia: atypical lymphocytes are noted in the peripheral smear. Jurcic, J. & Maslak, P., ASH Image Bank 2004: 101229. Copyright American Society of Hematology. All rights reserved. *See color plate section.*

by flow cytometry is considered pathologic [5]. Until recently an LGL count of greater than 2.0×10^9/L lasting for more than six months was considered the diagnostic criterion to define the disease [28,29]. Newer improved techniques to detect clonality have allowed diagnosis in patients with the appropriate clinical picture and low LGL counts (<500/µL) [30].

The majority of patients (80%) with T-LGL leukemia present with sustained neutropenia (ANC <1.5 $\times$ 10^9/L), with severe neutropenia (ANC <0.5 $\times$ 10^9/L) present in 45% of the cases [5]. Most, if not all, cases of the rare disorder of adult-onset cyclic neutropenia appear to be associated with T-LGL leukemia [31,32]. The mechanism for the neutropenia in T-LGL is incompletely understood. Marrow infiltration by LGL cells, although present in the majority of patients, is not extensive enough to account for the severe neutropenia. More recent evidence implicates apoptosis of neutrophils through the Fas/Fas ligand pathway as a potential pathogenic mechanism. T-LGL leukemic cells have been shown to constitutively express Fas ligand (FasL) gene transcripts [33]. High levels of circulating FasL have been detected in the serum of the majority of patients with T-LGL leukemia [34]. Serum from these patients was shown to trigger apoptosis of normal neutrophils. Also, resolution of neutropenia, after treatment with methotrexate, was associated with disappearance or marked reduction in FasL levels.

Mild to moderate anemia (hemoglobin <11 g/dL) is common (48%) in T-LGL leukemia, while 20% of patients are transfusion-dependent [4,6,9]. Coombs-positive autoimmune hemolytic anemia occurs occasionally [35], and PRCA is common. T-LGL leukemia has been identified as the most common cause of PRCA, accounting for 19% of cases [36]. The mechanism underlying PRCA in T-LGL leukemia appears to involve cytotoxicity of erythroid progenitors by the leukemic LGL [37,38].

Mild to moderate thrombocytopenia occurs in approximately 20% of patients with T-LGL and does not require platelet transfusions. Platelet counts <50 $\times$ 10^9/L are present in 5% of cases [4,6]. Rarely idiopathic thrombocytopenic purpura (ITP) can occur simultaneously with T-LGL leukemia [6].

Histological features

Bone-marrow involvement is present in up to 90% of patients, although it can be subtle and difficult to recognize. The most consistent finding is hypercellularity, occurring in more than 55% of cases. Left-shifted myeloid maturation is present in 20–45% of patients, and increased erythroid precursors are frequently observed. Marrow lymphocytosis is common and is usually interstitial and diffuse. Large reactive lymphoid aggregates are occasionally found. Immunohistochemical analysis of bone-marrow specimens demonstrate the presence of linear arrays of intravascular CD8(+), TIA-1(+), or granzyme B(+) lymphocytes in 67% of cases of T-LGL leukemia [39]. Staining for CD56 or CD57 on bone-marrow biopsies is not useful.

Spleen involvement demonstrates red pulp expansion with infiltration of the cords and sinuses by leukemic T-LGL, plasmacytosis, and reactive follicular hyperplasia of the germinal centers of the white pulp [40]. Lymph-node involvement is not observed. Liver biopsies are characterized by sinusoidal and portal infiltrates of T-LGL.

Serological features

Multiple serological abnormalities have been documented in T-LGL leukemia. Elevated titers of rheumatoid factor and antinuclear antibody are common, occurring in 60% and 40% of patients respectively [4,6,41]. Antineutrophil antibodies and circulating immune complexes are present in approximately half to two-thirds of cases, but their significance or relationship to neutropenia is uncertain. Serum protein electrophoresis often demonstrates a polyclonal hypergammaglobulinemia (45–63%), although a monoclonal gammopathy can rarely occur (<8%). Direct Coombs test is positive in 12% of patients but autoimmune hemolytic anemia is uncommon. Beta-2-microglobulin is elevated in 72% of cases [35] and antiplatelet antibodies are variably detected (25–60%). Soluble FasL is increased in >90% of patients and could be useful as a marker of disease activity [34,42].

Phenotype of T-LGL

T-LGL cells generally display an activated T-cell phenotype, although variations in phenotype between cases are common. The majority of T-LGL leukemic cells are CD3+, TCRαβ+, CD4−, CD8+, CD16+, CD57+, and CD94+ [4,9,43]. CD4+ with or without coexpression of CD8 occurs infrequently. Dual negativity of CD4/CD8 cells has rarely been described. CD57 positivity is present in nearly 100% of cases, but one-third of patients show partial CD57 expression similar to that seen in T cells from normal control subjects [44]. T-LGL cells also constitutively express CD2, CD45RA, HLA-DR, CD69, CD62L, and IL-2 receptor β but not IL-2 receptor α. CD56 is rarely expressed, but when present it has been associated with a more aggressive clinical course [45]. Further support that T-LGL cells are activated T cells is the fact that they express perforin, a component of cytoplasmic granules involved in cell cytotoxicity, granzyme B, and TIA-1 [46]. Virtually all T-LGL cases are TCRαβ, but a few TCRγδ cases have been reported and appear to behave clinically the same [47,48].

Establishment of clonality is the defining characteristic of T-LGL leukemia, and is accomplished through molecular analysis of the T-cell receptor (TCR). Demonstration of *TCR* β or γ gene rearrangement constitutes clonality and is most commonly assessed by Southern blot or polymerase chain reaction (PCR) respectively. PCR is more sensitive at detecting small clones due to selective amplification of desired gene fragments but has a higher false-negative rate than Southern blot due to incomplete primer sets. Southern blot has the drawback of a longer turnaround time and requires fresh tissue. Nevertheless, molecular techniques rarely fail to identify a clonal *TCR*αβ gene rearrangement. It is important to mention that monoclonal T-cell expansions can occur in benign disorders and healthy individuals [43,49], and some authors have questioned the true significance of these proliferations.

Etiology

The exact etiology of T-LGL leukemia is unknown but several pathophysiologic mechanisms have been proposed. Evidence suggests that an initial step is an antigen-driven mechanism resulting in clonal expansion. T-LGL cells express a cytotoxic phenotype consistent with antigen activation and, as mentioned earlier, they constitutively express perforin, which is seen only after activation [46]. Gene expression analysis in T-LGL cells using microarray technology has demonstrated upregulation of cytotoxic proteases and downregulation of proteolytic inhibitors consistent with activated cytotoxic T cells [50]. Also, T-LGL leukemia is frequently associated with other diseases, such as RA, that are involved in persistent antigenic stimulation.

Viral infection may represent a mechanism for antigen activation. Sera of 50% of patients with T-LGL leukemia show reactivity against human T-lymphotropic virus type 1 (HTLV-1) envelope protein p21e with the predominant immunoreactivity directed at the BA21 epitope. Despite this finding, the majority of patients are not infected with HTLV-1/2, suggesting a possible infection with a yet-to-be identified retrovirus with homology to HTLV [51].

Dysregulated apoptosis appears to play a central role in T-LGL leukemic cell expansions. CD95 (Fas)-induced apoptosis is critical in the elimination of activated lymphocytes and induction of peripheral tolerance. Despite expression of high levels of Fas and FasL, T-LGL leukemic cells are resistant to Fas-mediated apoptosis [52]. Signal transducers and activators of transcription (STAT) are inhibitors of apoptosis and represent an additional mechanism of dysregulated apoptosis in T-LGL. Leukemic T-LGL cells display high levels of activated STAT3. Inhibitors of STAT3 activation induce apoptosis of leukemic T-LGL cells, and diminished STAT3 expression resulted in restoration of Fas sensitivity [53].

Prognosis and treatment

T-LGL leukemia is a chronic lymphoproliferative disorder with an indolent clinical course. Morbidity and mortality is primarily the result of recurrent infections from chronic neutropenia and transfusion dependency from refractory anemia. Historical data reflecting the natural history of the disease is somewhat variable, reflecting differences in diagnostic criteria. An early large series demonstrated a survival rate of approximately 85% at a mean follow-up of 29 months [54]. A later series of 68 patients reported a median survival of greater than ten years [6]. Despite a chronic indolent clinical course, the majority of patients (69–73%) will require treatment, primarily due to recurrent infections [4,6]. Rare spontaneous remissions have been reported, including a case of $TCR\gamma\delta$ T-LGL leukemia [55,56]. Fever at diagnosis, low percentage of CD57+ cells, and a relatively low ($\leq 3000/\mu L$) LGL count have been identified as independent predictors of a poor clinical outcome [54].

Uncomplicated cytopenias can initially be observed. Indications for treatment include recurrent infections, profound neutropenia (ANC $<500/\mu L$), and symptomatic or transfusion-dependent anemia. Myeloid growth factors such as GM-CSF or G-CSF have been used for the treatment of isolated neutropenia with variable success [57,58]. Responses tend to be partial and transient, limiting its clinical utility. Prednisone alone can improve neutrophil counts in a few patients, but tapering universally results in recurrence of neutropenia [5]. One instance where steroid therapy alone may be sufficient is in patients with adult-onset cyclic neutropenia, where alternate-day steroids result in decreased LGL counts and resolution of neutrophil cycling [31]. Splenectomy is usually ineffective in resolving neutropenia and may actually increase circulating T-LGL cells [59]. Patients with autoimmune hemolytic anemia associated with LGL leukemia may benefit from splenectomy [60].

Methotrexate, which is also used to treat RA and Felty's syndrome, appears to be the most effective treatment for T-LGL leukemia. In a series of ten patients with T-LGL leukemia, low-dose oral methotrexate (10 mg/m^2/week) resulted in a 50% complete remission rate [61]. Disappearance of the TCR gene rearrangement occurred in 60% of the patients who achieved a complete remission. Anywhere from two weeks to four months of therapy were required before a response was observed. In patients who respond to methotrexate, treatment should be continued indefinitely to prevent a recurrence of disease [5]. The efficacy of low-dose methotrexate is probably due to its ability to selectively induce apoptosis of activated T cells by a Fas-independent pathway [62].

Cyclosporine A at a dose of 5–10 mg/kg/day has been shown to produce hematologic responses, with improvement in cytopenias in patients with T-LGL leukemia. In a study of 25 patients, the response rate to cyclosporine A was 56%, with a complete remission rate of 28% [63]. Multivariate analysis showed that the HLA-DR4 haplotype was highly predictive of response to cyclosporine A. Despite resolution of neutropenia, T-LGL clones persist on cyclosporine A therapy [64], suggesting that the therapeutic efficacy of cyclosporine A is related to decreased levels of FasL [5].

Oral cyclophosphamide 100 mg/day is an alternative regimen that has been shown to produce a response in T-LGL leukemia. It is typically used as second-line therapy in patients who fail to respond to methotrexate and/or cyclosporine A. Cyclophosphamide with prednisone is superior to prednisone alone [65] and may be the most effective treatment for PRCA associated with T-LGL leukemia [36].

Few data exist for other alternative therapies for T-LGL leukemia outside of small series and case reports. Purine analogs such as fludarabine, cladribine (2-chlorodeoxyadenosine), and deoxycoformycin have been used as second- and third-line therapies with some responses [6,8,66]. A case of successful treatment of refractory T-LGL leukemia with alemtuzumab (CAMPATH-1H) has recently been reported [67]. A few cases of allogeneic bone-marrow transplant have been described in the literature. This approach should be reserved for young patients with refractory disease and a sibling donor.

Combination chemotherapy is reserved for patients with the rare aggressive forms of T-LGL leukemia. These patients have a clinical course similar to aggressive NK-cell leukemia and often succumb to their disease within a year. Treatment typically involves a CHOP-like regimen (cyclophosphamide, doxorubicin, vincristine, prednisone) and overall response rate is poor. The refractoriness to cytotoxic chemotherapy is probably due to the leukemic T-LGL cells' constitutive expression of high levels of P-glycoprotein, the gene product of the multi-drug resistance gene (*MDR1*) [68].

Aggressive NK-cell leukemia

Overview

NK-cell expansions can be subdivided into two categories based on clinical presentation. Aggressive NK-cell leukemia is characterized by a rapidly progressive clinical course and is felt to represent the leukemic phase of extranodal NK/T-cell lymphoma [69,70]. Chronic NK-cell lymphocytosis is an indolent disease with a clinical course similar to T-LGL leukemia [71]. It is not clear whether chronic NK-cell lymphocytosis represents the malignant chronic phase of aggressive NK-cell leukemia or a benign reactive process.

Chronic NK-cell lymphocytosis

Approximately 5% of patients with an LGL proliferation have chronic NK-cell expansions [5]. The median age at diagnosis is 60 years old, with a slightly increased male-to-female ratio of 3 to 2. Patients experience an indolent clinical course with prolonged survival. No deaths occurred among ten patients after a median follow-up of five years [71]. Patients are often asymptomatic and lack lymphadenopathy, hepatomegaly, or splenomegaly. Associated diseases included PRCA, recurrent neutropenia, vasculitic syndromes, glomerulonephritis, and aplastic anemia [71,72]. In contrast to T-LGL leukemia, it is not associated with RA, and neutropenia, if present, tends to be moderate. The typical phenotype is CD3−, TCRαβ−, TCRγδ−, CD4−, CD8−, CD16+, CD56+, and variable expression of CD57. NK cells from these patients are distinguished by a skewed NK receptor expression characterized by loss of inhibitory KIR and high levels of activating receptors [73]. Such an altered ratio of activating to inhibitory NK receptors might impact disease pathogenesis by leading to inappropriate target lysis or cytokine production. A constitutively active Ras/MEK/ERK survival pathway has been found to contribute to NK expansion in these patients [74]. Treatment is usually not required, but in cases of severe neutropenia or recurrent infections immunosuppressive therapy can be effective [71].

Aggressive NK-cell leukemia

Aggressive NK-cell leukemia is more common in Asians than in whites [75]. Patients tend to be younger, with a median age at diagnosis of 39 years, but older patients can be affected as well (range 7–70 years) [4]. They often present very ill with B symptoms (fever, weight loss, night sweats) and hepatosplenomegaly. Lymphadenopathy is present in 27% of patients and marrow infiltration is universal. Gastrointestinal system involvement with jaundice and ascites [76] and central nervous system involvement with CSF infiltration [77] has been reported. A rapidly rising LGL count and a coagulopathy is common [78]. In contrast to T-LGL leukemia, neutropenia is usually moderate, while anemia and thrombocytopenia are more common and more severe [4]. Rheumatoid arthritis has not been described in association with NK-cell leukemia.

The usual immunophenotype is CD3−, TCRαβ−, TCRγδ−, CD4−, CD8+, CD16+, CD56+, and CD57+/−. NK cells do not express the T-cell receptor, and therefore *TCR* gene rearrangements are not useful to detect clonality. However, multiple cases of non-random chromosomal abnormalities have been described which provide evidence for clonality. The most common cytogenetic aberrations involve chromosomes 6q, 11q, 13q, and 17p [79–81]. Similar to extranodal NK/T-cell lymphoma, Epstein–Barr virus (EBV) can be detected in the majority of cases and has been implicated in the pathogenesis of the disease [82–84].

The prognosis of patients with NK-cell leukemia is extremely poor, with the majority of patients succumbing to the disease in weeks to months. In a series of eleven patients, nine died within two months of diagnosis [4]. The primary cause of death was multi-organ failure associated with coagulopathy and hemophagocytic syndrome. Response to combination chemotherapy is meager, and this may be due to resistance from increased expression of the *MDR1* gene product, P-glycoprotein [85]. Interleukin 4 (IL-4) has been shown to reverse expression and function of P-glycoprotein on leukemic NK cells, and may represent a potential immunomodulatory treatment mechanism [86]. A few case reports of successful treatment with allogeneic bone-marrow transplantation have been reported [87,88].

Extranodal NK/T-cell lymphoma, nasal type

Overview

Extranodal NK/T-cell lymphomas are rare, highly aggressive non-Hodgkin lymphomas that have a racial predilection for Asians, Mexicans, and South Americans [89–91] and a strong association with EBV [92]. It has a male predominance and typically presents in the sixth decade of life (range 21–76 years of age) [93,94]. This lymphoma is extranodal, with the most common location in the mid facial region, but other sites of disease can occur. It was formerly termed "angiocentric lymphoma" in the Revised European–American Lymphoma (REAL) classification, and is the cause of the syndrome known as "lethal midline granuloma."

Clinical features

The most common presentation is with a nasal or midline facial destructive tumor that results in nasal obstruction, discharge, and/or epistaxis. The tumor is locally destructive and frequently erodes into bones including the palatal, orbital, and maxillary bones [75]. The majority of patients (80–90%) present with localized stage I or II disease [95,96], but systemic progression occurs frequently and early. Other extranodal sites of involvement that have been described include skin, liver, upper aerodigestive tract, gastrointestinal tract, testis, and spleen [94,95]. Systemic symptoms of weight loss, fever, fatigue, and malaise are common. Hemophagocytic syndrome may occur throughout the course of disease [97].

Pathologic features

Extranodal NK/T-cell lymphomas exhibit a variable cytologic composition ranging from small or medium-sized cells to large transformed cells. Extensive necrosis is universal and angiocentric growth of tumor cells is frequently present [91]. The typical immunophenotype of the lymphoma cells is CD2+, CD3−, and CD56+. CD16 and CD57 are usually negative and the TCR is not rearranged. EBV is positive in nearly all cases [92] and detection may be helpful in diagnosis, prognosis, and disease monitoring [98]. The most common recurrent cytogenetic abnormalities in these disorders involve DNA losses at chromosomes 6q, 11q, 13q, and 17p [80].

Treatment and prognosis

Optimal treatment for extranodal NK/T-cell lymphoma has yet to be defined, which is due to the rarity of the disease and lack of prospective data. Radiotherapy is the mainstay of treatment for early-stage disease. Multiple studies have demonstrated no survival benefit for the addition of chemotherapy to radiotherapy in stage I disease [99,100]. However, there is a high systemic failure rate, and therefore combined-modality therapy with radiation and chemotherapy is often employed. As described earlier for other cytotoxic T-cell and NK-cell neoplasms, the resistance to conventional chemotherapy may be due to overexpression of P-glycoprotein, the product of the *MDR1* gene [101]. Anecdotal reports of autologous bone-marrow transplant and single-agent L-asparaginase as effective salvage treatment have been published [102,103].

Overall prognosis for extranodal NK/T-cell lymphoma is stage-dependent. There is a significant difference between stage I and II disease, with five-year overall survivals ranging from 42% to 75% for stage I disease, compared to 19–35% for stage II disease [99,100]. Disseminated disease has an extremely poor overall prognosis, with a median survival of two months [96].

Blastic NK-cell lymphoma

Overview

CD4+/CD56+ malignancies have recently been recognized as a unique entity with a specific clinical and pathological presentation. These neoplasms have been termed blastic NK-cell lymphomas in the WHO classification system. This term is somewhat of a misnomer in that there is mounting evidence that these tumors arise from type 2 dendritic cells (DC2) or plasmacytoid dendritic cells, and not NK cells [104,105].

Blastic NK-cell lymphoma is a rare disease that typically affects the elderly, with a median age of 69 years at diagnosis. There is a male-to-female predominance of 3 to 1, and the majority of patients present with cutaneous nodules. Lymphadenopathy and/or splenomegaly is frequent (61%), and cytopenias are common (91%). Circulating peripheral malignant cells are often detected, and marrow infiltration is the norm. Morphologic characteristics include a high frequency of vacuolation and cytoplasmic extensions. The phenotype consists of dual expression of CD4 and CD56 with the absence of typical B, T, and myeloid lineage markers [106]. Recurrent complex cytogenetic aberrations have been described involving chromosomes 5q, 12p, 13q, 6q, 15q, and 9 [107].

Blastic NK-cell lymphoma is an aggressive disease with a median survival of 12 months. The majority of patients achieve a complete response (86%) with combination chemotherapy but most of these patients (83%) will relapse within nine months. The most common sites of relapse are the bone marrow, skin, and central nervous system. Durable remissions have been reported with allogeneic bone-marrow transplantation [106].

Adult T-cell leukemia/lymphoma

Overview

Adult T-cell leukemia/lymphoma (ATLL) was first described in Japan in the late 1970s [108]. Discovery of HTLV-1 as the etiological agent followed a few years later [109]. HTLV-1 is a retrovirus that is endemic in Japan, the Caribbean basin, Africa, Central and South America, the southeastern USA, and eastern Europe. Most patients who develop ATLL live in endemic areas or originate from them [110]. Primary modes of transmission of HTLV-1 are sexual intercourse, neonatally via breast milk, needle sharing in intravenous drug use, and transfusion of cellular blood products. Despite high rates of infection in endemic areas, only 4% of chronic carriers will develop ATLL in their lifetime [111]. HTLV-1 has also been implicated as the causative agent of tropical spastic paresis/HTLV-1-associated myelopathy. The WHO classification system defines ATLL as a mature peripheral T-cell neoplasm associated with HTLV-1 [112].

Clinical features

ATLL has a median age of onset of 57 years, and is slightly more common in males than females [112]. Typical clinical manifestations are lymphadenopathy, skin lesions, peripheral-blood and bone-marrow involvement, splenomegaly, hypercalcemia, and lytic bone lesions. Pulmonary, central nervous system, and gastrointestinal tract infiltration also occur [112,113]. Hepatic involvement is common, occuring more frequently than in other non-Hodgkin lymphomas [114]. ATLL results in an immunodeficient state leading to serious bacterial, fungal, and opportunistic infections that are often fatal. Opportunistic malignancies such as Kaposi sarcoma have been described as well [115].

ATLL can have a variable clinical presentation, which can be divided into one of four clinical subtypes with prognostic value [112]. The acute subtype is the most common presentation, occurring in 57% of patients. It is characterized by an aggressive clinical course with leukemic manifestations and tumor lesions, often accompanied by hypercalcemia (70%). Prognosis is poor, with a median survival time of six months. The lymphoma type (19%) presents as lymphadenopathy with or without extranodal lesions, no lymphocytosis, and 1% or fewer abnormal peripheral T lymphocytes. Median survival time is 10 months. The chronic type (19%) is characterized by an absolute lymphocytosis, typically with 5% or more abnormal peripheral T lymphocytes. Organ involvement is limited to lymph nodes, skin, lung, liver, and spleen. No hypercalcemia is present, and median survival time is 24 months. The most indolent and least common (5%) is the smoldering type. No lymphocytosis or hypercalcemia is present, and disease is limited to skin or lung. Abnormal peripheral T lymphocytes may be 5% or more. Survival is frequently prolonged with a four-year survival rate of 63%. Progression from the chronic and smoldering types to the more aggressive acute type can occur and is associated with up- or downregulation of distinct sets of genes involved in cellular transformation [116].

Pathological features

The presence of highly pleomorphic and lobated lymphoid cells or "flower cells" in the peripheral blood is a morphologic characteristic feature of ATLL (Figs. 23.3, 23.4) [117]. These cells can resemble Sézary cells, and can be found in healthy carriers of HTLV-1. Blast-like cells with deep basophilic cytoplasm may also be present. The malignant cells of ATLL display the immunophenotype of a mature helper T lymphocyte. They typically are CD2+, CD3+, CD4+, CD5+, CD7−, CD8−, and CD25+. Rare cases have dual expression of CD4 and CD8, or dual negativity of both markers. Diagnosis is dependent on the demonstration of HTLV-1 antibodies and the presence of HTLV-1 DNA clonally integrated into the host genome.

Cytogenetic abnormalities are often present, but none is specific for ATLL. Reported abnormal karyotypes include trisomy 3, 7, and 21, changes

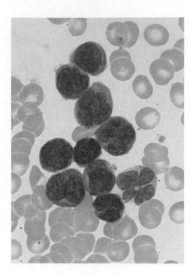

Figure 23.3 ATLL: peripheral blood smear showing abnormal lymphocytes with nuclear indentation or lobulation (Wright's stain). Myoshi, I. *et al.*, ASH Image Bank 2003: 100715. Copyright American Society of Hematology. All rights reserved. *See color plate section.*

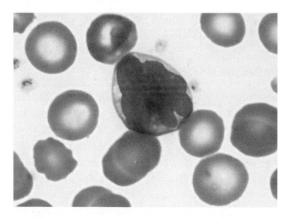

Figure 23.4 ATLL: "flower cells" can be described as having pleomorphic nuclei with deeply basophilic cytoplasm. Maslak, P., ASH Image Bank 2006: 6-00002. Copyright American Society of Hematology. All rights reserved. *See color plate section.*

in chromosomes 6 and 14, and loss of chromosome Y. Disease severity has been associated with the more complex chromosomal aberrations [118,119]. Recently, fine-scale deletional mapping of chromosome 6q identified a common deleted region

(6q15–21) present in 36% of patients with ATLL, suggesting a possible site for a putative tumor suppressor gene [120]. Also, deletion of the p16 gene or decreased p16 protein expression has been implicated in ATLL progression and shorter survival [121].

Treatment and prognosis

ATLL is a highly aggressive non-Hodgkin lymphoma characterized by a poor prognosis, with a median overall survival of eight months [122]. Survival differences exist within the disease as a whole depending on the clinical subtype, as described above. Other independent prognostic factors predicative of shortened survival include poor performance status, elevated lactate dehydrogenase, age greater than 40 years, increased tumor bulk, and hypercalcemia [112]. Expression of Ki-67 antigen on >18% of peripheral-blood lymphocytes portends a poor prognosis with a mean survival of three months. Conversely, low levels of Ki-67 antigen conferred a better prognosis with significantly improved survival [123]. High expression of lung resistance-related protein mRNA at diagnosis is another independent prognostic factor that correlates with shortened survival [124].

Treatment for ATLL remains unsatisfactory. Single-agent chemotherapy is generally ineffective. Combination chemotherapy regimens involving anthracyclines can induce fairly high response rates but patients invariably relapse and succumb to their disease. The lymphoma study group in Japan completed a trial involving 96 patients treated with three alternating combination regimens consisting of vincristine, cyclophosphamide, doxorubicin, prednisone, ranimustine, vindesine, etoposide, and carboplatin. Overall response rate was 81%, with a complete response rate of 35%. Median survival time was 13 months with a two-year survival of 31%. Hematologic toxicity was significant [125]. Allogeneic bone-marrow transplantation has been attempted in a few small series, with some patients achieving long-term survival [126]. Antiviral therapy with interferon gamma (IFN-γ) and zidovudine (AZT) has shown promising results [127,128].

One study demonstrated a response rate of 92% with a complete response rate of 58% when IFN-γ and AZT were used as initial treatment. Overall survival was 11 months but some patients showed long-term complete responses (42–84+ months) [127]. Other encouraging preclinical therapeutic strategies include arsenic trioxide and IFN-γ [129,130], all-trans retinoic acid [131], and inhibitors of NF-κB [132].

Cutaneous T-cell lymphoma

Overview

Cutaneous T-cell lymphoma (CTCL) includes mycosis fungoides (MF) and its leukemic variant, the Sézary syndrome (SS) (Figs. 23.5, 23.6). CTCL is a rare extranodal mature T-cell non-Hodgkin lymphoma characterized by primary skin infiltration with clonal T lymphocytes. [133–136]

Alibert, a French dermatologist, first described MF in 1806 as a mycotic-like plaque that developed into a mushroom-like tumor, hence the name [137]. MF is an uncommon disease, with an incidence of 2.9 per 100 000 per year, accounting for less than 0.5% of all new cases of non-Hodgkin lymphoma diagnosed in the USA each year [136]. However, it is the most common primary cutaneous lymphoma, accounting for 45% of all lymphomas presenting in the skin [138]. It has a predilection for older patients, with a peak incidence between 55 and 60 years of age at presentation, and a male-to-female ratio of 2 to 1. Although MF is mainly seen in older patients, it has been described in young patients, with similar clinical picture and course [139,140].

MF has an indolent course and long-term survival is fairly common. Diagnosis in early stage is difficult as it usually presents with scaly patches and plaques that resemble eczematous dermatitis or psoriasis. It usually takes multiple skin biopsies over several years to establish the diagnosis. SS has a more aggressive course, with circulating clonal T lymphocytes, generalized erythroderma, lymphadenopathy and splenomegaly, and carries a worse prognosis [139].

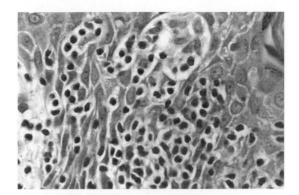

Figure 23.5 Mycosis fungoides: epidermotropism of atypical lymphocytes with cerebriform nuclei. Kadin, M., ASH Image Bank 2005: 101309. Copyright American Society of Hematology. All rights reserved. *See color plate section.*

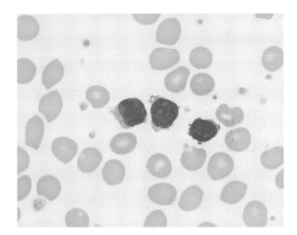

Figure 23.6 Sézary cells: the nuclear convolutions are most apparent in the cell in the center in this view. Lazarchick, J., ASH Image Bank 2004: 101081. Copyright American Society of Hematology. All rights reserved. *See color plate section.*

Etiology

The cause of CTCL remains unclear. MF may develop from an underlying benign reactive condition where chronic antigenic stimulation from environmental and/or occupational exposure to chemicals may incite neoplastic transformation [141,142].

Several case series support such a theory, including a large case–control study that showed a 4.3-fold increase in relative risk for individuals in manufacturing and construction industries [143–145]. However, two more recent case–control studies failed to support this hypothesis [146,147]. Hence, the role of environmental and/or occupational exposure to chemicals remains unclear. HTLV-1-related sequences have been detected from peripheral blood or cutaneous lesions of patients with MF and SS [148–150], suggesting that HTLV-1 may play a role in the etiology of CTCL. However, other studies failed to support a connection between the two [151–153]. Other viruses have also been implicated, including HTLV-2 and HIV [154–156]. A high incidence of seropositivity to cytomegalovirus has been reported, but the significance of such findings remains unclear [157].

Clinical picture

MF presents with patches, plaques, or fungating tumors, most commonly over the trunk and extremities, although any part of the skin may be involved. They are often associated with pruritis. Patients may progress from one stage to the other, or present with different types of lesions simultaneously. These lesions may wax and wane over a number of years, spontaneously or in response to topical steroids [158].

Evolution time from patch to plaque is variable, but it is usually a slow process that happens over years. At this stage, diagnosis is often difficult. In fact, the median duration from the onset of cutaneous lesions to the pathologic diagnosis of MF is about six years.

Patches are usually scaly, erythematous round or oval macular lesions that are very similar to eczematous dermatitis or psoriasis. Plaques are scaly, erythematous, well demarcated, with raised edges. Patches and plaques may start small, and then coalesce into larger patches or plaques. Rarely, progression to generalized erythroderma gives rise to the so-called "red man syndrome." Palms and soles are usually spared, but may become involved in a few

patients with the development of hyperkeratosis and deep fissures. Facial involvement is rare, but characteristic, giving rise to the so-called "leonine face" appearance.

Tumor stage usually presents as expanding nodules arising within pre-existing plaques. Rarely, patients may present with tumors without having pre-existing lesions, which is known as the "d'emblee" presentation. Tumors, and infrequently plaques, may ulcerate and become infected, giving rise to considerable morbidity in these patients.

At diagnosis, 42% of patients have limited plaques involving 10% or less of total body surface; 30% have extensive plaques; 16% have cutaneous tumors; and 12% have generalized erythroderma. Lymphadenopathy is uncommon in patients with limited plaque but occurs in approximately 50% of patients with extensive plaques, tumors, or erythroderma.

SS, the leukemic variant of MF, is characterized by the triad of generalized erythroderma, diffuse lymphadenopathy, and circulating malignant T lymphocytes with hyperconvoluted cerebriform nuclei, known as Sézary cells, in peripheral blood. Clinical manifestations also include alopecia, splenomegaly, intense pruritis, hyperkeratosis of the palms and soles, skin fissuring and ulceration with frequent cutaneous infections.

Extracutaneous involvement is rare in early-stage disease, but increases in frequency with disease progression, and correlates with the extent of skin manifestations. In a recent study, the risk for progression to extracutaneous disease at 20 years from diagnosis was 0% for limited patch/plaque (T1), 10% for generalized patch/plaque (T2), 35.5% for tumor stage (T3), and 41% for generalized erythroderma (T4) [159]. The lungs, spleen, liver, and gastrointestinal tract are among the more frequently affected organs.

Staging and prognosis

Staging for CTCL was established by the National Cancer Institute-sponsored Workshop on Cutaneous T-Cell Lymphomas in 1978, and follows

Table 23.1. Staging for cutaneous T-cell lymphoma. Adapted from Bunn PA Jr, Lamberg SI. Report of the Committee on Staging and Classification of Cutaneous T-cell Lymphomas. *Cancer Treat Rep* 1979; **63**: 725–8.

TNMB stage	Description
T: Skin tumor	
T0	Lesions clinically and/or histopathologically suggestive of CTCL
T1	Limited plaques or patches covering < 10% of skin surface
T2	Generalized plaques or patches covering > 10% of skin surface
T3	Cutaneous tumors
T4	Generalized erythroderma
N: Lymph nodes	
N0	No lymphadenopathy
N1	Palpable lymphadenopathy; lymph node pathology negative for CTCL
N2	No palpable lymphadenopathy, lymph node pathology positive for CTCL
N3	Palpable lymphadenopathy, lymph node pathology positive for CTCL
M: Viscera	
M0	No visceral involvement
M1	Visceral involvement with pathological confirmation
B: Blood	
B0	Atypical circulating cells not present (or <5%)
B1	Atypical circulating cells present (or >5%)

Staging	T	N	M
Ia	1	0	0
Ib	2	0	0
IIa	1–2	1	0
IIb	3	0–1	0
III	4	0–1	0
IVa	1–4	2–3	0
IVb	1–4	0–3	1

T, tumor; N, lymph nodes; M, metastasis; B, blood involvement.

the TNMB system [160]. It is based on the type and extent of skin involvement (T), lymph node involvement (N), visceral disease (M), and involvement of the blood (B) (Table 23.1).

In this classification, prognosis of T4 patients is better than that of T3 patients and the prognosis of patients with T2 patch and T2 plaque is significantly different [161]. In view of this, a modified staging classification was proposed in 2001 that split stage T2 into T2a (patches covering >10% skin surface) and T2b (plaques covering >10% skin surface) [162]. In 1988, Sausville *et al.* proposed stratifying patients

into early-stage, intermediate and advanced-stage disease based on prognostic outcome (Table 23.2) [163]. Notably, this system did not take into account blood involvement.

Recently, the International Society for Cutaneous Lymphomas (ISCL) has divided erythrodermic CTCL (stage III) into three subsets based on prognosis: SS, erythrodermic MF (secondary erythrodermic CTCL in pre-existing MF), and erythrodermic CTCL not otherwise defined [164].

SS is defined by one or more of the following: an absolute Sézary cell count of ≥1000 cells/mL; CD4/

Table 23.2. Staging of mycosis fungoides/Sézary syndrome. From Sausville *et al.* 1988 [163].

Early stage	
IA	<10% BSA patch or plaque (T1)
IB	≥10% BSA patch or plaque (T1)
IIA	T1–2, palpable adenopathy (node biopsy negative)
Intermediate stage	
IIB	Cutaneous tumors (T3)
III	Erythroderma (T4)
IVA	T1–4, node biopsy positive
Advanced stage	
IVB	T1–4, visceral involvement

CD8 ratio ≥10 by flow cytometry; increased lymphocyte counts with evidence of a T-cell clone in the blood by Southern blot or PCR; or the presence of a T-cell clone with chromosomal abnormalities.

Patients with stage IA disease have an overall life expectancy similar to an age-, sex-, and race-matched control population [165]. Only 9% of treated patients will progress to a more advanced stage of disease. Patients with stage IB or IIA disease have a median survival exceeding 11 years [161]. About one-quarter of these patients will progress, and nearly 20% will die of causes related to their disease. Patients with stage IIB and III without extracutaneous disease have median survivals of 3.2 and 4.6 years, respectively, and most patients will succumb to their disease.

Patients with erythroderma (T4) have highly variable outcomes ranging between one and ten years. Major adverse prognostic factors include age (<65 vs. >65 years), overall stage (III vs. IV), peripheral blood involvement (B0 vs. B1/2), and duration of symptoms [166,167]. Depending on the number of adverse prognostic factors (APF), three distinct subgroups were identified: favorable (no APF), intermediate (1 APF), and unfavorable (>1 APF), with median survivals of 10.2, 3.7, and 1.5 years respectively. Patients with stage IVA or IVB (extracutaneous disease) at presentation have a poor outcome with a median survival of about 13 months.

Transformation to large-cell lymphoma has been reported in as many as one-third of patients and carries a worse prognosis [168,169]. In one study, 39% of 115 patients with CTCL transformed into large-cell lymphoma, with a median time of 12 months from diagnosis of CTCL to transformation. Only 14% of those with stage I–IIA transformed into large-cell lymphoma, compared with 31% of those with stage IIB–IV disease. Survival was adversely impacted in patients who transformed, with a median survival of 37 months versus 163 months for the untransformed group. Transformation was especially common in patients with tumor-stage disease [170].

Diagnosis

As discussed earlier, diagnosing MF in early stage is difficult. Clinical presentation resembles eczematous dermatitis, psoriasis, and other inflammatory dermatoses. Histopathologically, CTCL is characterized by a lymphocytic infiltrate within the superficial dermis with atypical lymphocytes with dense, convoluted nuclei and scant cytoplasm. These cells tend to aggregate around Langerhans cells, forming the so-called Pautrier's microabscesses.

Frequently, there is migration of individual lymphocytes towards epidermal keratinocytes, which is referred to as epidermotropism. The epidermis is usually acanthotic, but lacks intercellular edema (spongiosis). The deep dermis and subcutis typically show no abnormalities [171].

Histopathologic criteria for the diagnosis are well established. Diagnostic categories include "diagnostic for CTCL," "consistent with CTCL," and "suggestive of CTCL." However, the false-negative and false-positive rates were as high as 40% and 44% respectively in the diagnosis of early MF based on histologic findings alone [172]. Hence, immunophenotyping and *TCR* gene rearrangement studies became important diagnostic tools.

Immunophenotypically, CTCL is a clonal proliferation of well-differentiated CD4+, CD45RO+ helper/memory T cells. Rarely, tumor cells may express a suppressor/cytotoxic CD8+ phenotype instead. Pan T-cell markers (e.g., CD2, CD3, and CD5) are usually expressed in early-stage disease, but this is lost as the disease progresses into the tumor stage and beyond. In over two-thirds of cases, tumor cells are negative for CD7, an antigen present on normal mature T cells. Deletion of CD7 is a fairly sensitive and specific marker for CTCL [171,173,174]. CTCL is often positive for activation markers including CD25 (IL-2 receptor) in about 60% of cases.

T-cell receptor gamma (TCR-γ) gene rearrangement studies by Southern blot analysis or the more sensitive PCR to establish clonality have been widely utilized in this disease and have proved invaluable, especially in cases with equivocal histopathology and immunophenotyping [175,176]. In one study, the combination of CD7 deletion and TCR-γ gene rearrangement by PCR on formalin-fixed, paraffin-embedded tissue demonstrated a sensitivity of 94% and a specificity of 96% [177].

Treatment

Several therapeutic interventions are currently available for the management of CTCL. The choice of treatment modality is guided primarily by the disease stage. Nevertheless, it is influenced by the patient's age, presenting symptoms, comorbidities, compliance, accessibility, socioeconomic factors, and the impact on quality of life. Symptomatic management with supportive measures such as emollients, local or systemic anti-pruritic therapy, and infection control measures are an integral part of treatment.

Patients with early-stage disease without extracutaneous involvement (T1 and T2) are usually treated with topical therapies, whereas those presenting with more advanced stage or extracutaneous involvement should receive systemic therapy as part of their treatment regimen. Currently, there is no evidence that systemic therapy is superior to conservative topical therapy in the management of early-stage disease [178,179].

Early-stage disease

Topical corticosteroids are commonly used as first-line topical therapy. Topical corticosteroid monotherapy can induce complete and partial remission in 31% and 63% of T1 patients, and in 25% and 57% of T2 patients, respectively [180]. Their therapeutic effect can be enhanced by the use of high-potency steroid preparations under occlusion, to further increase the response rate.

Phototherapy with ultraviolet B (UVB) has been used for stage I patch disease but may be less effective for plaques because of its limited penetration. Ultraviolet A (UVA) is more effective because of its greater penetration to the upper dermis. In 1974, the combined use of psoralen, a photosensitizer, with longwave UVA was described for the treatment of psoriasis and was adopted for CTCL [181]. The acronym PUVA has been used to describe this approach. PUVA is currently considered the front-line treatment for early-stage CTCL (stage I–IIa). It is also used in combination with other modalities in more advanced disease.

The efficacy of PUVA therapy is high, with complete response achieved in 60–90% of patients with early-stage disease, but response decreases with advanced-stage disease [182]. For patients with suboptimal response to PUVA, the addition of bexarotene or interferon alpha (IFN-α) to PUVA may be considered. A slight increase in the development of squamous and/or basal cell carcinoma after several years of PUVA therapy has been reported [182,183].

Total-skin electron-beam therapy (TSEBT) has been used with similar response in patients with tumor-stage (IIb) disease or those refractory to PUVA, albeit with a short duration of response. Adjuvant therapy (PUVA, topical chemotherapy, or low-dose systemic chemotherapy) is therefore recommended after completion of EBT [184,185]. Toxicity includes acute radiation dermatitis, nail dystrophy, and alopecia. Long-term complications include xerosis, hyperpigmentation, and telangiectasia.

Retinoic acid derivatives, including isotretinoin, etretinate, and acitretin, have demonstrated marginal potency against CTCL as monotherapy; however, they have been used mostly in combination with other modalities to enhance efficacy. The combination of any of these agents with PUVA gives comparable results to PUVA alone, but the UVA dose needed to induce remission appears lower. The use of these agents has been largely replaced by bexarotene in the treatment of CTCL.

Bexarotene, a novel selective retinoid-X-receptor (RXR) analog, available as a topical gel or an oral formulation, has demonstrated efficacy in the treatment of CTCL. Topical bexarotene 1% gel demonstrated a 23% complete response (CR) with an overall response rate (RR) of 63% and 50% in stage IA and IB, respectively, and a median time to progression of 149 days. These responses were more pronounced in patients with patch and plaque disease. Toxicities included rash and pruritis [186,187]. Oral bexarotene at a dosage of $300\,mg/m^2$/day also demonstrated a 48% RR [188]. Toxicities included headache, hyperlipidemia, and hypothyroidism. Due to its limited toxicity, oral bexarotene is often combined with other therapies including PUVA [189], extracorporeal photopheresis, and IFN-α with enhanced RRs and extended duration of response.

Topical chemotherapy with mechlorethamine (nitrogen mustard, HN2) has been successfully used in the treatment of early-stage disease. It takes 6–12 months to achieve remission in early patch and plaque disease. In a long-term follow-up of 203 patients, RR and CR rate were 93% and 65% in patch disease, and 72% and 34% in plaque disease [190]. With further maintenance therapy, remission in excess of two years has been achieved. Adverse effects include allergic or chemical dermatitis, urticaria, anaphylactoid reactions, and a small increase in the risk of development of skin cancer with prolonged use. Carmustine (BCNU) yields similar results, but its systemic absorption results in increased hematologic adverse effects. It can be used in patients allergic to HN2. Neither of these agents has had an impact on overall survival (OS) in early-stage disease.

Advanced disease

Extracorporeal photopheresis (ECP), a systemic form of PUVA therapy, was first described as a treatment for CTCL by Edelson *et al.* in 1987 [191]. ECP involves ingestion of a photosensitizer (8-methoxypsoralen or Uvadex) followed by leukopheresis of mononuclear leukocytes, which are exposed to UVA ex vivo and then reinfused into the patient. Although the exact mechanism is not fully understood, it involves the induction of host cytotoxic T-cell response against circulating tumor cells, which undergo apoptosis after DNA damage upon exposure to UVA in the presence of a radiosensitizer. ECP is currently the treatment of choice for patients with erythrodermic CTCL (stage III).

Although CR was only achieved in 21%, almost half of the patients showed >50% improvement and 83% had >25% disease response to therapy [191] and a prolonged survival compared with historical controls [192]. ECP is valuable, as it can achieve a significant improvement in the patient's quality of life with minimal side effects, namely transient nausea from the psoralen. ECP has been combined with IFN and retinoids with variable results [193]. Ongoing studies are exploring the combination of ECP and oral bexarotene.

Interferon alpha has direct immunomodulatory and anti-proliferative effects on CTCL when given at a dose of 3 MU three times weekly, with reported objective RR of 50–60% and CR rate about 10–20%, which are comparable to single-agent chemotherapy. Its combination with PUVA resulted in superior results, with widely varying response rates [194]. Although combined treatment with PUVA and IFN appears to have better clinical response rate and response duration when compared with either treatment alone, there are no randomized prospective clinical trials to confirm this impression.

Denileukin diftitox (DAB389IL-2, Ontak, DD) is a cytotoxic fusion protein combining the enzymatically active moiety of the diphtheria toxin to the receptor-binding domain of IL-2. It is currently used for patients with advanced disease (stage IIb–IVb), with tumors expressing CD25, who have failed other modalities. The CR and partial remission (PR) rates are 10–14% and 20–37% respectively [195–197]. Adverse effects include infusion-related hypersensitivity reactions and capillary leak syndrome in 69% and 23% of patients respectively. In one study where patients were premedicated with corticosteroids prior to DD, a 60% RR was reported in those with refractory CTCL. Moreover, the severity and frequency of infusion-related hypersensitivity reactions and capillary leak were significantly diminished [198]. DD in combination with various other active agents is currently undergoing investigation.

Systemic chemotherapy is reserved for patients with nodal or visceral involvement, and for those with disease resistant to other forms of therapy. Single-agent therapy can induce CR in about 30% and PR in up to 75% of patients. However, remissions are typically short-lived [160].

Methotrexate, cisplatin, etoposide, doxorubicin, bleomycin, pentostatin, gemcitabine, vinblastine, alkylating agents, purine analogs, topoisomerase II inhibitors, and systemic steroids have been used. Methotrexate produced the best outcome, with a CR rate around 60% and a duration of remission between 6 and 30 months in patients treated with a low to medium dose of weekly methotrexate [199]. In another cohort of 17 stage III patients treated with methotrexate, a five-year survival rate of 70% has been reported [200].

Purine analogs (fludarabine or cladribine) have demonstrated activity against CTCL. Cladribine was found to have RRs ranging from 20% to 40% in a small series of patients with refractory disease [201]. Gemcitabine is also an active agent, achieving CR and PR in 12% and 59% respectively in a phase II trial involving 44 patients with pretreated refractory or relapsed CTCL [202]. Pentostatin has been shown to have activity, with reported CR and PR of 25% and 71%, respectively, in a cohort of pretreated patients [203].

Liposomal doxorubicin is also an active agent with preferential uptake by cutaneous tumors versus normal skin. In a retrospective study of pegylated liposomal doxorubicin given every two to four weeks, RR of 88% was reported in patients with relapsed or refractory disease [204].

The most common combination chemotherapy regimen used is CHOP (cyclophosphamide, doxorubicin, vincristine, prednisone), but various regimens have been used including CVP (cyclophosphamide,

vincristine, prednisone), EPOCH (etoposide, vincristine, doxorubicin, cyclophosphamide, prednisone), and others. Analysis of several studies showed a 38% CR and 81% objective RR, with a duration of response ranging between 5 and 41 months [160]. Although RRs for combination regimens are better than that of single-agent chemotherapy, their efficacy must be balanced against increased toxicity, especially given that no significant survival benefit has been demonstrated with these therapies.

Novel therapies

Interleukin 12 (IL-12) has shown promising activity in patients with early-stage CTCL, with a 56% objective RR reported in one study [205]. IL-12 appears to work through stimulating IFN-γ release [206].

Interferon gamma appears promising, with a 31% objective RR in one study [206]. Several studies are currently underway to further explore the efficacy of IFN-γ and IL-12 alone or in combination with other agents.

Alemtuzumab (CAMPATH-1H), an anti-CD52 monoclonal antibody, has demonstrated activity in advanced CTCL, with an overall RR of 38%, which is short-lived [207]. Adverse effects include immunosuppression with significant infection, a high rate of grade 3–4 hematologic toxicity and cardiac toxicity. Because of this significant toxicity profile, alemtuzumab has not been widely used in CTCL, but studies with subcutaneous administration are currently under way.

Histone deactylase inhibitors are a novel class of agents that are capable of modulating gene expression by increasing the acetylation of histones. Depsipeptide (FK228) and suberoylanilide hydroxamic acid (SAHA) are two agents belonging to this class that are of interest in the treatment of CTCL. Depsipeptide has been shown to be active in CTCL and peripheral T-cell lymphoma [208,209]. Adverse effects include an infrequent propensity to cardiac arrhythmias. SAHA is an oral agent that has demonstrated activity in CTCL in phase I studies.

A phase II study is currently under way. The most significant adverse effect of SAHA was nausea.

BCX-1777, a novel agent that inhibits the purine nucleoside phosphorylase, appears to be an active agent. Phase I studies of BCX-1777 in patients with T-cell acute lymphocytic leukemia and CTCL have demonstrated responses. Further study of this molecule is under way.

A chimeric anti-CD4 monoclonal antibody was used as a single infusion in a phase I study in a small cohort of eight patients with CTCL. Seven of the eight patients responded to treatment, with an average freedom from progression of 25 weeks (range 6–52 weeks) [210]. Clinical trials using a fully human anti-CD4 antibody are currently in progress. Other T-cell targeted therapies include unmodified and ^{90}Y-anti-CD25 antibody and anti-Tac *Pseudomonas* exotoxin immunoconjugates. Radioimmunoconjugate therapy with ^{90}Y-T101 demonstrated activity in three of eight patients with CTCL [211].

A few reports of the use of autologous or allogeneic stem-cell transplantation for selected patients with CTCL have been published, showing varying degree of success [212–216]. Further studies are needed to delineate the role of stem-cell transplantation in the treatment of CTCL.

Peripheral T-cell lymphoma

Peripheral T-cell lymphomas (PTCL) are a group of aggressive non-Hodgkin lymphomas that arise from neoplastic T cells. They represent 10% of non-Hodgkin lymphoma worldwide [217], but are less common in North America [217,218]. Median age of presentation is 61 years. There is a slight male predilection, with a male-to-female ratio of 3 to 2 [217].

They have widely varying clinicopathologic features, but most present with generalized lymphadenopathy. Skin involvement may occur in the form of patches, plaques, or nodules. B symptoms including fever, weight loss, and night sweats are present in 40% of patients [217]. Most patients present with stage IV disease and have poor outcomes.

Peripheral T-cell lymphoma, unspecified (PTCL-U)

PTCL-U is the most common subtype, representing 3.7% of non-Hodgkin lymphomas [217]. It is a heterogeneous entity of T-cell neoplasms that usually manifests with predominantly nodal T-cell lymphomas. No consistent immunophenotypic, genetic, or clinical features have been associated with lymphomas in this category. Therefore, they are lumped under the PTCL-U category.

Clinically, 60% of these patients present with stage IV disease involving the lymph nodes, spleen, liver, skin, and other organs [217]. B symptoms, including fever, weight loss and pruritis, are present in 41% of patients [217]. Peripheral eosinophilia is not uncommon, and hemophagocytic syndromes may also be seen [219,220].

Histopathologically, PTCL-U contain a mixture of small, medium, and large atypical lymphocytes with variable amounts of eosinophils and histiocytes [221,222]. Immunophenotypically, these tumors have variable T-cell antigen expression, but are mostly CD2+, CD3+, CD4+, and less commonly CD5+ and CD7+ [217,221,223]. Conventional cytogenetics are usually abnormal, and TCR genes are rearranged in the majority of cases [224].

Multi-agent chemotherapy with an anthracycline-based regimen is the most commonly used frontline treatment. Spontaneous remissions have been rarely reported; however, prognosis is usually poor, with frequent relapses and a five-year OS rate of 26% in one study [217], even with multi-agent anthracycline-containing chemotherapy.

Angioimmunoblastic T-cell lymphoma

Angioimmunoblastic T-cell lymphoma (AITL) is a rare T-cell lymphoma accounting for approximately 2% of all non-Hodgkin lymphomas [217]. AITL is a disease of the elderly, with most patients presenting in the sixth and seventh decades of life, with no sex predilection [225].

Patients usually present with high fever, skin rash, generalized lymphadenopathy, and hepatosplenomegaly [225,226]. AITL is frequently associated with autoimmune disorders including Coombs-positive hemolytic anemia, cryoglobuline-mia, RA, vasculitis, and thyroid disease [225–227]. Polyclonal gammopathy is very common, with a marked increased risk of infection, which is a frequent cause of death in these patients [225–227]. Most cases demonstrate a moderately aggressive clinical behavior; however, a more protracted course or even spontaneous remission have been seen on rare occasions [225,226].

EBV viral particles could be identified in over 95% of patients with AITL, and a role for EBV in lymphomagenesis has been postulated [228]. However, more recent studies using double immunohisto-chemistry, in-situ hybridization, and microdissec-tion have shown that EBV-infected cells are B cells, and that EBV infection is unlikely to play a primary role in the lymphomagenesis of AITL [229,230].

Histopathologically, AITL is characterized by partial effacement of the lymph-node architecture with a pleomorphic infiltrate of atypical lymphocytes with clusters of follicular dendritic cells, epithelioid histiocytes, eosinophils, and plasma cells, accompanied by a proliferation of arborizing small vessels with thickened and occasionally hyalinized walls (Figs. 23.7, 23.8) [217,231].

Immunophenotypically, these cells are CD3+, CD4+. However, CD8+ cells are occasionally seen, and they are also frequently CD10+ [227,231]. Perivascular CD21+, CD23+ follicular dendritic cell clusters are useful in distinguishing AITL from other T-cell lymphomas [232]. T-cell receptor gene rearrangement is detectable in most cases [231,233].

Treatment options include single-agent steroids for early cases; however, this may increase the risk of infection. Several other therapeutic modalities have been tried with promising results in small cohorts of patients, including fludarabine [234], cladribine [235], low-dose methotrexate with steroids [236], and immunosuppression with cyclosporine.

Multi-agent chemotherapy with an anthracy-cline-containing regimen is superior to single-agent therapy, yielding a CR rate of 50–70%, albeit with frequent relapses and an increased risk of

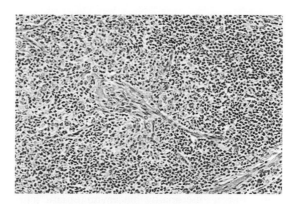

Figure 23.7 AITL: arborizing blood vessel(s). Kadin, M., ASH Image Bank 2003: 100652. Copyright American Society of Hematology. All rights reserved. *See color plate section.*

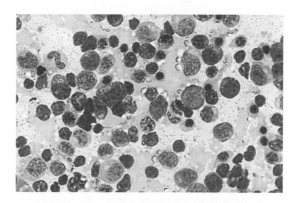

Figure 23.8 AITL: immunoblasts in bone-marrow aspirate stained with Giemsa. Kadin, M., ASH Image Bank 2003: 100652. Copyright American Society of Hematology. All rights reserved. *See color plate section.*

infection. Interferon alpha has been used as maintenance therapy to prolong chemotherapy-induced remissions [225,227]. Thalidomide has been tried in a small number of patients with relapsed or refractory disease, with promising results [237].

Prognosis is poor, with a median survival of less than 36 months and a five-year survival of around 30–35%, and most patients die of infectious complications rather than tumor progression [225,227].

Enteropathy-type T-cell lymphoma

Enteropathy-type T-cell lymphoma (ETL) is a rare form of T-cell lymphoma that accounts for less than 1% of all non-Hodgkin lymphomas and presents usually in the sixth and seventh decade in patients with gluten-sensitive enteropathy (GSE) or celiac disease.

ETL may occur in patients with a long history of GSE, but more commonly develops following a short history of adult GSE. It may occur in patients without prior clinical enteropathy, but asymptomatic jejunal villous atrophy and crypt hyperplasia are usually found upon excision [238]. Moreover, patients with ETL without clinical or pathologic evidence of GSE almost always have detectable anti-gliadin antibodies and/or the typical HLA type (DQA1 or DQB1) associated with GSE [239]. Treatment of GSE with a gluten-free diet usually prevents the development of ETL; however, the most typical presentation is the reappearance of symptoms of malabsorption and non-specific abdominal pain in a patient with a history of GSE who was responding to a gluten-free diet.

ETL most frequently involves the jejunum, with multiple circumferential ulcers that often perforate, resulting in significant morbidity and/or mortality. Microscopically, ulcers are surrounded by a variable mixture of small and medium atypical inflammatory cells, eosinophils, and large, sometimes anaplastic, malignant lymphocytes with pleomorphic nuclei (Fig. 23.9). In cases where there are more inflammatory cells, it may be hard to distinguish ETL from inflammatory bowel disease. Adjacent mucosa often shows villous atrophy with crypt hyperplasia, plasmacytosis, and a significant increase in the number of small intraepithelial lymphocytes that are part of the malignant clone [240,241].

Immunohistochemically, the tumor cells express CD3, CD7, the mucosal lymphoid antigen CD103, and cytotoxic proteins including granzyme B. In some cases, the cells may not express CD3 or, more often, may express CD8. CD30 is expressed in a subtype of ETL that is composed primarily of large anaplastic cells. In the subset of ETL comprised

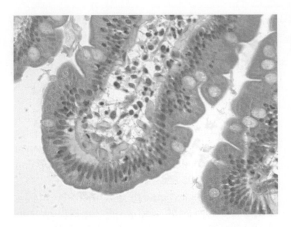

Figure 23.9 High magnification of normal duodenal mucosa for comparison to abnormal mucosa in enteropathy-type T-cell lymphoma. Kadin, M., ASH Image Bank 2003: 100846. Copyright American Society of Hematology. All rights reserved. *See color plate section.*

of sheets of small lymphocytes, the tumor cells express CD3, CD8, CD56, and granzyme B [242,243]. Genetically, the *TCR-γ* gene is often clonally rearranged [242].

A variety of chemotherapy regimens have been tried, including CHOP in small cohorts of patients, with variable responses (up to 58% RR in one study) [244]. However, these patients tend not to tolerate chemotherapy well and frequently develop gastrointestinal and septic complications.

Despite treatment, ETL usually exhibits aggressive behavior and poor prognosis, with one- and five-year OS rates of 38.7% and 19.7% respectively in one study [244]. Death is usually due to intestinal perforation caused by refractory malignant ulcers.

Subcutaneous panniculitis-like T-cell lymphoma

Subcutaneous panniculitis-like T-cell lymphoma (SPTCL) usually presents with multiple erythematous subcutaneous nodules primarily affecting the extremities [245]. In early stages, these lesions appear benign and are often confused with panniculitis [245]. It often requires multiple biopsies over a period of time to demonstrate progressive cytological atypia. As disease progresses, larger nodules may become necrotic. SPTCL may present with pancytopenia and hepatosplenomegaly. Fever, night sweats, weight loss, and malaise are common. Hemophagocytic syndrome is present in 37% of patients with SPTCL [246] and often signifies a more aggressive course and worse prognosis [245]. Dissemination to lymph nodes and other organs is rare. Median survival is about 32 months. There is a great deal of histopathologic variability in this disease. Lesions may show small atypical lymphocytes with clear cytoplasm, or larger cells with hyperchromatic nuclei. Fat necrosis often occurs and is usually surrounded by a histiocytic infiltrate. Mitotic figures, karyorrhexis, and necrosis are also common.

Immunophenotypically, these atypical lymphocytes express CD3, CD7, CD8, CD45RA, TIA-1, and perforins. They usually have clonal rearrangement of the β, and less frequently the γ, TCR gene [247]. Clinically, $\gamma\delta$ phenotype carries a worse prognosis [246,248].

SPTCL may have an indolent course for months to years, but frequently there is an acute aggression with the development of severe hemophagocytic syndrome, which is often fatal despite aggressive chemotherapy.

Prednisone is frequently used as initial therapy for cutaneous disease. In more advanced disease, multi-agent chemotherapy with an anthracycline-based regimen is most commonly used, with CR reported in about 30% of patients [246]. High-dose chemotherapy and stem-cell transplantation have been used in selected patients, with a 92% CR rate and median response duration of about 14 months [246].

REFERENCES

1. Non-Hodgkin's Lymphoma Classification Project. A clinical evaluation of the International Lymphoma Study Group classification of non-Hodgkin's lymphoma. *Blood* 1997; **89**: 3909–18.

2. Harris NL, Jaffe ES, Diebold J, *et al.* World Health Organization Classification of Neoplastic Diseases of the Hematopoietic and Lymphoid Tissues: Report of the Clinical Advisory Committee Meeting Airlie House, Virginia, November 1997. *J Clin Oncol* 1999; **17**: 3835–49.

3. Loughran TP Jr, Kadin ME, Starkebaum G, *et al.* Leukemia of large granular lymphocytes: association with clonal chromosomal abnormalities and autoimmune neutropenia, thrombocytopenia, and hemolytic anemia. *Ann Intern Med* 1985; **102**: 169–75.

4. Loughran TP Jr. Clonal diseases of large granular lymphocytes. *Blood* 1993; **82**: 1–14.

5. Lamy T, Loughran TP Jr. Clinical features of large granular lymphocyte leukemia. *Semin Hematol* 2003; **40**: 185–95.

6. Dhodapkar MV, Li CY, Lust JA, Tefferi A, Phyliky RL. Clinical spectrum of clonal proliferations of T-large granular lymphocytes: a T cell clonopathy of undetermined significance? *Blood* 1994; **84**: 1620–7.

7. Lamy T, Loughran TP. Large granular lymphocyte leukemia. *Cancer Control* 1998; **5**: 25–33.

8. Lamy T, Bauer FA, Liu JH, *et al.* Clinicopathological features of aggressive large granular lymphocyte leukaemia resemble Fas ligand transgenic mice. *Br J Haematol* 2000; **108**: 717–23.

9. Lamy T, Loughran TP Jr. Current concepts: large granular lymphocyte leukemia. *Blood Rev* 1999; **13**: 230–40.

10. Freimark B, Lanier L, Phillips J, Quertermous T, Fox R. Comparison of T cell receptor gene rearrangements in patients with large granular T cell leukemia and Felty's syndrome. *J Immunol* 1987; **138**: 1724–9.

11. Bowman SJ, Sivakumaran M, Snowden N, *et al.* The large granular lymphocyte syndrome with rheumatoid arthritis. Immunogenetic evidence for a broader definition of Felty's syndrome. *Arthritis Rheum* 1994; **37**: 1326–30.

12. Starkebaum G, Loughran TP Jr, Gaur LK, Davis P, Nepom BS. Immunogenetic similarities between patients with Felty's syndrome and those with clonal expansions of large granular lymphocytes in rheumatoid arthritis. *Arthritis Rheum* 1997; **40**: 624–6.

13. Burns CM, Tsai V, Zvaifler NJ. High percentage of CD8+, Leu-7+ cells in rheumatoid arthritis synovial fluid. *Arthritis Rheum* 1992; **35**: 865–73.

14. Molitor JL, Saint-Louis J, Louvet C, Vachon A, Vincent L, Beaulieu R. [Large granular T-cell lymphocytic leukemia disclosed by bilateral uveitis: association with celiac disease]. *Rev Med Interne* 1997; **18**: 237–9.

15. Shvidel L, Duksin C, Tzimanis A, *et al*. Cytokine release by activated T-cells in large granular lymphocytic leukemia associated with autoimmune disorders. *Hematol J* 2002; **3**: 32–7.

16. Go RS, Lust JA, Phyliky RL. Aplastic anemia and pure red cell aplasia associated with large granular lymphocyte leukemia. *Semin Hematol* 2003; **40**: 196–200.

17. Karadimitris A, Manavalan JS, Thaler HT, *et al*. Abnormal T-cell repertoire is consistent with immune process underlying the pathogenesis of paroxysmal nocturnal hemoglobinuria. *Blood* 2000; **96**: 2613–20.

18. Risitano AM, Maciejewski JP, Muranski P, *et al*. Large granular lymphocyte (LGL)-like clonal expansions in paroxysmal nocturnal hemoglobinuria (PNH) patients. *Leukemia* 2005; **19**: 217–22.

19. Saunthararajah Y, Molldrem JL, Rivera M, *et al*. Coincident myelodysplastic syndrome and T-cell large granular lymphocytic disease: clinical and pathophysiological features. *Br J Haematol* 2001; **112**: 195–200.

20. Papadaki T, Stamatopoulos K, Kosmas C, *et al*. Clonal T-large granular lymphocyte proliferations associated with clonal B cell lymphoproliferative disorders: report of eight cases. *Leukemia* 2002; **16**: 2167–9.

21. Lesesve JF, Feugier P, Lamy T, *et al*. Association of B-chronic lymphocytic leukaemia and T-large granular lymphocyte leukaemia. *Clin Lab Haematol* 2000; **22**: 121–2.

22. Hanada T, Ishida T, Kojima H, Tsuchiya T. Granular lymphocyte leukaemia in association with multiple myeloma. *Br J Haematol* 1992; **80**: 127–9.

23. Mohty M, Faucher C, Vey N, *et al*. Features of large granular lymphocytes (LGL) expansion following allogeneic stem cell transplantation: a long-term analysis. *Leukemia* 2002; **16**: 2129–33.

24. Gorochov G, Debre P, Leblond V, Sadat-Sowti B, Sigaux F, Autran B. Oligoclonal expansion of CD8+ CD57+ T cells with restricted T-cell receptor beta chain variability after bone marrow transplantation. *Blood* 1994; **83**: 587–95.

25. Dolstra H, Preijers F, Kemenade VDW-V, Schattenberg A, Galama J, De Witte T. Expansion of CD8+CD57+ T cells after allogeneic BMT is related with a low incidence of relapse and with cytomegalovirus infection. *Br J Haematol* 1995; **90**: 300–307.

26. Feher O, Barilla D, Locker J, Oliveri D, Melhem M, Winkelstein A. T-cell large granular lymphocytic leukemia following orthotopic liver transplantation. *Am J Hematol* 1995; **49**: 216–20.

27. Gentile TC, Hadlock KG, Uner AH, *et al*. Large granular lymphocyte leukaemia occurring after renal transplantation. *Br J Haematol* 1998; **101**: 507–12.

28. Semenzato G, Pandolfi F, Chisesi T, *et al*. The lymphoproliferative disease of granular lymphocytes. A heterogeneous disorder ranging from indolent to aggressive conditions. *Cancer* 1987; **60**: 2971–8.

29. Loughran TP Jr, Starkebaum G. Large granular lymphocyte leukemia. Report of 38 cases and review of the literature. *Medicine (Baltimore)* 1987; **66**: 397–405.

30. Semenzato G, Zambello R, Starkebaum G, Oshimi K, Loughran TP Jr. The lymphoproliferative disease of granular lymphocytes: updated criteria for diagnosis. *Blood* 1997; **89**: 256–260.

31. Loughran TP Jr, Clark EA, Price TH, Hammond WP. Adult-onset cyclic neutropenia is associated with increased large granular lymphocytes. *Blood* 1986; **68**: 1082–7.

32. Loughran TP Jr, Hammond WP. Adult-onset cyclic neutropenia is a benign neoplasm associated with clonal proliferation of large granular lymphocytes. *J Exp Med* 1986; **164**: 2089–94.

33. Perzova R, Loughran TP Jr. Constitutive expression of Fas ligand in large granular lymphocyte leukaemia. *Br J Haematol* 1997; **97**: 123–6.

34. Liu JH, Wei S, Lamy T, *et al*. Chronic neutropenia mediated by fas ligand. *Blood* 2000; **95**: 3219–22.

35. Gentile TC, Wener MH, Starkebaum G, Loughran TP Jr. Humoral immune abnormalities in T-cell large granular lymphocyte leukemia. *Leuk Lymphoma* 1996; **23**: 365–70.

36. Lacy MQ, Kurtin PJ, Tefferi A. Pure red cell aplasia: association with large granular lymphocyte leukemia and the prognostic value of cytogenetic abnormalities. *Blood* 1996; **87**: 3000–6.

37. Abkowitz JL, Kadin ME, Powell JS, Adamson JW. Pure red cell aplasia: lymphocyte inhibition of erythropoiesis. *Br J Haematol* 1986; **63**: 59–67.

38. Fisch P, Handgretinger R, Schaefer HE. Pure red cell aplasia. *Br J Haematol* 2000; **111**: 1010–22.

39. Morice WG, Kurtin PJ, Tefferi A, Hanson CA. Distinct bone marrow findings in T-cell granular lymphocytic leukemia revealed by paraffin section immunoperoxidase stains for CD8, TIA-1, and granzyme B. *Blood* 2002; **99**: 268–74.

40. Agnarsson BA, Loughran TP Jr, Starkebaum G, Kadin ME. The pathology of large granular lymphocyte leukemia. *Hum Pathol* 1989; **20**: 643–51.

41. Bassan R, Pronesti M, Buzzetti M, *et al.* Autoimmunity and B-cell dysfunction in chronic proliferative disorders of large granular lymphocytes/natural killer cells. *Cancer* 1989; **63**: 90–5.

42. Saitoh T, Karasawa M, Sakuraya M, *et al.* Improvement of extrathymic T cell type of large granular lymphocyte (LGL) leukemia by cyclosporin A: the serum level of Fas ligand is a marker of LGL leukemia activity. *Eur J Haematol* 2000; **65**: 272–5.

43. Bigouret V, Hoffmann T, Arlettaz L, *et al.* Monoclonal T-cell expansions in asymptomatic individuals and in patients with large granular leukemia consist of cytotoxic effector T cells expressing the activating CD94: NKG2C/E and NKD2D killer cell receptors. *Blood* 2003; **101**: 3198–204.

44. Morice WG, Kurtin PJ, Leibson PJ, Tefferi A, Hanson CA. Demonstration of aberrant T-cell and natural killer-cell antigen expression in all cases of granular lymphocytic leukaemia. *Br J Haematol* 2003; **120**: 1026–36.

45. Gentile TC, Uner AH, Hutchison RE, *et al.* CD3+, CD56+ aggressive variant of large granular lymphocyte leukemia. *Blood* 1994; **84**: 2315–21.

46. Oshimi K, Shinkai Y, Okumura K, Oshimi Y, Mizoguchi H. Perforin gene expression in granular lymphocyte proliferative disorders. *Blood* 1990; **75**: 704–8.

47. Foroni L, Matutes E, Foldi J, *et al.* T-cell leukemias with rearrangement of the gamma but not beta T-cell receptor genes. *Blood* 1988; **71**: 356–62.

48. Morikawa K, Oseko F, Hara J, Kobayashi S, Nakano A, Morikawa S. Functional analysis of clonally expanded CD8, TCR gamma delta T cells in a patient with chronic T-gamma lymphoproliferative disease. *Leuk Res* 1990; **14**: 581–92.

49. Posnett DN, Sinha R, Kabak S, Russo C. Clonal populations of T cells in normal elderly humans: the T cell equivalent to "benign monoclonal gammapathy". *J Exp Med* 1994; **179**: 609–18.

50. Kothapalli R, Bailey RD, Kusmartseva I, Mane S, Epling-Burnette PK, Loughran TP Jr. Constitutive expression of cytotoxic proteases and down-regulation of protease inhibitors in LGL leukemia. *Int J Oncol* 2003; **22**: 33–9.

51. Loughran TP Jr, Hadlock KG, Perzova R, *et al.* Epitope mapping of HTLV envelope seroreactivity in LGL leukaemia. *Br J Haematol* 1998; **101**: 318–24.

52. Lamy T, Liu JH, Landowski TH, Dalton WS, Loughran TP Jr. Dysregulation of CD95/CD95 ligand-apoptotic pathway in CD3(+) large granular lymphocyte leukemia. *Blood* 1998; **92**: 4771–7.

53. Epling-Burnette PK, Liu JH, Catlett-Falcone R, *et al.* Inhibition of STAT3 signaling leads to apoptosis of leukemic large granular lymphocytes and decreased Mcl-1 expression. *J Clin Invest* 2001; **107**: 351–62.

54. Pandolfi F, Loughran TP Jr, Starkebaum G, *et al.* Clinical course and prognosis of the lymphoproliferative disease of granular lymphocytes. A multicenter study. *Cancer* 1990; **65**: 341–8.

55. Shichishima T, Kawaguchi M, Ono N, Oshimi K, Nakamura N, Maruyama Y. Gamma delta T-cell large granular lymphocyte (LGL) leukemia with spontaneous remission. *Am J Hematol* 2004; **75**: 168–72.

56. Takeuchi M, Tamaoki A, Soda R, Takahashi K. Spontaneous remission of large granular lymphocyte T cell leukemia. *Leukemia* 1999; **13**: 313–14.

57. Lamy T, LePrise PY, Amiot L, *et al.* Response to granulocyte-macrophage colony-stimulating factor (GM-CSF) but not to G-CSF in a case of agranulocytosis associated with large granular lymphocyte (LGL) leukemia. *Blood* 1995; **85**: 3352–3.

58. Kaneko T, Ogawa Y, Hirata Y, *et al.* Agranulocytosis associated with granular lymphocyte leukaemia: improvement of peripheral blood granulocyte count with human recombinant granulocyte colony-stimulating factor (G-CSF). *Br J Haematol* 1990; **74**: 121–2.

59. Loughran TP Jr, Starkebaum G, Clark F, Wallace P, Kadin ME. Evaluation of splenectomy in large granular lymphocyte leukaemia. *Br J Haematol* 1987; **67**: 135–40.

60. Gentile TC, Loughran TP Jr. Resolution of autoimmune hemolytic anemia following splenectomy in CD3+ large granular lymphocyte leukemia. *Leuk Lymphoma* 1996; **23**: 405–8.

61. Loughran TP, Kidd PG, Starkebaum G. Treatment of large granular lymphocyte leukemia with oral low-dose methotrexate. *Blood* 1994; **84**: 2164–70.

62. Genestier L, Paillot R, Fournel S, Ferraro C, Miossec P, Revillard JP. Immunosuppressive properties of methotrexate: apoptosis and clonal deletion of activated peripheral T cells. *J Clin Invest* 1998; **102**: 322–8.

63. Battiwalla M, Melenhorst J, Saunthararajah Y, *et al.* HLA-DR4 predicts haematological response to cyclosporine in T-large granular lymphocyte lymphoproliferative disorders. *Br J Haematol* 2003; **123**: 449–53.

64. Sood R, Stewart CC, Aplan PD, *et al.* Neutropenia associated with T-cell large granular lymphocyte leukemia: long-term response to cyclosporine therapy despite persistence of abnormal cells. *Blood* 1998; **91**: 3372–8.

65. Go RS, Li CY, Tefferi A, Phyliky RL. Acquired pure red cell aplasia associated with lymphoproliferative disease of granular T lymphocytes. *Blood* 2001; **98**: 483–5.

66. Witzig TE, Weitz JJ, Lundberg JH, Tefferi A. Treatment of refractory T-cell chronic lymphocytic leukemia with purine nucleoside analogues. *Leuk Lymphoma* 1994; **14**: 137–9.

67. Rosenblum MD, LaBelle JL, Chang CC, Margolis DA, Schauer DW, Vesole DH. Efficacy of alemtuzumab treatment for refractory T-cell large granular lymphocytic leukemia. *Blood* 2004; **103**: 1969–71.

68. Lamy T, Drenou B, Fardel O, *et al.* Multidrug resistance analysis in lymphoproliferative disease of large granular lymphocytes. *Br J Haematol* 1998; **100**: 509–15.

69. Soler J, Bordes R, Ortuno F, *et al.* Aggressive natural killer cell leukaemia/lymphoma in two patients with lethal midline granuloma. *Br J Haematol* 1994; **86**: 659–62.

70. Jaffe ES, Harris NL, Stein H, Vardiman JW. *World Health Organization Classification of Tumours: Pathology and Genetics of Tumours of Haematopoietic and Lymphoid Tissues* (Lyon: IARC Press; 2001).

71. Tefferi A, Li CY, Witzig TE, Dhodapkar MV, Okuno SH, Phyliky RL. Chronic natural killer cell lymphocytosis: a descriptive clinical study. *Blood* 1994; **84**: 2721–5.

72. Rabbani GR, Phyliky RL, Tefferi A. A long-term study of patients with chronic natural killer cell lymphocytosis. *Br J Haematol* 1999; **106**: 960–6.

73. Epling-Burnette PK, Painter JS, Chaurasia P, *et al.* Dysregulated NK receptor expression in patients with lymphoproliferative disease of granular lymphocytes. *Blood* 2004; **103**: 3431–9.

74. Epling-Burnette PK, Bai F, Wei S, *et al.* ERK couples chronic survival of NK cells to constitutively activated Ras in lymphoproliferative disease of granular lymphocytes (LDGL). *Oncogene* 2004; **23**: 9220–9.

75. Cheung MM, Chan JK, Wong KF. Natural killer cell neoplasms: a distinctive group of highly aggressive lymphomas/leukemias. *Semin Hematol* 2003; **40**: 221–2.

76. Sheridan W, Winton EF, Chan WC, *et al.* Leukemia of non-T lineage natural killer cells. *Blood* 1988; **72**: 1701–7.

77. Ohno T, Kanoh T, Arita Y, *et al.* Fulminant clonal expansion of large granular lymphocytes. Characterization of their morphology, phenotype, genotype, and function. *Cancer* 1988; **62**: 1918–27.

78. Fernandez LA, Pope B, Lee C, Zayed E. Aggressive natural killer cell leukemia in an adult with establishment of an NK cell line. *Blood* 1986; **67**: 925–30.

79. Taniwaki M, Tagawa S, Nishigaki H, *et al.* Chromosomal abnormalities define clonal proliferation in CD3- large granular lymphocyte leukemia. *Am J Hematol* 1990; **33**: 32–8.

80. Siu LL, Chan JK, Kwong YL. Natural killer cell malignancies: clinicopathologic and molecular features. *Histol Histopathol* 2002; **17**: 539–54.

81. Wong KF, Zhang YM, Chan JK. Cytogenetic abnormalities in natural killer cell lymphoma/leukaemia: is there a consistent pattern? *Leuk Lymphoma* 1999; **34**: 241–50.

82. Kawa-Ha K, Ishihara S, Ninomiya T, *et al.* CD3-negative lymphoproliferative disease of granular lymphocytes containing Epstein–Barr viral DNA. *J Clin Invest* 1989; **84**: 51–5.

83. Hart DN, Baker BW, Inglis MJ, *et al.* Epstein–Barr viral DNA in acute large granular lymphocyte (natural killer) leukemic cells. *Blood* 1992; **79**: 2116–23.

84. Gelb AB, van de Rijn M, Regula DP Jr, *et al.* Epstein–Barr virus-associated natural killer-large granular lymphocyte leukemia. *Hum Pathol* 1994; **25**: 953–60.

85. Egashira M, Kawamata N, Sugimoto K, Kaneko T, Oshimi K. P-glycoprotein expression on normal and abnormally expanded natural killer cells and inhibition of P-glycoprotein function by cyclosporin A and its analogue, PSC833. *Blood* 1999; **93**: 599–606.

86. Tambur AR, Markham PN, Gebel HM. IL-4 inhibits P-glycoprotein in normal and malignant NK cells. *Hum Immunol* 1998; **59**: 483–7.

87. Ebihara Y, Manabe A, Tanaka R, *et al.* Successful treatment of natural killer (NK) cell leukemia following a long-standing chronic active Epstein–Barr virus (CAEBV) infection with allogeneic bone marrow transplantation. *Bone Marrow Transplant* 2003; **31**: 1169–71.

88. Takami A, Nakao S, Yachie A, *et al.* Successful treatment of Epstein–Barr virus-associated natural killer cell large granular lymphocytic leukaemia using allogeneic peripheral blood stem cell transplantation. *Bone Marrow Transplant* 1998; **21**: 1279–82.

89. Arber DA, Weiss LM, Albujar PF, Chen YY, Jaffe ES. Nasal lymphomas in Peru. High incidence of T-cell immunophenotype and Epstein–Barr virus infection. *Am J Surg Pathol* 1993; **17**: 392–9.

90. Elenitoba-Johnson KS, Zarate-Osorno A, Meneses A, *et al.* Cytotoxic granular protein expression, Epstein–Barr virus strain type, and latent membrane protein-1 oncogene deletions in nasal T-lymphocyte/natural killer cell lymphomas from Mexico. *Mod Pathol* 1998; **11**: 754–61.

91. Jaffe ES, Chan JK, Su IJ, *et al*. Report of the Workshop on Nasal and Related Extranodal Angiocentric T/ Natural Killer Cell Lymphomas. Definitions, differential diagnosis, and epidemiology. *Am J Surg Pathol* 1996; **20**: 103–11.

92. Chan JK, Yip TT, Tsang WY, *et al*. Detection of Epstein– Barr viral RNA in malignant lymphomas of the upper aerodigestive tract. *Am J Surg Pathol* 1994; **18**: 938–46.

93. Chan JK, Ng CS, Lau WH, Lo ST. Most nasal/nasopharyngeal lymphomas are peripheral T-cell neoplasms. *Am J Surg Pathol* 1987; **11**: 418–29.

94. Chan JK, Sin VC, Wong KF, *et al*. Nonnasal lymphoma expressing the natural killer cell marker CD56: a clinicopathologic study of 49 cases of an uncommon aggressive neoplasm. *Blood* 1997; **89**: 4501–13.

95. Cheung MM, Chan JK, Lau WH, *et al*. Primary non-Hodgkin's lymphoma of the nose and nasopharynx: clinical features, tumor immunophenotype, and treatment outcome in 113 patients. *J Clin Oncol* 1998; **16**: 70–7.

96. Kwong YL, Chan AC, Liang R, *et al*. CD56+ NK lymphomas: clinicopathological features and prognosis. *Br J Haematol* 1997; **97**: 821–9.

97. Takahashi N, Miura I, Chubachi A, Miura AB, Nakamura S. A clinicopathological study of 20 patients with T/natural killer (NK)-cell lymphoma-associated hemophagocytic syndrome with special reference to nasal and nasal-type NK/T-cell lymphoma. *Int J Hematol* 2001; **74**: 303–8.

98. Lei KI, Chan LY, Chan WY, Johnson PJ, Lo YM. Diagnostic and prognostic implications of circulating cell-free Epstein–Barr virus DNA in natural killer/ T-cell lymphoma. *Clin Cancer Res* 2002; **8**: 29–34.

99. Cheung MM, Chan JK, Lau WH, Ngan RK, Foo WW. Early stage nasal NK/T-cell lymphoma: clinical outcome, prognostic factors, and the effect of treatment modality. *Int J Radiat Oncol Biol Phys* 2002; **54**: 182–90.

100. Li YX, Coucke PA, Li JY, *et al*. Primary non-Hodgkin's lymphoma of the nasal cavity: prognostic significance of paranasal extension and the role of radiotherapy and chemotherapy. *Cancer* 1998; **83**: 449–56.

101. Yamaguchi M, Kita K, Miwa H, *et al*. Frequent expression of P-glycoprotein/MDR1 by nasal T-cell lymphoma cells. *Cancer* 1995; **76**: 2351–6.

102. Liang R, Chen F, Lee CK, *et al*. Autologous bone marrow transplantation for primary nasal T/NK cell lymphoma. *Bone Marrow Transplant* 1997; **19**: 91–3.

103. Nagafuji K, Fujisaki T, Arima F, Ohshima K. L-asparaginase induced durable remission of relapsed nasal NK/T-cell lymphoma after autologous peripheral blood stem cell transplantation *Int J Hematol* 2001; **74**: 447–50.

104. Bene MC, Feuillard J, Jacob MC. Plasmacytoid dendritic cells: from the plasmacytoid T-cell to type 2 dendritic cells CD4+CD56+ malignancies. *Semin Hematol* 2003; **40**: 257–66.

105. Chaperot L, Bendriss N, Manches O, *et al*. Identification of a leukemic counterpart of the plasmacytoid dendritic cells. *Blood* 2001; **97**: 3210–17.

106. Feuillard J, Jacob MC, Valensi F, *et al*. Clinical and biologic features of CD4(+)CD56(+) malignancies. *Blood* 2002; **99**: 1556–63.

107. Leroux D, Mugneret F, Callanan M, *et al*. CD4(+), CD56(+) DC2 acute leukemia is characterized by recurrent clonal chromosomal changes affecting 6 major targets: a study of 21 cases by the Groupe Francais de Cytogenetique Hematologique. *Blood* 2002; **99**: 4154–9.

108. Uchiyama T, Yodoi J, Sagawa K, Takatsuki K, Uchino H. Adult T cell leukemia: clinical and hematologic features of 16 cases. *Blood* 1977; **50**: 481–92.

109. Poiesz BJ, Ruscetti FW, Gazdar AF, Bunn PA, Minna JD, Gallo RC. Detection and isolation of type C retrovirus particles from fresh and cultured lymphocytes of a patient with cutaneous T-cell lymphoma. *Proc Natl Acad Sci USA* 1980; **77**: 7415–19.

110. Chadburn A, Athan E, Wieczorek R, Knowles DM. Detection and characterization of human T-cell lymphotropic virus type I (HTLV-I) associated T-cell neoplasms in an HTLV-I nonendemic region by polymerase chain reaction. *Blood* 1991; **77**: 2419–30.

111. Murphy EL, Hanchard B, Figueroa JP, *et al*. Modelling the risk of adult T-cell leukemia/lymphoma in persons infected with human T-lymphotropic virus type I. *Int J Cancer* 1989; **43**: 250–3.

112. Shimoyama M. Diagnostic criteria and classification of clinical subtypes of adult T-cell leukaemia-lymphoma. A report from the Lymphoma Study Group (1984–87). *Br J Haematol* 1991; **79**: 428–37.

113. Bunn PA Jr, Schechter GP, Jaffe E, *et al*. Clinical course of retrovirus-associated adult T-cell lymphoma in the United States. *N Engl J Med* 1983; **309**: 257–64.

114. Yamada Y, Kamihira S, Murata K, *et al*. Frequent hepatic involvement in adult T cell leukemia: comparison with non-Hodgkin's lymphoma. *Leuk Lymphoma* 1997; **26**: 327–35.

115. Greenberg SJ, Jaffe ES, Ehrlich GD, Korman NJ, Poiesz BJ, Waldmann TA. Kaposi's sarcoma in human T-cell leukemia virus type I-associated adult T-cell leukemia. *Blood* 1990; **76**: 971–6.

116. Tsukasaki K, Tanosaki S, DeVos S, *et al*. Identifying progression-associated genes in adult T-cell leukemia/lymphoma by using oligonucleotide micro-arrays. *Int J Cancer* 2004; **109**: 875–81.

117. Jaffe ES, Blattner WA, Blayney DW, *et al*. The pathologic spectrum of adult T-cell leukemia/lymphoma in the United States. Human T-cell leukemia/lymphoma virus-associated lymphoid malignancies. *Am J Surg Pathol* 1984; **8**: 263–75.

118. Sanada I, Tanaka R, Kumagai E, *et al*. Chromosomal aberrations in adult T cell leukemia: relationship to the clinical severity. *Blood* 1985; **65**: 649–54.

119. Itoyama T, Chaganti RS, Yamada Y, *et al*. Cytogenetic analysis and clinical significance in adult T-cell leukemia/lymphoma: a study of 50 cases from the human T-cell leukemia virus type-1 endemic area, Nagasaki. *Blood* 2001; **97**: 3612–20.

120. Hatta Y, Yamada Y, Tomonaga M, Miyoshi I, Said JW, Koeffler HP. Detailed deletion mapping of the long arm of chromosome 6 in adult T-cell leukemia. *Blood* 1999; **93**: 613–16.

121. Takasaki Y, Yamada Y, Sugahara K, *et al*. Interruption of p16 gene expression in adult T-cell leukaemia/lymphoma: clinical correlation. *Br J Haematol* 2003; **122**: 253–9.

122. Yamada Y, Kamihira S, Amagasaki T, *et al*. Adult T cell leukemia with atypical surface phenotypes: clinical correlation. *J Clin Oncol* 1985; **3**: 782–8.

123. Shirono K, Hattori T, Takatsuki K. A new classification of clinical stages of adult T-cell leukemia based on prognosis of the disease. *Leukemia* 1994; **8**: 1834–7.

124. Ohno N, Tani A, Uozumi K, *et al*. Expression of functional lung resistance: related protein predicts poor outcome in adult T-cell leukemia. *Blood* 2001; **98**: 1160–5.

125. Yamada Y, Tomonaga M, Fukuda H, *et al*. A new G-CSF-supported combination chemotherapy, LSG15, for adult T-cell leukaemia-lymphoma: Japan Clinical Oncology Group Study 9303. *Br J Haematol* 2001; **113**: 375–82.

126. Kami M, Hamaki T, Miyakoshi S, *et al*. Allogeneic haematopoietic stem cell transplantation for the treatment of adult T-cell leukaemia/lymphoma. *Br J Haematol* 2003; **120**: 304–9.

127. Hermine O, Allard I, Levy V, Arnulf B, Gessain A, Bazarbachi A. A prospective phase II clinical trial with the use of zidovudine and interferon-alpha in the acute and lymphoma forms of adult T-cell leukemia/lymphoma. *Hematol J* 2002; **3**: 276–82.

128. Gill PS, Harrington W Jr, Kaplan MH, *et al*. Treatment of adult T-cell leukemia-lymphoma with a combination of interferon alfa and zidovudine. *N Engl J Med* 1995; **332**: 1744–8.

129. Bazarbachi A, El Sabban ME, Nasr R, *et al*. Arsenic trioxide and interferon-alpha synergize to induce cell cycle arrest and apoptosis in human T-cell lymphotropic virus type I-transformed cells. *Blood* 1999; **93**: 278–83.

130. Mahieux R, Pise-Masison C, Gessain A, *et al*. Arsenic trioxide induces apoptosis in human T-cell leukemia virus type 1- and type 2-infected cells by a caspase-3-dependent mechanism involving Bcl-2 cleavage. *Blood* 2001; **98**: 3762–9.

131. Nawata H, Maeda Y, Sumimoto Y, Miyatake J, Kanamaru A. A mechanism of apoptosis induced by all-trans retinoic acid on adult T-cell leukemia cells: a possible involvement of the Tax/NF-kappaB signaling pathway. *Leuk Res* 2001; **25**: 323–31.

132. Mori N, Yamada Y, Ikeda S, *et al*. Bay 11-7082 inhibits transcription factor NF-kappaB and induces apoptosis of HTLV-I-infected T-cell lines and primary adult T-cell leukemia cells. *Blood* 2002; **100**: 1828–34.

133. Lutzner M, Edelson R, Schein P, Green I, Kirkpatrick C, Ahmed A. Cutaneous T-cell lymphomas: the Sezary syndrome, mycosis fungoides, and related disorders. *Ann Intern Med* 1975; **83**: 534–52.

134. Rappaport H, Thomas LB. Mycosis fungoides: the pathology of extracutaneous involvement. *Cancer* 1974; **34**: 1198–229.

135. Willemze R, Kerl H, Sterry W, *et al*. EORTC classification for primary cutaneous lymphomas: a proposal from the Cutaneous Lymphoma Study Group of the European Organization for Research and Treatment of Cancer. *Blood* 1997; **90**: 354–71.

136. Weinstock MA, Horm JW. Mycosis fungoides in the United States. Increasing incidence and descriptive epidemiology. *JAMA* 1988; **260**: 42–6.

137. Alibert J. Clinique de l'Hôpital Saint-Louis: ou, traité complet des maladies de la peau, contenant la description de ces maladies et leurs meilleurs modes de traitement. In Vincent JF, ed, *La Collection Medic@ Collection de Rééditions de Textes Anciens,*

vol. 2003 (Paris: Bibliothètheque Interuniversitaire de Médecine, 1833).

138. Foss F. Mycosis fungoides and the Sezary syndrome. *Curr Opin Oncol* 2004; **16**: 421–8.

139. Fink-Puches R, Zenahlik P, Back B, Smolle J, Kerl H, Cerroni L. Primary cutaneous lymphomas: applicability of current classification schemes (European Organization for Research and Treatment of Cancer, World Health Organization) based on clinicopathologic features observed in a large group of patients. *Blood* 2002; **99**: 800–5.

140. Crowley JJ, Nikko A, Varghese A, Hoppe RT, Kim YH. Mycosis fungoides in young patients: clinical characteristics and outcome. *J Am Acad Dermatol* 1998; **38**: 696–701.

141. Burg G, Kempf W, Haeffner A, *et al*. From inflammation to neoplasia: new concepts in the pathogenesis of cutaneous lymphomas. *Recent Results Cancer Res* 2002; **160**: 271–80.

142. Tan RS, Butterworth CM, McLaughlin H, Malka S, Samman PD. Mycosis fungoides: a disease of antigen persistence. *Br J Dermatol* 1974; **91**: 607–16.

143. Greene MH, Dalager NA, Lamberg SI, Argyropoulos CE, Fraumeni JF Jr. Mycosis fungoides: epidemiologic observations. *Cancer Treat Rep* 1979; **63**: 597–606.

144. Fischmann AB, Bunn PA Jr, Guccion JG, Matthews MJ, Minna JD. Exposure to chemicals, physical agents, and biologic agents in mycosis fungoides and the Sezary syndrome. *Cancer Treat Rep* 1979; **63**: 591–6.

145. Cohen SR, Stenn KS, Braverman IM, Beck GJ. Clinicopathologic relationships, survival, and therapy in 59 patients with observations on occupation as a new prognostic factor. *Cancer* 1980; **46**: 2654–66.

146. Whittemore AS, Holly EA, Lee IM, *et al*. Mycosis fungoides in relation to environmental exposures and immune response: a case–control study. *J Natl Cancer Inst* 1989; **81**: 1560–7.

147. Tuyp E, Burgoyne A, Aitchison T, MacKie R. A case–control study of possible causative factors in mycosis fungoides. *Arch Dermatol* 1987; **123**: 196–200.

148. Ghosh SK, Abrams JT, Terunuma H, Vonderheid EC, DeFreitas E. Human T-cell leukemia virus type I tax/rex DNA and RNA in cutaneous T-cell lymphoma. *Blood* 1994; **84**: 2663–71.

149. Hall WW, Liu CR, Schneewind O, *et al*. Deleted HTLV-I provirus in blood and cutaneous lesions of patients with mycosis fungoides. *Science* 1991; **253**: 317–20.

150. Pancake BA, Zucker-Franklin D. The difficulty of detecting HTLV-1 proviral sequences in patients with mycosis fungoides. *J Acquir Immune Defic Syndr Hum Retrovirol* 1996; **13**: 314–19.

151. Li G, Vowels BR, Benoit BM, Rook AH, Lessin SR. Failure to detect human T-lymphotropic virus type-I proviral DNA in cell lines and tissues from patients with cutaneous T-cell lymphoma. *J Invest Dermatol* 1996; **107**: 308–13.

152. Boni R, Davis-Daneshfar A, Burg G, Fuchs D, Wood GS. No detection of HTLV-I proviral DNA in lesional skin biopsies from Swiss and German patients with cutaneous T-cell lymphoma. *Br J Dermatol* 1996; **134**: 282–4.

153. Wood GS, Salvekar A, Schaffer J, *et al*. Evidence against a role for human T-cell lymphotrophic virus type I (HTLV-I) in the pathogenesis of American cutaneous T-cell lymphoma. *J Invest Dermatol* 1996; **107**: 301–7.

154. Biggar RJ, Engels EA, Frisch M, Goedert JJ. Risk of T-cell lymphomas in persons with AIDS. *J Acquir Immune Defic Syndr* 2001; **26**: 371–6.

155. Kaplan MH, Hall WW, Susin M, *et al*. Syndrome of severe skin disease, eosinophilia, and dermatopathic lymphadenopathy in patients with HTLV-II complicating human immunodeficiency virus infection. *Am J Med* 1991; **91**: 300–9.

156. Zucker-Franklin D, Pancake BA, Marmor M, Legler PM. Reexamination of human T cell lymphotropic virus (HTLV-I/II) prevalence. *Proc Natl Acad Sci USA* 1997; **94**: 6403–7.

157. Herne KL, Talpur R, Breuer-McHam J, Champlin R, Duvic M. Cytomegalovirus seropositivity is significantly associated with mycosis fungoides and Sezary syndrome. *Blood* 2003; **101**: 2132–6.

158. Smoller BR, Bishop K, Glusac E, Kim YH, Hendrickson M. Reassessment of histologic parameters in the diagnosis of mycosis fungoides. *Am J Surg Pathol* 1995; **19**: 1423–30.

159. de Coninck EC, Kim YH, Varghese A, Hoppe RT. Clinical characteristics and outcome of patients with extracutaneous mycosis fungoides. *J Clin Oncol* 2001; **19**: 779–84.

160. Bunn PA Jr, Hoffman SJ, Norris D, Golitz LE, Aeling JL. Systemic therapy of cutaneous T-cell lymphomas (mycosis fungoides and the Sezary syndrome). *Ann Intern Med* 1994; **121**: 592–602.

161. Kim YH, Chow S, Varghese A, Hoppe RT. Clinical characteristics and long-term outcome of patients with

generalized patch and/or plaque (T2) mycosis fungoides. *Arch Dermatol* 1999; **135**: 26–32.

162. Kashani-Sabet M, McMillan A, Zackheim HS. A modified staging classification for cutaneous T-cell lymphoma. *J Am Acad Dermatol* 2001; **45**: 700–6.

163. Sausville EA, Eddy JL, Makuch RW, *et al.* Histopathologic staging at initial diagnosis of mycosis fungoides and the Sezary syndrome: definition of three distinctive prognostic groups. *Ann Intern Med* 1988; **109**: 372–82.

164. Vonderheid EC, Bernengo MG, Burg G, *et al.* Update on erythrodermic cutaneous T-cell lymphoma: report of the International Society for Cutaneous Lymphomas. *J Am Acad Dermatol* 2002; **46**: 95–106.

165. Kim YH, Jensen RA, Watanabe GL, Varghese A, Hoppe RT. Clinical stage IA (limited patch and plaque) mycosis fungoides: a long-term outcome analysis. *Arch Dermatol* 1996; **132**: 1309–13.

166. Kim YH, Bishop K, Varghese A, Hoppe RT. Prognostic factors in erythrodermic mycosis fungoides and the Sézary syndrome. *Arch Dermatol* 1995; **131**: 1003–8.

167. Scarisbrick JJ, Whittaker S, Evans AV, *et al.* Prognostic significance of tumor burden in the blood of patients with erythrodermic primary cutaneous T-cell lymphoma. *Blood* 2001; **97**: 624–30.

168. Cerroni L, Rieger E, Hodl S, Kerl H. Clinicopathologic and immunologic features associated with transformation of mycosis fungoides to large-cell lymphoma. *Am J Surg Pathol* 1992; **16**: 543–52.

169. Dmitrovsky E, Matthews MJ, Bunn PA, *et al.* Cytologic transformation in cutaneous T cell lymphoma: a clinicopathologic entity associated with poor prognosis. *J Clin Oncol* 1987; **5**: 208–15.

170. Diamandidou E, Colome-Grimmer M, Fayad L, Duvic M, Kurzrock R. Transformation of mycosis fungoides/Sezary syndrome: clinical characteristics and prognosis. *Blood* 1998; **92**: 1150–9.

171. Hoppe RT, Wood GS, Abel EA. Mycosis fungoides and the Sezary syndrome: pathology, staging, and treatment. *Curr Probl Cancer* 1990; **14**: 293–371.

172. Glusac EJ, Shapiro PE, McNiff JM. Cutaneous T-cell lymphoma. Refinement in the application of controversial histologic criteria. *Dermatol Clin* 1999; **17**: 601–14.

173. Bergman R, Faclieru D, Sahar D, *et al.* Immunophenotyping and T-cell receptor [gamma] gene rearrangement analysis as an adjunct to the histopathologic diagnosis of mycosis fungoides. *J Am Acad Dermatol* 1998; **39**: 554–9.

174. Rappl G, Muche JM, Abken H, *et al.* CD4(+)CD7(-) T cells compose the dominant T-cell clone in the peripheral blood of patients with Sezary syndrome. *J Am Acad Dermatol* 2001; **44**: 456–61.

175. Weiss LM, Hu E, Wood GS, *et al.* Clonal rearrangements of T-cell receptor genes in mycosis fungoides and dermatopathic lymphadenopathy. *N Engl J Med* 1985; **313**: 539–44.

176. Ashton-Key M, Diss TC, Du MQ, Kirkham N, Wotherspoon A, Isaacson PG. The value of the polymerase chain reaction in the diagnosis of cutaneous T-cell infiltrates. *Am J Surg Pathol* 1997; **21**: 743–7.

177. Ormsby A, Bergfeld WF, Tubbs RR, Hsi ED. Evaluation of a new paraffin-reactive CD7 T-cell deletion marker and a polymerase chain reaction-based T-cell receptor gene rearrangement assay: implications for diagnosis of mycosis fungoides in community clinical practice. *J Am Acad Dermatol* 2001; **45**: 405–13.

178. Jorg B, Kerl H, Thiers BH, Brocker EB, Burg G. Therapeutic approaches in cutaneous lymphoma. *Dermatol Clin* 1994; **12**: 433–41.

179. Kaye F, Bunn PA, Steinberg S, *et al.* A randomized trial comparing combination electron-beam radiation and chemotherapy with topical therapy in the initial treatment of mycosis fungoides. *N Engl J Med* 1989; **321**: 1784–90.

180. Zackheim HS. Cutaneous T cell lymphoma: update of treatment. *Dermatology* 1999; **199**: 102–5.

181. Parrish JA, Fitzpatrick TB, Tanenbaum L, Pathak MA. Photochemotherapy of psoriasis with oral methoxsalen and longwave ultraviolet light. *N Engl J Med* 1974; **291**: 1207–11.

182. Herrmann JJ, Roenigk HH Jr, Honigsmann H. Ultraviolet radiation for treatment of cutaneous T-cell lymphoma. *Hematol Oncol Clin North Am* 1995; **9**: 1077–88.

183. Stern RS, Thibodeau LA, Kleinerman RA, Parrish JA, Fitzpatrick TB. Risk of cutaneous carcinoma in patients treated with oral methoxsalen photochemotherapy for psoriasis. *N Engl J Med* 1979; **300**: 809–13.

184. Holloway KB, Flowers FP, Ramos-Caro FA. Therapeutic alternatives in cutaneous T-cell lymphoma. *J Am Acad Dermatol* 1992; **27**: 367–78.

185. Jones GW, Wilson LD. Mycosis fungoides and total skin electron beam radiation. *Blood* 1997; **89**: 3062–4.

186. Heald P. The treatment of cutaneous T-cell lymphoma with a novel retinoid. *Clin Lymphoma* 2000; **1** (Suppl 1): S45–S49.

187. Breneman D, Duvic M, Kuzel T, Yocum R, Truglia J, Stevens VJ. Phase 1 and 2 trial of bexarotene gel for skin-directed treatment of patients with cutaneous T-cell lymphoma. *Arch Dermatol* 2002; **138**: 325–32.

188. Talpur R, Ward S, Apisarnthanarax N, Breuer-Mcham J, Duvic M. Optimizing bexarotene therapy for cutaneous T-cell lymphoma. *J Am Acad Dermatol* 2002; **47**: 672–84.

189. Stern DK, Lebwohl M. Treatment of mycosis fungoides with oral bexarotene combined with PUVA. *J Drugs Dermatol* 2002; **1**: 134–6.

190. Kim YH, Martinez G, Varghese A, Hoppe RT. Topical nitrogen mustard in the management of mycosis fungoides: update of the Stanford experience. *Arch Dermatol* 2003; **139**: 165–73.

191. Edelson R, Berger C, Gasparro F, *et al.* Treatment of cutaneous T-cell lymphoma by extracorporeal photochemotherapy. Preliminary results. *N Engl J Med* 1987; **316**: 297–303.

192. Heald P, Rook A, Perez M, *et al.* Treatment of erythrodermic cutaneous T-cell lymphoma with extracorporeal photochemotherapy. *J Am Acad Dermatol* 1992; **27**: 427–33.

193. Bisaccia E, Gonzalez J, Palangio M, Schwartz J, Klainer AS. Extracorporeal photochemotherapy alone or with adjuvant therapy in the treatment of cutaneous T-cell lymphoma: a 9-year retrospective study at a single institution. *J Am Acad Dermatol* 2000; **43**: 263–71.

194. Olsen EA. Interferon in the treatment of cutaneous T-cell lymphoma. *Dermatol Ther* 2003; **16**: 311–21.

195. Duvic M, Cather JC. Emerging new therapies for cutaneous T-cell lymphoma. *Dermatol Clin* 2000; **18**: 147–56.

196. Nichols J, Foss F, Kuzel TM, *et al.* Interleukin-2 fusion protein: an investigational therapy for interleukin-2 receptor expressing malignancies. *Eur J Cancer* 1997; **33** (Suppl 1): S34–S36.

197. Saleh MN, LeMaistre CF, Kuzel TM, *et al.* Antitumor activity of DAB389IL-2 fusion toxin in mycosis fungoides. *J Am Acad Dermatol* 1998; **39**: 63–73.

198. Foss FM, Bacha P, Osann KE, Demierre MF, Bell T, Kuzel T. Biological correlates of acute hypersensitivity events with DAB(389)IL-2 (denileukin diftitox, ONTAK) in cutaneous T-cell lymphoma: decreased frequency and severity with steroid premedication. *Clin Lymphoma* 2001; **1**: 298–302.

199. Rosen ST, Foss FM. Chemotherapy for mycosis fungoides and the Sezary syndrome. *Hematol Oncol Clin North Am* 1995; **9**: 1109–16.

200. Siegel RS, Pandolfino T, Guitart J, Rosen S, Kuzel TM. Primary cutaneous T-cell lymphoma: review and current concepts. *J Clin Oncol* 2000; **18**: 2908–25.

201. Kuzel TM, Hurria A, Samuelson E, *et al.* Phase II trial of 2-chlorodeoxyadenosine for the treatment of cutaneous T-cell lymphoma. *Blood* 1996; **87**: 906–11.

202. Zinzani PL, Baliva G, Magagnoli M, *et al.* Gemcitabine treatment in pretreated cutaneous T-cell lymphoma: experience in 44 patients. *J Clin Oncol* 2000; **18**: 2603–6.

203. Kurzrock R, Pilat S, Duvic M. Pentostatin therapy of T-cell lymphomas with cutaneous manifestations. *J Clin Oncol* 1999; **17**: 3117–21.

204. Wollina U, Dummer R, Brockmeyer NH, *et al.* Multicenter study of pegylated liposomal doxorubicin in patients with cutaneous T-cell lymphoma. *Cancer* 2003; **98**: 993–1001.

205. Rook AH, Wood GS, Yoo EK, *et al.* Interleukin-12 therapy of cutaneous T-cell lymphoma induces lesion regression and cytotoxic T-cell responses. *Blood* 1999; **94**: 902–8.

206. Kaplan EH, Rosen ST, Norris DB, Roenigk HH Jr, Saks SR, Bunn PA Jr. Phase II study of recombinant human interferon gamma for treatment of cutaneous T-cell lymphoma. *J Natl Cancer Inst* 1990; **82**: 208–12.

207. Kennedy GA, Seymour JF, Wolf M, *et al.* Treatment of patients with advanced mycosis fungoides and Sezary syndrome with alemtuzumab. *Eur J Haematol* 2003; **71**: 250–6.

208. Piekarz RL, Robey R, Sandor V, *et al.* Inhibitor of histone deacetylation, depsipeptide (FR901228), in the treatment of peripheral and cutaneous T-cell lymphoma: a case report. *Blood* 2001; **98**: 2865–8.

209. Sandor V, Bakke S, Robey RW, *et al.* Phase I trial of the histone deacetylase inhibitor, depsipeptide (FR901228, NSC 630176), in patients with refractory neoplasms. *Clin Cancer Res* 2002; **8**: 718–28.

210. Knox S, Hoppe RT, Maloney D, *et al.* Treatment of cutaneous T-cell lymphoma with chimeric anti-CD4 monoclonal antibody. *Blood* 1996; **87**: 893–9.

211. Foss FM, Raubitscheck A, Mulshine JL, *et al.* Phase I study of the pharmacokinetics of a radioimmunoconjugate, 90Y-T101, in patients with CD5-expressing leukemia and lymphoma. *Clin Cancer Res* 1998; **4**: 2691–700.

212. Herbert KE, Spencer A, Grigg A, Ryan G, McCormack C, Prince HM. Graft-versus-lymphoma effect in refractory cutaneous T-cell lymphoma after reduced-intensity HLA-matched sibling allogeneic stem cell

transplantation. *Bone Marrow Transplant* 2004; **34**: 521–5.

213. Guitart J, Wickless SC, Oyama Y, *et al.* Long-term remission after allogeneic hematopoietic stem cell transplantation for refractory cutaneous T-cell lymphoma. *Arch Dermatol* 2002; **138**: 1359–65.

214. Oyama Y, Guitart J, Kuzel TM, Burt RK, Rosen ST. High-dose therapy and bone marrow transplantation in cutaneous T-cell lymphoma. *Hematol Oncol Clin North Am* 2003; **17**: 1475–83, xi.

215. Bigler RD, Crilley P, Micaily B, *et al.* Autologous bone marrow transplantation for advanced stage mycosis fungoides. *Bone Marrow Transplant* 1991; **7**: 133–7.

216. Molina A, Nademanee A, Arber DA, Forman SJ. Remission of refractory Sezary syndrome after bone marrow transplantation from a matched unrelated donor. *Biol Blood Marrow Transplant* 1999; **5**: 400–4.

217. Rudiger T, Weisenburger DD, Anderson JR, *et al.* Peripheral T-cell lymphoma (excluding anaplastic large-cell lymphoma): results from the Non-Hodgkin's Lymphoma Classification Project. *Ann Oncol* 2002; **13**: 140–9.

218. Anderson JR, Armitage JO, Weisenburger DD. Epidemiology of the non-Hodgkin's lymphomas: distributions of the major subtypes differ by geographic locations. Non-Hodgkin's Lymphoma Classification Project. *Ann Oncol* 1998; **9**: 717–20.

219. Falini B, Pileri S, De Solas I, *et al.* Peripheral T-cell lymphoma associated with hemophagocytic syndrome. *Blood* 1990; **75**: 434–44.

220. Saragoni A, Falini B, Medri L, *et al.* [Peripheral T-cell lymphoma associated with hemophagocytic syndrome: a recently identified entity. Clinico-pathologic and immunohistochemical study of 2 cases]. *Pathologica* 1990; **82**: 359–69.

221. Weiss LM, Crabtree GS, Rouse RV, Warnke RA. Morphologic and immunologic characterization of 50 peripheral T-cell lymphomas. *Am J Pathol* 1985; **118**: 316–24.

222. Suchi T, Lennert K, Tu LY, *et al.* Histopathology and immunohistochemistry of peripheral T cell lymphomas: a proposal for their classification. *J Clin Pathol* 1987; **40**: 995–1015.

223. Borowitz MJ, Reichert TA, Brynes RK, *et al.* The phenotypic diversity of peripheral T-cell lymphomas: the Southeastern Cancer Study Group experience. *Hum Pathol* 1986; **17**: 567–74.

224. Weiss LM, Trela MJ, Cleary ML, Turner RR, Warnke RA, Sklar J. Frequent immunoglobulin and T-cell receptor gene rearrangements in "histiocytic" neoplasms. *Am J Pathol* 1985; **121**: 369–73.

225. Pautier P, Devidas A, Delmer A, *et al.* Angio-immunoblastic-like T-cell non Hodgkin's lymphoma: outcome after chemotherapy in 33 patients and review of the literature. *Leuk Lymphoma* 1999; **32**: 545–52.

226. Siegert W, Nerl C, Agthe A, *et al.* Angioimmunoblastic lymphadenopathy (AILD)-type T-cell lymphoma: prognostic impact of clinical observations and laboratory findings at presentation. The Kiel Lymphoma Study Group. *Ann Oncol* 1995; **6**: 659–64.

227. Dogan A, Attygalle AD, Kyriakou C. Angioimmunoblastic T-cell lymphoma. *Br J Haematol* 2003; **121**: 681–91.

228. Anagnostopoulos I, Hummel M, Finn T, *et al.* Heterogeneous Epstein–Barr virus infection patterns in peripheral T-cell lymphoma of angioimmunoblastic lymphadenopathy type. *Blood* 1992; **80**: 1804–12.

229. Brauninger A, Spieker T, Willenbrock K, *et al.* Survival and clonal expansion of mutating "forbidden" (immunoglobulin receptor-deficient) Epstein–Barr virus-infected B cells in angioimmunoblastic T cell lymphoma. *J Exp Med* 2001; **194**: 927–40.

230. Weiss LM, Jaffe ES, Liu XF, Chen YY, Shibata D, Medeiros LJ. Detection and localization of Epstein–Barr viral genomes in angioimmunoblastic lymphadenopathy and angioimmunoblastic lymphadenopathy-like lymphoma. *Blood* 1992; **79**: 1789–95.

231. Attygalle A, Al-Jehani R, Diss TC, *et al.* Neoplastic T cells in angioimmunoblastic T-cell lymphoma express CD10. *Blood* 2002; **99**: 627–33.

232. Lennert K. [Nature, prognosis and nomenclature of angioimmunoblastic (lymphadenopathy (lymphogranulomatosis X or T-zone lymphoma)]. *Dtsch Med Wochenschr* 1979; **104**: 1246–7.

233. Willenbrock K, Roers A, Seidl C, Wacker HH, Kuppers R, Hansmann ML. Analysis of T-cell subpopulations in T-cell non-Hodgkin's lymphoma of angioimmunoblastic lymphadenopathy with dysproteinemia type by single target gene amplification of T cell receptor-beta gene rearrangements. *Am J Pathol* 2001; **158**: 1851–7.

234. Tsatalas C, Margaritis D, Pantelidou D, Spanudakis E, Kaloutsi V, Bourikas G. Treatment of angioimmunoblastic lymphadenopathy with dysproteinemia-type T-cell lymphoma with fludarabine. *Acta Haematol* 2003; **109**: 110.

235. Sallah AS, Bernard S. Treatment of angioimmuno-blastic lymphadenopathy with dysproteinemia using 2-chlorodeoxyadenosine. *Ann Hematol* 1996; **73**: 295–6.

236. Gerlando Q, Barbera V, Ammatuna E, Franco V, Florena AM, Mariani G. Successful treatment of angio-immunoblastic lymphadenopathy with dysproteine-mia-type T-cell lymphoma by combined methotrexate and prednisone. *Haematologica* 2000; **85**: 880–1.

237. Strupp C, Aivado M, Germing U, Gattermann N, Haas R. Angioimmunoblastic lymphadenopathy (AILD) may respond to thalidomide treatment: two case reports. *Leuk Lymphoma* 2002; **43**: 133–7.

238. Isaacson PG, Du MQ. Gastrointestinal lymphoma: where morphology meets molecular biology. *J Pathol* 2005; **205**: 255–74.

239. Howell WM, Leung ST, Jones DB, *et al.* HLA-DRB, -DQA, and -DQB polymorphism in celiac disease and enteropathy-associated T-cell lymphoma. Common features and additional risk factors for malignancy. *Hum Immunol* 1995; **43**: 29–37.

240. Isaacson PG. Gastrointestinal lymphomas of T- and B-cell types. *Mod Pathol* 1999; **12**: 151–8.

241. Tallini G, West AB, Buckley PJ. Diagnosis of gastro-intestinal T-cell lymphomas in routinely processed tissues. *J Clin Gastroenterol* 1993; **17**: 57–66.

242. Murray A, Cuevas EC, Jones DB, Wright DH. Study of the immunohistochemistry and T cell clonality of enteropathy-associated T cell lymphoma. *Am J Pathol* 1995; **146**: 509–19.

243. Spencer J, Cerf-Bensussan N, Jarry A, *et al.* Enteropathy-associated T cell lymphoma (malignant histiocytosis of the intestine) is recognized by a monoclonal anti-body (HML-1) that defines a membrane molecule on human mucosal lymphocytes. *Am J Pathol* 1988; **132**: 1–5.

244. Gale J, Simmonds PD, Mead GM, Sweetenham JW, Wright DH. Enteropathy-type intestinal T-cell lym-phoma: clinical features and treatment of 31 patients in a single center. *J Clin Oncol* 2000; **18**: 795–803.

245. Gonzalez CL, Medeiros LJ, Braziel RM, Jaffe ES. T-cell lymphoma involving subcutaneous tissue. A clinicopathologic entity commonly associated with hemophagocytic syndrome. *Am J Surg Pathol* 1991; **15**: 17–27.

246. Go RS, Wester SM. Immunophenotypic and molecular features, clinical outcomes, treatments, and prognostic factors associated with subcutaneous panniculitis-like T-cell lymphoma: a systematic anal-ysis of 156 patients reported in the literature. *Cancer* 2004; **101**: 1404–13.

247. Salhany KE, Macon WR, Choi JK, *et al.* Subcutaneous panniculitis-like T-cell lymphoma: clinicopathologic, immunophenotypic, and genotypic analysis of alpha/beta and gamma/delta subtypes. *Am J Surg Pathol* 1998; **22**: 881–93.

248. Toro JR, Liewehr DJ, Pabby N, *et al.* Gamma-delta T-cell phenotype is associated with significantly decreased survival in cutaneous T-cell lymphoma. *Blood* 2003; **101**: 3407–12.

24

Chronic lymphocytic leukemia in the elderly

Alexander S. D. Spiers

Introduction

Definitions

Chronic lymphocytic leukemia (CLL) is a hematologic neoplasm of unknown etiology with a clinical course that is measured in years rather than in the weeks that used to characterize the clinical course of the acute leukemias. This distinction was made in the era before any effective therapy was available for the acute leukemias and rapid death was the usual outcome. As a result, the chronic leukemias were considered to be "favorable" diseases because of their longer prognosis. In young patients, advances in the treatment of the acute leukemias have been dramatic, frequently resulting in cure, and as a result the chronic leukemias are no longer considered so "favorable." In older patients, progress in treating the acute leukemias has been much more modest, and as a rule the prognosis of the chronic leukemias, particularly that of CLL, remains relatively favorable. The broad categories of the chronic leukemias that are encountered in the older person are listed in Table 24.1.

The *older person* is not so readily defined, because the concept of age is to many people, including physicians, highly subjective. A wry definition of "elderly" is "anyone significantly older than the observer," and psychologically there is much truth in this. From the viewpoint of the hematologist who treats leukemia by conventional means, the age of 70 years may be taken as the beginning of the older person's estate. A physician who treats by bone-marrow transplantation might draw the boundary at 60, or even 55, years.

Table 24.1. Chronic leukemias that are encountered in the older person.

Chronic lymphoid leukemias
   B-cell chronic lymphocytic leukemia (B-CLL)
   B-cell prolymphocytic leukemia (B-PLL)
   B-cell hairy-cell leukemia (B-HCL)
   B-cell lymphomas with blood involvement
   T-cell variants of the above disorders (uncommon)
Chronic myeloid leukemias
   Chronic granulocytic leukemia (CGL)
   Atypical myeloproliferative syndrome
   Chronic myelomonocytic leukemia (CMML)
   Rarer subvarieties of chronic myeloid neoplasia

Significance of older age in managing CLL

Older age has a significant impact on the management of most hematologic malignancies [1]. Its most obvious effect in the clinical situation is its strong association with the presence of *multiple medical problems*. Although disease should never be considered as an inevitable consequence of older age, the fact remains that as years accumulate, so do metabolic, degenerative, and neoplastic disorders, all of which may have a profound influence on the care of the patient when CLL must be managed. The most important medical conditions that affect the hematologist's approach to the older person with CLL are listed in Table 24.2.

Of almost equal importance is a physiologic change that inevitably accompanies aging: a *reduced functional reserve capacity* that affects all organ

Blood Disorders in the Elderly, ed. Lodovico Balducci, William Ershler, Giovanni de Gaetano.
Published by Cambridge University Press. © Cambridge University Press 2008.

Table 24.2. Concurrent medical problems that affect the management of chronic leukemia in the older person.

Problem	Consequences
Intellectual impairment	Problems with adherence to treatment
Chronic lung disease	Mortality from intercurrent infection; problems with some cytotoxic drugs
Hypertension	Cerebral hemorrhage when thrombocytopenic
Angina	Poor tolerance of anemia
Cardiac failure	Poor tolerance of transfusion, and of some drugs – e.g., anthracyclines
Atherosclerosis	Poor tolerance of anemia and leukocytosis
Arthritis	Medications promote GI hemorrhage
Diabetes mellitus	Exacerbations with corticosteroid therapy
Liver disease	Altered drug metabolism
Diverticulosis	Infection, perforation, sepsis
Renal impairment	Poor tolerance of hyperuricemia; problems with antibiotic therapy
Uterine prolapse	Urinary tract infections
Prostatomegaly	Urinary tract infections
Incontinence	Decubitus ulcers
Other primary cancers	Multiple problems, depending on site

This list is not exhaustive. Consideration must also be given to the psychological, social, environmental, and often pressing economic problems that have a profound impact on the practice of geriatric oncology.

systems. As a result of this natural and universal phenomenon, the healthy 80-year-old who looks twenty years younger is, in fact, much more frail than a genuine 60-year-old, and when subjected to stress may develop failure of one, and then multiple, organs in a fashion that would not occur in a younger person. Because of this major, though clinically occult, impairment in the elderly, certain types of therapy are fraught with risk (e.g., intensive chemotherapy) or may even be precluded (e.g., allogeneic bone-marrow transplantation).

In the older person with significant other disease, the prognosis of CLL may exceed the life expectancy

Table 24.3. Chronic lymphoid leukemias and related disorders.

B-cell chronic lymphocytic leukemia (B-CLL)
B-cell prolymphocytic leukemia (B-PLL)
B-cell hairy-cell leukemia (B-HCL)
B-cell non-Hodgkin lymphomas with blood involvement
    Small cleaved cell
    Lymphoplasmacytic
T-cell variants of the above disorders (uncommon)
Unique T-cell disorders
    Sézary syndrome
    Adult T-cell leukemia/lymphoma (ATLL)
    Large granular lymphocytic (LGL) leukemia

of the patient, and thus be of small importance, whereas a healthy 50-year-old with CLL will die from the disease unless it is cured, for example by bone-marrow transplantation. By contrast, in an elderly patient with severe coronary artery disease, the discovery of low-stage CLL has virtually no impact on life expectancy and there is no necessity to even treat the disease, let alone cure it. The reduced life expectancy that is an inevitable accompaniment of aging should not however be exaggerated. For example, a healthy woman of 75 has a life expectancy of 12 years; the diagnosis at age 75 of stage II CLL, with a prognosis of approximately seven years, therefore is not an unimportant event.

There are numerous subvarieties of chronic lymphoid leukemia and also several related disorders (Table 24.3), but the T-cell varieties are all so uncommon as to be of lesser importance clinically. Of the B-cell leukemias, chronic lymphocytic leukemia (B-CLL or simply CLL) is by far the most frequent and the most important.

For many years a relatively neglected disease, CLL has in the last decade been the focus of much important research that has increased our understanding of its biology and significantly improved its management, to the benefit of many older patients.

Terminology and classification

The terminology outlined in Table 24.3 is widely accepted, although some variations are encountered.

The nomenclature of the chronic lymphoid leukemias was until recently based mainly on morphologic considerations; descriptions of cells as "mature" or "differentiated" were based on their appearance. The ability to characterize cells by surface markers, antigenic determinants that are located on the cell membrane, led to major conceptual changes, the first and most fundamental of which was the recognition of T and B cells. With the advent of automated flow cytometry and the ability to study the surface markers of thousands of cells in every patient, subtle differences that are undetectable by morphologic methods alone are continually emerging. For example, the cells of B-CLL, despite their mature appearance, turn out to be more primitive than previously suspected. With the widespread application of flow cytometry, more accurate diagnoses of lymphoid neoplasms are now made, and ongoing revisions of current terminology can be anticipated. It remains to be seen to what extent these fine distinctions will be clinically important in selecting the most appropriate management for each patient.

Features of CLL

CLL is characterized by an absolute lymphocytosis in the bone marrow and peripheral blood. Cell proliferation is usually slow, but there is a remorselessly progressive accumulation of monoclonal, long-lived, mature-appearing B lymphocytes that are immunoincompetent and indeed produce immunosuppression. Whereas many other clinical features are regularly encountered in CLL, for example lymphadenopathy, splenomegaly, hepatomegaly, hematopoietic failure, hypogammaglobulinemia, and autoimmune phenomena, none is constant or essential to the diagnosis.

Epidemiology

CLL is the leukemia *par excellence* of the older person. It is rarely seen in patients aged less than 40 years, and its incidence increases steadily with advancing age, apparently without limit as it continues to rise in the ninth and tenth decades of life. The incidence of CLL increases 350-fold when ages 25 to 29 are compared with ages 80 to 84 [2]. A high *incidence* of CLL (approximately one-third of all new cases of leukemia) combines with a lengthy *survival* to produce a high *prevalence* of the condition: CLL comprises approximately half of all cases of leukemia in Western populations. It is safe to say that almost every geriatric practice or long-term care facility will have one or more patients with CLL, and physicians in every medical specialty will regularly encounter patients with this important disease. There is a male predominance that appears to have decreased with time; early in the twentieth century the male-to-female ratios for CLL in Western countries ranged from 2.5 to 3.0, whereas in more recent studies they are between 1.6 and 1.9. There are rare families that show clustering of cases of CLL, sometimes in association with cases of lymphoma or of immunologic diseases. Geographic and ethnic variation in incidence is greater for CLL than for any other type of leukemia [3]. The highest incidences of CLL are observed in whites in North America and in Europe. Lower rates are reported from South America and the Caribbean, and exceptionally low rates are found in India, Japan, China, and other areas of Asia, where B-CLL is a truly rare disease. This finding persists when adjustment is made for the lower average age of the population in some Asian countries. The reason for these fascinating variations that are peculiar to CLL is unknown. The geriatric oncologist who practices in North America or Europe is in an area where the incidence of CLL is already very high, and continues to increase as the average age of the population increases.

Symptoms

More than any other leukemia, CLL is apt to be diagnosed when it is still asymptomatic. A common scenario is the senior citizen who requires a surgical procedure for one of the conditions that are frequent in older age, for example inguinal hernia, uterine prolapse, or prostatomegaly. A routine preoperative blood count shows a marked absolute lymphocytosis, a follow-up bone-marrow examination shows infiltration with mature-appearing lymphocytes, and flow cytometry shows the circulating lymphocytes to be positive for surface membrane immunoglobulin (sIg) and the CD5 and CD21 antigens, findings typical for B-CLL. At one time, establishing the diagnosis of CLL would have led to the immediate cancellation of surgery, which might have been appropriate if acute leukemia had been diagnosed, but would be quite unnecessary for most patients with asymptomatic CLL. It is now widely recognized that the diagnosis of uncomplicated CLL does not preclude the provision of necessary surgery or other treatment, and indeed may not alter the patient's lifestyle or longevity in any way. Even open heart surgery can be successfully performed in elderly patients with CLL, although special attention must be paid to the high risk of serious infections [4].

Because routine physical examinations and blood tests in the absence of symptoms are becoming a regular feature of modern health care, increasing numbers of patients are being diagnosed with early CLL. Furthermore, flow cytometry has conferred the ability to diagnose CLL at a particularly early stage, when an absolute lymphocytosis has not become established, but a monoclonal lymphocytosis is unequivocally demonstrable. As a result of these advances, the survival of patients with CLL is likely to increase significantly, but it should be remembered that much of this "improvement" will be factitious and due to the statistical phenomenon of *lead time bias* – i.e. longer survival that is due solely to earlier diagnosis.

Some patients with CLL present with symptoms that are frequently associated with malignancy and with immunodeficiency disorders: malaise, weakness, night sweats, fever without apparent infection, and weight loss. Such constitutional symptoms are less frequent in CLL than they are in Hodgkin disease.

Other patients with CLL may present with symptoms of *anemia*: loss of energy, fatigue, dyspnea, anorexia, weight loss, and pallor. In the older person with cardiac disease or peripheral vascular disease, the symptoms of anemia may be angina, cardiac failure, or intermittent claudication. In an elderly patient with CLL, the anemia may be exacerbated by – or be entirely due to – intercurrent unrelated problems, for example gastrointestinal bleeding or a deficiency of vitamin B_{12} or folate. Such problems should be excluded before anemia is attributed to the leukemia itself, otherwise the disease may be erroneously upstaged.

A less frequent presentation of CLL is with symptoms attributable to *thrombocytopenia*: bruising, purpura, or hemorrhage. Presentation with *infection* is more common; patients with CLL are prone to infection by reason of hypogammaglobulinemia, decreased T-cell function, neutropenia, or combinations of these defects. Respiratory tract infection, particularly bronchitis and bronchopneumonia, may be the precipitating problem that leads to the diagnosis of CLL. Some patients present with the symptoms of one of the autoimmune disorders that are frequent in patients with CLL: immune thrombocytopenic purpura, autoimmune hemolytic anemia, or connective tissue disease.

Some patients with CLL initially present with symptoms that are due to organomegaly. *Lymphadenopathy* in the neck, axilla, or groin may become quite severe before it is symptomatic. In CLL, *splenomegaly* is less frequent and usually much less marked than it is in chronic granulocytic leukemia, and symptomatic enlargement of the spleen is rarely a cause of initial presentation. Similarly, *splenic infarction* is rare in CLL.

Although *leukocytosis* greater than $200 \times 10^9/L$ is not rare in untreated CLL, it is almost never symptomatic. Hyperviscosity of the blood and leukostatic lesions in the lungs and brain, frequent in acute myeloid leukemia (AML) with a high blast cell count, have been reported in CLL [5] but are very rare, even when the leukocyte count exceeds one million per microliter. This is because the lymphocyte of CLL, unlike the myeloblast, is small, readily deformable, relatively nonadherent, and does not invade blood vessel walls. Thus emergency treatment for hyperleukocytosis is rarely required in CLL, and the height of the leukocyte count per se is seldom an indication for treatment. Most patients, and not a few physicians, are difficult to convince that this is so.

Physical signs

The patient with CLL may not only be asymptomatic but also may have no physical signs that are referable to the disease. When abnormal findings are present, *pallor* and *lymphadenopathy* are the most frequent. Lymphadenopathy may be found in a single area or in multiple lymph-node fields. The nodes are typically soft, mobile, non-tender, and not matted together, and generally they are small, in the 1–2 cm range. Massive lymphadenopathy, with a bull neck or a severely distorted axilla, occurs but is uncommon. Lymphedema is rarely associated with the lymphadenopathy of CLL. Clinically, the enlarged lymph nodes of CLL are quite different from the hard, adherent nodes that characterize involvement by carcinoma. *Splenomegaly* is frequently absent, and when present is rarely massive; splenic enlargement that extends below the umbilicus or across the midline is more suggestive of chronic granulocytic leukemia, prolymphocytic leukemia (PLL), or hairy-cell leukemia. *Hepatomegaly*, if present at diagnosis, is usually mild. Bruises and purpura are not frequent features of newly diagnosed CLL, but both conditions may be observed in the older person in the absence of any hematologic disease, as a consequence of decreased elasticity of the skin. *Cutaneous infiltrates* may occur in B-CLL but are more frequent in the rare T-cell variant of the disease. Lesions of *herpes zoster* are not uncommon in CLL and are sometimes a presenting feature. Presentation with meningeal involvement [6] or with neurologic problems suggestive of progressive multifocal leukoencephalopathy [7] is rare but important to bear in mind, particularly in the older patient in whom central nervous system disorders of divers etiology are relatively frequent.

Laboratory findings

CLL is characterized by an absolute and sustained lymphocytosis in the peripheral blood, with predominantly mature-appearing lymphocytes, although some atypical forms can be detected in most cases and in a few instances 50% or more of the cells possess atypical morphologic features

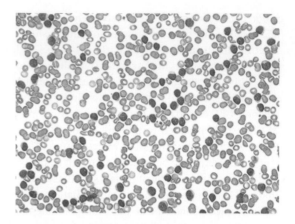

Figure 24.1 This peripheral smear shows that there can be heterogeneity in the appearance of the abnormal lymphocytes in CLL. Kadin, M., ASH Image Bank 2003: 100690. Copyright American Society of Hematology. All rights reserved. *See color plate section.*

(Fig. 24.1). There is an accompanying lymphocytosis in the bone marrow but evidence of bone-marrow failure – anemia, neutropenia, or thrombocytopenia – is frequently absent.

A Working Group sponsored by the National Cancer Institute has further specified typical cases of B-CLL that can be considered for protocol studies [8]. Marker studies should show sIg+, CD19+, CD20+, or CD24+. The cells must be CD5+ but negative for other pan-T markers, express either kappa or lambda light chains, and sIg must be present at low density. The minimum threshold for blood lymphocytes is 5×10^9/L and the blood lymphocytosis must be sustained over a period of at least four weeks upon repeated examinations. The lymphocytes must appear mature and no more than 55% may be atypical prolymphocytes or lymphoblasts. Patients with 11–55% prolymphocytes – thus resembling PLL – should be considered for special studies because the prognostic significance of their high incidence of cellular atypia is not well defined (Figs. 24.2, 24.3). The bone-marrow aspirate must contain ⩾30% lymphoid cells. The bone-marrow biopsy may show diffuse or nodular lymphocytic infiltration and the marrow must be normocellular or hypercellular.

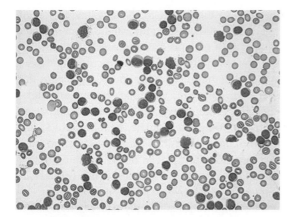

Figure 24.2 This mixed-cell variant of CLL contains a dimorphic population of cells. Kadin, M., ASH Image Bank 2003: 100935. Copyright American Society of Hematology. All rights reserved. *See color plate section.*

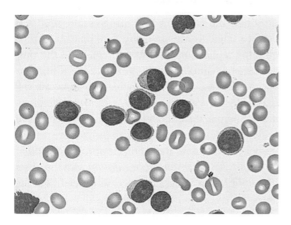

Figure 24.3 PLL variant of CLL: prominent nuclei characterize the prolymphocytes. Kadin, M., ASH Image Bank 2003: 100935. Copyright American Society of Hematology. All rights reserved. *See color plate section.*

The above specification is not universally accepted. Some hematologists will diagnose CLL when the lymphocytosis is less than 5×10^9/L if a B-cell monoclone with the appropriate surface markers is demonstrable. While such cases may indeed have CLL at an early stage, their inclusion in clinical studies may affect survival data by the mechanism of lead time bias referred to earlier.

Cytogenetic findings in CLL

This topic has been reviewed in depth [9], and only a few salient features will be considered here. Most types of chromosomal analysis require dividing cells that are in metaphase. Whereas this is no great problem in the acute leukemias or in chronic granulocytic leukemia (CGL), it is a major obstacle in CLL, since the tumor cells have a very low mitotic index and must be activated in vitro with mitogens that are effective for B cells (e.g., *Escherichia coli* lipopolysaccharide, Epstein–Barr virus). Cells from some patients with CLL do not respond to mitogens and evaluable metaphases cannot be obtained; in general it is not known if such unresponsive cells harbor any chromosomal anomalies. In some cases, fluorescent stains for specific chromosomes can be applied to interphase cells and may demonstrate numerical abnormalities – e.g., trisomies.

Cytogenetic techniques in CLL cells have shown two major chromosomal abnormalities with a probable pathogenetic role: trisomy 12 and deletions of the long arm of chromosome 13 (13q14). No relevant gene on chromosome 12, and no pathogenetic mechanism by which the occurrence of trisomy 12 may lead to the development of CLL, has been documented. Terminal deletions of the long arm of chromosomes 6 and 11 might also be significant in CLL. Additional material on the long arm of chromosome 14 (14q+) to form a marker chromosome is a common additional abnormality that does not appear to be of prognostic significance. Trisomy 12 has been associated with a poor survival, whereas 13q deletions or a normal karyotype indicate a good prognosis. Complex abnormal karyotypes in the CLL cells are more commonly found at diagnosis than developing during the course of the disease, and are adverse prognostic signs.

A large Danish study of 480 unselected newly diagnosed patients has produced new cytogenetic data in CLL and correlated them with immunophenotypic studies [10]. Of note, 25% of patients were considered to have an atypical immunophenotype. In patients with a typical CLL immunophenotype, chromosomal abnormalities were found in 22%, but they occurred in 48% of those with an atypical phenotype. Isolated trisomy 12 had no apparent prognostic effect, whereas anomalies of chromosome 17, and also multiple cytogenetic abnormalities, both correlated with shorter survival. In a multivariate survival analysis, chromosome 17 abnormalities were the only cytogenetic findings with independent prognostic value irrespective of immunophenotype.

A study by a German group showed improved detection of genomic aberrations when interphase CLL cells are studied by the technique of fluorescence in-situ hybridization (FISH) [11]. Chromosomal aberrations were found in 268 of 325 patients (82%) and patients could be divided into five cytogenetic categories: 17p−, 11q−, 12q trisomy, normal karyotype, and 13q−. The median survival times for patients in these groups were 32, 79, 114, 111, and 133 months, respectively. Patients with 17p− or 11q− had a significantly higher incidence of higher-stage CLL, while those with 13q− had the highest incidence of low-stage disease, so the correlation between cytogenetic and clinical findings was strong. Of special importance in this study is that because dividing cells were not required, all patients could be evaluated.

Despite their undoubted interest and prognostic significance, it has not been unequivocally shown that cytogenetic studies in CLL provide information significantly beyond that which is obtainable from clinically staging the disease (see below). If cytogenetic and immunophenotypic studies can be proved to identify the few poor-prognosis patients contained within a group with low-stage CLL, it will be possible to select these patients for earlier interventions that would not be indicated by the clinical stage alone.

Natural history and prognosis of CLL

General

While it is true that CLL may run a very long and extremely indolent course, there has been a strong tendency to overemphasize the supposedly benign nature of the disease, and to use this as a pretext for undertreatment. While some patients with CLL may live for more than 20 years, will never require treatment for leukemia, and will die from unrelated causes, most patients do far less well than this. The fact that most patients with CLL are elderly and many suffer from multiple medical problems means that in some instances the leukemia will not be the limiting factor in their survival and will not require treatment. However, many elderly people with CLL will die from the disease or its complications, and effective treatment for CLL can be expected to improve both the quality and the duration of life. This is especially so now that overall life expectancy in the elderly has improved significantly. If an elderly patient's life expectancy *without* CLL significantly exceeds their estimated survival *with* a diagnosis of CLL, the leukemia cannot be regarded as inconsequential.

The progression of CLL

Although the rate at which progression occurs is very variable, in almost every case of CLL there is ongoing replication of leukemia cells and the progressive accumulation of long-lived, immunoincompetent CLL cells. This increasing leukemic cell mass can induce *hematopoietic failure* with consequent anemia, thrombocytopenia, neutropenia, and their complications. There is also progressive *immunologic failure*, with deficient humoral and cellular immunity, and *immune dysregulation* with the onset of autoimmune diseases. In very advanced CLL, the *leukemic cell mass* causes problems directly: hypersplenism, compression of vital structures, hypermetabolism, and cachexia. Unless death occurs from an unrelated intercurrent disease, untreated CLL progresses inexorably to a fatal termination, whether this be in 12 months or 20 years.

Transformations of CLL

During its usually lengthy course, CLL may undergo a distinct transformation to a more adverse process; this is much less frequent than the disease evolution that is seen in almost every case of CGL. Transformations of CLL and some neoplastic complications of the disease are listed in Table 24.4. Acceleration of the disease to a more aggressive

Table 24.4. Transformations and complications in chronic lymphocytic leukemia.

Acceleration without morphologic change
Acquisition of multi-drug resistance
Prolymphocytoid acceleration
Richter's syndrome: non-Hodgkin lymphoma
Richter's syndrome: Hodgkin disease
Multiple myeloma
Acute lymphoblastic leukemia
Acute myeloid leukemia
Additional primary cancers

---

phase is relatively common, and its time of onset is unpredictable. The blood lymphocytosis increases rapidly and the lymph nodes, liver, and spleen enlarge progressively. The patient may develop constitutional symptoms, and hematopoietic failure and immunodeficiency appear for the first time, or worsen if already present. Although matters may be improved with a change of treatment, resistance to previously effective drug therapy usually appears and the patient dies from progressive and refractory CLL. In some patients, acceleration of CLL is accompanied by increasing numbers of prolymphocytoid cells in the peripheral blood, and this is termed *prolymphocytoid acceleration* [12]. Although the cells resemble prolymphocytes, their surface immunoglobulin density is low, like that of CLL cells, rather than high as in *de novo* prolymphocytic leukemia. The immunoglobulin type is the same as that of the original CLL cells, from which the prolymphocytoid cells are apparently evolved. Once prolymphocytoid acceleration has occurred, responsiveness to therapy declines and progressive clinical deterioration is the rule. New clinical findings may appear at this stage, for example increasing splenomegaly, soft-tissue masses [13], and malignant ascites and pleural effusion [14].

The evolution of a large-cell non-Hodgkin lymphoma in a patient with CLL was first described in 1928, and bears the eponym *Richter's syndrome* [15]. The literature relating to this development of CLL has recently been reviewed [16]. The clinical features of Richter's syndrome include fever, weight loss, increasing lymphadenopathy, splenomegaly, hepatomegaly, lymphocytopenia, and resistance to both chemotherapy and radiation therapy. Rapid clinical deterioration is the rule; many cases of Richter's syndrome have been diagnosed only at autopsy. This transformation occurs in less than 10% of patients with CLL; it appears to be more frequent in patients with multiple chromosome abnormalities in the CLL cells and a monoclonal gammopathy in the peripheral blood. In the older patient, Richter's syndrome is difficult to treat because aggressive therapies are apt to be poorly tolerated. Although Richter's syndrome usually involves a non-Hodgkin lymphoma, cases of *Hodgkin disease* have been reported. A very rare *myelomatous transformation* of CLL has been reported, with the heavy and light immunoglobulin chains of the myeloma cells identical to those of the original CLL cells [17]. After this transformation survival is reported as short.

Whereas transformation to a picture resembling acute myeloid leukemia occurs in over 75% of patients with CGL, transformation to *acute lymphoblastic leukemia* is seen in less than 1% of patients with CLL [18]. In most cases the lymphoblasts are of L2 morphology. *Acute myeloid leukemia* (AML) appears to occur with increased frequency in patients with CLL, even after adjusting for their older age. It is not thought that the AML is a direct development from the CLL cells. The reason for the association is unclear; whereas treatment of the CLL with ionizing irradiation or the leukemogenic alkylating agent chlorambucil may account for some cases of AML, the two diseases have been observed concurrently in patients with CLL who have never received any treatment. Reports on the occurrence of *additional primary cancers* in patients with CLL are conflicting [17], although Whipham first reported the association in 1878 [19]. Gunz and Angus reported that, except for an increased number of skin cancers, the incidence of other malignant diseases in CLL was not significantly higher [20]. A later study at Roswell Park Memorial Institute indicated an increased incidence of second cancers in patients with CLL; after skin cancers, lung cancer was the

Table 24.5. Immunologic complications of chronic lymphocytic leukemia.

Immunosuppression
    Hypogammaglobulinemia
    Decreased cellular immunity

Immune dysregulation
    Immune hemolytic anemia
    Immune thrombocytopenic purpura
    Immune neutropenia
    Pure red-cell aplasia
    Connective tissue diseases

---

most frequent (14/191 patients) [21]. The confounding effects of age and smoking make firm interpretation of the data difficult, but it seems reasonable to recommend that the physician caring for a patient with CLL should always be attentive to symptoms that might indicate a lung cancer.

Immunologic complications of CLL

The immunologic complications of CLL are outlined in Table 24.5. The *immunosuppression* that is characteristic of this disease is of great clinical importance. Patients with CLL are prone to infections with tuberculosis, yeasts, and other vegetative organisms because of defective cellular immunity, and are also liable to respiratory and other mucosal infections because of defective antibody production. In the older patient with CLL, opportunistic infections are productive of much morbidity and mortality, even when there is no neutropenia. The immunosuppression of CLL is very rarely improved by treatment of the leukemia and may be made worse by it, particularly if severe neutropenia is induced by cytotoxic agents, or the inflammatory response is suppressed by corticosteroids, thus impairing two additional body defenses. *Immune dysregulation* in CLL may be the result of attempts by the immune system to control the neoplastic production of B cells, with resultant exhaustion of the system of regulatory T cells. Immune cytopenias are frequent in CLL and should always be sought when the blood count deteriorates, as they generally respond well to

treatment with glucocorticoid drugs. *Pure red-cell aplasia* is characterized by severe and progressive anemia with reticulocytopenia, a negative Coombs test, and severe hypoplasia or complete absence of red-cell precursors in the bone marrow. This condition usually responds very well to immunosuppressive therapy; it is therefore important to distinguish it from the anemia that results when erythropoiesis is compromised by progression of the CLL itself.

Prognosis of CLL

The survival from diagnosis of patients with B-CLL varies from a few months to over 20 years. For many years the survival of individual patients appeared to be unpredictable, and this made treatment decisions difficult: to treat a patient who is destined to live for years without significant progression of the disease is clearly inappropriate, while to withhold therapy until deterioration is severe is probably leaving things too late. In the absence of reliable indicators of prognosis, recommendations regarding the timing of treatment for CLL were based largely on personal opinions. There existed both "interventionist" and "watch and wait" schools of thought, and the overall results of these approaches were not very different, except that the interventionists treated many patients who would have done as well (or better) had they been left alone. Many studies identified factors that were thought to possess some prognostic significance, and these are summarized in Table 24.6.

Careful study of these factors indicates that some are without prognostic value (e.g., age or sex), while others (e.g., β2-microglobulin, total body potassium) do not provide any information beyond that provided by the clinical stage. Certain other observations (e.g., lymphocyte doubling time, cytogenetics, tritiated thymidine uptake) may provide information that is of independent prognostic value after correction for the stage of disease, but this remains to be proved by a multivariate analysis of a large patient database. The most significant advance in assigning prognoses to patients with CLL was the development of a useful staging system.

Table 24.6. Proposed prognostic factors in chronic lymphocytic leukemia.

Older age	multivariate analysis shows no effect [22]
Sex	multivariate analysis shows no effect [22]
Performance status (PS)	poor PS associated with poor survival [23]
Neutropenia at diagnosis	does not correlate with prognosis [22]
Gammaglobulin	low IgA indicates poor prognosis [24]
Anemia at diagnosis	strong indicator of poor prognosis [25]
Coombs test +	no prognostic effect [26]
Lymphocyte count	poor prognosis over 50×10^9/L [16]
Lymphocyte doubling	short doubling time is adverse [27,28]
Lymphocyte atypia	disputed; atypia possibly adverse [16]
Marrow histology	diffuse CLL infiltrate adverse [16,29]
High serum LDH	not if corrected for stage [16]
Cell phenotype	sIg phenotype not prognostic [16,30]
β2-microglobulin (β2M)	high serum β2M in advanced CLL [31,32]
^{3}H-thymidine uptake	high uptake means early progression [33]
deoxythymidine kinase	elevated serum level: progressive CLL [34]
total body K^+	increases with advancing CLL [35]
cytogenetics	poor prognosis if complex changes [9,10]

Clinical staging of CLL

Endeavors to identify groups of patients with CLL and different prognoses were made in the 1960s by Galton [27], Boggs and his coworkers [36], and Dameshek [37]. Rai and his colleagues devised a five-stage system in 1968 and tested it retrospectively on a series of their own patients and on two published series; they then tested the system prospectively on another group of patients who were at that time undergoing therapy or observation. In all these analyses the Rai staging system proved to be simple and easy to use and accurately predicted the survival

Table 24.7. The Rai system for clinical staging of CLL [38].

Stage	Extent of disease
0	Lymphocytosis in blood and bone marrow
I	Lymphocytosis plus lymphadenopathy (local or generalized, small nodes or bulky)
II	Lymphocytosis plus enlarged spleen and/or liver (nodes may or may not be enlarged)
III	Lymphocytosis plus anemia (Hb <11 g/dL; enlarged nodes, spleen, or liver may or may not be present)
IV	Lymphocytosis plus thrombocytopenia (<100 × 10^9/L; anemia and enlarged nodes, spleen, and liver may or may not be present)

Unlike many other staging systems, a higher stage does not necessarily include all the features of the preceding stage.

Table 24.8. Median survival time according to Rai stage [38].

Clinical stage	Median survival in months
0	>150
I	101
II	71
III	19
IV	19
All patients	71

time of patients with CLL. The system was published in 1975 [38] and is set out in Table 24.7. The survival times that were reported in the original series [38] are shown in Table 24.8; more recent series have shown broadly similar results, although in some the survivals in Stage III and Stage IV are somewhat longer.

From inspection of Table 24.8 it is at once apparent that stage 0 or I CLL is a relatively benign disease and stage III or IV CLL is a life-threatening condition with a prognosis that is only a little better than that of acute leukemia in an adult. Perhaps most importantly, it is seen that stage II CLL – the largest category – has a median survival of under six years and should not be considered in any sense a "benign" disease. This is particularly so in patients whose age and overall health would confer a prognosis of 12, 18, or more years if they did not suffer from CLL.

Other staging systems have been formulated by Binet and his colleagues [22] and by the International Workshop on CLL [39]; they differ from the Rai system in detail but not in principle and they produce similar clinical results. In North America the Rai system is the most widely used.

Management of the older patient with CLL

General principles

In past years the approach to management of CLL varied considerably between different centers and also between individual physicians, and there was no standard policy. The recent advances in clinical staging, and thus in assessing each patient's prognosis, have made it possible to formulate an approach that is more generally accepted.

Younger patients (40–60 years old) with CLL are a special problem because (a) they will almost certainly die of the disease, and (b) they will suffer a major loss of life expectancy because they have developed CLL. In these patients, trials of innovative and aggressive therapies, in the setting of a formal clinical study, should always be considered.

The geriatric oncologist can and should be more conservative for the following reasons. Many patients are asymptomatic at the time of diagnosis, in many the disease will pursue an indolent course for long periods, and the available treatment for elderly patients is palliative rather than curative. Currently there is no demonstrated advantage to the early, as opposed to the later, exhibition of antileukemic drugs in CLL. In very elderly or infirm patients, the diagnosis of CLL may not affect the life expectancy and treatment for CLL could not be expected to produce benefit, although it could still do harm by virtue of its side effects. In asymptomatic patients, who usually will have stage 0, I, or II CLL, it is good practice to observe without treatment, whereas in stage III or IV disease, treatment is generally begun at once. Patients who are observed without treatment may be seen every 6 to 12 weeks; the features that are followed are indicated in Table 24.9.

Table 24.9. Follow-up of an untreated patient with CLL.

Symptoms	Night sweats, fever, weight loss, malaise, infections, declining performance status
Signs	Development of, or change in, enlarged lymph nodes, liver, or spleen
Laboratory	Hemoglobin, platelet count, neutrophil count, lymphocyte doubling time, serum immunoglobulin level, Coombs test, bone-marrow biopsy

The above represents the desirable minimum. Other investigations are done as indicated.

An extremely important factor in the care of the elderly patient with CLL is the provision of a high standard of *general medical care* for any coexisting diseases; the geriatric oncologist is thoroughly familiar with this special aspect of his or her field. Put simply, patients with CLL who receive excellent general care, and frequently no antileukemic therapy, will have a longer duration and a better quality of life than those who do not.

Indications for active treatment

The indications for the institution of active therapy in CLL have been widely discussed [16,40–46]. They are summarized in Table 24.10. Most oncologists would concur with these recommendations, although the threshold for considering that splenomegaly is massive or that lymphadenopathy is bulky must be subject to individual variation.

Some oncologists would add other indications, for example a short lymphocyte doubling time, usually taken as under six months. This indicates progressive disease and the likelihood that the patient's disease will shortly progress to a higher Rai stage. Treatment as soon as rapid doubling of the lymphocyte count is documented may prevent this occurrence, but no formal study has been reported that tests this hypothesis. Han and Rai [16] have recommended active treatment for progressive hyperlymphocytosis, basing their recommendation on three reports of hyperleukocytosis-associated

Table 24.10. Indications for active treatment in CLL.

(1) Significant disease-related symptoms
(2) Anemia or thrombocytopenia due to progressive leukemia (stage III or IV CLL)
(3) Autoimmune hemolysis or thrombocytopenia; pure red-cell aplasia
(4) Progressive massive splenomegaly, with or without hypersplenism
(5) Progressive bulky lymphadenopathy, with or without pressure effects or cosmetic problems
(6) Increasing frequency of bacterial infections

With increasing improvements in treatment, the above conservative indications are becoming outdated.

hyperviscosity syndrome in patients with CLL. They suggest instituting therapy when the total leukocyte count is between 100 and 150×10^9/L. This threshold was set empirically and it seems unlikely that the recommendation will be widely accepted unless a clinical study is done that supports it, since problems with hyperviscosity are rare and treatment for CLL is far from innocuous, particularly in the older patient.

Available treatments for CLL

Over the past half-century, many agents and very numerous schedules of administration have been employed in the management of CLL, and these have been extensively reviewed [16,41–46]. Some regimens are now of mainly historical interest, and only the treatments that are most important in current clinical practice will be considered here. Aggressive therapies that are not appropriate for the older patient – for example, allogeneic bone-marrow transplantation – will not be discussed at length.

Radiation therapy

Since the advent of cytotoxic chemotherapy, radiation therapy has had only a restricted role in the management of CLL. It is no longer employed for the systemic treatment of the disease, but it is of value in the control of local problems [47]. When a patient with CLL has a dominant lymph-node mass that is symptomatic, local irradiation is the palliative

treatment of choice. Response rates to modest doses of radiation (e.g., 15 Gy) approach 100% and local and systemic toxic effects are generally minimal. Usually the dose of radiation administered is much smaller than the doses that are administered when a lymphoma is treated with curative intent, and therefore the same area can be irradiated again at a later date should the lymph-node mass recur. If a patient is receiving chemotherapy but there is a large mass – lymph node, tonsil, or spleen – that is not responding satisfactorily to the chemotherapy, the addition of local irradiation improves the response without significant toxicity. Irradiation of the spleen in CLL usually reduces splenomegaly and sometimes there is an improvement in lymphocytosis, anemia, and thrombocytopenia. However, in many patients the hemoglobin level and platelet count decline significantly, and splenic irradiation must be administered with caution, particularly in patients who have received much chemotherapy.

Allopurinol

The xanthine oxidase inhibitor allopurinol prevents the conversion of xanthine to the less soluble uric acid. When lymphoid malignancies are treated with effective chemotherapy or radiation, massive lysis of tumor tissue sometimes takes place in a very short period, resulting in the production of large amounts of urate. This may lead to renal calculi, or more seriously to urate nephropathy with renal tubular obstruction and renal failure, which is sometimes fatal. When treatment for CLL is begun, good hydration of the patient must be ensured, and consideration should be given to concurrent therapy with allopurinol, 300 mg daily for 21 days, to prevent hyperuricemia and the resultant hyperuricosuria. This is particularly important in the elderly, who are more likely to have reduced renal function. It is also advisable in the presence of bulky disease, or a uric acid level that is elevated *before* therapy, or if there is a history of renal disease or gout. Treatment with allopurinol is generally well tolerated, but occasional patients develop drug-sensitivity rashes which can be very severe.

Table 24.11. The side effects of adrenal corticosteroids.

General	Particularly important in the elderly
Psychosis	Hypertension
Acne	Sodium and water retention
Excessive appetite	Dependent edema
Cutaneous striae	Cardiac failure
Hirsutism	Osteoporosis
Liability to infection	Reactivation of tuberculosis
Obesity	Hyperglycemia, diabetes
Masking of infection	Peptic ulceration
	Hypokalemia
	Hyperuricemia

Adrenal corticosteroids

The adrenal corticosteroids, usually in the form of prednisone, prednisolone, or dexamethasone, are used extensively in the treatment of CLL. They are modestly immunosuppressive and also are potent lympholytic agents, occasionally producing a response so brisk that hyperuricemia results (see above). Unfortunately, steroids produce a galaxy of adverse effects, listed in Table 24.11. Many of these unwanted effects – for example diabetes mellitus, osteoporosis, and hypertension – are particularly serious in older people, who are prone to these conditions even in the absence of corticosteroid therapy. Single-agent treatment with a corticosteroid is indicated when CLL is complicated by autoimmune hemolytic anemia or idiopathic thrombocytopenic purpura (ITP), or when the disease has become unresponsive to other agents. In a previously untreated patient with severe hemopoietic failure, it is common practice to begin therapy with a corticosteroid alone, because these agents can bring about improvement without inducing further myelosuppression. Corticosteroids are frequently administered in combination with an alkylating agent in the management of CLL, although it is questionable if the addition of a steroid actually improves the results when the alkylating agent is administered intensively. Long-term therapy with corticosteroids should be avoided, because the adverse effects (Table 24.11) are much

more frequent and more severe when treatment is given for an extended period.

Intermittent pulses of a corticosteroid, for example 5–7 days per month, even in substantial doses, are better tolerated. *High-dose* corticosteroid therapy, for example methylprednisolone $1 \text{g/m}^2/\text{day}$ by the intravenous route for five days at monthly intervals, is well tolerated and has produced partial remissions with a median duration of eight months (range 6–78 months) in approximately 50% of heavily pretreated patients with refractory CLL [48]. This is a useful stratagem in carefully selected patients.

Androgens and estrogens

Androgens and other anabolic steroids have occasionally been used in CLL when there is bone-marrow failure that has not responded to prednisone with or without an alkylating agent. Improvements in anemia and thrombocytopenia have been reported [49–51], but these agents should be used with caution because most of them are hepatotoxic and they may exacerbate pre-existing prostatic hypertrophy. It is probable that erythropoietin will prove to be more effective than anabolic steroids for improving bone-marrow failure in CLL; clinical studies are currently addressing this question. It is of considerable interest that some patients with CLL and carcinoma of the prostate, treated for the latter condition with diethylstilbestrol, showed rapid reductions in their peripheral blood lymphocytosis [52,53]. Unfortunately, the severe cardiovascular side effects of estrogens are a relative contraindication to their use in an elderly patient with CLL.

Alkylating agents

Many alkylating agents, including nitrogen mustard, triethylenemelamine, busulfan, chlorambucil, and cyclophosphamide, have been used in the treatment of CLL, but only chlorambucil and cyclophosphamide have remained in regular, widespread use [46]. Chlorambucil [27,41,54,55] is reliably absorbed from the gastrointestinal tract, has some selective cytotoxicity for lymphoid cells, and is relatively free of side effects such as nausea, vomiting, alopecia, and cystitis. However, it should not be forgotten that chlorambucil is mutagenic, leukemogenic, and a potent stem-cell poison that can permanently impair the function of the bone marrow. Long-term myelosuppression is particularly likely to occur when low doses of chlorambucil are administered every day for many weeks or months; this is probably also the best way to induce resistance of CLL to the drug, and perhaps is the mode of administration that is most likely to induce AML. Fortunately, in recent years most physicians have adopted a high-dose intermittent schedule for the administration of chlorambucil [56–58]. This schedule is at least as effective as low-dose daily chlorambucil, patient compliance is excellent, and the hematologic toxicity is less: dose reductions are required less frequently than with a daily dosing regimen. This suggests that the dose of chlorambucil on an intermittent regimen could be *escalated* and a higher response rate might be obtained. My practice is to administer chlorambucil at night, in a dose of 20 mg, for 4–7 consecutive nights, at an interval of 28 days, usually beginning with a four-dose course. If tolerance is good, as reflected in serial blood counts, the total dose can be increased, usually by increasing the number of nightly administrations per course. Nausea and vomiting are very rare, and progressive hematologic toxicity is avoided because the substantial interval enables the full effects of each course to be seen before another course is prescribed. A practical point worth noting is that chlorambucil should not be taken with orange juice or other vitamin-C-containing vehicle, as the ascorbic acid is a reducing agent and can inactivate the alkylating agent.

Two randomized trials conducted in France have addressed the value of treatment in indolent (Binet stage A) CLL [59]. In the first study, 609 patients were randomly assigned to receive no treatment or daily chlorambucil, and in the second trial, 926 patients received either no treatment or combined chlorambucil and prednisone in pulses for five days every month. Although 76% of patients in the first trial and 69% in the second trial had a response to therapy, there was no prolongation of survival compared to the patients who were initially observed and received

treatment only if disease progression occurred. In the untreated group in the first trial, 49% of patients did not have progression to more advanced disease and did not need treatment after follow-up of more than 11 years; however 27% of patients with stage A CLL died of causes related to the disease. This important study confirms the relatively good survival of low-stage CLL when untreated, and shows convincingly that early treatment does not improve the prognosis. It appears that the addition of prednisone to treatment with chlorambucil confers no advantage. The failure of early treatment with chlorambucil to improve the overall prognosis suggests that, even when good hematologic responses are obtained, the treatment is ineffective in a biological sense.

While it is well known that the alkylating agents busulfan and cyclophosphamide possess pulmonary toxicity, it is less widely recognized that chlorambucil, also an alkylating agent, can induce severe and sometimes fatal pulmonary fibrosis [60]. The key factor may be that for all of these agents, by virtue of chronic low-dose administration or large intermittent doses, very high total doses are frequently achieved. Elderly patients with reduced lung function are particularly vulnerable to respiratory compromise and thus are at special risk when chlorambucil is administered for long periods to high lifetime doses. Withdrawal of the drug is followed by improvement in some cases. The administration of steroids in high doses is commonly practiced, but there is no compelling evidence of the efficacy of this treatment.

Like other alkylating agents, chlorambucil is mutagenic, and probably leukemogenic and carcinogenic as well. There are numerous instances of chronic bone-marrow failure, AML, or myelodysplasia occurring in patients with CLL after prolonged exposure to chlorambucil; this may be cited as an additional reason not to begin treatment with this agent unnecessarily early. On the other hand, most patients with CLL are of an age when neoplastic diseases, including AML and myelodysplastic syndrome (MDS), are relatively frequent, and it is unreasonable to blame chlorambucil – or other treatment – for all these instances. This is underlined by a recent review in which five men with *untreated*

CLL developed AML (three patients), presented with concurrent AML (one patient), or concurrent MDS (one patient); numerous other cases were cited from the literature [61]. Thus, in patients who have received it, the leukemogenic role of chlorambucil is easily overestimated.

Cyclophosphamide is also widely used in the treatment of CLL. Unlike chlorambucil, cyclophosphamide is available in an intravenous as well as an oral form. It has the disadvantages that it causes alopecia and also hemorrhagic cystitis. This complication, well recognized with high-dose parenteral cyclophosphamide, can also occur with chronic low doses given by mouth [62]. The principal indications for the use of cyclophosphamide in CLL are when chlorambucil is not well tolerated (which is rare) or when a multiple-agent chemotherapeutic regimen is administered.

Multiple-agent regimens

Several multi-drug regimens have been employed in the treatment of CLL. The most frequently used are CVP (cyclophosphamide + vincristine + prednisone) [63], CHOP (cyclophosphamide + doxorubicin [in low dose] + vincristine + prednisone) [63], M-2 (vincristine + carmustine + cyclophosphamide + melphalan + prednisone) [64], and POACH (prednisone + vincristine + cytarabine + cyclophosphamide + doxorubicin) [65]. All of these regimens were originally devised for the treatment of non-Hodgkin lymphoma or myeloma, and they all contain vincristine, a drug that has not shown any single-agent activity in CLL. Since vincristine causes both constipation and peripheral neuropathy, both of which are frequent problems in older people even in the absence of drug therapy, it should be *omitted* from these regimens as a toxic agent of unproved value in CLL. The value of multiple-drug regimens in CLL is controversial. A large French study [63] showed that CVP was more toxic, but no more effective, than single-agent chlorambucil. The same group found that in advanced CLL, the survival of patients who were treated with CHOP was markedly superior to CVP (and possibly to chlorambucil, although this

was not directly tested). The anthracycline antibiotics have not been particularly active as single agents in CLL, and this apparent superior survival with CHOP has not always been confirmed by other workers [46]. In a study of the POACH regimen at the M. D. Anderson Cancer Center [65], 19 of 34 (56%) previously untreated patients responded, with a 21% complete remission rate, while 8 of 31 (26%) previously treated patients responded, with a complete remission rate of 7%. Mortality was very much higher in the previously treated patients. As this was a single-arm study, it is not possible to assess the merits of the POACH regimen relative to other therapies. It is certainly active in CLL, but appears to be dangerous and not very effective for previously treated patients.

Splenectomy

Although splenectomy has been widely studied in CLL [66–70], there have been no formal trials to compare it with systemic chemotherapy or with splenic irradiation. The usual indications for splenectomy are autoimmune hemolysis or autoimmune thrombocytopenia that have responded inadequately to corticosteroids or immunosuppressive drugs, and hypersplenism in the absence of autoimmune disease. Splenectomy has occasionally been performed for the relief of massive, symptomatic splenomegaly. In the older patient a careful evaluation must be made to determine their suitability for general anesthesia and surgery. As with other elective splenectomies, pneumococcal vaccine should be administered before surgery, but the patient with CLL may fail to mount a satisfactory antibody response, and long-term penicillin prophylaxis after splenectomy may be a more effective preventive measure.

Evaluation of response to therapy

Definitions of a complete response to therapy in CLL have been proposed in two sets of guidelines [8,71]. Both require normalization of the peripheral blood and the bone marrow, together with disappearance of symptoms and physical signs of the disease. One group [71] recommends determining by further tests if the complete remission is a "clonal" one, by demonstrating normalization of the T : B cell ratio in the blood and normalization of the kappa : lambda light chain ratio among B cells, and decrease of CD5-positive B cells to less than 25%. The completeness of remission can be tested even further by demonstrating the resolution of markers of the neoplastic clone – idiotype, immunoglobulin gene rearrangement, and chromosomal abnormalities. From the viewpoint of the clinician, the most relevant criteria of response are the relief of symptoms, the correction of physical and hematologic abnormalities, the resolution of any transfusion needs, and freedom from infections. Most important, the patient's *performance status* should improve and be brought as close to normal as the patient's age and the presence of other illnesses permit. In the case of a *partial response*, the *stage of disease* should improve – for example from stage III to stage 0. It seems probable that a patient who is stage 0 as a result of treatment may not have the excellent prognosis of an untreated stage 0 patient: this is a subject for further study.

Modern purine antagonists: fludarabine, cladribine, and pentostatin

Fludarabine

Fludarabine monophosphate is the most recent drug to find a major role in the treatment of CLL, and is the most effective single agent ever to be tested in that disease. It is a purine analog with a substituted fluorine atom that confers resistance to deamination and consequent inactivation by the cellular enzyme adenosine deaminase [72]. Following injection it is dephosphorylated in plasma to form arabinosyl-2-fluoroadenine [73,74]. It is actively taken up by cells and phosphorylated to its 5'-triphosphate, F-ara-ATP, which is the active form of the drug. F-ara-ATP inhibits DNA synthesis by competing with deoxy-ATP for incorporation into DNA, and also by inhibiting ribonucleotide reductase. F-ara-ATP is also incorporated into RNA and is an inhibitor of DNA repair. The major toxicity of fludarabine is myelosuppression; it is well tolerated subjectively, with little nausea or vomiting

and almost no alopecia [75]. In early studies, significant neurotoxicity was encountered, but this occurred at doses approximately four times greater than are now employed [76]. Fludarabine was evaluated in CLL by Grever and his colleagues [77]. Of 22 previously treated patients, 19 showed some response, with one complete remission and three excellent partial remissions. A study by Keating and colleagues in 68 previously treated patients with CLL demonstrated complete remission in 15% and a partial response in 44% [78]. These are astonishingly good results, particularly for previously treated patients, when it is recalled that in previously *untreated* patients who receive chlorambucil and corticosteroids, complete remissions are seen in perhaps 5–10% of patients at best. The major toxic effects associated with fludarabine therapy were myelosuppression and episodes of fever and infection. Ten patients died during the study, seven of them during the first three courses of treatment, and it was clear that this potent agent must be handled with caution.

When a drug performs well in patients with a previously treated neoplastic disease, results are usually even better when the drug is administered to previously untreated patients. Keating and his colleagues [79] administered fludarabine, 30 mg/m^2/day by the intravenous route for five days every four weeks, to 33 previously untreated patients with advanced or progressive CLL. The complete remission rate using the National Cancer Institute's guidelines, which permit the presence of residual lymphoid nodules in the bone marrow, was a remarkable 75%. Six of the 33 patients (18%) failed to respond and three died of infection during the first three cycles of treatment. It is very important to note that all three of these patients were aged over 75 years and all had Rai stage III–IV disease. In a three-year follow-up of this study [80], there were 35 previously untreated patients with a complete remission rate of 74% and partial remissions in 6% of patients, for an overall response rate of 80%. The median duration of response was 33 months. These results are far superior to any that have been reported in previously untreated patients for alkylating agents, with or without corticosteroids or additional cytotoxic drugs.

In another study by the same group, previously treated patients with CLL received fludarabine combined with prednisone [81]. The results of treatment were not better than those obtained with fludarabine alone, but as all the patients had received prednisone previously, this study did not completely rule out any synergistic effect of the drug combination if it were used in untreated patients, but later studies appeared to do so.

Keating and his colleagues have reported on the long-term follow-up of patients with CLL who received fludarabine-based regimens as initial therapy [82]. Three different fludarabine studies were included; patients began treatment between 1986 and 1993 and the results were reported in 1998, with 5–12 years of follow-up in a total of 174 patients with progressive or advanced CLL. The overall response rate was 78% and the median survival was 63 months. No difference in response rate or survival was noted in the 71 patients who received fludarabine as a single agent compared with the 103 patients who received prednisone in addition. The median time to progression of responders was 31 months, and the overall median survival was 74 months. Age over 70 years and disease that was Rai stage III or IV were associated with shorter survival. Over 50% of patients who relapsed after fludarabine therapy responded to salvage treatment, usually with a fludarabine-based regimen. During treatment there was severe suppression of both CD4+ and CD8+ T lymphocytes in the blood, and recovery towards normal levels was slow, but despite this the incidence of infections was low for patients in remission. Richter's syndrome occurred in nine patients, and eight of these died. These results indicate that fludarabine is a potent regimen for initial induction therapy in previously untreated CLL, and the safety profile of the treatment compares well with that of other therapies.

Four randomized studies [83–86] have shown fludarabine to have a higher response rate than chlorambucil, CAP (cyclophosphamide + doxorubicin + prednisone), or French CHOP (cyclophosphamide + low-dose doxorubicin + vincristine + prednisone). Treatment with fludarabine yields higher response rates than chlorambucil and a longer duration of remission and progression-free survival, but no overall survival advantage has as yet been demonstrated. When fludarabine was compared with chlorambucil and with CAP, there was no increase in toxicity or early death when fludarabine was given as initial therapy.

Combinations of fludarabine with other agents

It is important to determine if combination with other agents can increase the effectiveness of fludarabine. The combination of cyclophosphamide and fludarabine induced complete responses in 3/6 patients with CLL, despite unsatisfactory responses to fludarabine alone [87]; this combination merits further evaluation. A randomized controlled trial of fludarabine versus chlorambucil versus fludarabine with chlorambucil in previously untreated patients with CLL showed that single-agent fludarabine was superior to single-agent chlorambucil, while the combination of the two drugs was not superior to fludarabine alone and was more toxic, leading to the closure of that arm of the study [87]. In Germany the combination of fludarabine with epirubicin was studied in 44 patients; of the 38 patients who were evaluable for response, 25 were previously untreated [88]. For the whole group the overall response rate was 82%, with 32% complete remissions; for the untreated patients the corresponding figures were 92% and 40%. These results do not definitely indicate superiority of the regimen to single-agent fludarabine, but they might justify a randomized trial of the two treatments. In a small non-randomized study in previously untreated patients with CLL, induction therapy with fludarabine was followed by consolidation with high-dose cyclophosphamide [89]. Before the consolidation 16% of patients achieved a complete or a nodular complete response in the bone marrow, and following consolidation this fraction increased threefold to 48%. These interesting results require confirmation, and might not apply to older patients, as all the participants in this study were aged less than 69 years.

There is much scope for further therapeutic studies in CLL. With the advent of fludarabine, should the value of earlier treatment be reappraised? Is there a place for maintenance therapy with fludarabine? Is there an optimal combination – and sequencing – for administering fludarabine and an alkylating agent as combined therapy? The National Cancer Institute has sponsored revised guidelines for diagnosis and treatment of CLL [90], and further revisions are to be expected.

Cladribine

The purine analog cladribine (2-chlorodeoxyadenosine) has demonstrable activity in CLL, including refractory cases, but does not appear to be as effective as fludarabine [46]. Recently, a European group reported their experience with patients aged 70 years and older with CLL that was untreated (33 patients) or relapsed (10 patients) [91]. They received a median of three 5-day courses of cladribine and 13 (30%) had a complete response, Only one previously treated patient responded, but with the small numbers there was no significant difference between the groups. No patient had received fludarabine as previous treatment. Thrombocytopenia and infection were frequent and six patients (14%) died. This study shows that cladribine is active in CLL but does not suggest that it is as effective or as safe as fludarabine.

Pentostatin

The anti-tumor antibiotic 2′-deoxycoformycin, or pentostatin, is an antagonist of adenosine deaminase and an intensely lymphocytotoxic purine antagonist. Pentostatin has demonstrable activity in CLL, including refractory cases [92], but does not appear to be as active as fludarabine [46]. A British group evaluated pentostatin in 29 patients with relapsed or refractory B-CLL [93]. Their ages ranged from 44 to 74, with a median of 60; thus they were younger than the average patient with CLL. Seventeen had received purine analogs (16 fludarabine, 1 cladribine). Pentostatin was administered as a daily bolus injection in a substantial dose ($2\,mg/m^2/day$ for 5 days). Of 24 patients who were evaluable for efficacy, two had a complete response (neither had previously received a purine analog) and five had a partial response (three had received a purine analog). Pentostatin in this schedule demonstrated salvage activity in previously treated patients with CLL and was not always cross-resistant with other purine analogs.

Complications of fludarabine therapy

Apart from corticosteroids, all the potent chemotherapeutic agents that are administered for CLL are *myelosuppressive*, and fludarabine is no exception. Thrombocytopenia and hemorrhage, and neutropenia and infection, are regular hazards, particularly when marrow function is significantly compromised before treatment is begun. These complications are more serious, and more frequently fatal, in the older patient with multiple medical problems.

Fludarabine also has a more unusual adverse effect: *autoimmune hemolytic anemia* or AIHA [94–97]. This can arise *de novo*, or as a recurrence or exacerbation of a previously diagnosed condition. It appears that patients with known AIHA may be more prone to this complication of treatment with fludarabine than other patients with CLL. The condition usually responds to corticosteroid therapy. A suggested mechanism for AIHA in this setting is the severe suppression of T cells that is induced by fludarabine; the inhibition of autoregulatory suppressor cells that maintain tolerance may trigger autoimmune hemolysis [96–98].

Since fludarabine antagonizes adenosine deaminase, there is accumulation of deoxyadenosine in erythrocytes during treatment with fludarabine; this damages the cells and may make them more susceptible to autoimmune destruction, thus accentuating a pre-existing process. A further possibility, that applies to other therapies also – e.g., chlorambucil – is that the myelotoxic activity of chemotherapeutic agents can simply *unmask* AIHA (rather than causing it) by suppressing the compensatory augmentation of erythropoiesis that may conceal the hemolytic process. It follows that before beginning fludarabine, or other cytotoxic therapy, in a patient with CLL, it is advisable to order a Coombs test, reticulocyte count, and serum folate level, to exclude the presence of AIHA.

The *tumor lysis syndrome* (TLS) of hyperuricemia, hyperkalemia, hypocalcemia, and frequently renal failure, has been anecdotally reported in patients with CLL after fludarabine therapy [99], but a study of 6137 patients with CLL who received fludarabine on a National Cancer Institute Group C protocol [100] disclosed only 20 patients (0.33%) with clinical and laboratory features of TLS; four died of renal failure and four of infection or congestive heart failure. Thus TLS is a rare complication of fludarabine therapy but is frequently fatal. Advanced CLL, organomegaly, and a high pretreatment WBC appeared to be risk factors for TLS.

There are isolated reports of AML or myelodysplasia arising in patients with CLL after treatment with fludarabine [101,102], but such instances are rare, and since *untreated* CLL has been associated with AML and also with MDS [103] the fludarabine treatment may not be to blame.

The current place of fludarabine in the therapy of CLL

If a patient cannot be entered into a formal therapeutic study, and an accepted indication for active treatment exists, should fludarabine be used as first-line therapy in previously untreated CLL? Although there is no universal agreement, I believe that on current evidence the answer is *yes*. This opinion is based on the high response rate (80–90%) and the extremely high incidence of complete remission (up to 75%), together with evidence of a remission duration that approaches three years and a median survival exceeding seven years. These results so far exceed those that are obtained with chlorambucil, with or without prednisone, or the more toxic anthracycline-containing regimens, that it may be a disservice to the patient *not* to administer fludarabine. My policy is to administer $25\,mg/m^2/day$ as a 30-minute intravenous infusion, daily for three days on the first occasion, and to repeat the treatment every four weeks, increasing its duration to four or five days if it is well tolerated. This cautious approach is appropriate for the elderly patient, particularly if the pretreatment blood count is poor, if comorbid

conditions are present, or if there is already a history of opportunistic infections.

Further support for the use of fludarabine as first-line therapy in CLL comes from the finding of a 64% response rate in patients with advanced CLL and genetic aberrations of the p53 protein, which have been associated with non-response to other therapies and short survival [104].

The merits of fludarabine are not beyond question. One comparison of fludarabine with conventional alkylating agent regimens found that fludarabine increases the incidence of complete response but does not increase survival [105].

Concern has been expressed about the responsiveness of CLL to salvage therapy after relapse in patients who receive fludarabine as initial therapy, but it has now been shown that most patients achieve a second remission, particularly if they achieved a complete remission with their first exposure to the drug [82].

Drug resistance in CLL

Like many other neoplastic diseases that respond well to initial chemotherapy, CLL frequently demonstrates the development of secondary resistance to previously effective drugs, evidenced by a failure of clinical and hematologic response. Although the patient whose disease has become refractory to alkylating agents and corticosteroids may in the short term do well with fludarabine as salvage therapy, the onset of drug resistance is always an ominous event that indicates a deteriorating prognosis. Further, CLL shows *primary* resistance to many drugs that are valuable in the chemotherapy of other diseases, for example methotrexate, vincristine, etoposide, and doxorubicin. The mechanisms of drug resistance in CLL have recently been reviewed [106]. Resistance to methotrexate and several other antimetabolite drugs that are specifically active in the S phase of the cell cycle appears to be attributable to the very low proliferative fraction in populations of CLL cells. Resistance to fludarabine, also an antimetabolite drug but for uncertain reasons active in CLL despite the low mitotic index, is mediated by loss of enzymes that activate the drug. Resistance to chlorambucil and other alkylating agents appears to be due to enhanced mechanisms for repair of DNA and for the intracellular neutralization of alkylating molecules, while refractoriness to adrenal corticosteroids is associated with loss of the cellular receptors for these agents. Resistance to etoposide and doxorubicin may be due to the low expression of topoisomerase II, a major target of these drugs, in CLL cells [107] and/or to overexpression of the multi-drug resistance gene, *mdr1* [108]. Activation of mdr1 leads to synthesis of the glycoprotein gp-170, which acts as an efflux pump, removing the drugs from the intracellular environment. Studies of compounds – e.g., cyclosporine analogs, PSC-833 – that may reverse multiple drug resistance are in progress but these agents have not yet had a significant impact on hematologic practice. Numerous other measures to circumvent drug resistance in CLL have been proposed [106] but have not yet found a place in clinical practice.

There are several techniques for evaluating the activity of mdr1 in vitro, including the measurement of drug efflux and the assay of gp-170 with monoclonal antibodies [109]. The expression of gp-170 is more frequent with advancing stage but not with prior alkylating agent therapy. The functional expression of gp-170 increases with higher stage and previous treatment with agents of biological origin, e.g., vincristine and doxorubicin.

Sensitivity of CLL cells to fludarabine can be measured in vitro by the differential staining cytotoxicity (DiSC) assay [110]. Resistance to fludarabine was found in cells from 12/100 (12%) untreated patients and 45/143 (31%) patients who had received prior therapy, excluding fludarabine. Resistance was found in cells from 17/32 (53%) patients who had been treated with fludarabine. The clinical correlation of these tests was excellent: fludarabine was effective in 69% of patients whose cells were sensitive by DiSC assay, and in only 7% of those whose cells tested resistant. Of note, 81% of fludarabine-test-resistant patients were test-sensitive to other agents. The DiSC assay makes it possible to withhold fludarabine from patients who have a low likelihood of responding to it, thus saving the expense and toxic effects of an ineffective therapy and giving the patient the opportunity to receive an alternative and more effective therapy.

Management of autoimmune complications of CLL

Anemia in CLL always requires careful evaluation. It may be due to bone-marrow compromise induced by the disease, in which case the patient has stage III disease and an anticipated median survival of less than two years. The anemia may also be due to coexisting unrelated conditions, for example deficiencies of iron, vitamin B_{12}, or folate, gastrointestinal bleeding, or chronic diseases such as rheumatoid arthritis. All of these conditions are more frequent in the older patient. Finally, anemia may be due to AIHA; this is associated with the leukemia but does not make the patient's disease stage III. In such cases the direct antiglobulin (Coombs) test is usually positive and there is a reticulocytosis. It is not uncommon for active hemolysis to be complicated by folate deficiency because of the increased folate consumption, in which case macrocytosis may be observed and reticulocytosis may be suppressed. ITP also occurs in CLL and is less serious than the thrombocytopenia of bone-marrow failure; it does not make the patient's disease stage IV. The demonstration of antiplatelet antibodies is not a well-standardized test, and at many centers the diagnosis of ITP depends upon the finding of thrombocytopenia with adequate or increased megakaryocytes in the bone marrow (but this may not be the case if there is heavy marrow infiltration with CLL), and a response to corticosteroid therapy. AIHA and ITP may occur together (Evans syndrome). AIHA and ITP are usually treated with prednisone (100 mg/day) or dexamethasone (16 mg/day); these high doses can be tapered as soon as a response is seen. In the older patient it is wise to administer an H2-blocking drug (e.g., ranitidine) concurrently with the corticosteroid, and many would add anticandida prophylaxis with fluconazole. In the patient with AIHA, folate supplementation is recommended while there is active hemolysis. If the response to steroid therapy is inadequate, or only occurs at an unacceptably high dose that cannot be continued long-term, high-dose intravenous immunoglobulin should be added: 400 mg/kg/day for five days and then maintenance with the same daily dose administered once every 21 days. In occasional patients, splenectomy is necessary for the control of AIHA or ITP, and this operation carries increased risks in the older patient. Overall, the prognosis of patients with AIHA or ITP who respond to prednisone therapy is better than that of patients with anemia or thrombocytopenia that are due to stage III and stage IV CLL respectively. Many patients may also require chemotherapy for active CLL in addition to treatment for AIHA or ITP. It should be remembered that the administration of chlorambucil or other myelotoxic drugs may exacerbate the anemia of AIHA because any compensatory increase in erythropoiesis is suppressed. The rare autoimmune condition of pure red-cell aplasia (PRCA) is occasionally seen in CLL, and may be treated with corticosteroid, with or without the addition of cyclosporine.

Supportive care in CLL

Anemia in a patient with CLL, if due to the leukemia itself and not to hematinic factor deficiencies, blood loss, or chronic disease, is best treated by controlling the CLL and improving the function of the bone marrow. The transfusion of packed red blood cells is valuable during initial therapy, and also for patients whose erythrocyte production is not restored by treating the leukemia. Treatment with erythropoietin improves hemoglobin levels in some patients with CLL but it is not certain that this treatment is cost-effective when compared to transfusion, and in some patients it fails outright. Platelet transfusion in CLL is indicated only for hemorrhage, as it is in any chronic thrombocytopenic state.

For many years immunoglobulin replacement therapy has been employed empirically in patients with CLL for the prevention of infection, but it was only recently that a randomized, placebo-controlled study demonstrated conclusively that this therapy provides highly effective prophylaxis [111]. The recommended dose is 400 mg/kg, administered intravenously once every 21 days. This treatment is very expensive and should only be administered to a patient with CLL if there is hypogammaglobulinemia and a history of repeated infections. As patients with CLL frequently suffer from neutropenia, an excess of suppressor T cells over T helper cells, and deficient natural killer cells, immunoglobulin replacement is unlikely to fully restore immunocompetence. Infections in patients with CLL should be investigated aggressively and treated vigorously, and the physician must be alert to the possibility of infection with tuberculosis, or with unusual organisms, particularly yeasts and fungi [112].

Innovative treatment strategies for CLL

The introduction of fludarabine is the most significant advance in the management of CLL in four decades, but although fludarabine induces a high proportion of complete remissions in previously untreated patients with CLL, it has not demonstrated a potential for curing the disease. When patients with CLL become refractory to fludarabine, there is no fully accredited alternative therapy of comparable effectiveness, so there is a pressing need for further advances in treatment. Several innovative treatment strategies are under investigation [113,114]. Treatment with *monoclonal antibodies* (MoAbs) has been extensively studied in patients with CLL. Passive immunotherapy with *unconjugated* MoAbs turned out to be relatively safe but the clinical responses were minor in degree and usually transient, so this did not appear to be an effective treatment. A logical extension of MoAb therapy was to give the antibodies a warhead by conjugating them with *immunotoxins* before their administration. Studies have been carried out with single-chain immunotoxins – usually the A chain of ricin – and with two-chain immunotoxins consisting of ricin A and B chains but with the nonspecific galactose-binding sites of ricin blocked. These compounds have shown major activity against CLL cells in vitro, but clinical experience thus far is limited and responses have been relatively minor. Clinical studies are in progress with a *fusion protein* that has been produced by recombinant DNA technology, in which the receptor-binding domain of diphtheria toxin is replaced by the sequences of human interleukin 2 [113]. These compounds have significant anti-tumor activity but also significant toxicity, including elevated hepatic transaminases, hypoalbuminemia, fever, chest tightness, rashes, increased serum creatinine, and thrombocytopenia, and clearly would have to be administered with great caution in the older patient. Studies have also been done with *radioimmunoconjugates*, in which a MoAb is coupled to a radionuclide, ^{32}P or ^{131}I. By binding to CLL cells in the bone marrow as well as the peripheral blood, these compounds deliver radiation not only to their intended targets, but also to normal cells in the bone marrow, and myelosuppression results. Overall, MoAbs that are armed with immunotoxins or radionuclides do possess significant activity against CLL cells but their place – if any – in therapy is undetermined. Possibly they may be of value for the eradication of minimal residual disease – for example, after a complete remission has been obtained with fludarabine or other intensive chemotherapy.

Recent studies with two monoclonal antibodies, rituximab (anti-CD20) and alemtuzumab (anti-CD52) suggest that these more recent additions to the therapeutic armamentarium are capable of palliating CLL even after the onset of resistance to chemotherapeutic agents [114,115]. Although alemtuzumab is effective in fludarabine-refractory CLL, the treatment is associated with neutropenia and infection. In a recent study of 14 patients with refractory CLL, filgrastim was administered before and during treatment with alemtuzumab [116]. Both early (5/14) and delayed (4/14) neutropenia were observed, and reactivation of CMV infection occurred in six patients, with one death. There were five partial responses of CLL, but nine patients ceased treatment because of infection and hematologic toxicity; thus filgrastim did not render treatment with alemtuzumab safe.

Novel drug therapies continue to be studied in CLL. The macrocyclic lactone bryostatin 1 has shown activity in low-grade lymphoid neoplasms, and in patients with CLL has induced differentiation of the CLL cells to a hairy-cell phenotype [117]. A randomized study in 229 patients with untreated CLL compared cladribine + prednisone with chlorambucil + prednisone [118]. The rates of complete remission and of overall response were significantly higher in patients who received cladribine (47% and 87%, respectively) than in the patients who received chlorambucil (12% and 57%, respectively). Unfortunately, this higher rate of response did not translate into an improved overall survival for those who received cladribine. The apoptosis-inducing compound flavopiridol has demonstrated modest, schedule-dependent clinical activity in relapsed CLL and merits further investigation [119]. Advances in the use of monoclonal antibodies and novel drugs in the treatment of CLL have recently been reviewed [120,121].

Allogeneic transplantation of bone marrow (ABMT) or peripheral-blood stem cells (APBSCT) is generally felt to be too hazardous, or indeed lethal, for the older (over 70 years) patient with CLL. ABMT from unrelated donors has been described in a series of 38 younger patients with CLL [122]. The patients' median age was 45 years (range 26–57 years). After myeloablative therapy that included total-body irradiation the patients received bone marrow from matched unrelated donors. Prophylaxis against graft-versus-host disease (GVHD) consisted of methotrexate with cyclosporine or tacrolimus. Complete response was seen in 58% of patients, and partial response in 17%. Grade 2–4 acute GVHD occurred in 45% of patients at 100 days and chronic GVHD in 85% at five years. Failure-free survival was 30% at five years and treatment-related mortality was 38%. The data demonstrated that ABMT can secure lasting remissions in CLL, but the cost in terms of morbidity and mortality is very high, even in this selected group of unusually young patients with CLL.

Autologous stem-cell transplantation (ASCT) has fewer complications and is undergoing evaluation. A French group [123] has studied ASCT as salvage therapy in patients with refractory or relapsed CLL. Patients aged up to 66 years received intensive chemotherapy to induce remission and ASCT as consolidation treatment. Only 8/20 (40%) patients were able to complete the protocol, either because a new remission was not obtained or because not enough stem cells could be collected. Six of the eight grafted patients were alive and in complete clinical remission a median of 30 months after ASCT. The eight transplanted patients were aged 54 to 63 years, and these promising results cannot be extrapolated with confidence to patients aged over 70 years.

If ASCT is useful for salvage therapy it can be expected to be more effective when used earlier in the course of CLL, and a German group has tested this in 18 patients aged 29 to 61 years [124]. Only four patients had received no treatment, and 16 had recognized adverse prognostic features. Initial chemotherapy was followed by stem-cell harvesting, intensive chemotherapy and radiotherapy, and ASCT. Thirteen of 18 patients (72%) underwent ASCT and achieved complete remission; one relapsed at 36 months and 12 remained in remission at 12 to 48 months after ASCT. These early results are of great interest, particularly the absence of procedure-related deaths. If longer follow-up shows durable complete remissions, the procedure could be considered – as a formal randomized study – for carefully selected older patients with recently diagnosed CLL and poor prognostic features.

Transplantation with autologous peripheral-blood stem cells is increasingly practiced in patients with CLL who are in first remission after treatment with fludarabine. Unfortunately, the yield of stem cells is frequently poor after treatment with fludarabine. A recent study of stem-cell harvests after mobilization with cyclophosphamide and filgrastim showed a satisfactory yield in 23/56 (41%) patients [125]. Successful mobilization was associated with a longer interval from the last chemotherapy (>2 months). The harvest result was not affected by the number of fludarabine cycles.

Chemoimmunotherapy

It is logical to combine effective chemotherapeutic agents with monoclonal antibodies of proven efficacy in hope of securing an enhanced response. The combination of fludarabine, cyclophosphamide, and rituximab (FCR) has been studied in 177 patients with relapsed and refractory CLL [126]. The results were striking: 25% complete remission, 16% nodular partial remission, 32% partial remission, overall response rate 73%. Moreover, 12 (32%) of 37 complete responders who were tested had achieved a molecular remission in the bone marrow. The complete remission rate was exceptionally high for a group of previously treated patients.

As previously observed, regimens that are effective in relapsed patients frequently are even more effective in previously untreated patients. Keating and his colleagues administered the FCR combination to 224 previously untreated patients with advanced or progressive CLL [127]. The complete remission rate was 70%, nodular partial remission 10%, partial remission 15%, overall response rate 95%. Two-thirds of patients evaluated by flow cytometry after treatment had no detectable disease. The projected failure-free rate is 69% at four years. Two caveats apply to these very promising results: the median age of the patients was only 58 years, and only 33% had Rai stage III–IV disease. The results of long-term follow-up of the patients in this study will be of great interest.

Conclusion

CLL in the older person presents the geriatric hematologist–oncologist with many problems. Curative therapy with allogeneic bone-marrow transplantation is seldom an option for these patients, who cannot tolerate the severe morbidity of such intensive treatment. Similarly, intensive chemotherapy at levels below those used for transplantation is hazardous in the older patient and the risk increases with advancing age. Tolerance to many drugs, particularly anthracyclines and corticosteroids, is poor in older patients. The presence of multiple medical problems, particularly chronic degenerative diseases, complicates the care of many patients.

The correct approach is that which prevails in all of geriatric medicine – a detailed *global* assessment of each patient, careful attention to *all* of the patient's problems, and the assignment of a *priority* to the chronic leukemia in terms of its importance in the overall picture of performance status and life expectancy for that individual. That done, the individual and the leukemia are treated with the best skills, compassion, and insight that can be marshaled by the physician for the patient's benefit. We are singularly fortunate to be in an era when our ability to help the patient with CLL is already very great, and continues to increase year upon year.

REFERENCES

1. Quaglino D, Di Leonardo G, Furia N, *et al.* Therapeutic management of hematological malignances in elderly patients. Biological and clinical considerations. *Aging Clin Exp Res* 1997; **9**: 303–90.

2. Linet MS, Devesa SS. Descriptive epidemiology of the leukemias. In Henderson ES, Lister TA, eds, *Leukemia*, 5th edn (Philadelphia, PA: Saunders, 1990), 207–24.

3. Linet MS. *The Leukemias: Epidemiologic Aspects* (New York, NY: Oxford University Press, 1985).

4. Samuels LE, Kaufman MS, Morris RJ, *et al.* Open heart surgery in patients with chronic lymphocytic leukemia. *Leukemia Res* 1999; **23**: 71–5.

5. Baer MR, Stein RS, Dessypris EN. Chronic lymphocytic leukemia with hyperleukocytosis. The hyperviscosity syndrome. *Cancer* 1985; **56**: 2865–9.

6. Cash J, Fehir KM, Pollack MS. Meningeal involvement in early stage chronic lymphocytic leukemia. *Cancer* 1987; **59**: 798–800.

7. Case records of the Massachusetts General Hospital (Case 45-1988). *N Engl J Med* 1988; **319**: 1268.

8. Cheson BD, Bennett JM, Rai KR, *et al.* Guidelines for clinical protocols for chronic lymphocytic leukemia (CLL). Recommendations of the NCI-Sponsored Working Group. *Am J Hematol* 1988; **29**: 152–63.

9. Juliusson G, Gahrton G. Chromosome abnormalities in B-cell chronic lymphocytic leukemia. In Cheson BD, ed, *Chronic Lymphocytic Leukemia* (New York, NY: Dekker, 1993), 83–103.

10. Geisler CH, Philip P, Christensen BE, *et al.* In B-cell chronic lymphocytic leukaemia chromosome 17

11. Dohner H, Stilgenbauer S, Benner A, *et al.* Genomic aberrations and survival in chronic lymphocytic leukemia. *N Engl J Med* 2000; **343**: 1910–16.

12. Enno A, Catovsky D, O'Brien M, *et al.* "Prolymphocytoid" transformation of chronic lymphocytic leukemia. *Br J Haematol* 1979; **41**: 9–18.

13. Gujral S, Jain P, Bhutani M, *et al.* Prolymphocytic transformation in chronic lymphocytic leukemia presenting as bilateral periorbital swelling. *Am J Hematol* 1998; **58**: 98–9.

14. Shimoni A, Shvidel L, Shtalrid M, *et al.* Prolymphocytic transformation of B-chronic lymphocytic leukemia presenting as malignant ascites and pleural effusion. *Am J Hematol* 1998; **59**: 316–18.

15. Richter MN. Generalized reticular cell sarcoma of lymph nodes associated with lymphatic leukemia. *Am J Path* 1928; **4**: 285.

16. Han T, Rai KR. Chronic lymphocytic leukemia. In Henderson ES, Lister TA, eds, *Leukemia*, 5th edn (Philadelphia, PA: Saunders, 1990), 565–611.

17. Fermand JP, James JM, Herait P, *et al.* Associated chronic lymphocytic leukemia and multiple myeloma: origin from a single clone. *Blood* 1985; **66**: 291–3.

18. Laurent G, Gourdin MF, Flandrin G, *et al.* Acute blast crisis in a patient with chronic lymphocytic leukemia: immunoperoxidase study. *Acta Haematol* 1981; **65**: 60–6.

19. Whipham T. Splenic leukemia with carcinoma. *Trans Path Soc London* 1878; **29**: 313.

20. Gunz FW, Angus HB. Leukemia and cancer in the same patient. *Cancer* 1965; **18**: 145–52.

21. Moayeri H, Han T, Stutzman L, *et al.* Second neoplasms with chronic lymphocytic leukemia. *NY State J Med* 1976; **76**: 378–81.

22. Binet JL, Auquier A, Dighiero G, *et al.* A new prognostic classification of chronic lymphocytic leukemia derived from a multivariate survival analysis. *Cancer* 1981; **48**: 198–206.

23. Zippin C, Cutler SJ, Reeves WJ, *et al.* Survival in chronic lymphocytic leukemia. *Blood* 1973; **42**: 367–76.

24. Rozman C, Montserrat E, Vinolas N. Serum immunoglobulins in B-chronic lymphocytic leukemia. Natural history and prognostic significance. *Cancer* 1988; **61**: 279–83.

25. Rundles RW, Moore JO. Chronic lymphocytic leukemia. *Cancer* 1978; **42**: 941–5.

26. Hansen MM. Chronic lymphocytic leukemia clinical studies based on 189 cases followed for a long time. *Scand J Haematol Suppl* 1973; **18**: 1–286.

27. Galton DAG. The pathogenesis of chronic lymphocytic leukemia. *Can Med Assoc J* 1966; **94**: 1005–10.

28. Vinolas N, Reverter JC, Urbano-Ispizua A, *et al.* Lymphocyte doubling time in chronic lymphocytic leukemia: an update of its prognostic significance. *Blood Cells* 1987; **12**: 457–70.

29. Han T, Barcos M, Emrich L, *et al.* Bone marrow infiltration patterns and their prognostic significance in chronic lymphocytic leukemia: correlations with clinical, immunologic, phenotypic, and cytogenetic data. *J Clin Oncol* 1984; **6**: 562–70.

30. Baldini L, Mozzana R, Cortelezzi A, *et al.* Prognostic significance of immunoglobulin phenotype in B cell chronic lymphocytic leukemia. *Blood* 1985; **65**: 340–4.

31. Shatt B, Child JA, Karrgish SM, *et al.* Behaviour of serum beta 2-microglobulin and acute phase reactant proteins in chronic lymphocytic leukaemia. *Acta Haematol* 1980; **64**: 73.

32. Simonsson B, Wiw L, Nilsson K. Beta 2-microglobulin in chronic lymphocytic leukaemia. *Scand J Haematol* 1980; **24**: 174–80.

33. Juliusson G, Karl-Henrik R, Nilsson B, *et al.* Prognostic value of B-cell mitogen-induced and spontaneous thymidine uptake in vitro in chronic B-lymphocytic leukaemia cells. *Br J Haematol* 1985; **60**: 429–36.

34. Kallander CFR, Simonsson B, Hagberg H, *et al.* Serum deoxythymidine kinase gives prognostic information in chronic lymphocytic leukemia. *Cancer* 1984; **54**: 2450–5.

35. Chandra P, Sawitsky A, Chanana AD, *et al.* Correlation of total body potassium and leukemic cell mass in patients with chronic lymphocytic leukemia. *Blood* 1979; **53**: 594–603.

36. Boggs DR, Sofferman SA, Wintrobe MM, *et al.* Factors influencing the duration of survival of patients with chronic lymphocytic leukemia. *Am J Med* 1966; **40**: 243–54.

37. Dameshek W. Chronic lymphocytic leukemia – an accumulative disease of immunologically incompetent lymphocytes. *Blood* 1967; **29**: 566–84.

38. Rai KR, Sawitsky A, Cronkite EP, *et al.* Clinical staging of chronic lymphocytic leukemia. *Blood* 1975; **46**: 219–34.

39. International Workshop on CLL. Proposal for a revised prognostic staging system. *Br J Haematol* 1981; **48**: 365–7.

40. Spiers ASD. Chronic lymphocytic leukemia. In Gunz FW, Henderson ES, eds, *Leukemia*, 4th edn (New York, NY: Grune & Stratton, 1983), 709–40.

41. Rai KR, Sawitsky A, Jagathambal K, *et al.* Chronic lymphocytic leukemia. *Med Clin North Am* 1984; **68**: 697–711.

42. Sawitsky A, Rai KR. The chronic lymphoid leukaemias. In Whittaker JA, ed, *Leukaemia*, 2nd edn (Oxford: Blackwell, 1992), 468–94.

43. Rai KR. An outline of clinical management of chronic lymphocytic leukemia. In Cheson BD, ed, *Chronic Lymphocytic Leukemia* (New York, NY: Dekker, 1993), 241–51.

44. Digheiro G, Binet JL. When and how to treat chronic lymphocytic leukemia. *N Engl J Med* 2000; **343**: 1799–801.

45. Kalil N, Cheson BD. Management of chronic lymphocytic leukemia. *Drugs Aging* 2000; **16**: 9–27.

46. Keating MJ. Chemotherapy of chronic lymphocytic leukemia. In Cheson BD, ed, *Chronic Lymphocytic Leukemia* (New York, NY: Dekker, 1993), 297–336.

47. Kempin S, Shank B. Radiation in chronic lymphocytic leukemia. In Gale RP, Rai KR. eds, *Chronic Lymphocytic Leukemia: Recent Progress and Future Direction*. UCLA Symposia on Molecular and Cellular Biology, new series, Vol. 59 (New York, NY: Liss, 1987), 337.

48. Thornton PD, Hamblin M, Treleaven JG, *et al.* High dose methyl prednisolone in refractory chronic lymphocytic leukemia. *Leuk Lymphoma* 1999; **34**: 167–70.

49. Kennedy BJ. Androgenic hormone therapy in lymphatic leukemia. *JAMA* 1964; **190**: 1130–3.

50. Presant CA, Safdar SH. Oxymethalone in myelofibrosis and chronic lymphocytic leukemia. *Arch Intern Med* 1973; **132**: 175–8.

51. West WO. The treatment of bone marrow failure with massive androgen therapy. *Ohio State Med J* 1965; **61**: 347.

52. Narasimhan P, Amaral L. Lymphopenic response of patients presenting with chronic lymphocytic leukemia associated with carcinoma of the prostate to diethylstilbestrol: correlation of response to the in vitro synthesis of RNA by patient lymphocytes and its relationship to transcortin. *Am J Hematol* 1980; **8**: 369–75.

53. Narasimhan P, Glasberg S. Responses to diethylstilbestrol in a patient with refractory chronic lymphatic leukemia associated with non-Hodgkin's lymphoma

(Richter's syndrome). In *Proceedings of the Second International Congress on Hormones and Cancer* (New York, NY: Pergamon Press, 1983), abstract.

54. Galton DAG, Israel LG, Nabarro JDN, *et al*. Clinical trials of p(di-2-chloroethylamino)-phenylbutyric acid (CB1348) in malignant lymphoma. *Br Med J* 1955; **2**: 1172–6.

55. Han T, Ezdinli EZ, Shimaoka K, *et al*. Chlorambucil vs. combined chlorambucil-corticosteroid therapy in chronic lymphocytic leukemia. *Cancer* 1973; **31**: 502–8.

56. Huguley CM Jr. Treatment of chronic lymphocytic leukemia. *Cancer Treat Rev* 1977; **4**: 261–73.

57. Knospe WH, Loeb V Jr, Huguley CM Jr. Biweekly chlorambucil treatment of chronic lymphocytic leukemia. *Cancer* 1974; **33**: 555–62.

58. Sawitsky A, Rai KR, Glidewell O, *et al*. Comparison of daily versus intermittent chlorambucil and prednisone therapy in the treatment of patients with chronic lymphocytic leukemia. *Blood* 1977; **50**: 1049–59.

59. Digheiro G, Maloum K, Desablens B, *et al*. Chlorambucil in indolent chronic lymphocytic leukemia. *N Engl J Med* 1998; **338**: 1506–14.

60. Khong HT, McCarthy J. Chlorambucil-induced pulmonary disease: a case report and review of the literature. *Ann Hematol* 1998; **77**: 85–7.

61. Lai R, Arber DA, Brynes RK, *et al*. Untreated chronic lymphocytic leukemia concurrent with or followed by acute myelogenous leukemia or myelodysplastic syndrome. *Am J Clin Path* 1999; **111**: 373–8.

62. Spiers ASD, Chikkappa G, Wilbur HJ. (1983) Haemorrhagic cystitis after low-dose cyclophosphamide. *Lancet* 1983; **1**: 1213–14.

63. French Cooperative Group on Chronic Lymphocytic Leukaemia. Effectiveness of "CHOP" regimen in advanced untreated chronic lymphocytic leukaemia. *Lancet* 1986; **1**: 1346–9.

64. Kempin S, Lee BJ, Thaler HT, *et al*. Combination chemotherapy of advanced chronic lymphocytic leukemia: the M-2 protocol (vincristine, BCNU, cyclophosphamide, melphalan and prednisone). *Blood* 1982; **60**: 1110–21.

65. Keating MJ, Scouros M, Murphy S, *et al*. Multiple agent chemotherapy (POACH) in previously treated and untreated patients with chronic lymphocytic leukemia. *Leukemia* 1988; **2**: 157–64.

66. Delpero JR, Gastout JA, Letreut YP, *et al*. The value of splenectomy in chronic lymphocytic leukemia. *Cancer* 1987; **59**: 340–5.

67. Ferrant A, Michaux JL, Sokal G. Splenectomy in advanced chronic lymphocytic leukemia. *Cancer* 1986; **58**: 2130–5.

68. Merl SA, Theodarakis ME, Goldberg J, *et al*. Splenectomy for thrombocytopenia in chronic lymphocytic leukemia. *Am J Hematol* 1983; **15**: 253–9.

69. Pegourie B, Sotto J-J, Hollard D, *et al*. Splenectomy during chronic lymphocytic leukemia. *Cancer* 1987; **59**: 1626–30.

70. Stein RS, Weikert D, Reynolds V, *et al*. Splenectomy for end-stage chronic lymphocytic leukemia. *Cancer* 1987; **59**: 1815–18.

71. Binet JL, Catovsky D, Dighiero G, *et al*. Chronic lymphocytic leukemia: recommendations for diagnosis, staging and response criteria. *Ann Intern Med* 1989; **110**: 236–8.

72. Frederickson S. Specificity of adenosine deaminase toward adenosine and 2′-deoxyadenosine analogues. *Arch Biochem Biophys* 1966; **113**: 383.

73. Malspeis L, Grever MR, Staubus AE, *et al*. Pharmacokinetics of 2-F-ara-A (9-beta-D-arabinofuranosyl-2-fluoroadenine) in cancer patients during the Phase I clinical investigation of fludarabine phosphate. *Semin Oncol* 1990; **17**: 18–32.

74. Plunkett W, Huang P, Gandhi V. Metabolism and action of fludarabine phosphate. *Semin Oncol* 1990; **17** (5 Suppl. 8): 3–17.

75. Von Hoff DD. Phase I clinical trials with fludarabine phosphate. *Semin Oncol* 1990; **17** (5 Suppl. 8): 33–6.

76. Chun HG, Leyland-Jones B, Caryk SM, *et al*. Central nervous system toxicity of fludarabine phosphate. *Cancer Treat Rep* 1986; **70**: 1225–8.

77. Grever MR, Kopecky KJ, Coltman CA, *et al*. Fludarabine monophosphate: A potentially useful agent in chronic lymphocytic leukemia. *Nouv Rev Franc Hematol* 1988; **30**: 457.

78. Keating MJ, Kantarjian H, Talpaz M, *et al*. Fludarabine: a new agent with major activity against chronic lymphocytic leukemia. *Blood* 1989; **74**: 19–25.

79. Keating MJ, Kantarjian H, O'Brien S, *et al*. Fludarabine: a new agent with marked cytoreductive activity in untreated chronic lymphocytic leukemia. *J Clin Oncol* 1991; **9**: 44–9.

80. Keating MJ, O'Brien S, Kantarjian H, *et al*. Long-term follow-up of patients with chronic lymphocytic leukemia treated with fludarabine as a single agent. *Blood* 1993; **81**: 2878–84.

81. Keating MJ, Kantarjian H, O'Brien S, *et al*. Fludarabine (FLU)-Prednisone (PRED): a safe, effective combination

in refractory chronic lymphocytic leukemia. *Proc Am Soc Clin Oncol* 1989; **8**: 201 (abstract).

82. Keating MJ, O'Brien S, Lerner S, *et al.* Long-term follow-up of patients with chronic lymphocytic leukemia (CLL) receiving fludarabine regimens as initial therapy. *Blood* 1998; **92**: 1165–71.

83. French Cooperative Group on CLL. Multicentre prospective randomised trial of fludarabine versus cyclophosphamide, doxorubicin, and prednisone (CAP) for treatment of advanced-stage chronic lymphocytic leukaemia. *Lancet* 1996; **347**: 1432–8.

84. French Cooperative Group on CLL. Comparison of fludarabine (FDB), CAP and CHOP in previously untreated stage B chronic lymphocytic leukemia (CLL). First interim results of a randomized clinical trial in 247 patients. *Blood* 1994; **83**: 461a (abstract).

85. Rai KR, Peterson B, Elias L. A randomized comparison of fludarabine and chlorambucil for patients with previously untreated chronic lymphocytic leukemia. A CALGB, SWOG, CTG/NCI-C and ECOG inter-group study. *Blood* 1996; **88**: 141a (abstract).

86. Rai KR, Peterson BL, Appelbaum FR, *et al.* Fludarabine compared with chlorambucil as primary therapy for chronic lymphocytic leukemia. *N Engl J Med* 2000; **343**: 1750–7.

87. Zaja F, Rogato A, Russo D, *et al.* Combined therapy with fludarabine and cyclophosphamide in relapsed/resistant patients with B-cell chronic lymphocytic leukaemia and non-Hodgkin's lymphomas. *Eur J Haematol* 1997; **59**: 327–8.

88. Rummel MJ, Kafer G, Pfreundschuh M, *et al.* Fludarabine and epirubicin in the treatment of chronic lymphocytic leukaemia: a German multicenter phase II study. *Ann Oncol* 1999; **10**: 183–8.

89. Weiss MA, Glenn M, Maslak P, *et al.* Consolidation therapy with high-dose cyclophosphamide improves the quality of response in patients with chronic lymphocytic leukemia treated with fludarabine as induction therapy. *Leukemia* 2000; **14**: 1577–82.

90. Cheson BD, Bennett JM, Grever M, *et al.* National Cancer Institute-sponsored Working Group guidelines for chronic lymphocytic leukemia: revised guidelines for diagnosis and treatment. *Blood* 1996; **87**: 4990–7.

91. Robak T, Blasinska-Morawiec M, Blonsky JZ, *et al.* 2-chlorodeoxyadenosine (cladribine) in the treatment of elderly patients with B-cell chronic lymphocytic leukemia. *Leuk Lymphoma* 1999; **34**: 151–7.

92. Spiers ASD, Ruckdeschel JC, Horton J. Effectiveness of pentostatin (2'-deoxycoformycin) in refractory

lymphoid neoplasms. *Scand J Hematol* 1984; **32**: 130–4.

93. Johnson SA, Catovsky D, Child JA, *et al.* Phase I/II evaluation of pentostatin (2'-deoxycoformycin) in a five day schedule for the treatment of relapsed/refractory B-cell chronic lymphocytic leukaemia. *Invest New Drugs* 1998; **16**: 155–60.

94. Di Raimondo F, Giustolisi R, Cacciola E, *et al.* Autoimmune hemolytic anemia in chronic lymphocytic leukemia patients treated with fludarabine. *Leuk Lymphoma* 1993; **11**: 63–8.

95. Myint H, Copplestone A, Orchard J, *et al.* Fludarabine-related autoimmune haemolytic anaemia in patients with chronic lymphocytic leukaemia. *Br J Haematol* 1995; **91**: 341–4.

96. Gonzalez H, Leblond V, Azar N, *et al.* Severe autoimmune hemolytic anemia in eight patients treated with fludarabine. *Hematol Cell Ther* 1998; **40**: 113–18.

97. Taha HM, Narasihman P, Venkatesh L, *et al.* Fludarabine-related hemolytic anemia in chronic lymphocytic leukemia and lymphoproliferative disorders. *Am J Hematol* 1998; **59**: 316–19.

98. Rosenkrantz K, Dupont B, Flomenberg M. Relevance of autocytotoxic and autoregulatory lymphocytes in the maintenance of tolerance. *Concepts Immunopathol* 1987; **4**: 24–41.

99. List AF, Kummet TD, Adams JD, *et al.* Tumor lysis syndrome complicating treatment of chronic lymphocytic leukemia with fludarabine phosphate. *Am J Med* 1990; **89**: 388–90.

100. Cheson BD, Frame JN, Vena D, *et al.* Tumor lysis syndrome: an uncommon complication of fludarabine therapy of chronic lymphocytic leukemia. *J Clin Oncol* 1998; **16**: 2313–20.

101. Schlaifer D, Rigal-Huguet F, Pris J, *et al.* Secondary neoplasms in two patients treated with purine analogues. *Nouv Rev Franc Hematol* 1994; **36**: 341.

102. Frewin RJ, Provan D, Smith AG. Myelodysplasia occurring after fludarabine treatment for chronic lymphocytic leukaemia. *Clin Lab Haematol* 1997; **19**: 151–2.

103. Coppelstone JA, Mufti GJ, Hamblin TJ, *et al.* Immunological abnormalities in myelodysplastic syndromes II. Coexistent lymphoid or plasma cell neoplasms: a report of 20 cases unrelated to chemotherapy. *Br J Haematol* 1986; **63**: 149–59.

104. Valganon M, Giraldo P, Agirre X, *et al.* p53 aberrations do not predict individual response to fludarabine in patients with B-cell chronic lymphocytic leukaemia

in advanced stages Rai III/IV. *Br J Haematol* 2005; **129**: 53–9.

105. Richards S. Fludarabine increases complete response but not survival compared with conventional alkylator-based regimens for previously untreated chronic lymphocytic leukaemia. *Cancer Treat Rev* 2005; **31**: 332–5.

106. Silber R, Potmesil M. Drug resistance in chronic lymphocytic leukemia. In Cheson BD, ed, *Chronic Lymphocytic Leukemia* (New York, NY: Dekker, 1993), 221–39.

107. Potmesil M, Hsiang YH, Liu LF, *et al.* Resistance of human leukemic and normal lymphocytes to drug-induced DNA cleavage and low levels of DNA topo-isomerase II. *Cancer Res* 1988; **48**: 3537–43.

108. Holmes JA, Jacobs A, Carter G, *et al.* Is the mdr 1 gene relevant in chronic lymphocytic leukemia? *Leukemia* 1990; **4**: 216–18.

109. Friedenberg WR, Spencer SK, Musser C, *et al.* Multidrug resistance in chronic lymphocytic leukemia. *Leuk Lymphoma* 1999; **34**: 171–8.

110. Bosanquet AG, Johnson SA, Richards SM. Prognosis for fludarabine therapy of chronic lymphocytic leu kaemia based on ex vivo drug response by DiSC assay. *Br J Haematol* 1999; **106**: 71–7.

111. Cooperative Group for the Study of Immunoglobulin in Chronic Lymphocytic Leukemia. Intravenous immunoglobulin for the prevention of infection in chronic lymphocytic leukemia. A randomized, controlled clinical trial. *N Engl J Med* 1988; **319**: 902–7.

112. Kontoyianis DP, Anaissie EJ, Bodey GP. Infection in chronic lymphocytic leukemia: A reappraisal. In Cheson BD, ed, *Chronic Lymphocytic Leukemia* (New York, NY: Dekker, 1993), 399–417.

113. Rabinowe SN, Grossbard ML, Nadler LM. Innovative treatment strategies for chronic lymphocytic leukemia: monoclonal antibodies, immunoconjugates, and bone marrow transplantation. In Cheson BD, ed, *Chronic Lymphocytic Leukemia* (New York, NY: Dekker, 1993), 337–67.

114. Byrd JC, Rai KR, Weiss RB. What choices are available for treatment of the patient with chronic lymphocytic leukemia who is fludarabine-refractory? *Semin Oncol* 2000; **27**: xii-xvi.

115. Herold M, Schulze A, Hartwig K, *et al.* Successful treatment and re-treatment of resistant B-cell chronic lymphocytic leukemia with the monoclonal anti-CD 20 antibody rituximab. *Ann Hematol* 2000; **79**: 332–5.

116. Lin TS, Flinn IW, Lucas MS, *et al.* Filgrastim and ale-mtuzumab (Campath-1H) for refractory chronic lymphocytic leukemia. *Leukemia* 2005; **19**: 1207–10.

117. Varterasian ML, Mohammad RM, Shurafa MS, *et al.* Phase II trial of Bryostatin 1 in patients with relapsed low-grade non-Hodgkin's lymphoma and chronic lymphocytic leukemia. *Clin Cancer Res* 2000; **6**: 825–8.

118. Robak T, Blonski JZ, Kasznicki M, *et al.* Cladribine with prednisone versus chlorambucil with prednisone as first-line therapy in chronic lymphocytic leukemia: report of a prospective, randomized, multicenter trial. *Blood* 2000; **96**: 2723–9.

119. Byrd JC, Peterson BL, Gabrilove J, *et al.* Treatment of relapsed chronic lymphocytic leukemia by 72-hour continuous infusion or 1-hour bolus infusion of fla-vopiridol: results from Cancer and Leukemia Group B study. *Clin Cancer Res* 2005; **11**: 4176–81.

120. Lundin J, Osterborg A. Advances in the use of mono-clonal antibodies in the therapy of chronic lymphocytic leukemia. *Semin Hematol* 2004; **41**: 234–45.

121. Wendtner CM, Eichhorst BF, Hallek MJ. Advances in chemotherapy for chronic lymphocytic leukemia. *Semin Hematol* 2004; **41**: 224 33.

122. Pavletic S, Khouri IF, Haagenson M, *et al.* Unrelated donor bone marrow transplantation for B-cell chronic lymphocytic leukemia after using myeloablative conditioning: results from the Center for International Blood and Marrow Transplant Research. *J Clin Oncol* 2005; **23**: 5788–94.

123. Sutton L, Maloum K, Gonzalez H, *et al.* Autologous hematopoietic stem cell transplantation as salvage treatment for advanced B cell chronic lymphocytic leukemia. *Leukemia* 1998; **12**: 1699–707.

124. Dreger P, von Neuhoff N, Kuse R, *et al.* Early stem cell transplantation for chronic lymphocytic leukaemia: a chance for cure? *Br J Cancer* 1998; **77**: 2291–7.

125. Lysak D, Koza V, Jindra P, *et al.* Mobilization of peripheral blood stem cells in CLL patients after front-line fludarabine treatment. *Ann Hematol* 2005; **84**: 456–61.

126. Wierda W, O'Brien S, Wen S, *et al.* Chemoimmu-notherapy with fludarabine, cyclophosphamide, and rituximab for relapsed and refractory chronic lymphocytic leukemia. *J Clin Oncol* 2005; **23**: 4070–8.

127. Keating M, O'Brien S, Albitar M, *et al.* Early results of a chemoimmunotherapy regimen of fludarabine, cyclophosphamide, and rituximab as initial therapy for chronic lymphocytic leukemia. *J Clin Oncol* 2005; **23**: 4079–88.

25

Polycythemia vera and idiopathic myelofibrosis in the elderly

Jerry L. Spivak

Introduction

The chronic myeloproliferative disorders, polycythemia vera (PV), idiopathic myelofibrosis (IMF) and essential thrombocytosis (ET), are acquired clonal stem-cell disorders involving a multipotent hematopoietic progenitor cell, and are characterized by overproduction of one or more of the formed elements of the blood, a tendency to develop extramedullary hematopoiesis, and, in a small percentage of patients, transformation to acute leukemia. Although uncommon, these disorders are not rare, and recent scientific advances have shed new light on their pathogenesis. The current World Health Organization (WHO) classification scheme for the chronic myeloproliferative diseases places PV, IMF, and ET in the same category as chronic myelogenous leukemia (CML), chronic neutrophilic leukemia (CNL), chronic eosinophilic leukemia (CEL), and the hypereosinophilic syndrome [1]. However, this classification scheme ignores that fact that other than bone-marrow hyperactivity, PV, IMF, and ET are totally different from CML, CNL, and CEL with respect to clinical course and molecular pathogenesis, but closely related to each other. Indeed, PV, IMF, and ET have occurred in different members of the same family [2] and their clinical and molecular features are sufficiently similar (Table 25.1) that, rather than being separate disorders, they could well be different manifestations of the same disorder. Moreover, given the body's limited biologic repertoire, both possibilities are likely. PV, IMF, and ET are very rare in children and while they spare no

age group amongst adults, their incidence increases greatly with aging such that they are most frequent in individuals older than 60 years, in whom they can no longer be considered uncommon illnesses [3]. This review will focus on PV and IMF, with an emphasis on patients aged 60 years and older.

Epidemiology

Polycythemia vera is the commonest of the chronic myeloproliferative disorders, with a frequency of approximately 2/100 000 [4] and a progressive increase with age such that in men older than 80 years the incidence was as high as 18.3/100 000, and in women older than 70 years the incidence was 14.6/100 000 [5]. The onset is most common in the fifth decade in women and the sixth decade in men. Although there is a slight male predominance overall, below age 40, women predominate. Polycythemia vera spares no ethnic group but is most common in whites, particularly in individuals of Ashkenazi extraction, and infrequent in those of African descent. Familial expression is well documented but uncommon. By contrast, idiopathic myelofibrosis is the least common of the chronic myeloproliferative disorders, with an overall incidence of approximately 1/100 000 and a peak frequency at age 60 with no gender bias [3].

Pathogenesis

The etiology of the chronic myeloproliferative disorders remains an enigma. Unlike some other

Blood Disorders in the Elderly, ed. Lodovico Balducci, William Ershler, Giovanni de Gaetano.
Published by Cambridge University Press. © Cambridge University Press 2008.

Table 25.1. Features common to the chronic myeloproliferative disorders, polycythemia vera, idiopathic myelofibrosis, and essential thrombocytosis.

Involvement of a multipotent hematopoietic progenitor cell

Dominance of the abnormal clone over normal polyclonal hematopoiesis

Abnormalities of chromosomes 1, 8, 9, 13, and 20

Marrow hypercellularity and megakaryocyte dysplasia

Growth-factor-independent (endogenous) colony formation

Altered production of one or more of the formed elements of the blood

Thrombosis and hemorrhage

Myelofibrosis

Extramedullary hematopoiesis

Transformation to acute leukemia but at low and differing frequencies

Expression of *JAK2* V617F, over expression of granulocyte PRV-1 mRNA, and impaired expression of Mpl, but not in all patients

---

hematologic malignancies, irradiation exposure has not proved to be an inciting factor.

Cytogenetic abnormalities occur in 30% of polycythemia vera patients [6] and approximately 50% of idiopathic myelofibrosis patients [7], but none is specific for either illness and they often appear to be secondary abnormalities, occurring during the course of the illness, enhanced in expression by chemotherapy, and sometimes evanescent [8]. All of the chronic myeloproliferative disorders share in common growth-factor-independent in-vitro hematopoietic progenitor-cell colony formation, and recently the basis for this was identified to be constitutive activity of the hematopoietic tyrosine kinase JAK2 [9].

JAK2 is the cognate tyrosine kinase for the erythropoietin receptor, the thrombopoietin receptor, Mpl, and the granulocyte colony-stimulating factor receptor. In over 90% of polycythemia vera patients and approximately 40% of idiopathic myelofibrosis and essential thrombocytosis patients, a point mutation in the autoinhibitory pseudokinase domain of the *JAK2* gene (V617F) results in constitutive JAK2

activation [10]. Such activation can account for the growth-factor independence or growth-factor hypersensitivity in these disorders, but because of their clinical differences it cannot be the only genetic abnormality involved in their pathogenesis. In both polycythemia vera and idiopathic myelofibrosis patients, homozygosity for the mutation occurs due to uniparental disomy of chromosome 9 [11] or reduplication of chromosome 9 [12], but to date homozygosity for *JAK2* V617F has not been identified in essential thrombocytosis. Importantly, no significant clinical differences have been observed between patients who are homozygous for the *JAK2* mutation and those who are heterozygous. Similarly, there have been no significant clinical differences between polycythemia vera patients who expressed the mutation and those who do not. The situation is less clear with respect to idiopathic myelofibrosis, since in one large retrospective study those patients who expressed *JAK2* V617F had a shorter survival than those who did not [13], while in another study those who expressed the mutation were older and had a higher incidence of thrombosis but not a difference in survival [14].

Myelofibrosis is a hallmark of idiopathic myelofibrosis but can also occur not only during the course of polycythemia vera but as a presenting manifestation of that disease, in which case it does not confer a bad prognosis [15]. Indeed, the concept that myelofibrosis per se is associated with impaired bone-marrow function in polycythemia vera in the absence of exposure to myelotoxic drugs has not been substantiated [16]. As a corollary, it has been demonstrated that idiopathic myelofibrosis can have a prefibrotic cellular phase characterized primarily by thrombocytosis [17], and that thrombocytosis can also be the presenting manifestation of polycythemia vera [18]. These shared characteristics strongly suggest a common etiology for these disorders; the occurrence of both disorders as well as essential thrombocytosis in the same family supports this contention [19].

In this regard, it is important to note that myelofibrosis in the chronic myeloproliferative disorders is a reactive process [20], in contrast to the hematopoietic cell abnormalities, which are the consequence of a clonal process. Normally, in adults, hematopoiesis is extravascular in location and requires support from accessory cells including adipocytes, macrophages, endothelial cells, and fibroblasts residing in an extracellular matrix that is rich in collagen, glycosoaminoglycans that bind soluble colony-stimulating factors, and adhesive proteins such as fibronectin and vitronectin. Myelofibrosis is defined as a marked increase in collagen deposition, as demonstrated by a positive stain for reticulin. Reticulin is actually collagen that is coated with extracellular matrix substances that are argyrophilic and bind silver [21]. When the amount of collagen increases, the fibrils are not as coated with matrix substances and can bind to classical stains for collagen [22]. As marrow cellularity increases, the quantity of collagen increases compensatorily; this is physiologic not pathologic. However, when the quantity of collagen exceeds the degree of cellularity, true myelofibrosis can be said to be present. This is manifest by contiguous, thickened fibrils, as opposed to the thinner and non-contiguous fibrils associated with increased marrow cellularity, and inability to aspirate marrow. It is important to remember that as a reactive process myelofibrosis is also a reversible one.

Osteosclerosis is a part of the continuum of myelofibrosis, and in the chronic myeloproliferative disorders does not occur in the absence of myelofibrosis. It represents the deposition of mineral in the bony trabeculae of the marrow without the remodeling that occurs in metabolic bone disease, and it is thought to be due in part to overproduction of the osteoclast inhibitor osteoprotegerin [23]. The stimulus for myelofibrosis and osteosclerosis is unknown, but both megakaryocytes and mononuclear cells are involved, since both overexpression of thrombopoietin [24] and *JAK2* V617F [25] is associated with myelofibrosis in animal models and TGF-β appears to be an important cytokine in this process [26].

An increase in bone-marrow vascularity is another feature associated with myelofibrosis, but its mechanism is unknown. It correlates best with the degree of marrow cellularity rather than the extent of the myelofibrosis [27]. Another characteristic histologic feature of myelofibrosis is marrow sinusoidal dilation associated with intrasinusoidal hematopoiesis, a process that is distinctly unphysiologic and accounts for the increase in circulating CD34+ cells in idiopathic myelofibrosis [28]. Interestingly, there is also an increase in circulating endothelial precursor cells that appears to precede the increase in CD34+ cells in this disorder [29].

Clinical features

With the advent of electronic particle counters, hematologic illnesses are being recognized at an earlier stage in their natural history. Thus both polycythemia vera and idiopathic myelofibrosis are being discovered at an asymptomatic stage with only blood-count abnormalities. These disorders may also be first recognized because of a disease complication. In the case of polycythemia vera, this may be a thrombotic or hemorrhagic event or unremitting pruritus; idiopathic myelofibrosis may come to recognition because of easy satiety due to splenic enlargement or constitutional symptoms such as fever, night sweats, and weight loss. Table 25.2 lists the symptoms of polycythemia vera, and Table 25.3 lists those of idiopathic myelofibrosis. None of these symptoms are disease-specific, and must be combined with laboratory studies to distinguish these disorders from the many benign and malignant diseases that they mimic (Tables 25.4 and 25.5).

Laboratory abnormalities

Polycythemia vera is unique amongst the chronic myeloproliferative disorders because in this disorder there is overproduction of red cells, white cells, and platelets. However, less than 50% of patients present with a panmyelopathy involving all three cell lines [5]. In approximately 15% of patients, isolated erythrocytosis will be the sole presenting abnormality; in

Table 25.2. Presenting symptoms in polycythemia vera (in more than 10% of patients).

Weakness or fatigue
Headache
Dizziness or vertigo
Bleeding or bruising
Dyspnea
Abdominal pain
Visual symptoms
Paresthesias or extremity pain
Pruritus
Thrombosis
Dyspepsia

Table 25.3. Presenting symptoms in idiopathic myelofibrosis (in more than 10% of patients).

Fatigue
Weight loss
Abdominal pain
Dyspnea
Bleeding
Night sweats
Bone pain
Gout or renal stones
Fever

Table 25.4. Causes of relative and absolute erythrocytosis.

Relative erythrocytosis	Hemoconcentration secondary to dehydration, diuretics, hypertension, androgens or tobacco abuse
Absolute erythrocytosis	
Hypoxia	Carbon monoxide intoxication
	High-affinity hemoglobin
	High altitude
	Pulmonary disease
	Right-to-left shunts
	Sleep apnea syndrome
	Neurologic disease
Renal disease	Renal artery stenosis
	Focal sclerosing or membranous glomerulonephritis
	Renal transplantation
Tumors	Hypernephroma
	Hepatoma
	Cerebellar hemangioblastoma
	Uterine fibromyoma
	Adrenal tumors
	Meningioma
	Pheochromocytoma
Drugs	Androgens
	Recombinant erythropoietin
Familial (with abnormal hemoglobin function; Chuvash, EPO receptor mutations)	
Idiopathic (primary)	
Polycythemia vera	

another 5–10%, thrombocytosis alone is the first laboratory abnormality. Erythrocytosis and leukocytosis, or erythrocytosis and thrombocytosis, are other combinations that have been observed. Iron-deficiency anemia may be present if there has been gastrointestinal hemorrhage. The serum cholesterol may be low and the leukocyte alkaline phosphatase high. The latter abnormality, as well as elevation of the serum vitamin B_{12} level and serum B_{12} binding capacity due to neutrophil release of transcobalamin III, reflects leukocyte activation due to the *JAK2* V617F mutation. If there is extensive liver extramedullary hematopoiesis, the serum alkaline phosphatase will be elevated, and with significant leukocytosis there will be hyperuricemia.

Classically, the serum erythropoietin level is lower in polycythemia vera than in any other form of erythrocytosis. However, a low serum erythropoietin level can also be seen in essential thrombocytosis at an equivalent hematocrit [30], while the serum erythropoietin level can also be normal in both polycythemia vera and hypoxic forms of erythrocytosis [31]. Erythropoietin-independent in-vitro erythroid colony is another hallmark of polycythemia vera, though not specific for it amongst the chronic

Table 25.5. Causes of myelofibrosis.

Clonal
  Acute leukemia (lymphocytic, myelogenous,
    megakaryocytic)
  Chronic myelogenous leukemia
  Hairy-cell leukemia
  Hodgkin disease
  Idiopathic myelofibrosis
  Lymphoma
  Multiple myeloma
  Myelodysplasia
  Metastatic carcinoma
  Polycythemia vera
  Systemic mastocytosis
Nonclonal
  HIV infection
  Hyperparathyroidism
  Renal osteodystrophy
  Systemic lupus erythematosus
  Tuberculosis
  Vitamin D deficiency
  Thorium dioxide exposure
  Gray platelet syndrome

Table 25.6. Sites of extramedullary hematopoiesis in idiopathic myelofibrosis (in order of frequency).

Spleen
Liver
Lymph nodes
Kidneys and ureters
Retroperitoneum
Peritoneum and mesentery
Lungs and pleura
Adrenals
Skin
Heart
Dura mater
Breasts
Ovaries

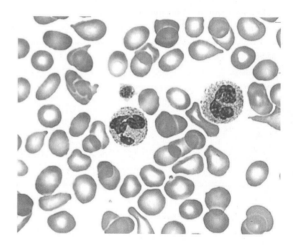

Figure 25.1 Idiopathic myelofibrosis: a typical picture in the peripheral blood may include dacrocytes, dysplastic granulocytes and large platelets. Maslak, P., ASH Image Bank 2004: 101216. Copyright American Society of Hematology. All rights reserved. *See color plate section.*

myeloproliferative disorders [32]. The assay is also not widely available and has been superseded by the assay for *JAK2* V617F, which is present in over 90% of polycythemia vera patients.

In idiopathic myelofibrosis, in contrast to its companion chronic myeloproliferative disorders, there is impaired blood-cell production as well as blood-cell overproduction. Thus anemia, usually normochromic and normocytic, is the most common abnormality, and in approximately 25% of patients thrombocytopenia occurs. Extramedullary hematopoiesis, manifest by circulating nucleated red cells and immature leukocytes, is a characteristic feature of idiopathic myelofibrosis, though not specific for it (Table 25.6); teardrop-shaped red cells are caused by splenomegaly (Fig. 25.1) [33]. The leukocyte alkaline phosphatase level can be normal, elevated, or low, and the serum alkaline phosphatase will be elevated if there is hepatic extramedullary hematopoiesis. An increase of circulating CD34+ cells is a unique early feature of idiopathic myelofibrosis, and is seen only later in the course of polycythemia vera [28].

Bone-marrow histology

Marrow hypercellularity with loss of the fat spaces is a characteristic of myeloproliferative disorders. Classically, there is a panmyelosis with trilineage

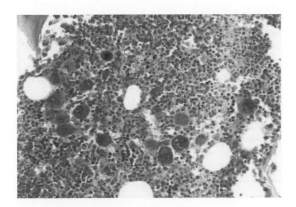

Figure 25.2 Bone-marrow biopsy showing clustering of megakaryocytes with mature cytoplasm, and variable nuclear lobulations. Lazarchick, J., ASH Image Bank 2001: 100172. Copyright American Society of Hematology. All rights reserved. *See color plate section.*

hematopoietic cell hyperplasia and an increase in megakaryocytes (Fig. 25.2), usually large with hyperchromatic and cloud-like nuclei and generally in clusters, and stainable iron may be absent. However, in polycythemia vera, marrow cellularity may be normal, and in some patients there may be significant myelofibrosis at the time of diagnosis [15]. As a corollary, a prefibrotic, cellular phase of idiopathic myelofibrosis has been recognized [34]. In more advanced stages of idiopathic myelofibrosis, marrow is unaspirable and there is a thick network of collagen fibers with clusters of megakaryocytes and dilated sinuses and increased capillarity. In advanced stages there may be a diminution in hematopoietic cells as well as osteosclerosis. However, the histologic picture in idiopathic myelofibrosis is frequently heterogeneous and marrow histology should not be relied upon for staging purposes.

Coagulation abnormalities

Coagulation abnormalities are common in all the chronic myeloproliferative disorders, are largely limited to the platelets, and reflect both intrinsic and acquired abnormalities of platelet structure and function and the effect of platelet number. There is a storage pool defect defined by loss of alpha granules and dense bodies and reduced intraplatelet levels

of ADP, 5HT, and fibrinogen [35,36], and increased surface expression of thrombospondin, P-selection, CD41, and GPIV [37]. Paradoxically, there is impaired aggregation in response to ADP, epinephrine, or collagen as well as evidence of platelet activation in the form of increased thromboxane synthesis and spontaneous platelet aggregation [38]. A prolonged bleeding time is observed in 20% of patients without correlation with platelet function defects. If the platelets exceed 1000×10^9/L, there is adsorption and destruction of the highest-molecular-weight von Willebrand factor multimers by the platelets. Anatomic abnormalities of the platelet canalicular and dense tubular systems probably represent intrinsic platelet abnormalities [39], as does impaired expression of the thrombopoietin receptor, Mpl [40]. Other abnormalities, however, may be acquired due to platelet interactions with red cells, leukocytes, or endothelial cells [41], since in polycythemia vera phlebotomy can improve platelet function [42]. Interestingly, a hemorrhagic tendency appears to be most common in idiopathic myelofibrosis [43].

Cytogenetic abnormalities

Non-random chromosomal abnormalities are present in approximately 30% of polycythemia vera patients at the time of diagnosis [6] and in over 50% of idiopathic myelofibrosis patients [44]. Chemotherapy or irradiation increases their incidence [8]. No chromosomal abnormality is specific for a particular myeloproliferative disorder. The most frequently observed abnormalities are trisomies of 1q, 8, 9 and 9p, 13q–, and 20q–. Loss of heterozygosity on chromosome 9p is probably the most common abnormality and involves the *JAK2* locus [6]. Trisomy 8 and 12q– appear to confer a poorer prognosis in idiopathic myelofibrosis [45], while complex chromosome abnormalities have been associated with a poor prognosis in both polycythemia vera and idiopathic myelofibrosis.

Radiologic abnormalities

Osteosclerosis can be identified radiologically as an increase in medullary bone density, and can be particularly striking in the ribs and vertebral bodies. The X-ray presence of osteosclerosis suggests at least 40% involvement of the marrow space with myelofibrosis [46]. There may also be hypertrophic osteoarthropathy with tibial onion-skinning.

Immunologic abnormalities

Immunologic abnormalities appear to be unique to idiopathic myelofibrosis amongst the chronic myeloproliferative disorders. These include antinuclear and smooth muscle antibodies, rheumatoid factor, hypocomplementemia, circulating immune complexes, and Coombs positivity [47,48]. It is of interest in this regard that myelofibrosis can complicate systemic lupus [49]. Usually, the expression of immune complexes is associated with constitutional symptoms in idiopathic myelofibrosis.

Diagnosis

Establishing the diagnosis of a chronic myeloproliferative disorder is not easy. These disorders clinically mimic each other as well as the other benign and malignant disorders that can cause erythrocytosis, leukocytosis, thrombocytosis, or myelofibrosis. Furthermore, the chronic myeloproliferative disorders change their clinical manifestations during their natural history and there is as yet no specific clinical marker for any of them. Erythrocytosis is the hallmark of polycythemia vera, the one feature that distinguishes it from its companion myeloproliferative disorders, and the clinical feature that is responsible for its most frequent serious complications, thrombosis and hemorrhage. Unfortunately, unless the hematocrit is $\geqslant 60\%$ (hemoglobin $\geqslant 20\,\mathrm{g/dL}$) in a man or $\geqslant 48\%$ (hemoglobin $\geqslant 17\,\mathrm{g/dL}$) in a woman, it is not possible to determine from the hematocrit, hemoglobin, or red cell count whether there is an absolute elevation of the red cell mass as opposed to plasma volume contraction [50]. Since the red cell mass and plasma volume vary independently of each other, it is also not possible to calculate the red cell mass from a plasma volume measurement [51]. Attempts to use

Table 25.7. PVSG diagnostic criteria for polycythemia vera. From Wasserman 1971 [55].

Elevated red cell mass
Normal arterial oxygen saturation

Splenomegaly
Plus any two below if no splenomegaly
    Leukocytosis $>12 \times 10^9/\mathrm{L}$
    Thrombocytosis $>400 \times 10^9/\mathrm{L}$
    LAP >100
    Elevated B_{12} $>900\,\mathrm{pg/mL}$ or $uB_{12}BC$ $>2200\,\mathrm{pg/mL}$

formulas for estimating the red cell mass or creating hemoglobin or hematocrit thresholds as suggested by the WHO have also proved futile [52]. In addition, establishing the size of the red cell mass provides an indication of how much blood must be removed by phlebotomy to restore the red cell mass to normal. Thus a simple diagnostic test becomes a therapeutic guide. Polycythemia vera is, of course, unique since as the red cell mass increases in that disorder, the plasma volume expands [53]. This, as well as the development of splenomegaly, has the effect of masking the red cell mass expansion [54] and this is particularly true in women. Although *JAK2* V617F is present in over 90% of polycythemia vera patients, it is not specific for that disorder. Therefore, if polycythemia vera is a diagnostic consideration, red cell mass and plasma volume measurements are mandatory. Figure 25.3 provides a diagnostic approach to the evaluation of a patient suspected of having erythrocytosis, which it should be emphasized is not synonymous with polycythemia vera, and which incorporates *JAK2* V617F analysis, in contrast to the classical diagnostic criteria of the Polycythemia Vera Study Group (PVSG; Table 25.7).

A bone-marrow examination is not necessary for the diagnosis of polycythemia vera because the test lacks specificity, and in some patients marrow morphology is actually normal [15], but it is mandatory for the diagnosis of idiopathic myelofibrosis. Whether the diagnosis of this disorder can be made in the absence of myelofibrosis is currently under scrutiny [17]. To improve diagnostic accuracy,

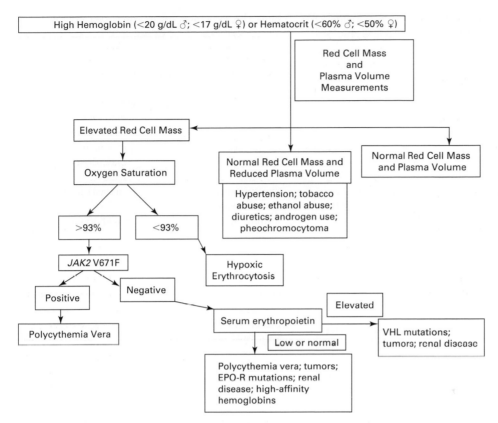

High Hemoglobin (<20 g/dL ♂; <17 g/dL ♀) or Hematocrit (<60% ♂; <50% ♀)

Red Cell Mass
and
Plasma Volume
Measurements

Elevated Red Cell Mass

Normal Red Cell Mass and
Reduced Plasma Volume

Normal Red Cell Mass
and Plasma Volume

Oxygen Saturation

Hypertension; tobacco
abuse; ethanol abuse;
diuretics; androgen use;
pheochromocytoma

>93%   <93%

JAK2 V671F

Hypoxic
Erythrocytosis

Positive   Negative

Elevated

Serum erythropoietin

VHL mutations;
tumors; renal disease

Polycythemia Vera

Low or normal

Polycythemia vera; tumors;
EPO-R mutations; renal
disease; high-affinity
hemoglobins

Figure 25.3 An algorithm for the evaluation of suspected erythrocytosis when the hematocrit is ≤60% (hemoglobin ≤20 g/dL) in a man or ≤50% (≤17 g/dL) in a woman. Above these values, it can be presumed that the red cell mass is elevated.

criteria have been proposed for idiopathic myelofibrosis but these lack specificity, since they really only define myelofibrosis with myeloid metaplasia [56] and these are histologic processes common to many diseases (Table 25.8). Furthermore, since splenomegaly is present at the time of diagnosis in over 90% of patients with idiopathic myelofibrosis, considering it an optional criterion appears inappropriate. *JAK2* V617F is of some help but it is not expressed in the majority of idiopathic myelofibrosis patients.

The inability to aspirate bone marrow in idiopathic myelofibrosis also makes it difficult to distinguish this disorder from a number of other illnesses causing myelofibrosis, many of which have an increased incidence in the elderly. These include chronic myelogenous leukemia, myelodysplasia, acute myelofibrosis, bone marrow lymphoma, hairy-cell leukemia, multiple myeloma, metastatic carcinoma in the marrow, polycythemia vera, and systemic mastocytosis. Thus, if *JAK2* V617F is absent, the diagnostic evaluation should include peripheral blood bcr-abl and MDS FISH and conventional cytogenetics, flow cytometry for peripheral blood CD34+ cells, and marrow immunohistochemistry for CD34+ cells.

Natural history

The natural history of polycythemia vera as presented in standard hematology textbooks assumes

Table 25.8. Diagnostic criteria for myelofibrosis with myeloid metaplasia (MMM). From Barosi *et al.*, The Italian Consensus Conference on Diagnostic Criteria for Myelofibrosis with Myeloid Metaplasia, 1999 [65].

Necessary criteria
  (A) Diffuse bone-marrow fibrosis
  (B) Absence of the Philadelphia chromosome or BCR-ABL rearrangement in peripheral blood cells

Optional criteria
  (1) Splenomegaly of any grade
  (2) Anisopoikilocytosis with teardrop erythrocytes
  (3) Presence of circulating immature myeloid cells
  (4) Presence of circulating erythroblasts
  (5) Presence of clusters of megakaryocytes and anomalous megakaryocytes in bone-marrow biopsy sections
  (6) Myeloid metaplasia

A diagnosis of MMM is acceptable if the following combinations are present:

Splenomegaly present	The two necessary criteria plus any other two optional criteria
Splenomegaly absent	The two necessary criteria plus any four optional criteria

Table 25.9. The complications of polycythemia vera.

Complication	Cause
Thrombosis, hypertension, hemorrhage	Elevated red mass
Organomegaly	Elevated red cell mass or extramedullary hematopoiesis
Pruritus, acid-peptic disease	Inflammatory mediators or elevated red cell mass
Hyperuricemia, gout, renal stones	Increased cell turnover
Erythromelalgia or ocular migraine	Thrombocytosis
Hemorrhage	Elevated red cell mass or acquired von Willebrand disease
Myelofibrosis	Reaction to the neoplastic clone
Wasting syndrome	Disease acceleration
Acute leukemia	Therapy-related or clonal evolution

that the disorder is monolithic, when in fact it is variable with respect to its clinical course. Furthermore, the conventionally accepted natural history was derived from a small number of patients, whose treatment would be considered inadequate according to today's standards. Of course, it also needs to be emphasized that the diagnosis of polycythemia vera is being made earlier in its course than ever before. What is clear is that the disease can be very indolent or very aggressive, and this usually becomes evident within the first five years after diagnosis. The complications of polycythemia vera are listed in Table 25.9. With respect to age, the potential complications from either erythrocytosis or thrombocytosis take on particular significance, since an older vasculature or diminished cardiac reserve will only serve to magnify these, while their remedies may not be tolerated as easily in the elderly. Although one epidemiologic study suggested that polycythemia

vera patients had a normal lifespan [57], others have suggested that their lifespan is shorter [58]. No studies to date, however, have identified specific risk factors other than a history of thrombosis or age >60 years [59] and, with respect to acute leukemia (which occurs in approximately 2% of patients not exposed to mutagenic agents) older age [60,61].

By contrast, until recently, prognosis in idiopathic myelofibrosis had been considered to be grim, with a median survival of five years. However, recent epidemiologic studies have demonstrated that idiopathic myelofibrosis is also not a monolithic illness, and have established risk stratification schemes that permit identification of patients with an indolent illness and those with aggressive disease [62–64]. The most important risk factors are age ≥65 years, anemia, leukocytosis, circulating blast cells, constitutional symptoms, and cytogenetic abnormalities (Table 25.10). For example, an

Table 25.10. Three risk stratification strategies for idiopathic myelofibrosis.

Reference	Prognostic factors	Number of prognostic factors	Risk group	Median survival (months)
Dupriez *et al.* 1996 [71]	Hemoglobin <10 g/dL	0	Low	93
	WBC <4 or >30 × 10⁹/L	1–2	High	17
Cervantes *et al.* 1998 [72]	Hemoglobin <10 g/dL	0–1	Low	99
	Constitutional symptoms	2–3	High	21
	Blast cells >1%			
Reilly 2006 [73]	Age >65 years			
	Hemoglobin ≤10 g/dL			
	Karyotype normal		Low	44
	Karyotype abnormal		High	16
	Age >65 years			
	Hemoglobin >10 g/dL			
	Karyotype normal		Low	70
	Karyotype abnormal		High	78

idiopathic myelofibrosis patient less than 65 years old without anemia or cytogenetic abnormalities had a median life expectancy of 180 months, while his older counterpart had a life expectancy of just 70 months [64]. *JAK2* V617F expression was also noted to confer a poorer prognosis in one study [13], but in another the mutation only correlated with older age and a history of thrombosis [14]. The consequences of idiopathic myelofibrosis reflect the extent of extramedullary hematopoiesis, which can cause extreme enlargement of the liver and spleen with the attendant portal hypertension, hyperuricemia, anemia, thrombocytopenia, and cachexia. No organ or tissue is immune to the development of extramedullary hematopoiesis, and when aggressive it may be a harbinger of transformation to acute leukemia, which appears to occur ten times more frequently than in polycythemia vera [65]. Pulmonary hypertension is an unusual complication, which could be due either to pulmonary extramedullary hematopoiesis or possibly to myelofibrosis [66].

Treatment

In most patients, the chronic myeloproliferative disorders are indolent illnesses, whose clinical course can be measured in decades. Furthermore, since these disorders are being recognized much earlier and since we now understand the toxicities of many therapies that were once standard for these disorders, previous estimates of longevity are no longer valid. Given the chronicity of these illnesses, the first rule of therapy should be that treatment must be safe as well as effective, and the second rule should be that the treatment must not be worse than the disease. Treatment also needs to be tailored to the patient's medical status [67]. This is particularly important because, with the exception of bone-marrow transplantation, there is no curative therapy for polycythemia vera or idiopathic myelofibrosis.

With respect to polycythemia vera, the first line of therapy is to reduce the red cell mass by phlebotomy, to a gender-specific hematocrit level of no more than 42% (hemoglobin 12 g/dL) in a woman or 45% (hemoglobin 14 g/dL) in a man [68]. This will prevent thrombosis or hemorrhage, reduce the blood pressure and often spleen size, and in some patients alleviate pruritus. Additionally, there will be an improvement in platelet hemostatic function. The extent of phlebotomy can be judged from the initial red cell mass determination. This does not need to be repeated, since the target hematocrit will always be that reached after the excess red cells have been removed. If a red cell mass cannot be performed, the hematocrit and hemoglobin guidelines stated above should be followed. It must be emphasized that in the presence of splenomegaly, with the attendant increase in plasma volume, even a hematocrit of 40% may be too high in a woman. It is also not widely appreciated that if there is a thrombosis, the higher the hematocrit, the greater the degree of tissue damage.

Early studies of phlebotomy therapy used too high a hematocrit threshold and failed to distinguish between genders with respect to this [68]. They also failed to appreciate that phlebotomy has two goals: first to mechanically reduce intravascular volume overload and hyperviscosity, and second to keep the red cell mass normal by inducing iron deficiency. It has been well demonstrated in adults, even those over age 60, that iron deficiency in the absence of anemia does not impair aerobic function [69]. The induction of iron deficiency also does not cause a significant increase in the platelet count because hematopoietic progenitor cells are autonomous in polycythemia vera. Any increase in the platelet count is a consequence of the natural history of the disease, and in this regard it must emphasized that the principal cause of thrombosis in polycythemia vera is the elevated red cell mass, not the platelet count [67]. Although phlebotomy induces a rapid increase in plasma volume, some heart-disease or elderly patients cannot tolerate the volume loss initially [70]. In these patients, replacement of the volume loss with crystalloid is appropriate.

Thrombocytosis in either polycythemia vera or idiopathic myelofibrosis can cause microvascular symptoms such as ocular migraine, erythromelalgia, and even digital gangrene. In such patients, aspirin is the initial drug of choice. Exceptions include patients with very high platelet counts in whom acquired von Willebrand disease is present or who have other risk factors for hemorrhage, and those suffering from transient ischemic attacks. In these patients, a platelet-lowering agent should be used. Anagrelide is the safest drug but probably should not be used when there are significant cardiovascular risk factors unless the patient has failed other remedies; hydroxyurea has been demonstrated to be the initial drug of choice for transient ischemic attacks [71], presumably because it is a nitric oxide donor [72]. However, hydroxyurea is a proven tumor promoter and potentiates the effects of UV light in producing skin cancer [73]. It also potentiates the leukemogenic and carcinogenic effects of alkylating agents and irradiation [74–76] and should not be used in combination with them if at all possible. Interferon alpha is another agent that should be considered for the treatment of thrombocytosis because, like anagrelide, it is not a mutagen [77]. Unfortunately, the side effects of interferon alpha are such that many patients, particularly older ones, cannot tolerate it. There is no correlation between the platelet count and thrombosis in polycythemia vera and it is probably unnecessary to lower the platelet count any more than is necessary to reduce symptoms or the risk of hemorrhage. Although it has been recommended that daily aspirin be used in polycythemia vera [78], the patients studied were inadequately phlebotomized [79].

Asymptomatic leukocytosis requires no treatment; nor does the hyperuricemia unless the uric acid is $\geq 10\,mg/dL$. In this regard, it is important to remember that low-dose aspirin blocks uric acid excretion. Generally, a rapidly rising or very high leukocyte count in the absence of infection suggests the development of extramedullary hematopoiesis, which warrants therapy.

The most difficult therapeutic problem in polycythemia vera and idiopathic myelofibrosis is exuberant extramedullary hematopoiesis leading to the development of splenomegaly and hepatomegaly with the attendant mechanical discomfort, easy satiety, weight loss, and portal hypertension. Fortunately this is not the lot of all patients with polycythemia vera, but it is probably the most common problem in idiopathic myelofibrosis. Hydroxyurea is not an effective drug in many patients, and interferon alpha is the drug of choice in polycythemia vera; interferon alpha has not been as effective in idiopathic myelofibrosis. In these patients, low-dose thalidomide and prednisone has been effective [80].

Splenectomy is the next consideration in patients who fail drug therapy for control of extramedullary hematopoiesis. It is a major surgical procedure that may be complicated by splanchnic vein thrombosis [81] or substantial hepatomegaly, and it may not alleviate the portal hypertension. In patients unable to tolerate a major surgical procedure, the choices of therapy include low-dose alkylating therapy, ^{32}P, or splenic irradiation. The latter is usually effective, but at a substantial risk of neutropenia and infection, and is at best temporizing, though it may be successful on more than one occasion [82]. Extramedullary hematopoiesis can develop in any organ or tissue of the body, and when localized can be treated effectively with localized irradiation. Widespread extramedullary hematopoiesis suggests disease acceleration. In some patients pulmonary extramedullary hematopoiesis can cause pulmonary hypertension [66].

Anemia and thrombocytopenia are features unique to idiopathic myelofibrosis amongst the chronic myeloproliferative disorders, and are often difficult to manage. In patients with a serum erythropoietin level less than 125 mIU/mL, recombinant erythropoietin has proved effective [83], but the hormone can cause enlargement of the liver or spleen. Splenectomy is not an effective remedy in most patients for correction of anemia or thrombocytopenia, but low-dose thalidomide has proved effective in some patients. If anemia is associated with constitutional symptoms in the absence of infection, a trial of prednisone may be worthwhile. Some authors have suggested the use of impeded androgens such as danazol for the treatment of anemia in idiopathic myelofibrosis [84]. While effective in some patients, these agents when used chronically can have significant side effects such as fluid retention, hepatocellular injury, and priapism.

As mentioned above, marrow transplantation is the only curative therapy for the chronic myeloproliferative disorders, but given the longevity of most patient with polycythemia vera, the median age of onset of 60 years, and the initial mortality associated with the transplantation procedure, there is little role for the procedure in this disease. In idiopathic myelofibrosis, however, where longevity is more restricted, bone-marrow transplantation is a serious consideration. This treatment has been most effective in patients under age 45 with low-risk disease [85]. Transplantation-related mortality was high at approximately 30%, with a five-year survival of more than 60% under age 45 but only 14% for patients older than this. Recently, reduced-intensity conditioning regimens have reduced transplantation-related mortality and survival rates as high as 70% have been obtained [86]. However, more studies are needed with respect to this approach before it can be routinely recommended.

REFERENCES

1. Vardiman JW, Harris NL, Brunning RD. The World Health Organization (WHO) classification of the myeloid neoplasms. *Blood* 2002; **100**: 2292–302.
2. Perez-Encinas M, Bello JL, Perez-Crespo S, De Miguel R, Tome S. Familial myeloproliferative syndrome. *Am J Hematol* 1994; **46**: 225–9.
3. Wallis PJ, Skehan JD, Newland AC, *et al*. Effects of erythrapheresis on pulmonary haemodynamics and oxygen transport in patients with secondary polycythaemia and cor pulmonale. *Clin Sci* 1986; **70**: 91–8.
4. Ania BJ, Suman VJ, Sobell JL, *et al*. Trends in the incidence of polycythemia vera among Olmsted County, Minnesota residents, 1935–1989. *Am J Hematol* 1994; **47**: 89–93.
5. Berglund S, Zettervall O. Incidence of polycythemia vera in a defined population. *Eur J Haematol* 1992; **48**: 20–6.
6. Najfeld V, Montella L, Scalise A, Fruchtman S. Exploring polycythaemia vera with fluorescence in situ hybridization: additional cryptic 9p is the most frequent abnormality detected. *Br J Haematol* 2002; **119**: 558–66.
7. Lim CS, Jung KH, Kim YS, *et al*. Secondary polycythemia associated with idiopathic membranous nephropathy. *Am J Nephrol* 2000; **20**: 344–6.
8. Swolin B, Weinfeld A, Westin J. A prospective long-term cytogenetic study in polycythemia vera in relation to treatment and clinical course. *Blood* 1988; **72**: 386–95.
9. James C, Ugo V, Le Couedic JP, *et al*. A unique clonal JAK2 mutation leading to constitutive signalling causes polycythaemia vera. *Nature* 2005; **434**: 1144–8.

10. Jones AV, Kreil S, Zoi K, *et al.* Widespread occurrence of the JAK2 V617F mutation in chronic myeloproliferative disorders. *Blood* 2005; **106**: 2162–8.

11. Kralovics R, Guan Y, Prchal JT. Acquired uniparental disomy of chromosome 9p is a frequent stem cell defect in polycythemia vera. *Exp Hematol* 2002; **30**: 229–36.

12. Chen Z, Notohamiprodjo M, Guan XY, *et al.* Gain of 9p in the pathogenesis of polycythemia vera. *Genes Chromosomes Cancer* 1998; **22**: 321–4.

13. Campbell PJ, Griesshammer M, Dohner K, *et al.* V617F mutation in JAK2 is associated with poorer survival in idiopathic myelofibrosis. *Blood* 2006; **107**: 2098–100.

14. Tefferi A, Lasho TL, Schwager SM, *et al.* The JAK2(V617F) tyrosine kinase mutation in myelofibrosis with myeloid metaplasia: lineage specificity and clinical correlates. *Br J Haematol* 2005; **131**: 320–8.

15. Ellis JT, Peterson P, Geller SA, Rappaport H. Studies of the bone marrow in polycythemia vera and the evolution of myelofibrosis and second hematologic malignancies. *Semin Hematol* 1986; **23**: 144–55.

16. Roberts BE, Miles DW, Woods CG. Polycythaemia vera and myelosclerosis: a bone marrow study. *Br J Haematol* 1969; **16**: 75–85.

17. Thiele J, Kvasnicka HM. Hematopathologic findings in chronic idiopathic myelofibrosis. *Semin Oncol* 2005; **32**: 380–94.

18. Jantunen R, Juvonen E, Ikkala E, *et al.* Development of erythrocytosis in the course of essential thrombocythemia. *Ann Hematol* 1999; **78**: 219–22.

19. Perez-Encinas M, Bello JL, Perez-Crespo S, De Miguel R, Tome S. Familial myeloproliferative syndrome. *Am J Hematol* 1994; **46**: 225–9.

20. Jacobson RJ, Salo A, Fialkow PJ. Agnogenic myeloid metaplasia: a clonal proliferation of hematopoietic stem cells with secondary myelofibrosis. *Blood* 1978; **51**: 189–94.

21. Puchtler H, Waldrop FW. Silver impregnation methods for reticulum fibers and reticulin: a re-investigation of their origins and specificity. *Histochemistry* 1978; **57**: 177–87.

22. Charron D, Robert L, Couty MC, Binet JL. Biochemical and histological analysis of bone marrow collagen in myelofibrosis. *Br J Haematol* 1979; **41**: 151–61.

23. Bock O, Loch G, Schade U, *et al.* Osteosclerosis in advanced chronic idiopathic myelofibrosis is associated with endothelial overexpression of osteoprotegerin. *Br J Haematol* 2005; **130**: 76–82.

24. Yan XQ, Lacey D, Hill D, *et al.* A model of myelofibrosis and osteosclerosis in mice induced by overexpressing thrombopoietin (mpl ligand): reversal of disease by bone marrow transplantation. *Blood* 1996; **88**: 402–9.

25. Wernig G, Mercher T, Okabe R, *et al.* Expression of Jak2V617F causes a polycythemia vera-like disease with associated myelofibrosis in a murine bone marrow transplant model. *Blood* 2006; **107**: 4274–81.

26. Rameshwar P, Chang VT, Thacker UF, Gascon P. Systemic transforming growth factor-beta in patients with bone marrow fibrosis: pathophysiological implications. *Am J Hematol* 1998; **59**: 133–42.

27. Mesa RA, Hanson CA, Rajkumar SV, Schroeder G, Tefferi A. Evaluation and clinical correlations of bone marrow angiogenesis in myelofibrosis with myeloid metaplasia. *Blood* 2000; **96**: 3374–80.

28. Barosi G, Viarengo G, Pecci A, *et al.* Diagnostic and clinical relevance of the number of circulating CD34+ cells in myelofibrosis and myeloid metaplasia. *Blood* 2001; **98**: 3249–55.

29. Massa M, Rosti V, Ramajoli I, *et al.* Circulating CD34+, CD133+, and vascular endothelial growth factor receptor 2-positive endothelial progenitor cells in myelofibrosis with myeloid metaplasia. *J Clin Oncol* 2005; **23**: 5688–95.

30. Andreasson B, Lindstedt G, Kutti J. Plasma erythropoietin in essential thrombocythaemia: at diagnosis and in response to myelosuppressive treatment. *Leuk Lymphoma* 2000; **38**: 113–20.

31. Haga P, Cotes PM, Till JA, Minty BD, Shinebourne EA. Serum immunoreactive erythropoietin in children with cyanotic and acyanotic congenital heart disease. *Blood* 1987; **70**: 822–6.

32. Zwicky C, Theiler L, Zbaren K, Ischi E, Tobler A. The predictive value of clonogenic stem cell assays for the diagnosis of polycythaemia vera. *Br J Haematol* 2002; **117**: 598–604.

33. DiBella NJ, Silverstein MN, Hoagland HC. Effect of splenectomy on teardrop-shaped erythrocytes in agnogenic myeloid metaplasia. *Arch Intern Med* 1977; **137**: 380–1.

34. Thiele J, Kvasnicka HM, Boeltken B, *et al.* Initial (prefibrotic) stages of idiopathic (primary) myelofibrosis (IMF): a clinicopathological study. *Leukemia* 1999; **13**: 1741–8.

35. Pareti FI, Gugliotta L, Mannucci L, Guarini A, Mannucci PM. Biochemical and metabolic aspects of platelet dysfunction in chronic myeloproliferative disorders. *Thromb Haemost* 1982; **47**: 84–9.

36. Wehmeier A, Sudhoff T, Meierkord F. Relation of plate-let abnormalities to thrombosis and hemorrhage in chronic myeloproliferative disorders. *Semin Thromb Hemost* 1997; **23**: 391–402.

37. Jensen MK, de Nully BP, Lund BV, Nielsen OJ, Hasselbalch HC. Increased platelet activation and abnormal membrane glycoprotein content and redistribution in myeloproliferative disorders. *Br J Haematol* 2000; **110**: 116–24.

38. Berger S, Aledort LM, Gilbert HS, Hanson JP, Wasserman LR. Abnormalities of platelet function in patients with polycythemia vera. *Cancer Res* 1973; **33**: 2683–7.

39. Barnhart MI, Kim TH, Evatt BL, *et al*. Essential thrombocythemia in a child: platelet ultrastructure and function. *Am J Hematol* 1980; **8**: 87–107.

40. Moliterno AR, Hankins WD, Spivak JL. Impaired expression of the thrombopoietin receptor by platelets from patients with polycythemia vera. *N Engl J Med* 1998; **338**: 572–80.

41. Falanga A, Marchetti M, Evangelista V, *et al*. Polymorphonuclear leukocyte activation and hemostasis in patients with essential thrombocythemia and polycythemia vera. *Blood* 2000; **96**: 4261–6.

42. Wehmeier A, Fricke S, Scharf RE, Schneider W. A prospective study of haemostatic parameters in relation to the clinical course of myeloproliferative disorders. *Eur J Haematol* 1990; **45**: 191–7.

43. Wehmeier A, Daum I, Jamin H, Schneider W. Incidence and clinical risk factors for bleeding and thrombotic complications in myeloproliferative disorders. A retrospective analysis of 260 patients. *Ann Hematol* 1991; **63**: 101–6.

44. Tefferi A, Mesa RA, Schroeder G, *et al*. Cytogenetic findings and their clinical relevance in myelofibrosis with myeloid metaplasia. *Br J Haematol* 2001; **113**: 763–71.

45. Tefferi A, Mesa RA, Schroeder G, *et al*. Cytogenetic findings and their clinical relevance in myelofibrosis with myeloid metaplasia. *Br J Haematol* 2001; **113**: 763–71.

46. Pettigrew JD, Ward HP. Correlation of radiologic, histologic, and clinical findings in agnogenic myeloid metaplasia. *Radiology* 1969; **93**: 541–8.

47. Rondeau E, Solal-Celigny P, Dhermy D, *et al*. Immune disorders in agnogenic myeloid metaplasia: relations to myelofibrosis. *Br J Haematol* 1983; **53**: 467–75.

48. Gordon BR, Coleman M, Kohen P, Day NK. Immunologic abnormalities in myelofibrosis with activation of the complement system. *Blood* 1981; **58**: 904–10.

49. Kaelin WG Jr, Spivak JL. Systemic lupus erythematosus and myelofibrosis. *Am J Med* 1986; **81**: 935–8.

50. Pearson TC, Botterill CA, Glass UH, Wetherley-Mein G. Interpretation of measured red cell mass and plasma volume in males with elevated venous PCV values. *Scand J Haematol* 1984; **33**: 68–74.

51. Balga I, Solenthaler M, Furlan M. Should whole-body red cell mass be measured or calculated? *Blood Cells Mol Dis* 2000; **26**: 25–31.

52. Johansson PL, Safai-Kutti S, Kutti J. An elevated venous haemoglobin concentration cannot be used as a surrogate marker for absolute erythrocytosis: a study of patients with polycythaemia vera and apparent polycythaemia. *Br J Haematol* 2005; **129**: 701–5.

53. Spivak JL. Polycythemia vera: myths, mechanisms, and management. *Blood* 2002; **100**: 4272–90.

54. Lamy T, Devillers A, Bernard M, *et al*. Inapparent polycythemia vera: an unrecognized diagnosis. *Am J Med* 1997; **102**: 14–20.

55. Wasserman LR. The management of polycythemia vera. *Br J Haematol* 1971; **21**: 371–6.

56. Barosi G, Ambrosetti A, Finelli C, *et al*. The Italian Consensus Conference on Diagnostic Criteria for Myelofibrosis with Myeloid Metaplasia. *Br J Haematol* 1999; **104**: 730–7.

57. Rozman C, Giralt M, Feliu E, Rubio D, Cortes MT. Life expectancy of patients with chronic nonleukemic myeloproliferative disorders. *Cancer* 1991; **67**: 2658–63.

58. Passamonti F, Rumi E, Pungolino E, *et al*. Life expectancy and prognostic factors for survival in patients with polycythemia vera and essential thrombocythemia. *Am J Med* 2004; **117**: 755–61.

59. Finazzi G, Barbui T. Risk-adapted therapy in essential thrombocythemia and polycythemia vera. *Blood Rev* 2005; **19**: 243–52.

60. Finazzi G, Caruso V, Marchioli R, *et al*. Acute leukemia in polycythemia vera: an analysis of 1638 patients enrolled in a prospective observational study. *Blood* 2005; **105**: 2664–70.

61. Marchioli R, Finazzi G, Landolfi R, *et al*. Vascular and neoplastic risk in a large cohort of patients with polycythemia vera. *J Clin Oncol* 2005; **23**: 2224–32.

62. Dupriez B, Morel P, Demory JL, *et al*. Prognostic factors in agnogenic myeloid metaplasia: a report on 195 cases with a new scoring system. *Blood* 1996; **88**: 1013–18.

63. Cervantes F, Barosi G, Demory JL, *et al*. Myelofibrosis with myeloid metaplasia in young individuals: disease characteristics, prognostic factors and identification of risk groups. *Br J Haematol* 1998; **102**: 684–90.

64. Reilly JT. Idiopathic myelofibrosis: pathogenesis to treatment. *Hematol Oncol* 2006; **24**: 56–63.

65. Cervantes F, Tassies D, Salgado C, *et al*. Acute transformation in nonleukemic chronic myeloproliferative disorders: actuarial probability and main characteristics in a series of 218 patients. *Acta Haematol* 1991; **85**: 124–7.

66. Dingli D, Utz JP, Krowka MJ, Oberg AL, Tefferi A. Unexplained pulmonary hypertension in chronic myeloproliferative disorders. *Chest* 2001; **120**: 801–8.

67. van Genderen PJ, Troost MM. Polycythaemia vera and essential thrombocythaemia in the elderly. *Drugs Aging* 2000; **17**: 107–19.

68. Pearson TC, Weatherly-Mein G. Vascular occlusive episodes and venous haematocrit in primary proliferative polycythaemia. *Lancet* 1978; **2**: 1219–21.

69. Rector WG, Fortuin NJ, Conley CL. Non-hematologic effects of chronic iron deficiency. A study of patients with polycythemia vera treated solely with venesections. *Medicine (Baltimore)* 1982; **61**: 382–9.

70. Kiraly JF, Feldmann JE, Wheby MS. Hazards of phlebotomy in polycythemic patients with cardiovascular disease. *JAMA* 1976; **236**: 2080–1.

71. Harrison CN, Campbell PJ, Buck G, *et al*. Hydroxyurea compared with anagrelide in high-risk essential thrombocythemia. *N Engl J Med* 2005; **353**: 33–45.

72. King SB. Nitric oxide production from hydroxyurea. *Free Radic Biol Med* 2004; **37**: 737–44.

73. Sanchez-Palacios C, Guitart J. Hydroxyurea-associated squamous dysplasia. *J Am Acad Dermatol* 2004; **51**: 293–300.

74. Finazzi G, Ruggeri M, Rodeghiero F, Barbui T. Second malignancies in patients with essential thrombocythaemia treated with busulphan and hydroxyurea: long-term follow-up of a randomized clinical trial. *Br J Haematol* 2000; **110**: 577–83.

75. Najean Y, Rain J. Treatment of polycythemia vera: use of 32p alone or in combination with maintenace therapy using hydroxyurea in 461 patients greater than 65 years of age. *Blood* 1997; **89**: 2319–27.

76. Cameron YC, Cortes J, Barkoh B, *et al*. t(3; 21)(q26; q22) in myeloid leukemia: an aggressive syndrome of blast transformation associated with hydroxyurea or antimetabolite therapy. *Cancer* 2006; **106**: 1730–8.

77. Silver RT. Interferon alfa: effects of long-term treatment for polycythemia vera. *Semin Hematol* 1997; **34**: 40–50.

78. Landolfi R, Marchioli R, Kutti J, *et al*. Efficacy and safety of low-dose aspirin in polycythemia vera. *N Engl J Med* 2004; **350**: 114–24.

79. Spivak J. Daily aspirin: only half the answer. *N Engl J Med* 2004; **350**: 99–101.

80. Mesa RA, Steensma DP, Pardanani A, *et al*. A phase 2 trial of combination low-dose thalidomide and prednisone for the treatment of myelofibrosis with myeloid metaplasia. *Blood* 2003; **101**: 2534–41.

81. Tefferi A, Mesa RA, Nagorney DM, Schroeder G, Silverstein MN. Splenectomy in myelofibrosis with myeloid metaplasia: a single-institution experience with 223 patients. *Blood* 2000; **95**: 2226–33.

82. Elliott MA, Tefferi A. Splenic irradiation in myelofibrosis with myeloid metaplasia: a review. *Blood Rev* 1999; **13**: 163–70.

83. Cervantes F, Alvarez-Larran A, Hernandez-Boluda JC, *et al*. Erythropoietin treatment of the anaemia of myelofibrosis with myeloid metaplasia: results in 20 patients and review of the literature. *Br J Haematol* 2004; **127**: 399–403.

84. Cervantes F, Hernandez-Boluda JC, Alvarez A, Nadal E, Montserrat E. Danazol treatment of idiopathic myelofibrosis with severe anemia. *Haematologica* 2000; **85**: 595–9.

85. Guardiola P, Anderson JE, Bandini G, *et al*. Allogeneic stem cell transplantation for agnogenic myeloid metaplasia: a European Group for Blood and Marrow Transplantation, Societe Francaise de Greffe de Moelle, Gruppo Italiano per il Trapianto del Midollo Osseo, and Fred Hutchinson Cancer Research Center Collaborative Study. *Blood* 1999; **93**: 2831–8.

86. Rondelli D, Barosi G, Bacigalupo A, *et al*. Allogeneic hematopoietic stem-cell transplantation with reduced-intensity conditioning in intermediate- or high-risk patients with myelofibrosis with myeloid metaplasia. *Blood* 2005; **105**: 4115–19.

PART V

Disorders of hemostasis in the elderly

26

Acquired hemophilia in the elderly

Francesco Baudo, Francesco de Cataldo

Introduction

The acquired hemophilia syndrome occurs more frequently in advanced age: the majority of the patients are over 60 years, and comorbidities are frequent. Acquired hemophilia is a rare clinical syndrome characterized by acute bleeding, either spontaneous or related to surgery or trauma, in patients with negative family and personal history, and it may be severe and fatal [1–4]. The depletion of factor VIII (FVIII:C), or much less frequently of other factors, is mediated by specific autoantibodies, directed against functional epitopes with neutralization and/or accelerated clearance of the factor from the plasma [5].

The clinical information discussed in this chapter is retrieved from reports including more than ten patients and from a survey of the Italian hemophilia centers.

Epidemiology

The incidence of acquired hemophilia varies between 0.1 and 1.0 cases per million population per year, but it is likely that not all affected patients are included in the published surveys [1,2,6,7]. The median age at presentation varies between 55 and 78 years (Table 26.1) [1,4,7–25], with equal distribution between the sexes except in the younger age groups because of the cases related to pregnancy (Table 26.2) [1,4,7–9,11–26]. Acquired hemophilia is commonly associated with a variety of clinical conditions: autoimmune diseases (systemic lupus erythematosus, rheumatoid arthritis, asthma), solid tumors, lymphoproliferative diseases, and

pregnancy, but in 50% it is idiopathic (Table 26.3) [1,7,8,11,12,14,15,17–20,22–26]. Drug association is very rare (Table 26.4) [1,10,12,14,15,20,22,23,27–32]. The association with malignancy is three times higher in men than in women, without a definite relation to tumor type, although acquired hemophilia is more common in solid tumors than in lymphoproliferative diseases [3,14,33–35]. Occasionally

Table 26.1. Acquired hemophilia: age (median and range) at presentation.

Author	Patients (n)	Age (years)	Patients >60 years old (%)
Green [1]	163	—	91 (55.8%)
Di Bona [4]	17	59.0 (21–78)	5 (29.4%)
Lottenberg [7]	16	68.0 (35–61)	12 (75%)
Spero [8]	18	63.7 (19–86)	—
Lian [9]	12	65.0 (19–76)	8 (66%)
Morrison [10]	65	62.0 (11–90)	38 (58.4%)
Green [11]	31	68.0 (25–82)	26 (83.9%)
Schwartz [12]	19	66.4 (24–88)	12 (63.1%)
Söhngen [13]	10	63.5 (24–80)	6 (60%)
Bossi [14]	34	69.0 (22–93)	20 (58.8%)
Yee [15]	24	69.0 (2–92)	—
Grünewald [16]	10	72.0 (55–87)	9 (90%)
Delgado [17]	17	67.0 (8–86)	10 (58.8%)
Baudo [18]	96	65.0 (2–88)	—
Nemes [19]	26	63.0 (22–85)	16 (61.5%)
Huang [20]	15	55.0 (21–80)	7 (46.8%)
Baudo [21]	15	72.0 (62–81)	15 (100%)
Collins [22]	18	70.0 (38–87)	12 (66.6%)
Sallah [23]	34	57.5 (26–82)	15 (44.1%)
Holme [24]	14	78.0 (58–94)	12 (85.7%)
Zeitler [25]	35	65.0 (28–81)	23 (65.7%)

Blood Disorders in the Elderly, ed. Lodovico Balducci, William Ershler, Giovanni de Gaetano.
Published by Cambridge University Press. © Cambridge University Press 2008.

Table 26.2. Acquired hemophilia: sex distribution.

Author	Patients (n)	Male (n)	Female (n)	Pregnancy-related (n)
Green [1]	205	108	97	13
Di Bona [4]	17	8	9	5
Lottenberg [7]	16	11	5	1
Spero [8]	18	9	9	1
Lian [9]	12	3	9	1
Green [11]	31	15	16	2
Schwartz [12]	19	7	12	1
Söhngen [13]	10	4	6	1
Bossi [14]	34	15	19	3
Yee [15]	28	11	17	4
Grünewald [16]	10	5	5	0
Delgado [17]	17	9	8	4
Baudo [18]	96	38	58	20
Nemes [19]	26	13	13	2
Huang [20]	15	7	8	3
Baudo [21]	15	9	6	0
Collins [22]	18	12	6	0
Sallah [23]	34	18	16	3
Holme [24]	14	6	8	0
Zeitler [25]	35	15	20	4
Kessler [26]	65	32	33	7
Total (%)	735	355 (48.3%)	380 (51.7%)	75 (10.2%)

disappearance of the inhibitor is associated with therapy [33,34].

Characteristics of the inhibitors

The inhibitor is an anti-FVIII:C in over 98% of the cases. Therefore the characteristics of the inhibitor and the laboratory diagnosis refer to anti-FVIII:C antibodies. Readers interested in acquired hemophilia with antibodies with other specificities can find further details in the relevant publications [36–46].

FVIII:C is a protein ($\sim$300 kDa) constituted by a heavy chain (HC) and a light chain (LC) and 2332 amino acid residues. The complex FVIIIa-phospholipid-Ca is the cofactor of activated FIX (FIXa) in the activation reaction of factor X (FX) to FXa (Fig. 26.1) [47]. The FVIII:C molecule is structured in domains carrying the fuctional sites [48]. The binding sites of the major FVIII ligands and the targets of the inhibitory antibodies are depicted in Fig. 26.2.

The antibodies arising in congenital hemophilia are IgG antibodies acting with a first-order kinetics reaction. The antibodies in the acquired hemophilia syndrome are IgG1 and IgG4 autoantibodies acting with a second-order kinetics reaction. This difference is relevant to the laboratory diagnosis and to the therapy. The binding sites of the FVIII:C ligands have been mapped by the use of antibodies. The main antigenic regions are the A_2 and C_2 domains: in 62% of the patients with acquired hemophilia the dominant inhibitor is directed either against A_2 or C_2 domains, in contrast to congenital hemophilia, where the majority of the inhibitors have both anti-A_2 and anti-C_2 epitope specificity [49–51]. The time and temperature of the neutralization reaction are important features in reference to the laboratory tests. No complement fixation occurs; therefore no organ damage ensues [5]. Autoantibodies have less cross-reactivity with heterologous FVIII compared to alloantibodies; the therapeutic use of porcine FVIII concentrate may be warranted (if re-marketed).

Clinical picture

The diagnosis of acquired hemophilia is suggested by the clinical picture and confirmed by laboratory tests. Acute bleeding occurs in patients without a family and personal history. The onset may be spontaneous but quite frequently is related to a trivial trauma or intervention (intramuscular injection or positioning of a venous catheter) or to a surgical procedure (about 25% of the cases) [4,11–18,20, 22–24]. Occasionally patients with an overlooked prolonged APTT (activated partial thromboplastin time) before surgery are referred to specialized centers because of critical perioperative bleeding. In the Italian survey the preoperative APTT, when measured, was always prolonged [18]. Critical bleeding may occur during procedures carried out because of misdiagnosed compartmental syndromes: retropharyngeal and retroperitoneal hemorrhages, extensive muscular hematomata with compression

Table 26.3. Acquired hemophilia: underlying conditions (percentage of patient number with each condition)

	Green [1]	Lotten- berg [7]	Spero [8]	Green [11]	Schwartz [12]	Bossi [14]	Yee [15]	Delgado [17]	Baudo [18]	Nemes [19]	Huang [20]	Collins [22]	Sallah [23]	Holme [24]	Zeitler [25]	Kessler [26]
Patients (n)	178	16	18	31	19	34	24	17	96	26	15	18	34	14	35	65
Idiopathic (%)	46.1	68.8	77.8	38.7	21	47.2	45.9	41.2	46.8	53.8	26.7	77.8	26.5	71.4	68.5	52.4
Autoimmune disorders (%)	18	0	0	29	21	20.6	20.9	17.6	16.6	7.7	6.7	5.5	29.5	7.2	10.5	17
Drug- related (%)	5.6	0	0	0	5.4	2.9	4.1	0	0	0	6.6	5.5	11.7	0	0	3
Pregnancy (%)	7.3	6.2	5.5	6.5	5.3	8.8	16.6	23.5	21	7.7	20	0	5.9	0.0	10.5	11
Malignancies (%)	6.7	25	0	3.2	21	14.7	12.5	17.7	9.4	19.2	26.7	11.2	17.6	21.4	7.8	13.5
Dermatologic disorders (%)	4.5			0	0	2.9	0	0	1	7.7	0	0	0	0	0	2
Other (%)	11.8	0	16.7	22.6	26.3	2.9	0	0	5.1	3.8	13.3	0	8.8	0	2.7	1.5

Other: diabetes, hepatitis, glomerulonephritis, MGUS, blood transfusion, cytomegalovirus infection, surgery, Gram-negative sepsis, nephrotic syndrome, thrombotic thrombocytopenic purpura, chronic obstructive pulmonary disease, herpes zoster, ischemic heart disease.

Table 26.4. Drugs associated with acquired hemophilia.

Antibiotics	penicillins, ampicillin, sulphonamides, chloramphenicol, ciprofloxacin, cephalosporin [10,14,23,27]
Antifungal	griseofulvin [12]
Antithrombotic	clopidogrel [28]
Anticonvulsants	diphenylhydantoin, phenytoin [1,29]
Antidepressant	thioxanthenes, flupenthixol, fluphenazine [20,22,30]
Antineoplastic	fludarabine [31]
Antimalarial	[15,32]
Antiangina	hydralazine [32]
Immunological agent	interferon alpha [31]

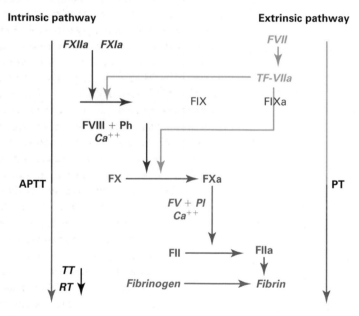

Figure 26.1 Simplified scheme of the coagulation cascade and laboratory tests; intrinsic (in blue), extrinsic (in green), and common (in red) pathway. TF, tissue factor; Ph, phospholipid; APTT, activated partial thromboplastin time; PT, prothrombin time; RT, reptilase time. *See color plate section.*

of nervous and vascular structures. Hematomata of the iliopsoas muscle, in particular, are often unrecognized, leading to unnecessary diagnostic invasive procedures (Fig. 26.3). Intracranial hemorrhages in the clinical course are a rare but catastrophic event (Italian survey 2%).

At presentation major bleeding, although variable in the different series, occurs in the majority (66.5%) of patients (Table 26.5) [1,4,7,13,14,16–18,20,22–25]. We have classified bleeding as major or minor according to the author's definition, when available, or following personal interpretation of the clinical data as

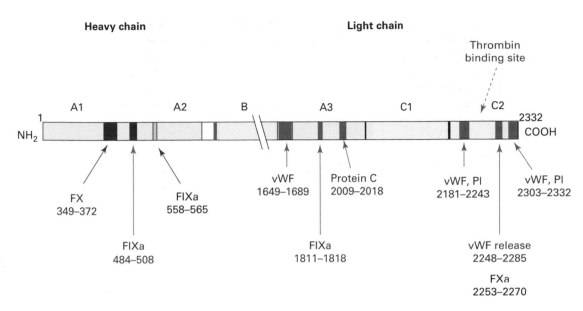

Figure 26.2 FVIII structure (simplified as relevant to the present discussion). Heavy chain (A1, A2, B domains) and light chain (A3, C1, C2 domains). Arrows indicate the binding sites of the major FVIII ligands as mapped by the use of alloantibodies: FIXa, FX, FXa, vWF, phospholipids (Pl), and protein C. Blue indicates target of FVIII inhibitors. Dotted arrow indicates that the inhibitor target is not mapped to date. From Saenko *et al.* 2002 [48], reproduced with permission of the author. *See color plate section.*

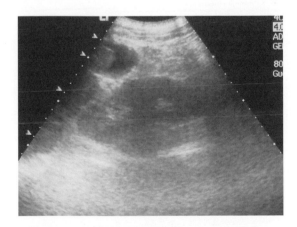

Figure 26.3 A 69-year-old man with severe abdominal pain and clinical signs of acute abdomen; on prednisone for 12 months for polymyalgia. Echography interpreted as aneurysm of the iliac artery: PT ratio 1.05, APTT ratio 1.9. At surgery: iliopsoas hematoma, severe intra- and postoperative bleeding; transferred to our department. PT ratio 1.29, APTT ratio 2.3; FVIII 2.5% human and porcine anti-FVIII inhibitor, 63 and 3 BU/mL respectively.

Table 26.5. Acquired hemophilia: number of patients with major bleeding at presentation.

Author	Patients (n)	Bleeding (n)	Major bleeding (n)
Green [1]	189	189	164
Di Bona [4]	17	17	6
Lottenberg [7]	16	16	5
Söhngen [13]	10	10	2
Bossi [14]	34	34	18
Grünewald [16]	10	10	8
Delgado [17]	17	17	8
Baudo [18]	96	96	50
Huang [20]	34	34	21
Collins [22]	15	15	8
Sallah [23]	14	14	6
Holme [24]	18	18	5
Zeitler [25]	35	35	35
Total (%)	505	505	336 (66.5%)

reported. A definition of severe bleeding is shown in Table 26.6 [52], and sites of bleeding are reported in Table 26.7 [4,7,8,11–20,22–26]. Common sites of less dramatic but serious bleeding are the skin (ecchymoses and hematomata), muscles and mucosae (melena, hematuria, metrorrhagia, epistaxis, gingivorrhagia). Hemarthroses are less frequent than in

Table 26.6. Definition of severe bleeding. From Sallah and Aledort 2005 [52].

Decrease in hemoglobin >3 g/dL
Need for transfusion with packed red blood cells
Bleeding into the retropharyngeal or retroperitoneal
   regions
Compartment-syndrome
Intracranial hemorrhage
Periorbital bleeding
Any hemorrhagic event requiring admission to the
   intensive care unit

congenital hemophilia, occurring in the Italian survey either as a presenting sign (7.3% of 96 patients) or at relapse (16.1% of 31 patients) [18]. Bleeding may be mild: in the analysis of eight reports with definition of bleeding severity [4,14,16–18,22–24] 66 patients (28.8%) did not require treatment at presentation (no further details are given), but management may be very demanding because of the intensity of the bleeding and the comorbidities. Hypovolemia and circulating failure may be life-threatening. In the series of Green and Lechner bleeding was defined as severe in 87% of the patients and was particularly common in the first few weeks from presentation [1]. By contrast, Collins and colleagues reported severe bleeding in 5 out of 18 patients [22]. Bleeding-related mortality overall is 12.5% including the old reports.

Bleeding is correlated neither with the inhibitor titer nor with the FVIII:C levels. In an analysis of 15 reports [11–14,17,19,20,22,24,32,35,53–56] no correlation was found by univariate and bivariate

Table 26.7. Acquired hemophilia. Clinical manifestation (number) at presentation. Data derived from the original reports; some patients have multiple sites.

Author	Patients (n)	Bleeding (n)	Muscle	CNS	Deep[a]	Joint	Mucosa[b]	Skin
Di Bona [4]	17	17	8	1	4	0	6	8
Lottenberg [7]	16	16	2	2	3	1	6	12
Spiro [8]	18	18	9	1	5	7	9	0
Green [11]	65	64	17	0	5	2	5	2
Schwartz [12]	19	19	1	0	3	1	9	8
Söhngen [13]	10	10	5	0	0	2	1	4
Bossi [14]	34	34	32	0	7	4	20	32
Yee [15]	24	23	2	0	2	0	11	23
Grünewald [16]	10	10	7	2	1	0	0	10
Delgado [17]	17	17	3	1	2	0	9	3
Baudo [18]	96	96	59	0	8	7	31	36
Nemes [19]	26	26	9	1	6	0	2	7
Huang [20]	15	15	4	0	4	3	1	9
Collins [22]	18	18	5	2	2	0	7	16
Sallah [23]	34	34	9	2	2	1	13	15
Holme [24]	14	14	5	1	1	0	5	8
Zeitler [25]	35	35	32	0	6	0	2	0
Kessler [26]	65	65	21	0	12	1	12	15

[a] Deep = retroperitoneal, pleural, ocular, abdominal.
[b] Mucosa = gingivorrhagia, epistaxis, hematuria, metrorrhagia, GI tract bleeding.

analysis between clinical and laboratory data: severe bleeding in 97/230 patients, FVIII:C median value 2% (range 0–30), inhibitor titer median value 22 BU/mL (range 0.5–4750). Therefore, at variance with patients with congenital hemophilia, they are not valuable in guiding therapy.

Laboratory diagnosis

A simplified scheme of the coagulation cascade is represented in Fig. 26.1 to clarify the meaning of the relevant laboratory tests. FXa is pivotal in the activation of prothrombin to thrombin. The complex FVIII, phospholipids, and calcium ions is the cofactor in the activation reaction of FX to FXa by FIXa.

The APTT explores the intrinsic (blue) and common (red) pathways; it is prolonged because of the inhibition of the involved factor by the inhibitor: the APTT of the mixture of normal and patient plasma is also prolonged. The prothrombin time is normal because it explores the extrinsic (green) and common (red) pathways, which are not affected by the inhibitor, and because a complete thromboplastin is added. The interaction of FVIII:C and inhibitor is a second-order kinetics reaction. The relationship between inhibitor and factor concentration is not expressed by a straight line (first-order reaction) but is curvilinear, indicating that residual factor activity may be recovered (Fig. 26.4). This reaction is time- and temperature-dependent. The behavior of the inhibitor carries practical implications. The APTT

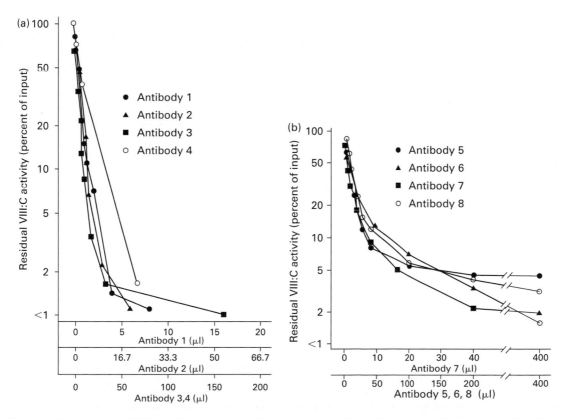

Figure 26.4 Inactivation of FVIII:C activity by (a) type I alloantibodies and (b) type II autoantibodies. From Grawril and Hoyer 1982 [57], reproduced with permission of the authors.

of the patient/normal plasma mixture requires a two-hour incubation at 37 °C; the factor VIII:C assay should be carried out at 0 and 120 minutes. FVIII:C activity (median 4, range 1–30%) is usually recovered in approximately 70% of the patients. The same principles apply to the quantification of the inhibitor. The normal plasma is mixed with different dilutions of the patient plasma. After two hours' incubation the residual factor is quantified. The inhibitor strength is expressed in units according to the recovery of the factor (Bethesda method): 1 unit = 50% reduction of the concentration of the factor. The quantification of the units is related to the dilution that induces a 50% reduction of the factor (e.g., 50% reduction with a dilution 1 : 20 of the patient plasma = 20 BU). The concentration of the factor is calculated by interpolating the value of the study sample in a reference standard curve. In over 99% of cases the inhibitor is FVIII:C-specific, but in rare cases it is specific for another component of the coagulation cascade. Measurement of the antiporcine FVIII:C inhibitor will be required when the porcine concentrate is again on the market.

The APTT is also prolonged in the antiphospholipid syndrome (lupus anticoagulant) and during therapy with unfractionated heparin. These clinical situations are readily excluded in the history because of the lack of hemorrhages and the knowledge of heparin therapy respectively. Further details are given by Brandt *et al.* [58]. A laboratory diagnostic algorithm is presented in Fig. 26.5.

Management of acquired hemophilia

The management is directed to the control of the bleeding and the suppression of the inhibitor. The sudden onset of clinically significant bleeding without family and personal history with a prolonged APTT and normal prothrombin time requires urgent consultation and eventual transfer of the patient to the reference center. The published studies are retrospective and include a limited number of patients with different primary clinical conditions. No prospective randomized trial comparing the

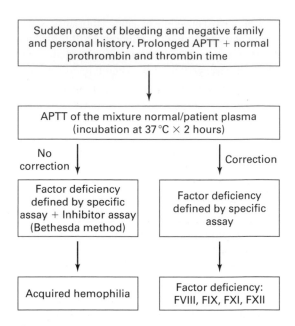

Figure 26.5 Laboratory diagnosis algorithm for acquired hemophilia.

efficacy of the various antihemorrhagic or immunosuppressive agents has been carried out to date; none of the available agents is effective in all the patients [59–64].

Control of hemorrhage

Efficient hemostasis can be achieved with a variety of methods (Table 26.8): normalization/correction of FVIII:C deficiency (human plasma-derived or recombinant FVIII concentrates, porcine FVIII concentrate, desmopressin), bypassing the inhibitor activity (activated prothrombin-complex concentrate [APCC], recombinant activated FVII [rFVIIa]), neutralization of the inhibitor by idiotypic anti-FVIII antibodies (high-dose immunoglobulins), removal of the inhibitor by immunoadsorption or plasmapheresis. Combined modalities may be necessary. The criteria for the antihemorrhagic therapy are the site and the entity of bleeding, age and comorbities, underlying disorders, inhibitor titer. Clinically the most significant are site and intensity (Tables 26.6, 26.7). Guidelines to define the entity

Table 26.8. Agents used and recommended dose in the treatment of acute bleeding in acquired hemophilia.

Agents	Initial dose	Subsequent doses
Human FVIII concentrate	50–100 IU/kg	50–100 IU/kg 2–3 times/day or 5–15 U/kg/h by continuous infusion
Recombinant FVIII concentrate	50–100 IU/kg	50–100 IU/kg 2–3 times/day or 5–15 U/kg/h by continuous infusion
Porcine FVIII concentrate	50–100 IU/kg	50–100 IU/kg 2–3 times/day or 5–15 U/kg/h by continuous infusion
DDAVP (Desmopressin; 1-deamino-8-D-arginine)	0.3 μg/kg[a]	0.3 μg /kg/day[a]
APCC (activated prothombin complex concentrate)	50–100 IU/kg	50–100 IU/kg 2–3 times/day or continuous infusion
rFVIIa (recombinant activated factor VII)	90 μg/kg	90 μg /kg every 3–6 hours as bolus or 10–20 μg/kg/h by continuous infusion
High-dose immunoglobulin	1 or 0.4 g/kg	1 or 0.4 g/kg for 2 or 5 consecutive days

[a] Recommended doses for intravenous or subcutaneous infusion; fixed doses of 300 mg in adults and 150 mg in children by intranasal spray.

of bleeding are published [65]. The categorization of bleeding as minor, moderate, or severe depends largely on clinical evaluation by the physician. In minor bleeding (e.g., ecchymoses) initial observation without intervention is justified. But the overall bleeding-related mortality rate approaches 12.5% (survey of the literature), mainly due to early hemorrhagic complications. Therefore strict observation and early intervention are essential in every patient.

Factor VIII replacement

FVIII replacement is the treatment of choice when the bleeding is minor and the inhibitor titer is low (<5 BU/mL) [60,62,63]. A loading dose is given as a bolus to neutralize the inhibitor and to achieve the hemostatic level, followed by subsequent doses given by bolus or by continuous infusion for maintenance [66,67]. The recovery and half-life of the infused FVIII:C cannot be predicted because of the variable kinetics of FVIII:C [2] (second-order kinetics reaction; see Laboratory diagnosis, above). Nevertheless the determination of recovery is clinically useful. FVIII:C recovery is monitored by determining its concentration before the infusion and 30 minutes and 6 hours after it, and the dose to be infused is calculated accordingly [68–70]. FVIII concentrates are plasma-derived or recombinant, and both have a

high efficacy and a very low risk of transmitting viral infections [71]. In acquired hemophilia the anamnestic response is a rare event [18,52,66,67,72–74]. FVIII autoantibodies have a low cross-reactivity with porcine FVIII; therefore a satisfactory hemostatic level may be obtained even in patients with high inhibitor titer [10,26,75,76]. Pyrexia, flushing, urticaria, severe anaphylactic reactions, thrombocytopenia are the possible adverse effects [10,26,77–79]. The porcine FVIII concentrate is out of the market but its re-marketing is being considered. A phase II study of a recombinant product in hemophilia A is under way in the USA, Canada, and South Africa.

Desmopressin (DDAVP; 1-deamino-8-D-arginine), a synthetic vasopressin analog, releases FVIII/von Willebrand factor from the vascular endothelium [80]. When infused intravenously or administered subcutaneously [81] or intranasally [82], FVIII:C increases three- to fivefold above the baseline value [82,83], sufficient to treat minor bleeding. The tachyphylaxis phenomenon limits it use to three or four consecutive days. The anti-diuretic and vasomotor side effects require caution in older patients [62,84]. DDAVP is indicated in the treatment of mild congenital hemophilia and von Willebrand disease [82]. The experience in acquired hemophilia, very limited and anecdotal [84–86], indicates that DDAVP may be used in the treatment of patients with mild bleeding and low-titer acquired FVIII:C inhibitor (<5 BU/mL) [87].

High-dose immunoglobulins

The response has been attributed to the presence of anti-idiotype antibodies in the pooled immunoglobulins [88,89]. In a prospective multi-center study, 19 patients with low-titer inhibitor were treated with 400 mg/kg for five consecutive days or 1000 mg/kg for two days, with a response rate (complete and partial remission) of 25% [90]. Multiple courses are needed to obtain a sustained response.

FVIII-inhibitor bypassing concentrate

Concentrates with FVIII inhibitor-bypassing activity are a plasma-derived "prothrombin complex" of activated factors (FIX and FVIIa in particular) (APCC), bypassing the intrinsic pathway of the coagulation cascade (Fig. 26.1). The mechanism of action is not completely understood. APCCs are used in the treatment of FVIII inhibitors in congenital hemophilia [91,92], but experience in acquired hemophilia is quite limited (Table 26.9) [16,23,24]. The standard dose is between 50 and 100 IU/kg every 8–12 hours. Efficacy is not predictable by laboratory tests [93–95]. Clinical endpoints are used to monitor treatment. When APCC is used as first-line therapy, response rate in severe and moderate bleeding ranges from 76% to 100% [16,23,24]. Normal hemostasis was also observed in two patients undergoing surgery [96]. Adverse effects are mild (pruritus, rash, back pain, diarrhea). Thromboembolic complications were reported in patients with other risk factors [97–99].

Recombinant activated FVII (rFVIIa) is produced by genetic engineering and activated during the purification process. At high concentration it activates FX (see Fig. 26.1), bypassing the intrinsic pathway (FVIII/IX) via a tissue-factor-dependent or independent reaction [100]. "Its action is localized to the site of bleeding since systemic activation, if it occurs, appears to be minimal despite the administration of large doses of the factor even in people without coagulopathy" [101]. Its efficacy has been

Table 26.9. Acquired hemophilia: APCC in patients with severe bleeding.

Author	Episodes (n)	Severe/ moderate	Complete response
Grünewald [16][a]	6	6/0	6
Sallah [23][b]	34	21/13	16/13
Holme [24][b]	7	6/1	6/1

[a] prospective study.
[b] retrospective study.

demonstrated in hemophilic patients with inhibitor, but its use is not well defined in acquired hemophilia. Two studies have been reported, using rFVIIa either as first-line or as salvage therapy, and the data are summarized in Table 26.10. Hay *et al.* reported on the use of rFVIIa in 74 episodes in 38 patients registered in 32 centers between 1990 and 1995 (NovoSeven® compassionate use program) [102]: 6 patients (14 episodes) as first-line therapy, 32 patients (60 episodes) as salvage therapy. Treatment was carried out at the standard dose (90 μg/kg every 2–6 hours, median duration 3.9 days, median number of doses 28). The clinical efficacy was assessed at 8 hours, 24 hours, and at the end of treatment and "was categorized by the supervising physician as effective, partial response, or ineffective, based on clinical examination of the bleed, careful monitoring of vital signs, full blood count and ultrasonography or CT scanning where appropriate." An effective response was observed in all 14 episodes in which rFVIIa was used as first-line therapy. An effective response was observed in 75% and a partial response in 17% of the episodes when it was used as salvage therapy. The response to treatment was in general rapid: bleeding was controlled within 8–24 hours in 92% of the episodes. Three patients died because of bleeding: GI tract and CNS bleeding occurred in one patient each, one and seven days after discontinuation of treatment; one patient, who failed rFVIIa, died of retroperitoneal hemorrhage. One patient had an episode of DIC concomitant to hypovolemic shock; no other thromboembolic complications occurred.

Table 26.10. Acquired hemophilia: rFVIIa as first-line or as salvage therapy.

Author	Fist-line therapy		Salvage therapy		Bleeding-related deaths
	Episodes (n)	Efficacy (E/P)	Episodes (n)	Efficacy (E/P)	Patients (n)
Baudo [21][a]	19	17/1	1	1	1/15
Hay [102][b]	14	14	60	45/10	3/38

[a] prospective study.

[b] retrospective study.

Clinical efficacy evaluated as effective (E) or partially effective (P).

A prospective study was carried out in Italy in 2001. Fourteen patients (20 bleeding episodes), selected according to the severity of bleeding, received rFVIIa as first-line therapy and one patient after failure of DDAVP and porcine FVIII. Treatment was very effective or effective in 13/15 patients (87%) and in 18/20 bleeding episodes (90%), in the majority of the cases within 24 hours, with no difference between intermittent and continuous infusion [21].

Management relies on clinical evaluation because of the lack of laboratory monitoring, and the short half-life (6 hours) necessitates frequent administrations. Thromboembolic complications are rare [21,102–105], and their relation to rFVIIa administration is controversial because of confounding factors (e.g., stroke, cancer, surgery, pregnancy, liver failure, congestive heart failure, coronary artery disease) [106–112].

Removal of the inhibitor

The inhibitor can be removed by plasmapheresis or by immunoadsorption (staphylococcal protein A bound to sepharose or to silica matrix, sepharose-bound polyclonal sheep antihuman antibodies). This technique is useful in particular clinical conditions (e.g., prior to surgery) and in severe bleeding may be life-saving. Extracorporeal methods have only temporary effect and need replacement therapy with FVIII concentrates immediately after the procedure. Simultaneous immunosuppression is needed because of the subsequent rebound. The need for special equipment and expertise limit these methods to specialized centers [113–117].

Immunosuppressive therapy

The aim of immunosuppressive therapy is the suppression of the inhibitor. To carry out sufficiently powered prospective controlled studies to evaluate the efficacy of the different therapeutic agents would be difficult. Efficacy is also difficult to assess because of the possibility of spontaneous remissions: in children, in postpartum women, and in drug associated cases spontaneous complete disappearance of the inhibitor was reported in up to 36% of the patients [7], but this occurrence is unpredictable and the patients remain at great risk of severe bleeding if the inhibitor persists [11]. Therefore immunosuppressive therapy should be initiated as soon as the diagnosis is established (grade B recommendation based on level IIb evidence [8,54,68]). Prednisone as monotherapy or in combination with cyclophosphamide and other immunosuppressive agents is the standard intervention: prednisone at a dose of ≥1 mg/kg per day for a minimum of three weeks; cyclophosphamide (2 mg/kg per day), vincristine, azathioprine (standard doses) alone or in combination. The therapy should be carried out with adequate doses and duration [8,62,63,118]. Previous experience in hemophiliacs suggests the importance of carrying out the treatment according to hematologic tolerance [119]. Complete remission rate and overall mortality are significantly lower in the treated patients (Table 26.11) [120]. The data, pooled from non-homogeneous studies (Table 26.12) and the meta-analysis of Delgado (Table 26.13), indicate a high response rate with prednisone alone, but sustained remission after

Table 26.11. Acquired hemophilia. Response to immunosuppressive therapy: complete response and mortality rate. Meta-analysis by Delgado *et al.* 2003 [120].

Immunosuppressive therapy	Complete response (%)	Mortality rate (%)	Disease related-mortality (%)
Yes	79	20	10
No	41	41	19
p	<0.001	0.023	0.198

Table 26.12. Acquired hemophilia. Immunosuppressive therapy (pregnancy excluded): first-line or after steroid failure.

Therapy	Papers (*n*)	Patients (*n*)	CR (%)	CR or PR (%)	F (%)	Follow-up in CR (months)
Steroids [a]	11	98	57 (58.2)	7 (7.1)	34 (34.7)	10.5 (0.5–190) (28 patients)
Chemotherapy ± steroids [b]	13	130	90 (69.2)	12 (9.3)	28 (21.5)	12 (1–216) (46 patients)

CR, complete remission (specifically reported disappearance of the inhibitor); PR, partial remission (disappearance or decrease of the inhibitor not specified); F, failure.

[a] dose and duration variable (1–2 mg/kg/d).

[b] Cyclophosphamide, azathioprine, vincristine (dose and duration variable).

Table 26.13. Acquired hemophilia. Response to immunosuppressive therapy (IST): steroids and combined therapy. Meta-analysis by Delgado *et al.* 2003 [120].

Immunosuppressive therapy	Complete response (%)	Mortality rate (%)	Disease-related mortality (%)
Steroids	70	26	18
Cyclophosphamide + steroids	89	16	6
No therapy	41	41	19
p	<0.0001	0.031	0.041

prednisone discontinuation is rare. Conclusive data on the follow-up duration and relapse cannot be retrieved because of the limited information. Positive predictive factors are a low initial inhibitor level and a short interval between the appearance of the inhibitor and the start of therapy [61–63,118]. The problem of infectious complications and mortality related to the immunosuppressive therapy has been addressed but data are scanty [120].

In a randomized prospective multi-center trial 31 patients with newly diagnosed acquired hemophilia were treated with prednisone 1 mg/kg/day for three weeks; 20 non-responders were randomized: four patients prednisone (1 mg/kg/day), six patients cyclophosphamide 2 mg/kg/day, ten patients prednisone + cyclophosphamide for an additional six weeks. The inhibitor disappeared in three patients (75%) treated with prednisone and in eight patients (50%) treated with cyclophosphamide or cyclophosphamide + prednisone. No information on the follow-up were given [11].

In the Italian study 65 out of the 90 patients are evaluable for immunosuppressive therapy [18]. Three patients died before starting treatment, one because of bleeding, two from the underlying disease. Eight patients with a low inhibitor titer

Table 26.14. Acquired hemophilia. Results of immunosuppressive therapy in the Italian study. From Baudo *et al.* 2003 [18].

Therapy	Induction: final results				Relapse			
	n	CR	PR	F	*n*	CR	PR	F
Steroid + immunoglobulins	32	27	2	3	5	3	1	1
Chemo + combined therapy	31	23	4	4	6	4	2	0
Cyclosporine	2	2	0	0	0	0	0	0
Total	65	52	6	7	11	7	3	1

Chemotherapy: cyclophosphamide, azathioprine, melphelan

CR, complete remission; PR, partial remission; F, failure

Table 26.15. Cyclosporine A alone or in combination with steroids as salvage therapy.

Author	Patients (*n*)	Baseline inhibitor	CR/PR/F	Time to CR (months)	Therapy duration (months)	CR follow-up (months)
Schulman [121]	7	320 (15 –>1000)	5/1/1	NA	NA	NA
Brox [122]	2	14.4–7.4	2/0/0	NA	NA	20–24
Maclean [123]	1	40	1/0/0	3	14	10[a]

CR, complete remission; PR, partial remission; F, failure; Cyclosporine plasma level 200–250 mg/L.

[a] Follow-up after cyclosphorine discontinuation.

(<10 BU) did not receive immunosuppressive therapy; three of them died because of bleeding complications. Information relevant to the response to immunosuppressive therapy was missing in 14 patients. Results of the initial immunosuppressive therapy showed complete remission in 46 cases (70.7%), partial remission in 13 (20%), failure in 6 (9.3%). Four patients in partial remission achieved a complete remission after discontinuation of treatment. The other patients, including the failures, received further treatment with alternative modalities. The figures reported in Table 26.14 refer to the final results including the outcome of relapse. Patients with low (<10 BU) or high (>10 BU) inhibitor titer did not differ in the rate of complete remission (30 and 22 patients, respectively). Eleven patients (21%) relapsed; eight were rescued with additional therapy. One patient died because of bleeding; two patients achieved a spontaneous complete remission.

Other modalities have been introduced, and promising results have been reported with cyclosporine A [121–123] and 2-chlorodeoxyadenosine (cladribine) [124]. The limited experience is summarized in Tables 26.15, 26.16. The use of anti CD-20 antibody (rituximab) is recent. We have retrieved information from recent reviews, abstracts of meetings, and a Medline search. The reports deal with single patients or small groups (4–10 patients), and are not clear on the modalities of treatment. Our interpretation was that rituximab was either associated with other antihemorrhagic therapy or administered after resolution of bleeding. Therefore we considered only the efficacy on FVIII and inhibitor behavior (Table 26.17). Rituximab was administered at a dose of 375 mg/m^2 per week per 4–8 weeks. A complete remission and a partial remission were achieved in 75.5 and 6.6% respectively with a time to response from 1 week to 21 months. Complete

Table 26.16. 2-chlorodeoxyadenosine (2CDA, cladribine) in acquired hemophilia [124].

Number of patients	6
Number of cycles	1 in 5 patients; 2 in 1 patient
Inhibitor titer before treatment (BU/mL, median and range)	51 (18–162)
Nadir inhibitor titer (BU/mL)	1–4
Time to inhibitor nadir (days, median and range)	137 (102–280)
FVIII:C maximum level (%, median and range)	70 (54–87)
Follow-up	NA

Prospective study; no bleeding during treatment; no major toxicities. 2CDA dose: 0.1 mg/kg per day by continuous infusion for a total of 7 days

remission at two years was 94% [125,126]. More experience with rituximab is needed.

Immunotolerance is an accepted and effective treatment of hemophilic patients with inhibitor but has been rarely applied in acquired hemophilia (Table 26.18). Evidence of its effectiveness and safety has been demonstrated in patients treated by the Budapest protocol (human FVIII combined with cyclophosphamide and methylprednisolone) [19]. A complete and sustained remission has been obtained in 19/20 patients (95%). Similar results have been reported with a modified Malmö protocol (immunoadsorption, high doses of FVIII, high-dose immunoglobulin, cyclophosphamide and corticosteroids) [127–129]. Bleeding was rapidly controlled with one or two apheresis sessions without recurrence. Inhibitor decreased to undetectable

Table 26.17. Anti-CD20 monoclonal antibody (rituximab) in patients with acquired hemophilia.

Patients (n)	Resolution of bleeding	Normalization of FVIII	Disappearance of inhibitor	Increase of FVIII	Decrease of inhibitor	Time to response
45	42	34	34	3	3	1 week–21 months

Table 26.18. Immunotolerance in acquired hemophilia. Critical bleeding controlled rapidly during one or two apheresis sessions.

Author	Protocol	Patients (n)	Baseline inhibitor (BU/mL)	CR/PR	Time to CR	Relapse	Final CR	Follow-up (months)	Bleeding-related deaths
Nemes [19]	Budapest	20	25 (2.2–1128)	19	3 (2–12) weeks	2	19	21.2 (2–93)	0
Zeitler [129][a]	Bonn–Malmö	35	146 (6–3600)	31/4 [b]	3 (2–4) days	2[c]	31	44 (5–86)	0

Budapest protocol: FVIII + cyclophosphamide + methylprednisolone.

Bonn–Malmö protocol: immunoadsorption + high-dose immunoglobulin + FVIII concentrate + cyclophosphamide + prednisolone.

CR = complete remission defined as normal FVIII:C with undetectable inhibitor during a minimum follow-up of 12 months.

PR, partial remission defined as FVIII:C recovery up to 30%, inhibitor titer <5 BU/mL or both.

[a] Severe side effects: infections (3), neutropenia (1), mucositis (1) successfully managed by antibiotics without discontinuation of Bonn–Malmö.

[b] 2 patients discontinued therapy for concomitant diseases.

[c] CR after apheresis and immunosuppression.

levels: median 3 days; median of therapy duration 14 days; complete response 88%; median follow-up 44 months.

Conclusion

The majority of cases of acquired hemophilia occur in the general hospitals, with bleeding that may be life-threatening. In the presence of an unexplained and often severe hemorrhage with abnormally prolonged APTT it is important to seek immediate specialist advice. A prolonged APTT is often overlooked. Because of the rarity of the disorder, the complexity of treatment, and the potential risk of death related to severe bleeding, these patients should be managed in the hemophilia centers or under their supervision.

REFERENCES

1. Green D, Lechner K. A survey of 215 non-haemophilic patients with inhibitors to factor VIII. *Thromb Haemost* 1981; **45**: 200–3.

2. Hoyer LW. Factor VIII inhibitors. *Curr Opin Hematol* 1995; **2**: 365–71.

3. Morrison AE, Ludlam CA. Acquired haemophilia and its treatment. *Br J Haematol* 1995; **89**: 231–6.

4. Di Bona E, Schiavoni M, Castaman G, Ciavarella N, Rodeghiero F. Acquired hemophilia: experience of two Italian centers with 17 new cases. *Haemophilia* 1997; **3**: 183–8.

5. Hoyer LW, Gawryl MS, de la Fuente B. Immunological characterization of factor VIII inhibitors. In Hoyer LW, ed, *Factor VIII Inhibitors* (New York, NY: Liss, 1984), 73–85.

6. Shapiro SS, Hultin M. Acquired inhibitors to blood coagulation factors. *Semin Thromb Hemost* 1975; **1**: 336–85.

7. Lottenberg R, Kentro TB, Kitchens CS. Acquired haemophilia: a natural history study of 16 patients with factor VIII inhibitors receiving little or no therapy. *Arch Intern Med* 1987; **147**: 1077–81.

8. Spero JA, Lewis JH, Hasiba U. Corticosteroid therapy for acquired FVIII: C inhibitors. *Br J Haematol* 1981; **48**: 636–42.

9. Lian EC, Larcada AF, Chiu AY. Combination immunosuppressive therapy after factor VIII infusion for acquired factor VIII inhibitor. *Ann Intern Med* 1989; **110**: 774–8.

10. Morrison AE, Ludlam CA, Kessler CM. Use of porcine factor VIII in the treatment of patients with acquired hemophilia. *Blood* 1993; **81**: 1513–20.

11. Green D, Rademaker AW, Briet E. A prospective randomized trial of prednisolone and cyclophosphamide in the treatment of patients with factor VIII antibodies. *Thromb Haemost* 1993; **70**: 753–7.

12. Schwartz RS, Gabriel DA, Aledort LM, Green D, Kessler CM. A prospective study of acquired (autoimmune) factor VIII inhibitors with high-dose intravenous gammaglobulin. *Blood* 1995; **86**: 797–804.

13. Söhngen D, Specker C, Bach D, *et al.* Acquired factor VIII inhibitors in nonhemophilic patients. *Ann Hematol* 1997; **74**: 89–93.

14. Bossi P, Cabane J, Ninet J, *et al.* Acquired hemophilia due to factor VIII inhibitors in 34 patients. *Am J Med* 1998; **105**: 400–8.

15. Yee TT, Taher A, Pasi KJ, Lee CA. A survey of patients with acquired haemophilia in a hemophilia centre over 28-year period. *Clin Lab Haematol* 2000; **22**: 275–8.

16. Grünewald M, Beneke H, Güthner C, Germowitz A, Brommer A, Griesshammer M. Acquired haemophilia: experiences with a standardized approach. *Haemophilia* 2001; **7**: 164–9.

17. Delgado J, Villar A, Jimenez-Yuste V, Gago J, Quintana M, Hernandez-Navarro F. Acquired hemophilia: a single-center survey with emphasis on immunotherapy and treatment-related side-effects. *Eur J Haematol* 2002; **69**: 158–64.

18. Baudo F, Mostarda G, de Cataldo F. Acquired factor VIII and factor IX inhibitors: survey of the Italian haemophilia centers (AICE). *Haematologica* 2003; **88** (Suppl 12): 93–9.

19. Nemes L, Pitlik E. Ten years experience with immunotolerance induction therapy in acquired hemophilia. *Haematologica* 2003; **88** (Suppl 12): 106–10.

20. Huang YW, Saidi P, Philipp C. Acquired factor VIII inhibitors in non-haemophilic patients: clinical experience of 15 cases. *Haemophilia* 2004; **10**: 713–21.

21. Baudo F, de Cataldo F, Gaidano G. Treatment of acquired factor VIII inhibitor with recombinant activated factor VIIa: data from the Italian registry of acquired hemophilia. *Haematologica* 2004; **89**: 759–61.

22. Collins P, Macartney N, Davies R, Lees S, Giddins J, Majer R. A population based, unselected, consecutive

cohort of patients with acquired haemophilia A. *Br J Haematol* 2004; **124**: 86–90.

23. Sallah S. Treatment of acquired hemophilia with factor eight inhibitor bypassing activity. *Haemophilia* 2004; **10**: 169–73.

24. Holme PA, Brosstad F, Tjønnfjord GE. Acquired haemophilia: management of bleeds and immune therapy to eradicate autoantibodies. *Haemophilia* 2005; **11**: 510–15.

25. Zeitler H, Ulrich-Merzenich G, Hess L, *et al.* Treatment of acquired hemophilia by the Bonn–Malmö Protocol: documentation of an in vivo immunomodulating concept. *Blood* 2005; **105**: 2287–93.

26. Kessler CM, Ludlam. The treatment of acquired factor VIII inhibitors: worldwide experience with porcine factor VIII concentrate. *Semin Hematol* 1993; **30** (Suppl 1): 22–7.

27. Hultin MB, Shapiro SS, Bowman HS, *et al.* Immunosuppressive therapy of factor VIII inhibitors. *Blood* 1976; **48**: 95–108.

28. Haj M, Dasani H, Kundu S, Mohiti U, Collins PW. Acquired haemophilia A may be associated with clopidogrel. *BMJ* 2004; **329**: 323.

29. O'Reilly RA, Hamilton RD. Acquired hemophilia, meningioma and diphenylhydantoin therapy. *J Neurosurg* 1980; **53**: 600–5.

30. Stewart AJ, Manson LM, Dasani H, Beddall A, Collins P, Shima M. Acquired haemophilia in recipients of depot thioxanthenes. *Haemophilia* 2000; **6**: 709–12.

31. Sallah S, Wan JY. Inhibitors against factor VIII associated with the use of interferon-alpha and fludarabine. *Thromb Haemost* 2001; **86**: 1119–21.

32. Burnet SP, Duncan EM, Lloyd JV, Han P. Acquired haemophilia in South Australia: a case series. *Intern Med J* 2001; **31**: 556–9.

33. Hauser I, Lechner K. Solid tumors and FVIII antibodies. *Thromb Haemost* 1999; **82**: 1005–7.

34. Sallah S, Nguten NP, Abdallah JM, Hanrahan LR. Acquired hemophilia in patients with hematologic malignancies. *Arch Pathol Lab Med* 2000; **124**: 730–4.

35. Sallah S, Wan JY. Inhibitors against factor VIII in patients with cancer. *Cancer* 2001; **91**: 1067–74.

36. Bajaj SP, Rapaport SI, Barclay S, Herbst KD. Acquired hypoprothrombinemia to non-neutralizing antibodies to prothrombin; mechanism and management. *Blood* 1985; **65**: 1538–43.

37. Wong RS, Lau FY, Cheng G. Successful treatment of acquired hypoprothrombinemia without associated lupus anticoagulant using intravenous immunoglobulin. *Haematologica* 2001; **86**: 551.

38. Favaloro EJ, Posen J, Ramakrishna R, *et al.* Factor V inhibitors: rare or not uncommon? A multi-laboratory investigation. *Blood Coag Fibrinolysis* 2004; **15**: 637–47.

39. Collins HW, Gonzalez MF. Acquired factor IX inhibitor in a patient with adenocarcinoma of the colon. *Acta Haematol* 1984; **71**: 49–52.

40. Miller K, Neely JE, Krivit W, Edson JR. Spontaneous acquired factor IX inhibitor in a nonhemophiliac child. *J Pediatr* 1978; **93**: 232–4.

41. Largo R, Sigg P, von Felten A, Straub PW. Acquired factor IX inhibitor in a nonhaemophilic patient with autoimmune disease. *Br J Haematol* 1974; **26**: 129–40.

42. Mulhare PE, Tracy PB, Golden EA, Branda RF, Bovill EG. A case of acquired factor X deficiency with in vivo and in vitro evidence of inhibitor activity directed against factor X. *Am J Clin Pathol* 1991; **96**: 196–200.

43. Smith SV, Liles DK, White GC 2nd, Brecher ME. Successful treatment of transient acquired factor X deficiency by plasmapheresis with concomitant intravenous immunoglobulin and steroid therapy. *Am J Hematol* 1998; **57**: 245–52.

44. Bern MM, Sahud M, Zhukov O, Qu K, Mithchell W. Treatment of factor XI inhibitor using recombinant activate factor VIIa. *Haemophilia* 2005; **11**: 20–5.

45. Goodrick MJ, Prentice AG, Copplestone JA, Pamphilon DH, Boon RJ. Acquired factor XI inhibitor in chronic lymphocytic leukaemia. *J Clin Pathol* 1992; **45**: 352–3.

46. Reece EA, Clyne LP, Romero R, Hobbins JC. Spontaneous factor XI inhibitors. Seven additional cases and review of the literature. *Arch Intern Med* 1984; **144**: 525–9.

47. van Dieijen G, Tans G, Rosing J, Hemker HC. The role of phospholipids and factor VIIIa in the activation of bovine factor X. *J Biol Chem* 1981; **256**: 3433–42.

48. Saenko EL, Ananyeva NM, Kouiavskaia DV, *et al.* Hemophilia A: effects of inhibitory antibodies on factor VIII functional interactions and approaches to prevent their action. *Haemophilia* 2002; **8**: 1–11.

49. Scandella D, Mattingly M, de Graaf S, Fulcher CA. Localization of epitopes for human factor VIII inhibitor antibodies by immunoblotting and antibody neutralization. *Blood* 1989; **74**: 1618–26.

50. Scandella D, Gilbert GE, Shima M, *et al.* Some factor VIII inhibitor antibodies recognize a common epitope corresponding to C2 domain amino acids 2248–2312 which overlap a phospholipids binding site. *Blood* 1995; **86**: 1811–19.

51. Prescott R, Nakai H, Saenko EV, *et al.* The inhibitor antibody response is more complex in hemophilia A patients than in most nonhemophiliacs with factor VIII autoantibodies. Recombinate and Kogenate Study Groups. *Blood* 1997; **89**: 3663–71.

52. Sallah S, Aledort L. Treatment of patients with acquired inhibitors. *J Thromb Haemost* 2005; **3**: 595–7.

53. Dykes AC, Walker ID, Lowe GDO, Tait RC. Combined prednisolone and intravenous immunoglobulin treatment for acquired factor VIII inhibitors: a 2-year review. *Haemophilia* 2001; **7**: 160–3.

54. Rubinger M, Houston DS, Schwetz N, Woloschuk DMM, Israel SJ, Johnston JB. Continuous infusion of porcine factor III in the management of patients with factor VIII inhibitors. *Am J Hematol* 1997; **56**: 112–18.

55. Saxena R, Mishra DK, Kashyap R, Choudhry VP, Mahapatra M, Bhargava M. Acquired haemophilia: a study of ten cases. *Haemophilia* 2000; **6**: 78–83.

56. Lindgren A, Wadenvik H, Tengborn L. Characterization of inhibitors to FVIII with an ELISA in congenital and acquired haemophilia A. *Haemophilia* 2002; **8**: 644–8.

57. Grawril NS, Hoyer LW Inactivation of factor VIII coagulant activity by two different types of human antibodies. *Blood* 1982; **60**: 1103–9.

58. Brandt JT, Triplett DA, Alving B, Scharrer I. Criteria for the diagnosis of lupus anticoagulant: an update. *Thromb Haemost* 1995; **74**: 1185–90.

59. Ludlam CA, Morrison AE, Kessler C. Treatment of acquired hemophilia. *Semin Hematol* 1994; **31** (Suppl 4): 16–19.

60. Cohen AJ, Kessler CM. Acquired inhibitors. *Baillieres Clin Haematol* 1996; **9**: 331–54.

61. Hay CRM. Acquired hemophilia. *Baillieres Clin Haematol* 1998; **11**: 287–303.

62. Kessler CM, Nemes L. Acquired inhibitors to factor VIII. In Rodriguez-Merchan EC, Lee CA, eds, *Inhibitors in Patients with Haemophilia* (Oxford: Blackwell, 2002), 98–112.

63. Ewenstein BM, Putnam KG, Bohn RL. Nonhemophilic inhibitors of coagulation. In Kitchens CS, Alving BM, Kessler CM, eds, *Consultative Hemostasis and Thrombosis* (Philadelphia, PA: Saunders, 2002), 75–90.

64. Baudo F, de Cataldo F. Acquired hemophilia: a critical syndrome. *Haematologica* 2004; **89**: 96–100.

65. Palareti G, Leali N, Coccheri S, *et al.* Bleeding complications of oral anticoagulant treatment: an inception-cohort, prospective collaborative study (ISCOAT). Italian Study on Complications of Oral Anticoagulant Therapy. *Lancet* 1996; **348**: 423–8.

66. Kasper CK. The therapy of factor VIII inhibitors. *Prog Hemostas Thromb* 1989; **9**: 57–86.

67. Lusher JM. Use of factor VIII by-passing agents to control bleeding in patients with acquired factor VIII inhibitors. In Kessler CM, ed, *Acquired Hemophilia*, 2nd edn (Princeton, NJ: Excerpta Medica, 1995), 113–29.

68. Hay CRM, Baglin TP, Collins PW, Hill FGH, Keeling DM. The diagnosis and management of factor VIII and IX inhibitors: a guideline from the UK Haemophilia Centre Doctors Organization (UKHCDO). *Br J Haematol* 2000; **111**: 78–90.

69. Association of Hemophilia Clinic Directors of Canada. Suggestions for the management of factor VIII inhibitors. *Haemophilia* 2000; **6** (Suppl 1): 52–9.

70. Gringeri A, Mannucci PM. Italian guidelines for the diagnosis and treatment of patients with haemophilia and inhibitors. *Haemophilia* 2005; **11**: 611–19.

71. Ludlam CA, Mannucci PM, Powderly WG on behalf of the European Interdisciplinary Working Group. Addressing current challenges in haemophilia care: consensus recommendations of a European Interdisciplinary Working Group. *Haemophilia* 2005; **11**: 433–7.

72. Blatt PM, White GC 2nd, McMillan CW, Roberts HR. Treatment of antifactor VIII antibodies. *Thromb Haemost* 1977; **38**: 514–23.

73. Kessler CM. An introduction to factor VIII inhibitors. The detection and quantitation. *Am J Med* 1991; **91** (Suppl 5A): 33–6.

74. Solymoss S. Post partum acquired factor VIII inhibitors: results of a survey. *Am J Hematol* 1998; **59**: 1–4.

75. Bona RD, Ribeno M, Klatsky AV, Panek S, Magnifico H, Rickles FR. Continuous infusion of porcine FVIII for the treatment of patients with factor VIII inhibitors. *Semin Hematol* 1993; **30** (Suppl 1): 32.

76. Gribble J, Garvey MB. Porcine factor VIII provides clinical benefit to patients with high levels of inhibitors to human and porcine factor VIII. *Haemophilia* 2000; **6**; 482–6.

77. Gatti L, Mannucci PM. Use of porcine factor VIII in the management of seventeen patients with factor VIII antibodies. *Thromb Haemost* 1984; **51**: 379–84.

78. Hay CRM, Bolton-Maggs P. Porcine factor VIIIC in the management of patients with factor VIII inhibitors. *Transf Med Rev* 1991; **5**: 145–51.

79. Gringeri A, Santagostino E, Tradati F. Adverse effects of treatment with porcine FVIII. *Thromb Haemost* 1991; **65**: 245–7.

80. Kaufmann JE, Oksche A, Wollheim CB, Günther G, Rosenthal W, Vischer UM. Vasopressin induced von Willebrand factor secretion from endothelial cells involves V2 receptors and cAMP. *J Clin Invest* 2000; **106**: 107–16.

81. Rodeghiero F, Castaman G, Mannucci PM. Prospective multicenter study on subcutaneous concentrated desmopressina for home treatment of patients with von Willebrand disease and mild or moderate hemophilia A. *Thromb Haemost* 1996; **76**: 692–6.

82. Mannucci PM, Canciani MT, Rota L, Donovan BS. Response of factor VIII/von Willebrand factor to DDAVP in healthy subjects and patients with haemophilia A and von Willebrand disease. *Br J Haematol* 1981; **47**: 283–93.

83. Mannucci PM, Aberg M, Nilsson IM, Robertson B. Mechanism of plasminogen activator and factor VIII increase after vasoactive drugs. *Br J Haematol* 1975; **30**: 81–93.

84. Muhm M, Grois N, Kier P, et al. 1-Deamino-8-d-arginine vasopressin in the treatment of non-haemophilic patients with acquired factor VIII inhibitor. *Haemostasis* 1990; **20**: 15.

85. De la Fuente, Panek S, Hoyer LW. The effect of 1-deamino 8 D-arginine vasopressin (DDAVP) in non haemophilic patient with an acquired type II inhibitor. *Br J Haematol* 1985; **59**: 127.

86. Naorose-Abidi SM, Bond LR, Chitolie A, Bevan DH. Desmopressin therapy in patients with acquired factor VIII inhibitors. *Lancet* 1988; **1**: 366.

87. Mudad R, Kane WH. DDAVP in acquired haemophilia A: case report and review of the literature. *Am J Hematol* 1993; **43**: 295–9.

88. Sultan Y, Maisonneuve P, Kazatchkine MD, Nydegger UE. Anti-idiotypic suppression of auto-antibodies to factor VIII (anti-haemophilic factor) by high-dose intravenous gammaglobulin. *Lancet* 1984; **2**: 765–8.

89. Sultan Y. Acquired hemophilia and its treatment. *Blood Coagul Fibrinolysis* 1997; **8** (Suppl 1): S15–S18.

90. Schwartz RS, Gabriel DA, Aledort LM, Green D, Kessler CM. A prospective study of acquired (autoimmune) factor VIII inhibitors with high-dose intravenous gammaglobulin. *Blood* 1995; **86**: 797–804.

91. Negrier C, Goudemand J, Sultan Y, et al. Multicentre retrospective study on the utilization of FEIBA in France in patients with factor VIII and factor IX inhibitors. *Thromb Haemost* 1977; **77**: 1113–19.

92. Sjamsoedin LJ, Heijen L, Mauser-Bunschoten EP, et al. The effect of activated prothrombin-complex (FEIBA) on joint and muscle bleeding in patients with hemophilia and antibodies for factor VIII. A double blinded clinical trial. *N Engl J Med* 1981; **305**: 717–21.

93. Lusher JM, Shapiro SS, Palascek JE, et al. Efficacy of prothrombin complex concentrates in haemophiliacs with antibodies to factor VIII. A multicentre therapeutic trial. *N Engl J Med* 1980; **303**: 421–5.

94. Turecek PL, Varadi K, Gritsch H et al. Factor Xa and prothrombin: mechanism of action of FEIBA. *Vox Sang* 1999; **77** (Suppl 1): 72S–79S.

95. White GC. Seventeen years' experience with Autoplex/Autoplex T. Evaluation of inpatients with severe haemophilia A and factor VIII inhibitors at a major haemophilia center. *Haemophilia* 2000; **6**; 508–12.

96. Tjønnfjord GE, Brinch L, Gedde-Dahl III T, Brosstad FR. Activated prothrombin complex concentrate (FEIBA®) treatment during surgery in patients with inhibitors to FVIII/IX. *Haemophilia* 2004; **10**: 174–8.

97 Chavin SI, Siegel DM, Rocco TA, Olson JP. Acute myocardial infarction during treatment with an activated prothrombin complex concentrate in a patient with factor VIII deficiency and a factor VIII inhibitor. *Am J Med* 1988; **85**: 245–9.

98. Mizon P, Goudemand J, Jude B, Marey A. Myocardial infarction after FEIBA therapy in a hemophilia-B patient with a factor IX inhibitor. *Ann Hematol* 1992; **64**: 309–11.

99. Lusher JM. Use of prothrombin complex concentrates in management of bleeding in hemophiliacs with inhibitors: benefit and limitations. *Semin Hematol* 1994; **31**: 49–52.

100. Lisman T, De Groot G. Mechanism of action of recombinant factor VIIa. *J Thromb Haemost* 2003; **1**: 1138–9.

101. Robert HR, Monroe DM, White G. The use of recombinant factor VIIa in the treatment of bleeding disorders. *Blood* 2004; **104**: 3858–64.

102. Hay CR, Negrier C, Ludlam CA. The treatment of bleeding in acquired haemophilia with recombinant factor VIIa: a multicenter study. *Thromb Haemost* 1997; **78**: 1463–7.

103. Arkin S, Cooper HA, Hutter JJ, et al. Activated recombinant human coagulation factor VII therapy for intracranial hemorrhage in patients with Haemophilia A or B with inhibitors. *Haemostasis* 1998; **28**: 93.

104. Scharrer I. Recombinant factor VIIa for patients with inhibitors to factor VIII or IX deficiency. *Hemophilia* 1999; **5**: 253–9.

105. Baudo F, Redaelli R, Caimi TM, Mostarda G, Somaini G, de Cataldo F. The continuous infusion of

recombinant activated factor VIIa (rFVIIa) in patients with factor VIII inhibitors activates the coagulation and the fibrinolytic systems without clinical complications. *Thromb Res* 2000; **99**: 21–4.

106. Hay CRM. Thrombosis and recombinant factor VIIa. J *Thromb Haemost* 2004; **2**: 1698–9.

107. Abshire T, Kenet G. Recombinant factor VIIa: review of efficacy, dosing regimens and safety in patients with congenital and acquired factor VIII or IX inhibitors. J *Thromb Haemost* 2004; **2**: 899–909.

108. Aledort LM. Comparative thrombotic event incidence after infusion of recombinant factor VIIa versus factor VIII inhibitory bypass activity. *J Thromb Haemost* 2004; **2**: 1700–8.

109. Abshire T. The safety of recombinant factor VIIa: a reply to rebuttal. *J Thromb Haemost*. 2004; **2**: 2079.

110. Sallah S, Isaksen M, Seremetis S, Payne Rojkjaer L. Comparative thrombotic event incidence after infusion of recombinant factor VIIa vs factor VIII inhibitory bypass activity. A rebuttal. *J Thromb Haemost* 2005; **3**: 820–2.

111. Aledort LM. Comparative thrombotic event incidence after infusion of recombinant factor VIIa vs factor VIII inhibitory bypass activity: a rebuttal. *J Thromb Haemost* 2005; **3**: 822.

112. O'Connell KA, Wood JJ, Wise RP, Lozier JN, Braun MM. Thromboembolic adverse events after use of recombinant human coagulation factor VII. *JAMA* 2006; **295**: 293–8.

113. Nilsson I, Sundqvist SB, Freiburghaus C. Extracorporeal protein A sepharose and specific affinity chromatography for removal of antibodies. In Hoyer LW, ed, *Factor VIII Inhibitors* (New York, NY: Liss, 1984), 225–41.

114. Négrier C, Dechavanne M, Alfonsi F, Tremisi PJ. Successful treatment of acquired factor VIII antibody by extracorporeal immunoadsorption. *Acta Haematol* 1991; **85**: 107–10.

115. Gjörstrup P, Berntorp E, Larsson L, Nilsson IM. Kinetic aspects of removal of IgG and inhibitors in hemophiliacs using protein A immunoadsorption. *Vox Sang* 1991; **61**: 244–50.

116. Knöbl P, Derfler K. Extracorporeal immunoadsorption for the treatment of haemophilic patients with inhibitors to factor VIII or IX. *Vox Sang* 1999; **77** (Suppl 1): 57S–64S.

117. Jansen M, Schmaldienst S, Banyai, *et al.* Treatment of coagulation inhibitors with extracorporeal immunoadsorption (Ig Therasorb). *Br J Haematol* 2001; **112**: 91–7.

118. Feinstein DI, Green D, Federici AB, Goodnight SH. Diagnosis and management of patients with spontaneously acquired inhibitors of coagulation. *Hematology* 1999; American Society of Hematology Education Program Book, 192–208.

119. Bussi L, Baudo F, de Cataldo F. Factor VIII concentrate and cyclophosphamide in patients with factor VIII inhibitors. *Blood* 1974; **44**: 767.

120. Delgado J, Jimenez-Yuste V, Hernandez-Navarro F, Villar A. Acquired hemophilia: review and meta-analysis focused on therapy and prognostic factors. *Br J Haematol* 2003; **121**: 21–35.

121. Schulman S, Langevitz P, Livneh A, Martinowitz U, Seligsohn U, Varon D. Cyclosporine therapy for acquired factor VIII inhibitor in a patient with systemic lupus erythematosus. *Thromb Haemost* 1995; **76**: 344–6.

122. Brox AG, Laryea H, Pelletier M. Successful treatment of acquired factor VIII inhibitors with cyclosporin. *Am J Hematol* 1998; **57**: 87–8.

123. Maclean PS, Tait RC, Lowe GDO, Walker ID, McColl MD. Successful elimination of factor VIII inhibitors using cyclosporin. *Br J Haematol* 2003; **122**: 1024–6.

124. Sallah S, Wan JY. Efficacy of 2-chlorodeoxyadenosine in refractory factor VIII inhibitors in persons without hemophilia. *Blood* 2003; **101**: 943–5.

125. Stachnik JM. Rituximab in the treatment of acquired hemophilia. *Ann Pharmacother* 2006; **40**: 1151–7.

126. Sperr WR, Lechner K, Pabinger I. Rituximab for the treatment of acquired antibodies to factor VIII. *Haematologica* 2007; **92**: 66–71.

127. Huth-Kuhne A, Ehrenforth S, Scharrer I, Zimmermann R. A new treatment option for patients with acquired hemophilia A: the modified Malmö–Heidelber protocol. *Thromb Haemost* 2001; **86**: 3364a.

128. Hess L, Zeitler H, Unkrig C, *et al.* Modified Bonn–Malmö protocol (MBM-P). *Haematologica* 2003; **88** (Suppl. 12): 78–85.

129. Zeitler H, Ulrich-Merzenich G, Hess L, *et al.* Treatment of acquired hemophilia by the Bonn–Malmö protocol: documentation of an in vivo immunomodulating concept. *Blood* 2005; **105**: 2287–93.

27

Blood coagulation and aging

Jozef Vermylen, Marc F. Hoylaerts

Introduction

The incidence of thrombotic complications increases with age. This is the case not only for arterial disease, in which thrombotic occlusion is the major complication of an unstable atherosclerotic plaque, but also for venous thromboembolism. Indeed, the risk of venous thrombosis increases sharply with age, from roughly 1 per 10 000 people per year before age 40 to 1 in 100 per year for those over age 75 years [1,2]. The purpose of this chapter is to describe the pathophysiology of blood coagulation and to attempt to identify the changes associated with aging.

The pathophysiology of blood coagulation

Blood coagulation plays a fundamental role in the arrest of bleeding. When a vessel is severed, blood loss is stopped by the development within the wound of a "hemostatic plug" consisting of tightly packed platelets held together by fibrin fibers. The coagulation process refers to the formation of these fibrin fibers. Whereas this physiologic response to trauma mainly takes place within the vessel wall and around the damaged vessel, the same process may occur pathophysiologically within the vessel lumen, when for instance the endothelium is disrupted. The plug then no longer has a hemostatic function, but potentially encroaches on the flow of blood; this intravascular plug is called a thrombus and again consists of cellular elements (platelets, leukocytes, and red cells) held together by fibrin. We shall now discuss how insoluble fibrin fibers are formed.

Fibrin formation

Fibrin fibers are formed locally by the action of thrombin on fibrinogen. Fibrinogen is an elongated symmetrical molecule (Fig. 27.1), that consists of three pairs of peptide chains (α, β, γ) linked together by their aminoterminal ends in a central disulfide knot. Fibrinogen is relatively abundant in plasma (2–4 g/L) and its concentration increases with aging, as shall be discussed later. Thrombin is a proteolytic enzyme that, besides other functions to be discussed further, removes the central aminoterminal parts of the α and β chains, thereby releasing fibrinopeptides A and B [3,4]. Fibrinogen with removed fibrinopeptides is called fibrin monomer. As a result of fibrinopeptide removal, two central polymerization sites become exposed, which can interact with complementary polymerization sites at the extremity of fibrinogen or fibrin monomer molecules, mainly by hydrophobic bonding. Staggered interaction of fibrin monomers, as illustrated in Fig. 27.1, leads to the initial fibrin fiber (polymer). Thrombin also transforms the proenzyme, factor XIII, into a transglutaminase that covalently links glutamic acid and lysine residues of adjacent fibrin monomers, thereby markedly increasing the cohesion of the fibrin fibers [5].

Thrombin generation

Coagulation as a surface-mediated process

Let us now move to the local generation of thrombin. In contrast to fibrinogen, the other clotting factors are present in plasma at relatively low concentrations; they must first be assembled on a surface for

Blood Disorders in the Elderly, ed. Lodovico Balducci, William Ershler, Giovanni de Gaetano.
Published by Cambridge University Press. © Cambridge University Press 2008.

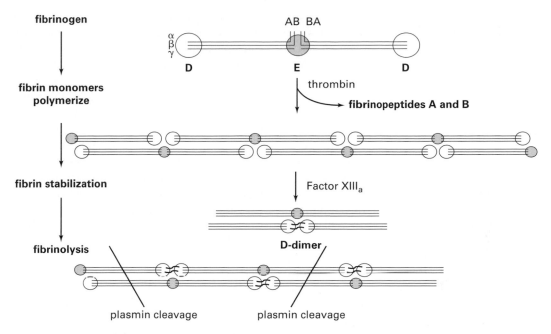

Figure 27.1 Fibrin formation and dissolution. A, B represent fibrinopeptides A and B; α, β, γ, the three pairs of chains composing fibrinogen; D, the C-terminal ends of the chains; E, the central N-terminal disulfide knot; D-dimer, the epitope resulting from cross-linking of adjacent D domains by factor XIIIa.

efficient interactions; blood coagulation must be considered a surface-catalyzed process. This surface is provided by platelets that have become activated by the vessel wall damage (see Chapter 28). Activated platelets have altered membrane characteristics. Normally, negative phospholipids, such as phosphatidylserine, are sequestered in the inner leaflet of the phospholipid bilayer; upon platelet activation, possibly as a consequence of the mobilization of surface membrane microdomains known as lipid rafts [6], membrane asymmetry is perturbed and phosphatidylserine becomes exposed on the surface. It then serves as a ligand for numerous clotting factors. Prothrombin, factor VII, factor IX, and factor X are proenzymes that bind in a calcium ion-dependent manner to phosphatidylserine through gammacarboxyglutamic acid residues at their aminoterminal ends (the so-called gla-domain). These related proenzymes have evolved through gene duplication [7]. The gammacarboxyglutamic acid residues result from the additional carboxylation

of glutamic acid residues in a vitamin K-dependent manner [8]. In the absence of vitamin K absorption (e.g., obstructive jaundice) or following intake of a vitamin K antagonist (e.g., warfarin) this posttranslational modification does not occur and as a result these proteins, although secreted into the bloodstream, can no longer gather and interact on a surface; as a result, coagulation is prevented.

Besides proenzymes, the coagulation system also involves a number of protein cofactors that help in the assembly of the (pro)enzymes. Two major cofactors are factors V and VIII; both have six sequential domains arranged in the order A_1–A_2–B–A_3–C_1–C_2. They too are the result of an ancient gene duplication [7]. Both bind to phospholipids through the C_2 domain by the burial of hydrophobic residues within the phospholipid bilayer; these hydrophobic residues are surrounded by positively charged residues that interact with negatively charged phospholipid head groups, again concentrating these cofactors in membrane areas that expose phosphatidylserine [9].

Additional mechanisms localize factor V and factor VIII to the surface of activated platelets. Factor V is synthesized by hepatocytes and in part actively endocytosed from plasma by megakaryocytes; it is then cleaved into a partially active form [10] and stored in the platelet α-granules. Upon platelet activation, these granules fuse with the platelet membrane, to which active factor V remains attached. Factor VIII is transported in the circulation bound to a much larger multimeric protein called von Willebrand factor (the largest multimers may have a molecular weight over 20 000 000). von Willebrand factor switches from a globular to an elongated conformation upon exposure to shear [11]. Shear develops when the flow path is restricted by the accumulation of activated platelets. Once elongated, von Willebrand factor strongly binds to the glycoprotein Ibα and IIb/IIIa receptors on the activated platelets; the cotransported factor VIII thereby indirectly accumulates on these platelets [12]. Finally, the proenzyme factor XI also binds to glycoprotein Ibα [13].

The origin of tissue factor

The coagulation factors thus assemble on the surface of activated platelets, but what starts their interaction? It is now generally accepted that tissue factor initiates the coagulation cascade in vivo. Tissue factor is an integral membrane protein that is normally present on the surface of most cells *outside* the vasculature, in particular vascular adventitia, implying that tissue factor represents a "hemostatic envelope" ready to activate coagulation when vascular integrity is disrupted [14]. But how could tissue factor contribute to thrombus formation within a vessel?

Endothelial cells can be induced to express tissue factor in vitro, but whether this phenomenon occurs in pathologic conditions in vivo has been doubted. Atheromatous plaques are rich in tissue factor, which mainly originates from macrophages [15]. However, platelets adhering to the ruptured plaque effectively prevent contact between the plaque tissue factor and the blood [16]. In 1999, the unexpected concept of blood-borne tissue factor emerged [17]. When native human blood is allowed to flow over a glass coverslip at high shear, platelets adhere to the coverslip via von Willebrand factor, and tissue-factor-containing microparticles adhere to the platelet layer; the adherent tissue factor is biologically active, as evidenced by fibrin formation. Further information on the possible origin of these tissue-factor-containing microparticles has recently been forthcoming. Using bone-marrow transplantation in transgenic mice, Chou and colleagues [18] demonstrated that the microparticles are of bone-marrow origin, leading to the major implication that the bone marrow contributes to hemostasis by releasing not only platelets but also blood-borne tissue factor into the bloodstream. These microparticles may result from leukocyte fragmentation, since they express not only tissue factor but also P-selectin glycoprotein ligand 1 [19]. The latter allows the binding of the microparticles to activated platelets [20]; indeed, the membrane of the platelet α-granule contains P-selectin, which is exposed on the platelet surface upon fusion of the granule membrane with this surface. This interaction between circulating tissue-factor-bearing microparticles and adhering activated platelets explains how the coagulation process is localized: it is only on the surface of activated platelets that tissue factor encounters the accumulated clotting factors with which it can interact. The tissue-factor-bearing microvesicles may even fuse with the membrane of activated platelets [21].

The stage is now set to describe thrombin formation in detail. It can be separated into an initiation and a propagation phase.

The initiation of coagulation

Tissue factor is a transmembrane protein cofactor, not an enzyme. Blood always contains small amounts of factor VIIa (factor VII refers to the proenzyme, VIIa to the active enzyme). Tissue factor binds both factor VII and factor VIIa and promotes the autocatalytic activation of factor VII. This reaction requires that the tissue-factor/factor-VIIa and tissue-factor/factor-VII complexes encounter each other by lateral diffusion in the plane of the membrane [22]. This process of interaction by limited lateral diffusion [23] is fundamental for all membrane-bound coagulation reactions. Tissue factor/factor VIIa activates both factor X and factor IX [24]. Factor X activation is responsible for the initiation phase, factor IX activation for the propagation phase. Factor Xa activates prothrombin on the platelet surface, with active factor V provided by the platelet α-granules as surface-bound cofactor. The cleavage of prothrombin is sequential. In the first stage, meizothrombin is generated [25]; this active enzyme remains attached to the phospholipid surface and, by lateral diffusion, may activate plasma factor V adsorbed onto this surface [26]. Subsequent removal of fragments including the gla-domain of prothrombin results in soluble thrombin, which diffuses away from the catalytic phospholipid surface.

The propagation of coagulation

Thrombin binds with high affinity to glycoprotein Ibα on human platelets [27]. This allows further platelet activation via thrombin cleavage of protease-activated receptors [28]. Since the von Willebrand factor/factor VIII also binds to glycoprotein Ibα, this spatial organization allows thrombin to activate factor VIII and to dissociate it from von Willebrand factor [29]. This activated factor VIII can then join factor IXa on the phospholipid surface; the factor-IXa/factor-VIIIa complex then activates factor X; this constitutes the basis for the propagation

phase of blood coagulation, which ultimately results in a further explosive generation of thrombin.

As mentioned previously, not only thrombin but also factor XI binds to platelet glycoprotein Ibα, where thrombin efficiently activates factor XI [30]. Factor IX is activated by factor XIa in addition to the previously mentioned activation by the tissue-factor/factor-VIIa complex; this explains why some patients with factor XI deficiency have a bleeding tendency [31].

Figure 27.2 summarizes the blood coagulation process, while Fig. 27.3 illustrates thrombin generation when blood flow deposits tissue-factor-bearing microparticles and coagulation factors upon a layer of activated platelets, overlying for instance a ruptured atherosclerotic plaque.

Stasis and thrombin generation

Thrombus development, however, occurs not only in diseased arteries, but also in areas of blood stasis. Examples are the development of deep vein thrombosis in an immobilized limb or the growth of a thrombus in the left atrium in the case of atrial fibrillation, pathologies frequently present in elderly subjects.

Twenty years ago it had already been found that when veins are ligated and left *in situ* for 24 to 72 hours, deposition of leukocytes, platelets, and fibrin can be observed [32]. Kawasaki *et al.* [33] studied fibrin formation within the mouse common carotid artery, which had simply been ligated proximal to the

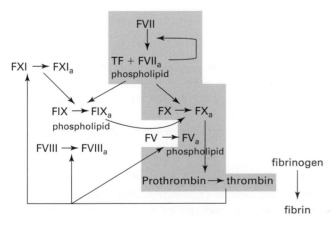

Figure 27.2 A current scheme of blood coagulation. The propagation phase is to the left of the figure. F, factor; TF, tissue factor.

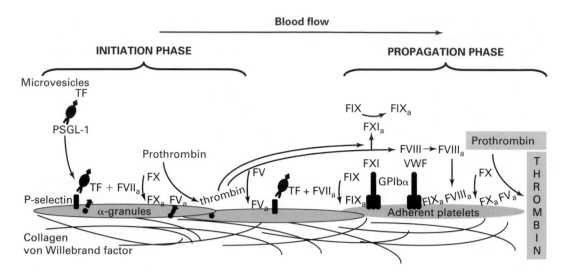

Figure 27.3 Thrombin generation in blood flowing over activated platelets on a damaged vessel wall. PSGL-1, P-selectin glycoprotein ligand 1; GPIbα, glycoprotein Ibα; F, factor; TF, tissue factor; VWF, von Willebrand factor.

bifurcation, thereby resulting in a column of stagnant blood. After one day, platelet–leukocyte conjugates started to line the endothelium. They were associated with the appearance of tissue-factor-positive fibrin deposits. This observation is compatible with mutual activation of platelets and leukocytes [34] when they reside in areas of stasis. Polymorphonuclear leukocytes activate platelets by releasing cathepsin G [35]. The activated platelets expose P-selectin on their surface, inducing cell–cell adhesion via P-selectin glycoprotein ligand 1 on leukocytes. Engagement of P-selectin glycoprotein 1 by P-selectin induces signal transduction in leukocytes [36], resulting in tissue factor expression on monocytes [37] and also neutrophils [38]. The conjugation of leukocytes expressing tissue factor with activated platelets binding clotting factors allows thrombin generation to occur. In view of the presence of stasis, thrombin is not rapidly diluted or swept away; as a result, a fibrin-rich thrombus forms. Thrombin also induces the exocytosis of Weibel–Palade bodies, containing P-selectin and von Willebrand factor, from endothelial cells. Expression of P-selectin on the endothelial surface causes further leukocyte activation and tissue factor expression [39]. In the model used by Kawasaki *et al.* [33], fibrin formation within the ligated carotid artery

provides the scaffold for neointima formation. As a result, reducing plasma fibrinogen levels or inducing thrombocytopenia resulted in significantly less neointima development. The same was observed in factor VIII-knockout mice, indicating that also in areas of stasis the propagation phase of blood coagulation plays a major role [33]. The carotid artery ligation model had originally been developed by Kumar and Lindner [40], who then observed that neointima formation was markedly reduced in P-selectin deficient mice [41], again implying a major role for platelet–leukocyte interaction in this process.

Thromboembolism secondary to atrial fibrillation accounts for approximately one-quarter of all strokes. Wysokinski and colleagues [42] performed quantitative immunohistochemistry to define the composition of atrial thrombi. These thrombi were fibrin-rich; tissue factor colocalized to areas rich in platelets and granulocytes, again implying that tissue factor expression results from platelet–leukocyte interaction in areas of stasis.

Regulation of thrombin generation

We have so far described how thrombin is generated in areas of flow and of stasis. We have also

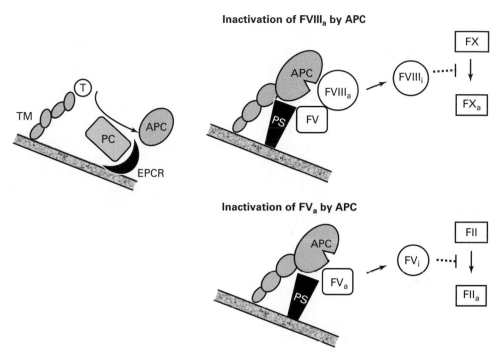

Figure 27.4 The thrombomodulin/protein-C/protein-S system. TM, thrombomodulin; T, thrombin; PC, protein C; EPCR, endothelial protein C receptor; APC, activated protein C; PS, protein S; FVIIIi, inactivated factor VIII; FVi, inactivated factor V; FII, prothrombin.

mentioned a number of positive feedback mechanisms through which thrombin enhances its own generation: thrombin induces further platelet activation and activates plasma factors V, VIII, and XI. To keep the coagulation process under control, there must also be negative feedback mechanisms. Again these processes are surface-linked, with normal endothelium playing here a major role, thereby preventing extension of the thrombus into healthy vessels. We shall discuss in succession antithrombin, the thrombomodulin/protein-C/protein-S system, and tissue factor pathway inhibitor.

Antithrombin is a proteinase inhibitor that blocks not only thrombin but also factor Xa and to some extent also factors IXa and XIa. Antithrombin is a slow inhibitor in vitro. Its efficiency is increased more than 1000-fold following binding to heparan-containing proteoglycans on healthy endothelium (or following injection of heparin as anticoagulant).

A specific pentasaccharide sequence within heparan induces a conformational change in antithrombin that allows efficient interaction with the target proteinase. Antithrombin complexed to endothelial cell proteoglycan thus protects against extension of thrombosis. Congenital heterozygous antithrombin deficiency predisposes to venous thrombosis [43].

The *thrombomodulin/protein-C/protein-S* system is illustrated in Fig. 27.4. Thrombomodulin is a transmembrane endothelial surface protein that efficiently binds thrombin. Once bound, thrombin loses its procoagulant properties but instead activates protein C, attached to the endothelial protein C receptor [44,45]. Activated protein C is a vitamin K-dependent proteinase; it has an aminoterminal gla-domain; it therefore can efficiently translocate to the phosphatidylserine-exposing phospholipid bilayer of activated platelets. On this surface, activated protein C cleaves and inactivates factor

VIIIa and factor Va, thereby turning down further thrombin generation. To efficiently cleave these cofactors, activated protein C itself requires a cofactor, protein S [46]. Protein S also is a vitamin K-dependent protein that binds to phosphatidylserine-containing surfaces through its gla-domain, but it is not an enzyme. Factor Va is inactivated in part by cleavage at Arg506. Congenital protein C and S deficiencies and mutation of factor V at Arg506 (the factor V Leiden mutation) have been associated with an increased tendency to venous thrombosis also in the heterozygous state [47–49].

Tissue factor pathway inhibitor is a protein that is bound to the endothelium, and that is also present in plasma in free form or linked to lipoproteins [50,51]. It consists of three tandem repeated serine protease inhibitor domains homologous in structure to Kunitz trypsin inhibitor. The first Kunitz domain (Kunitz 1) binds to the tissue-factor/factor-VIIa complex, whereas the Kunitz 2 domain forms a complex with factor Xa. In this way a quaternary complex is formed (Fig. 27.5) that effectively blocks the initiation phase of blood coagulation. The Kunitz 3 domain and the basic carboxy-terminal domain are involved in cell surface binding [52].

Fibrinolysis

We have now addressed fibrin formation and its control. Let us now briefly concentrate on fibrin removal. Thrombosis should indeed be viewed as a dynamic process, the thrombus growing or shrinking depending on whether fibrin deposition or fibrin removal (fibrinolysis) predominates. Fibrinolysis (Fig. 27.6) once more is a surface-mediated process, in which the fibrin strands orchestrate their own degradation. The fibrin-cleaving protease is plasmin, formed through activation of plasminogen. The latter proenzyme contains five homologous triple-loop structures or "kringles" [53], constituting lysine-binding sites, that mediate the specific binding of plasminogen to fibrin. On the fibrin surface, plasminogen is transformed into plasmin by plasminogen activators, in blood mainly tissue-type plasminogen activator; this serine protease also contains kringle domains that allow specific binding to fibrin [54]. Tissue-type plasminogen activator is mainly secreted by irritated endothelial cells [55]. In the absence of fibrin, tissue-type plasminogen activator is a poor enzyme, but the presence of fibrin strikingly enhances the activation rate of plasminogen, by assembly of these components on the fibrin surface via their lysine-binding sites [56]. Plasmin enhances its own generation by exposing new carboxy-terminal lysine residues as a result of the fibrin chain cleavage, thereby allowing additional binding of plasminogen and its activator [57]. The action of plasmin on fibrin leads to the formation of soluble fibrin degradation products; degradation of cross-linked fibrin results in fragments consisting of the cross-linked carboxy-terminal ends of adjacent fibrin

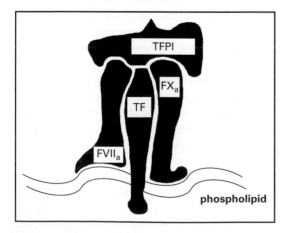

Figure 27.5 Tissue factor/factor VIIa and factor Xa inhibition by tissue factor pathway inhibitor (TFPI).

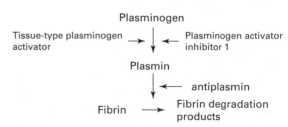

Figure 27.6 The physiologic fibrinolytic system in plasma.

molecules, and containing the so-called D-dimer epitope (Fig. 27.1) [58]. D-dimer epitope measurement is a sensitive means of detecting fibrin formation and degradation in vivo in man.

The fibrinolytic system again is kept under control at three levels. The first level is the inhibition of fibrinolysis by high concentrations of thrombin. Thrombin transforms a procarboxypeptidase into an active enzyme that efficiently removes carboxy-terminal lysine residues from fibrin and thereby impedes further binding of plasminogen and tissue-type plasminogen activator to fibrin and therefore plasmin generation. This proenzyme is known as procarboxypeptidase U or *thrombin-activatable fibrinolysis inhibitor* (TAFI) [59,60].

The second level is provided by α_2-*antiplasmin*; this serine protease inhibitor contains a secondary binding site that reacts with the lysine-binding sites of plasminogen and plasmin [61]. Plasmin formed at the fibrin surface has both its lysine-binding sites and active site occupied, and is thus only slowly inactivated by α_2-antiplasmin (half-life about 10–100 seconds); in contrast free plasmin is rapidly inhibited by α_2-antiplasmin (half-life 0.1 seconds) [62]. Alpha$_2$-antiplasmin thus prevents plasmin from digesting proteins at a distance from the fibrin surface.

The third level of regulation is provided by *plasminogen activator inhibitor 1*, the physiologic inhibitor of tissue-type plasminogen activator. The plasma levels of this serine protease inhibitor, synthesized by the liver, adipocytes and the endothelium, are positively associated with obesity and insulin resistance (the "metabolic syndrome"), itself a risk factor for cardiovascular events [63].

A few additional remarks

Many people have been awed by the apparent complexity of the coagulation system. As our knowledge has increased, we start to realize how the system has evolved to allow a delicate balance that permits efficient fibrin formation at the level of vascular damage, while preventing uncontrolled extension of fibrin deposition in blood flowing through healthy vessels. We have also become aware of the marked difference between blood clotting in vitro and in vivo. In a glass tube, factor XII and high-molecular-weight kininogen carrying prekallikrein adsorb onto the surface. Mutual activation of factor XII and prekallikrein then occurs, resulting in factor XIIa and kallikrein. Factor XIIa then activates factor XI, and the coagulation cascade is initiated. Subjects with factor XII, or prekallikrein, or high-molecular-weight kininogen deficiency have blood that fails to clot in a glass tube and have an extremely prolonged activated partial thromboplastin time (APTT), yet they have no bleeding problem and are not protected against thrombosis. We now know that the physiological activator of factor XI is thrombin. The factor XII system even does not seem to be of importance in the clotting of extracorporeal circuits [64]. It more likely is involved in inflammation [65].

Modification of clotting factors with aging

The level of a number of clotting factors is known to change with aging, usually in the direction that would seem to facilitate thrombosis. The origin may be multifactorial: the aging process per se, a low-grade chronic inflammation, even decreased mobility. These various aspects will briefly be mentioned.

Perhaps the most striking study is that of Mari and colleagues in centenarians [66]. These authors measured parameters of coagulation and fibrinolysis in 25 healthy centenarians, 25 healthy adults between 18 and 50 years, and 25 between 51 and 69 years of age as controls. Older controls had, in general, slightly higher values of several coagulation and fibrinolysis measurements than younger controls. Centenarians had striking signs of heightened coagulation enzyme activity, as assessed directly by measuring factor VIIa in plasma ($p < 0.01$, compared with either control group) or indirectly by measuring the peptides released following activation of prothrombin, or factor IX, or factor X (all $p < 0.001$). In addition, circulating complexes of thrombin with antithrombin were increased, confirming increased thrombin generation. Thrombin activity was accompanied by signs of enhanced formation of fibrin, as evidenced by high circulating levels of fibrinopeptide A ($p < 0.001$), and of increased breakdown of fibrin, as reflected by elevated levels of D-dimer and of plasmin complexed to α_2-antiplasmin (both $p < 0.001$). Plasma concentrations of fibrinogen and of factor VIII were higher than in controls, whereas other coagulation factors were not elevated. The authors concluded that the very elderly do not escape the state of hypercoagulability associated with aging, but that this phenomenon is compatible with health and longevity. Their conclusion is compatible with Virchow's famous triad, implying that hypercoagulability by itself does not cause thrombosis, provided vessel wall and blood flow are intact. The increased levels of factor VIIa may indicate that exposure to (blood-borne) tissue factor is increased with age.

Meade *et al.* [67] had already noted in 1979 that plasma *fibrinogen* concentrations increase with age, but also with obesity or smoking; alcohol consumption decreases the fibrinogen level. A raised plasma fibrinogen level is now recognized as a strong and independent predictor of the risk of coronary death and myocardial infarction [68]. The risk of venous thrombosis associated with high plasma fibrinogen levels is mainly apparent in older individuals [69]. High levels of plasma fibrinogen may increase the thrombus size or make the thrombus more resistant to fibrinolysis [70]. *Factor XIII* also rises with age [71], and also increases resistance to fibrinolysis [72].

Balleisen and colleagues [73] observed that not only fibrinogen but also *factor VIII* increase with age. Raised factor VIII levels are clearly associated with thrombosis. In the prospective cardiovascular health study [74], elevated factor VIII levels were associated with cardiovascular disease and mortality in elderly men. An elevated factor VIII also significantly increased the risk of ischemic stroke in the Atherosclerosis Risk in Communities study [75]. An elevated factor VIII level in addition is a risk factor for venous thrombosis [76], also in the elderly [77]. The association of thrombosis with high factor VIII levels is not surprising, since the normal concentration of factor VIII in plasma is extremely low (0.7 nM, compared to, e.g., 90 nM for factor IX), and therefore the level of factor VIII is the rate-limiting step in the propagation phase of blood coagulation [78]. An animal model of thrombophilia has confirmed that high plasma factor VIII levels are thrombogenic [12].

An interesting finding was made by Wannamethee *et al.* [79]. They observed in a study involving 3 810 elderly men that physical activity was significantly and inversely dose–response-related to plasma fibrinogen level, factors VIII and IX, D-dimer level (indicating less fibrin formation), tissue-type plasminogen activator antigen (indicating reduced endothelial irritation), even after adjustment for possible confounders. These men had also been screened 20 years before (baseline). An examination of changes in physical activity between baseline and 20 years later showed that inactive men who took up at least light physical activity had levels of blood variables approaching those who remained at least lightly active. Those who became inactive showed levels more similar to those who remained inactive. The authors conclude that the benefit of physical activity on cardiovascular disease may be at least partly a result of effects on blood coagulation.

The effect of age on the vitamin K-dependent proteins is variable. *Factor VII* [73] and *factor IX* [80] increase with age, while *protein C* levels remain unchanged [81]. A rise in factor VII has been associated with an increased risk of ischemic heart disease [82]. Besides age, factor VII levels are modulated by polymorphisms in the factor VII gene [83,84] and by dietary fat and blood lipids [85]: the factor VII gene 353R polymorphism and serum triglyceride levels are positively associated with higher factor VII levels. In older women, the strength of the association of factor VII with serum triglycerides varies according to genotype of the R/Q353 polymorphism, whereas in older men the association of factor VII with triglycerides was weaker [86]. A dietary study in over 3000 elderly subjects indicated that total fat intake is positively related to the factor VII level in elderly women only, saturated fat intake being positively related to the factor VII level in both elderly men and women. Fiber intake was inversely related to the factor VII level in both sexes, indicating that a diet low in saturated fat and high in fiber may reduce the factor VII-mediated hypercoagulability associated with old age [87].

An increased plasma level of factor IX constitutes a risk factor for venous thrombosis [88]. Making use of the age-dependent increase of factor IX and the age-independence of the protein C level, the Kurachis have attempted to identify the molecular mechanisms of the age-related regulation of genes. Using lines of human factor IX minigenes in transgenic mice, they identified two genetic elements, ASE (age stable expression) and AIE (age increased expression), to be essential for generating age-related stable and increased factor IX gene expression patterns respectively [89]. ASE is located at a small 5′ upstream region (−802 to −784) of the human factor IX gene, AIE was identified in the middle of the human factor IX 3′–untranslated region. Deletion of ASE led to a decline of human factor IX levels in the mice. On the other hand, the human protein C minigene, while possessing an ASE element, lacks an AIE element, resulting in a stable unchanging expression in transgenic mice; addition of the factor IX AIE element to the protein C minigene converted the stable expression to an age-related increased expression of protein C [90]. This pioneering work on age-related gene regulation has been elegantly reviewed [91]. In this review the Kurachis emphasize that, while the coagulation factors increase with age, the protease inhibitors remain essentially unchanged, thereby tilting the balance between enzymes and inhibitors towards a hypercoagulable state.

Plasminogen activator inhibitor 1 (PAI-1) however is an exception to this rule. Bonfigli and colleagues [92] have studied the influence of the 4G/5G polymorphism in the promoter region of the *PAI-1* gene on the age-related expression. They observed that the presence of the 4G allele increases the level of PAI-1 in plasma from the age of 20 years onwards, while this is not the case in 5G/5G subjects. Perhaps 4G in this area of the promoter constitutes an age-increase element, to use the Kurachi terminology. Alternatively, the 4G allele may be more responsive than the 5G allele to a transcription signal that increases with age.

An increased level of PAI-1 would delay fibrin removal and thereby promote thrombosis. Eriksson *et al.* [93] found the prevalence of the 4G allele to be significantly higher in patients with myocardial infarction. Paradoxically, Mannucci and colleagues [94] found in centenarians a significantly higher frequency of the 4G allele of *PAI-1* and of the homozygous 4G/4G genotype than in young healthy controls. So homozygosity for the 4G allele, despite its association with impaired fibrinolysis, is compatible with successful aging, provided one has healthy vessels and blood flow.

From this brief overview of changes in the coagulation system in elderly subjects, one may conclude that old age is a hypercoagulable state that may contribute to arterial and venous thrombosis in areas of vessel wall disease and of stasis. On the other hand, light exercise and a healthy diet appear to have a beneficial effect on this hypercoagulability and should therefore be encouraged.

REFERENCES

1. Nordström M, Lindblad B, Bergqvist D, Kjellström T. A prospective study of the incidence of deep-vein thrombosis within a defined urban population. *J Intern Med* 1992; **232**: 155–60.
2. Anderson FA, Wheeler HB, Goldberg RJ, *et al.* A population based perspective of the hospital incidence and case-fatality rate of deep vein thrombosis and pulmonary embolism. The Worcester DVT study. *Arch Intern Med* 1991; **151**: 933–8.
3. Blombäck B. Fibrinogen and fibrin-proteins with complex roles in hemostasis and thrombosis. *Thromb Res* 1996; **83**: 1–75.
4. Mosesson MW. Fibrinogen and fibrin structure and functions. *J Thromb Haemost* 2005; **3**: 1894–904.
5. Lorand L. Factor XIII and the clotting of fibrinogen: from basic research to medicine. *J Thromb Haemost* 2005; **3**: 1337–48.
6. Lopez JA, Del Conde I, Shrimpton CN. Receptors, rafts, and microvesicles in thrombosis and inflammation. *J Thromb Haemost* 2005; **3**: 1737–44.
7. Davidson CJ, Tuddenham EG, McVey JH. 450 million years of hemostasis. *J Thromb Haemost* 2003; **1**: 1487–94.
8. Stenflo J, Fernlund P, Egan W, Roepstorff P. Vitamin K dependent modifications of glutamic acid residues in prothrombin. *Proc Natl Acad Sci USA* 1974; **71**: 2730–3.
9. Pratt KP, Shen BW, Takeshima K, Davie EW, Fujikawa K, Stoddard BL. Structure of the C2 domain of human factor VIII at 1.5 A resolution. *Nature* 1999; **402**: 439–42.

10. Gould WR, Simioni P, Silveira JR, Tormene D, Kalafatis M, Tracy PB. Megakaryocytes endocytose and subsequently modify human factor V in vivo to form the entire pool of a unique platelet-derived cofactor. *J Thromb Haemost* 2005; **3**: 448–9.

11. Siedlecki CA, Lestini BJ, Kottke-Marchant KK, Eppel SJ, Wilson DL, Marchant RE. Shear-dependent changes in the three-dimensional structure of human von Willebrand factor. *Blood* 1996; **88**: 2939–50.

12. Kawasaki T, Kaida T, Arnout J, Vermylen J, Hoylaerts MF. A new animal model of thrombophilia confirms that high plasma factor VIII levels are thrombogenic. *Thromb Haemost* 1999; **81**: 306–11.

13. Baglia FA, Shrimpton CN, Emsley J, *et al*. Factor XI interacts with the leucine-rich repeats of glycoprotein Ib alpha on the activated platelet. *J Biol Chem* 2004; **279**: 49323–9.

14. Drake TA, Morrissey JH, Edgington TS. Selective cellular expression of tissue factor in human tissues. Implications for disorders of hemostasis and thrombosis. *Am J Pathol* 1989; **134**: 1087–97.

15. Fuster V, Fallon JT, Badimon JJ, Nemerson Y. The unstable atherosclerotic plaque: clinical significance and therapeutic intervention. *Thromb Haemost* 1997; **78**: 247–55.

16. Mathcock JJ, Nemerson Y. Platelet deposition inhibits tissue factor activity: in vitro clots are impermeable to factor Xa. *Blood* 2004; **104**: 123–7.

17. Giesen PL, Rauch U, Bohrmann B, *et al*. Blood-borne tissue factor: another view of thrombosis. *Proc Natl Acad Sci USA* 1999; **96**: 2311–15.

18. Chou J, Mackman N, Merrill-Skoloff G, Pedersen B, Furie BC, Furie B. Hematopoietic cell-derived microparticle tissue factor contributes to fibrin formation during thrombus propagation. *Blood* 2004; **104**: 3190–7.

19. Furie B, Furie BC. The molecular basis of platelet and endothelial cell interaction with neutrophils and monocytes: role of P-selectin and the P-selectin ligand, PSGL-1. *Thromb Haemost* 1995; **74**: 224–7.

20. Falati S, Liu Q, Gross P, *et al*. Accumulation of tissue factor into developing thrombi in vivo is dependent upon microparticle P-selectin glycoprotein ligand 1 and platelet P-selectin. *J Exp Med* 2003; **197**: 1585–98.

21. Del Conde I, Shrimpton CN, Thiagarajan P, Lopez JA. Tissue-factor-bearing microvesicles arise from lipid rafts and fuse with activated platelets to initiate coagulation. *Blood* 2005; **106**: 1604–11.

22. Neuenschwander PF, Fiore MM, Morrissey JH. Factor VII autoactivation proceeds via interaction of distinct protease-cofactor and zymogen-cofactor complexes. Implications of a two-dimensional enzyme kinetic mechanism. *J Biol Chem* 1993; **268**: 21489–92.

23. Singer SJ, Nicholson GL. The fluid mosaic model of the structure of cell membranes. *Science* 1972; **175**: 720–31.

24. Almus FE, Rao LVM, Rapaport SI. Functional properties of factor VIIa/tissue factor formed with purified tissue factor and with tissue factor expressed on cultured endothelial cells. *Thromb Haemost* 1989; **62**: 1067–73.

25. Krishnaswamy S, Mann KG, Nesheim ME. The prothrombinase-catalyzed activation of prothrombin proceeds through the intermediate meizothrombin in an ordered, sequential reaction. *J Biol Chem* 1986; **261**: 8977–84.

26. Tans G, Nicolaes GA, Thomassen MC, *et al*. Activation of human factor V by meizothrombin. *J Biol Chem* 1994; **269**: 15969–72.

27. De Marco L, Mazzucato M, Masotti A, Fenton JW 2nd, Ruggeri ZM. Function of glycoprotein Ib alpha in platelet activation induced by alpha-thrombin. *J Biol Chem* 1991; **266**: 23776–83.

28. Coughlin SR. Protease-activated receptors in hemostasis, thrombosis and vascular biology. *J Thromb Haemost* 2005; **3**: 1800–14.

29. Vlot AJ, Koppelman SJ, Bouma BN, Sixma JJ. Factor VIII and von Willebrand factor. *Thromb Haemost* 1998; **79**: 456–65.

30. Yun TH, Baglia FA, Myles T, *et al*. Thrombin activation of factor XI on activated platelets requires the interaction of factor XI and glycoprotein Ib alpha with thrombin anion-binding exosites I and II, respectively. *J Biol Chem* 2003; **278**: 48112–19.

31. Walsh PN. Roles of platelets and factor XI in the initiation of blood coagulation by thrombin. *Thromb Haemost* 2001; **86**: 75–82.

32. Schaub RG, Simmons CA, Koets MH, Romano PJ, Stewart GJ. Early events in the formation of a venous thrombus following local trauma and stasis. *Lab Invest* 1984; **51**: 218–24.

33. Kawasaki T, Dewerchin M, Lijnen HR, Vreys I, Vermylen J, Hoylaerts MF. Mouse carotid artery ligation induces platelet-leukocyte-dependent luminal fibrin, required for neointima development. *Circ Res* 2001; **88**: 159–66.

34. Makino A, Glogauer M, Bokoch GM, Chien S, Schmid-Schönbein GW. Control of neutrophil pseudopods by fluid shear: role of the Rho family GTPases. *Am J Physiol Cell Physiol* 2005; **288**: C863–C871.

35. Evangelista V, Piccardoni P, White JG, de Gaetano G, Cerletti C. Cathepsin G-dependent platelet stimulation by activated polymorphonuclear leukocytes and

inhibition by antiproteinases: role of P-selectin-mediated cell–cell adhesion. *Blood* 1993; **81**: 2947–52.

36. Hidari KI, Weyrich AS, Zimmerman GA, McEver RP. Engagement of P-selectin glycoprotein ligand-1 enhances tyrosine phosphorylation and activates mitogen-activated kinases in human neutrophils. *J Biol Chem* 1997; **272**: 28750–6.

37. Celi A, Pellegrini G, Lorenzet R, *et al.* P-selectin induces the expression of tissue factor on monocytes. *Proc Natl Acad Sci USA* 1994; **91**: 8767–71.

38. Maugeri N, Brambilla M, Camera M, *et al.* Human polymorphonuclear leukocytes produce and express functional tissue factor upon stimulation. *J Thromb Haemost* 2006; **4**: 1323–30.

39. Polgar J, Matsukova J, Wagner DD. The P-selectin, tissue factor, coagulation triad. *J Thromb Haemost* 2005; **3**: 1590–6.

40. Kumar A, Lindner V. Remodeling with neointima formation in the mouse carotid artery after cessation of blood flow. *Arterioscler Thromb Vasc Biol* 1997; **17**: 2238–44.

41. Kumar A, Hoover JL, Simmons CA, Lindner V, Shebuski RJ. Remodeling and neointimal formation in the carotid artery of normal and P-selectin-deficient mice. *Circulation* 1997; **96**: 4333–42.

42. Wysokinski WE, Owen WG, Fass DN, Patrzalek DD, Murphy L, McBane RD. Atrial fibrillation and thrombosis: immunohistochemical differences between *in situ* and embolized thrombi. *J Thromb Haemost* 2004; **2**: 1637–44.

43. Rosenberg RD, Aird WC. Vascular-bed-specific hemostasis and hypercoagulable states. *N Engl J Med* 1999; **340**: 1555–64.

44. Fukudome K, Esmon CT. Identification, cloning and regulation of a novel endothelial protein C/activated protein C receptor. *J Biol Chem* 1994; **269**: 26486–91.

45. Esmon CT. Thrombomodulin as a model of molecular mechanisms that modulate protease specificity and function at the vessel surface. *FASEB J* 1995; **9**: 946–55.

46. Rosing J, Hoekema L, Nicolaes GA, *et al.* Effects of protein S and factor Xa on peptide bond cleavages during inactivation of factor Va and factor VaR506Q by activated protein C. *J Biol Chem* 1995; **270**: 27852–8.

47. Griffin JH, Evatt B, Zimmerman TS, Kleiss AJ, Wideman C. Deficiency of protein C in congenital thrombotic disease. *J Clin Invest* 1981; **68**: 1370–3.

48. Comp PC, Esmon CT. Recurrent venous thromboembolism in patients with a partial deficiency of protein S. *N Engl J Med* 1984; **311**: 1525–8.

49. Bertina RM, Koeleman BP, Koster T, *et al.* Mutation in blood coagulation factor V associated with resistance to activated protein C. *Nature* 1994; **369**: 64–7.

50. Broze GJ Jr, Miletich JP. Isolation of the tissue factor inhibitor produced by HepG2 hepatoma cells. *Proc Natl Acad Sci USA* 1987; **84**: 1886–90.

51. Wun TC, Kretzmar KK, Girard TJ, Miletich JP, Broze GJ Jr. Cloning and characterization of a cDNA coding for the lipoprotein-associated coagulation inhibitor shows that it consists of three tandem Kunitz-type inhibitory domains. *J Biol Chem* 1988; **263**: 6001–4.

52. Piro O, Broze GJ Jr. Role of the Kunitz-3 domain of tissue factor pathway inhibitor-alpha in cell surface binding. *Circulation* 2004; **110**: 3567–72.

53. Claeys H, Sottrup-Jensen L, Zajdel M, Petersen TE, Magnusson S. Multiple gene duplication in the evolution of plasminogen. Five regions of sequence homology with the two internally homologous structures of prothrombin. *FEBS Lett* 1976; **61**: 20–4.

54. Pennica D, Holmes WE, Kohr WJ, *et al.* Cloning and expression of human tissue-type plasminogen activator cDNA in *E. coli. Nature* 1983; **301**: 214–21.

55. Amery A, Vermylen J, Maes H, Verstraete M. Enhancing the fibrinolytic activity in human blood by occlusion of blood vessels. I. The appearance of the phenomenon. *Thromb Diath Haemorrh* 1962; **7**: 70–85.

56. Hoylaerts M, Rijken DC, Lijnen HR, Collen D. Kinetics of the activation of plasminogen by human tissue plasminogen activator: role of fibrin. *J Biol Chem* 1982; **257**: 2912–19.

57. Thorscn S. The mechanism of plasminogen activation and the variability of the fibrin effector during tissue-type plasminogen activator-mediated fibrinolysis. *Ann NY Acad Sci* 1992; **667**: 52–63.

58. Declerck PJ, Mombaerts P, Holvoet P, De Mol M, Collen D. Fibrinolytic response and fibrin fragment D-dimer levels in patients with deep vein thrombosis. *Thromb Haemost* 1987; **58**: 1024–9.

59. Bajzar L, Manuel R, Nesheim ME. Purification and characterization of TAFI, a thrombin-activable fibrinolysis inhibitor. *J Biol Chem* 1995; **270**: 14477–84.

60. Willemse JL, Lears JR, Hendriks DF. Fast kinetic assay for the determination of procarboxypeptidase U (TAFI) in human plasma. *J Thromb Haemost* 2005; **3**: 2353–5.

61. Holmes WE, Nelles L, Lijnen HR, Collen D. Primary structure of human alpha2-antiplasmin, a serine protease inhibitor (serpin). *J Biol Chem* 1987; **262**: 1659–64.

62. Wiman B, Collen D. On the kinetics of the reaction between human antiplasmin and plasmin. *Eur J Biochem* 1978; **84**: 573–8.

63. Alessi MC, Peiretti F, Morange P, Henry M, Nalbone G, Juhan-Vague I. Production of plasminogen activator inhibitor-1 by human adipose tissue: possible link between visceral fat accumulation and vascular disease. *Diabetes* 1997; **46**: 860–7.

64. Frank RD, Weber J, Dresbach H, Thelen H, Weiss C, Floege J. Role of contact system activation in hemodialyzer-induced thrombogenicity. *Kidney Int* 2001; **60**: 1972–81.

65. Sainz IM, Isordia-Salas I, Castaneda JL, *et al.* Modulation of inflammation by kininogen deficiency in a rat model of inflammatory arthritis. *Arthritis Rheum* 2005; **52**: 2549–52.

66. Mari D, Mannucci PM, Coppola R, Bottasso B, Bauer KA, Rosenberg RD. Hypercoagulability in centenarians: the paradox of successful aging. *Blood* 1995; **85**: 3144–9.

67. Meade TW, Chakrabarti R, Haines AP, North WR, Stirling Y. Characteristics affecting fibrinolytic activity and plasma fibrinogen concentrations. *Br Med J* 1979; **1**: 153–6.

68. Danesh J, Collins R, Appleby P, Peto R. Association of fibrinogen, C-reactive protein, albumin, or leukocyte count with coronary heart disease: meta-analysis of prospective studies. *JAMA* 1998; **279**: 1477–82.

69. Van Hylckama Vlieg A, Rosendaal FR. High levels of fibrinogen are associated with the risk of deep venous thrombosis mainly in the elderly. *J Thromb Haemost* 2003; **1**: 2677–8.

70. Koenig W. Fibrin(ogen) in cardiovascular disease: an update. *Thromb Haemost* 2003; **89**: 601–9.

71. Ariens RA, Kohler HP, Mansfield MW, Grant PJ. Subunit antigen and activity levels of blood coagulation factor XIII in healthy individuals: relation to sex, age, smoking and hypertension. *Arterioscler Thromb Vasc Biol* 1999; **19**: 2012–16.

72. Siebenlist KR, Mosesson MW. Progressive cross-linking of fibrin γ-chains increases resistance to fibrinolysis. *J Biol Chem* 1994; **269**: 28414–19.

73. Balleisen L, Bailey J, Epping PH, Schulte H, van de Loo J. Epidemiological study on factor VII, factor VIII and fibrinogen in an industrial population. I. Baseline data in regard to age, gender, body-weight, smoking, alcohol, pill-using, and menopause. *Thromb Haemost* 1985; **54**: 475–9.

74. Tracy RP, Arnold AM, Ettinger W, Fried L, Meilahn E, Savage P. The relationship of fibrinogen and factors VII and VIII to incident cardiovascular disease and death in the elderly. *Arterioscler Thromb Vasc Biol* 1999; **19**: 1776–83.

75. Folsom AR, Rosamond WD, Shakar E, *et al.* Prospective study of markers of hemostatic function with risk of ischemic stroke. The Atherosclerosis Risk in Communities (ARIC) study investigators. *Circulation* 1999; **100**: 736–42.

76. Koster T, Blann AD, Briet E, Vandenbroucke JP, Rosendaal FR. Role of clotting factor VIII in effect of von Willebrand factor on occurrence of deep-vein thrombosis. *Lancet* 1995; **345**: 152–5.

77. Oger E, Lacut K, Van Dreden P, *et al.* High plasma concentration of factor VIII coagulant is also a risk factor for venous thromboembolism in the elderly. *Haematologica* 2003; **88**: 465–9.

78. Jones KC, Mann KG. A model for the tissue factor pathway to thrombin. II. A mathematical simulation. *J Biol Chem* 1994; **269**: 23367–73.

79. Wannamethee SG, Lowe GD, Whincup PH, Rumley A, Walker M, Lennon L. Physical activity and hemostatic and inflammatory variables in elderly men. *Circulation* 2002; **105**: 1785–90.

80. Sweeney JD, Hoernig LA. Age-dependent effect on the level of factor IX. *Am J Clin Pathol* 1993; **99**: 687–8.

81. Bauer K, Weiss LM, Sparrow D, Vokonas PS, Rosenberg RD. Aging-associated changes in indices of thrombin generation and protein C activation in humans. Normative aging study. *J Clin Invest* 1987; **80**: 1527–34.

82. Meade TW, Mellows S, Brozovic M, *et al.* Haemostatic function and ischaemic heart disease: principal results of the Northwick Park Heart Study. *Lancet* 1986; **2**: 533–7.

83. Di Castelnuovo A, D'Orazio A, Amore C, *et al.* Genetic modulation of coagulation factor VII plasma levels: contribution of different polymorphisms and gender-related effects. *Thromb Haemost* 1998; **80**: 592–7.

84. Lane DA, Grant PJ. Role of hemostatic gene polymorphisms in venous and arterial thrombotic disease. *Blood* 2000; **95**: 1517–32.

85. Mennen LI, Schouten EG, Grobbee DE, Kluft C. Coagulation F VII, dietary fat and blood lipids: a review. *Thromb Haemost* 1996; **76**: 492–9.

86. Mennen LI, de Maat MP, Schouten EG, *et al.* Coagulation factor VII, serum-triglycerides and the R/Q 353 polymorphism: differences between older men and women. *Thromb Haemost* 1997; **78**: 984–6.

87. Mennen LI, Witteman JC, den Breeijen JH, *et al.* The association of dietary fat and fiber with coagulation

factor VII in the elderly: the Rotterdam study. *Am J Clin Nutr* 1997; **65**: 732–6.

88. van Hylckama Vlieg A, van der Linden IK, Bertina RM, Rosendaal FR. High levels of factor IX increase the risk of venous thrombosis. *Blood* 2002; **95**: 3678–82.

89. Kurachi S, Deyashiki Y, Takeshita J, Kurachi K. Genetic mechanisms of age regulation of human blood coagulation factor IX. *Science* 1999; **285**: 739–43.

90. Zhang K, Kurachi S, Kurachi K. Genetic mechanisms of age regulation of protein C and blood coagulation. *J Biol Chem* 2002; **277**: 4532–40.

91. Kurachi K, Kurachi S. Molecular mechanisms of age-related regulation of genes. *J Thromb Haemost* 2005; **3**: 909–14.

92. Bonfigli AR, Sirolla C, Cemerelli S, *et al.* Plasminogen activator inhibitor-1 plasma level increases with age in subjects with the 4G allele at position –675 in the promoter region. *Thromb Haemost* 2004; **92**: 1164–5.

93. Eriksson P, Kallin B, van't Hooft FM, Bavenholm P, Hamsten A. Allele-specific increase in basal transcription of the plasminogen activator inhibitor 1 gene is associated with myocardial infarction. *Proc Natl Acad Sci USA* 1995; **92**: 1851–5.

94. Mannucci PM, Mari D, Merati G, *et al.* Gene polymorphisms predicting high plasma levels of coagulation and fibrinolysis proteins: a study in centenarians. *Arterioscler Thromb Vasc Biol* 1997; **17**: 755–9.

28

Platelet disorders in the elderly

Laura Terranova, Giancarla Gerli, Marco Cattaneo

Thrombocytopenia

Platelets are derived from megakaryocytes in the bone marrow, but they can also be released from circulating megakaryocytes that regularly inhabit the capillaries of the lung [1]. Platelet turnover is about 2×10^{11} per day; the platelet lifespan is 8–10 days. Platelets distribute between the circulation and the spleen. In normal individuals, the splenic pool, which corresponds to approximately 30–40% of the total, is in dynamic equilibrium with the circulating pool and is proportional to the splenic mass. Splenic enlargement from a variety of causes is associated with a great increase in the proportion of platelets sequestered in the spleen, which is presumed to represent slower transit of platelets through the enlarged or congested splenic pulp. Platelet destruction results from phagocytosis by macrophages of the hepatic and splenic reticuloendothelial system.

Thrombocytopenia can be defined as a persistent fall in the platelet count below 150×10^9/L. It can be "mild," when the platelet count is between 100 and 150×10^9/L, "moderate" (50–99×10^9/L), "severe" (20–49×10^9/L), and "extremely severe" ($<20 \times 10^9$/L). Given that automated particle counters may give spuriously low results, especially in the presence of giant platelets, it is important to confirm low platelet counts by examining a well-prepared peripheral blood smear. It is important to note that in many instances a decrease in the platelet count may be due to an artifact caused by the chelation of cations by EDTA, which is the commonly used anticoagulant to collect blood samples for platelet count. This phenomenon, known by the term *pseudothrombocytopenia*, is due to in-vitro platelet agglutination or platelet satellitosis around granulocytes, mediated by platelet-specific antibodies that react with platelets only at very low concentrations of Ca^{2+}, such as in EDTA-treated blood samples. The condition can be easily recognized by inspecting a smear of EDTA blood from the patient (which should always be examined when facing any type of hematologic disorder), which will show platelet agglutinates or platelets resetting the granulocytes, instead of the normal-appearing isolated platelets in a proportion of approximately 1 : 20 with red blood cells. Measurement of platelet count in blood samples anticoagulated with different anticoagulants (such as citrate or heparin) or in native blood could also be useful, but probably superfluous. Further evaluation of the patient should always be postponed until pseudothrombocytopenia has been excluded.

Thrombocytopenia is a frequent hematologic disorder in the elderly, although no definite data are available on its real prevalence. The normal range of platelet count (150–450×10^9/L) does not change as people age [2]; therefore the presence of thrombocytopenia, even in mild forms, always deserves careful evaluation. Evaluation of an elderly patient with thrombocytopenia is the same as that of an adult, younger patient, but usually more cumbersome because of the potential multifactorial pathogenesis of the condition in the elderly. A careful clinical history should be particularly focused on the use of drugs. The blood count, if carefully examined, paying particular attention to morphometric platelet

Blood Disorders in the Elderly, ed. Lodovico Balducci, William Ershler, Giovanni de Gaetano.
Published by Cambridge University Press. © Cambridge University Press 2008.

parameters (MPV, mean platelet volume; PDW, platelet distribution width), can help to explain the pathogenesis of the condition: low MPV and PDW values are typical of decreased or ineffective megakaryocytopoiesis, while high values are more typical of thrombocytopenia due to increased platelet destruction. Furthermore, careful morphological examination of a peripheral blood smear is essential for the correct diagnosis. Bone-marrow aspiration, which can usually be withheld in the young patient affected by thrombocytopenia, is mandatory in the case of elderly patients.

The clinical presentation of patients with thrombocytopenia may vary widely, according to its pathogenesis, the severity of the decrease in platelet count, and the coexistence of other risk factors for bleeding. Usually, thrombocytopenia due to increased platelet destruction is associated with fewer bleeding complications than those caused by decreased megakaryocytopoiesis. This phenomenon is usually interpreted as due to the presence of larger and younger platelets in the circulation of patients with increased platelet destruction. Bleeding complications are extremely rare for platelet counts above 50×10^9/L, while they become much more frequent at platelet counts below 20×10^9/L. The most important risk factor for bleeding in thrombocytopenic patients is age: the older the patient, the higher the bleeding risk. Other common risk factors include trauma, fever, infections, and anemia. Mucocutaneous bleeding (nose, gum, gastrointestinal bleeds, hematuria, purpura) are typical bleeding manifestations of thrombocytopenia. Bleeds in the central nervous system are very rare in young patients, but increase in frequency with age. A relatively high incidence of retinal bleeding has been described in elderly patients [3].

Classification

Thrombocytopenia can be due to:

- decreased platelet production
- increased platelet destruction (immune- or non-immune-mediated)

- abnormalities of platelet distribution
- disorders of dilution

Disorders of platelet production

In the elderly, disorders of platelet production include:

- decreased megakaryocytopoiesis
- ineffective platelet production

A decrease in the number of marrow megakaryocytes is characteristic of bone-marrow damage caused by radiation, alcohol (which has an inhibitory effect on the marrow megakaryocytes), chemicals, and drugs. Drugs that most frequently associate with thrombocytopenia include immunosuppressive agents, thiazide diuretics, anticonvulsants, gold salts, non-steroidal anti-inflammatory drugs, and interferon. Viruses, such as HCV, HIV, and CMV, can selectively inhibit megakaryocytopoiesis [4]. Disorders of stem cells can also cause ineffective thrombopoiesis. Thrombocytopenia due to ineffective platelet production is often the first clinical picture of myelodysplastic syndromes (MDSs), a group of clonal stem-cell diseases characterized by ineffective hematopoiesis, multilineage blood cell dysplasia, and peripheral cytopenia with normocellular or hypercellular marrow. MDSs predominantly affect older populations, with a median age of onset of 60 to 70 years: their annual incidence is approximately 3.5 to 10 per 100 000 in the general population and 15 to 50 per 100 000 in the elderly population [5]. The presence and the severity of thrombocytopenia is correlated to the MDS subtype, being more frequent and more severe in the most advanced and high-risk forms. The presence of thrombocytopenia at presentation is considered a negative prognostic factor in MDSs and has therefore been included in the International Prognostic Scoring System (IPSS) [6]. The diagnosis of MDSs is based on peripheral-blood cell counts and morphologic examination of peripheral blood and bone marrow. Additional studies, useful in establishing diagnosis, include immunophenotyping and cytogenetic analysis [6].

Other disorders associated with ineffective platelet production include vitamin B_{12} or folate deficiency, which are particularly frequent in the elderly, due to inadequate dietary intake or gastrointestinal diseases associated with malabsorption [4]. Vitamin B_{12} and folate deficiencies are characterized by asynchronous maturation of the cellular nucleus due to defective DNA synthesis, resulting in megaloblastic anemia. Thrombocytopenia is present in about 20% of patients with megaloblastic anemia and is usually mild. Macrocytes and hypersegmented neutrophils can be observed in the peripheral blood smear, while bone-marrow examination reveals hypercellularity, presence of large erythroblasts with immature nuclei (presence of fine, primitive chromatin), and normal hemoglobin formation.

Increased platelet destruction

Increased platelet destruction is the most common cause of thrombocytopenia. Typically, platelet survival is decreased and the number of megakaryocytes in the bone marrow is increased. Increased platelet destruction can be mediated by immune and non-immune mechanisms.

Immune thrombocytopenia

Immune platelet destruction may be mediated by autoantibodies against a platelet antigen, antibodies against a platelet alloantigen, antibodies against an autologous or heterologous antigen absorbed into the platelet surface, or by immune complexes. Platelet destruction results from phagocytosis of the opsonized platelets by macrophages of the reticuloendothelial system, especially in the spleen. Immune thrombocytopenias include:

- autoimmune (idiopathic) thrombocytopenic purpura (ITP)
- thrombocytopenias associated with autoimmune diseases
- drug-induced thrombocytopenia
- post-transfusion purpura

Autoimmune (idiopathic) thrombocytopenic purpura (ITP)

ITP is an autoimmune disorder characterized by low platelet count and mucocutaneous bleeding. The diagnosis of ITP is based on the exclusion of concomitant diseases that could account for the decrease in platelet count [7]. Systemic symptoms, organomegaly, enlarged lymph nodes and abnormalities of the other blood cell lines must be ruled out. When autoimmune thrombocytopenia is associated with autoimmune hemolytic anemia it is known as Evans syndrome.

The interaction of platelets with an autoantibody (usually of the IgG class) results in their premature removal from the circulation by macrophages of the reticuloendothelial system, especially the spleen. In many cases the antibody is directed against antigen sites on the glycoprotein IIb/IIIa or Ib/IX/V complexes.

ITP is the most common type of thrombocytopenia in the elderly, accounting for 20–25% of all bleeding disorders; it usually affects women more frequently than men. Frederiksen and Schmidt, in a study on 221 patients with ITP in a Danish county, estimated an annual incidence of 4.62 per 100 000 in persons over 60 years of age, whereas in younger people it was 1.94 per 100 000 persons [8].

Laboratory investigation at the time of presentation should be kept to a minimum. Platelet kinetic studies and detection of platelet-associated antibodies are not recommended.

Thrombocytopenia associated with autoimmune diseases

Immune thrombocytopenia is associated with a variety of autoimmune diseases. Symptoms and signs are generally those of the underlying disease. The major disease of interest in this category is systemic lupus erythematosus (SLE), whose annual incidence rate in the elderly is approximately 7.5 per 100 000 [9]. Viral infections, most commonly caused by HIV or HCV, are often associated with immune thrombocytopenia. Immune-mediated thrombocytopenia is commonly observed in patients with lymphoproliferative disorders, particularly chronic lymphocytic leukemia and non-Hodgkin lymphomas [10]. Signs and symptoms generally reflect the severity of the primary disease.

Drug-induced thrombocytopenia

Drug-induced thrombocytopenia is very common in elderly people, who are often on multi-drug treatment. Drugs that are most commonly associated with thrombocytopenia are listed in Table 28.1; however,

it must be borne in mind that any drug or chemical has the potential to cause thrombocytopenia. Several potential pathogenic mechanisms may be involved in drug-induced thrombocytopenia (Table 28.2) [11]. Despite the fact that the relative risk of developing thrombocytopenia may be high for some drugs (Table 28.1), the global incidence of drug-induced thrombocytopenia is relatively low [12].

A particular type of drug-induced thrombocytopenia is that caused by heparin (heparin-induced thrombocytopenia, HIT), which can associate with severe thrombotic manifestations. This syndrome results from the generation of an IgG antibody directed against a complex of heparin and platelet factor 4 (PF4), which causes platelet activation. The same antibodies are not specific for heparin, but also interact with the PF4/glycosaminoglycan complex that is present on the vascular wall. Occupancy of the platelet FcγRIIa receptor by PF4/heparin/IgG immune complex leads to receptor clustering and platelet activation. Activated platelets release additional PF4, leading to a vicious cycle of progressive

Table 28.1. Drugs most strongly associated with autoimmune thrombocytopenic purpura.

Drug	Estimated relative risk of thrombocytopenia on multivariate analysis (95% CI)
Quinidine/quinine	101 (31–324)
Sulfonamide antibiotics	40 (10–62)
Dipyridamole	14 (3.5–54)
Sulfonylureas	4.8 (1.5–16)
Furosemide	2.8 (0.8–10)
Sodium salicylate	2.6 (1.3–5.0)
Digoxin	1.5 (0.4–5.5)

Table 28.2. Mechanisms of drug-induced immune thrombocytopenia.

Type	Mechanism	Examples
Hapten-induced antibody	Drug binds covalently to membrane glycoprotein and functions as hapten to induce antibody response	Penicillin
"Quinine-type" thrombocytopenia	Drug binds non-covalently to platelet membrane glycoprotein to produce "compound" epitopes or induce conformational changes for which the antibody is specific	Quinidine, quinine, sulfonamide antibiotics
Autoantibody induction	Drug induces true autoantibodies that bind to platelet membrane glycoproteins	Gold salts, procainamide
Immune complex-mediated	Drug binds to a normal protein to form immunogenic complexes; antibody reacts with these complexes to form immune complexes which activate platelets via Fc receptors	Heparin
Fibrinogen receptor antagonist (FRA)	Drug binds to the platelet fibrinogen receptor (GPIIb–IIIa) to induce conformational changes (LIBS) that are recognized by the antibody	Tirofiban, epitifabatide
Drug-specific	The antibody recognizes a platelet-specific monoclonal antibody that is bound to its target	Abciximab

platelet and coagulation activation. HIT can be viewed as an acquired hypercoagulable state, with increased thrombin generation and increased risk for arterial and venous thrombosis [13]. Its prevalence in heparin-treated patients is about 1–3% with unfractionated heparin, but may be lower with low-molecular-weight heparins. The clinical picture is characterized by thrombocytopenia, usually severe, occurring 5–10 days after starting heparin treatment or earlier when the patient has been previously exposed to the drug. The diagnosis of HIT may be difficult and should be based on [14]:

(1) a fall in platelet count below 150×10^9/L, or greater than 50% of baseline, 5–10 days after starting heparin treatment
(2) normalization in the platelet count within few days (5–7) after discontinuation of heparin
(3) no clinically apparent alternative explanation for thrombocytopenia

Confirmatory laboratory tests are now available. A mild lowering of the platelet count may occur in the first 24 hours as a result of platelet clumping; this condition, which is usually referred to as "type 1" HIT, has no major clinical impact and often recovers spontaneously, without discontinuing heparin [15].

Post-transfusion purpura

Post-transfusion purpura is a rare and severe thrombocytopenia, which usually occurs approximately 10 days after a blood transfusion. It has been attributed to antibodies in the recipient developing against the human platelet antigen 1a (HPA-1a). Severe thrombocytopenia may occur some hours after a blood or plasma transfusion, due to involuntary transfusion of specific antibodies against the platelet antigen HPA-1a [16].

Non-immune thrombocytopenia

Among non-immune disorders of platelet destruction, the most common in elderly patients are thrombotic thrombocytopenic purpura and disseminated intravascular coagulation.

Thrombotic thrombocytopenic purpura

Thrombotic thrombocytopenic purpura (TTP) and hemolytic–uremic syndrome (HUS) are rare disorders whose varied clinical manifestations result from the formation of platelet-rich thrombi within the microvasculature, consequent tissue ischemia, and thrombocytopenia. In the elderly, TTP is much more common than HUS, which mostly affects children. The identification, characterization, and clinical observation of ADAMTS13 (a disintegrin and metalloprotease with thrombospondin-1-like domains) have provided important insights into the pathogenesis of TTP. ADAMTS13 is a plasma enzyme essential for postsecretion proteolytic processing of von Willebrand factor (VWF). Absence of ADAMTS13 is associated with the occurrence of abnormally large multimers of VWF and is also associated with the occurrence of TTP. Initial assumptions that absent ADAMTS13 was itself the cause of TTP have been tempered by subsequent observations that ADAMTS13 activity can be severely deficient without clinical abnormalities and that patients can have characteristic clinical features of TTP without severe ADAMTS13 deficiency. A current interpretation of these observations is that ADAMTS13 deficiency is a major risk factor for the development of TTP, but it is neither always necessary nor sufficient to cause TTP. This interpretation is consistent with other vascular and thrombotic disorders in which multiple risk factors and associated conditions contribute to the etiology of acute events [17–19]. ADAMTS13 deficiency may be congenital or acquired, immune-mediated, associated with metastases, bone-marrow transplantation, drugs, HIV infection, and *Escherichia coli* O157 infection.

Very-high-molecular-weight multimers of VWF in plasma, which are normally cleaved by ADAMTS13, induce in-vivo platelet aggregation, resulting in microthrombi formation in small vessels, causing infarction of the perfused organ. The clinical presentation is usually characterized by fever, neurologic abnormalities, uremia, asthenia, nausea, arthralgias, and myalgias, and may be heterogeneous based on the multiplicity of the districts involved [20]. The neurological syndrome is characterized by headache, sensorial deficit and/or focal motorial deficit (central and/or peripheral), paresthesia, convulsions, coma.

The diagnosis of TTP is based upon clinical signs and symptoms as well as on laboratory findings. Principal features are thrombocytopenia, microangiopathic hemolytic anemia (with reticulocytosis, increased bilirubin and LDH levels, reduction in haptoglobin levels, anisopoikilocytosis, schistocytosis, and negative Coombs test), neurological syndrome, and/or renal failure. Disseminated intravascular coagulation, triggered by tissue damage and increase of circulating tissue factor, may complicate the clinical and laboratory presentation [20].

Disseminated intravascular coagulation (DIC)
Disseminated intravascular coagulation is an acquired disorder characterized by the in-vivo widespread activation of coagulation, which results in the intravascular deposition of fibrin and consumption of coagulation factors and platelets. It may be associated with a fulminant hemorrhagic or thrombotic syndrome or have a less severe and chronic course. DIC occurs as a consequence of many disorders that are associated with the release of procoagulant material into the circulation or that cause widespread endothelial damage or platelet aggregation. The most common causes of DIC are listed in Table 28.3 [21].

Widespread endothelial damage or entry of procoagulant material into the circulation leads to intravascular thrombin generation, which leads to the formation of fibrin, which can deposit in the microcirculation or complex with circulating fibrinogen. The presence of thrombi on the vascular walls stimulates the fibrinolytic system, with the formation of fibrin and fibrinogen degradation products, which interfere with fibrin polymerization, thus contributing to the coagulation defect. The combined action of thrombin and plasmin normally causes depletion of fibrinogen, prothrombin, and factors V and VIII. Intravascular thrombin also causes widespread platelet aggregation, which leads to consumption of platelets, aggravating the bleeding risk of the patient.

Table 28.3. Common clinical conditions associated with disseminated intravascular coagulation.

Sepsis
Trauma
Cancer (myeloproliferative diseases, solid tumors)
Vascular disorders (giant hemangioma, aortic aneurysm)
Reaction to toxins (e.g., snake venom, drugs, amphetamines)
Immunologic disorders (severe allergic reaction, hemolytic transfusion reaction, transplant rejection)

The clinical presentation is characterized by bleeding, particularly from venipuncture sites or recent wounds. There may be generalized bleeding in the gastrointestinal tract, the oropharynx, into the lungs and urogenital tract. Less frequently microthrombi may cause skin lesions, renal failure, gangrene of the fingers or toes, or cerebral ischemia [22]. Laboratory findings include thrombocytopenia, prolonged PT and APTT, deficiency of fibrinogen and high levels of fibrinogen and fibrin degradation products. Many patients present with microangiopathic hemolytic anemia, due to fragmentation of the red blood cells in the microcirculation: typically, fragmented red blood cells can be observed in peripheral blood smears.

Disorders of platelet distribution

Under physiological conditions, the splenic platelet pool accounts for about one-third of the total platelet mass, while under pathological conditions characterized by enlarged spleen, it can reach 90% of the platelet mass, thus causing a decrease in circulating platelets. Under these conditions, thrombocytopenia is usually mild or moderate and associated with anemia and/or leukopenia [16].

Disorders of platelet distribution can be found in the giant hemangioma syndrome or during prolonged hypothermia (e.g., extracorporeal circulation for cardiac surgery). Hypothermia is also the cause of the transient thrombocytopenia that can be observed in elderly patients who have remained unconscious in a cold environment for a long period [23].

Disorders of platelet dilution

These thrombocytopenias are the result of blood dilution that occurs as a consequence of massive blood or plasma transfusions [23].

Pseudothrombocytopenia

As already mentioned, pseudothrombocytopenia is a rare condition (0.07–0.11% of all blood samples [24]) in which platelet counts are reported to be decreased. This phenomenon is due to the reaction of platelet-specific antibodies with platelets in the presence of EDTA. It can be excluded through a platelet count in a different anticoagulant and an inspection of a blood smear. The most frequent cause of pseudo-thrombocytopenia is in-vitro platelet clumping in EDTA-anticoagulated blood. The mechanism of this reaction appears to involve antiplatelet antibodies, more frequently IgM or IgG. Platelet agglutinates develop in vitro within some minutes from blood collection and keep forming in the following 60 to 90 minutes. In 10–20% of cases, pseudothrombo-cytopenia may also be seen in samples containing citrate as anticoagulant. Inhibitors of the glycoprotein GPIIb/IIIa complex, which are used in patients undergoing percutaneous coronary intervention, may cause pseudothrombocytopenia [24].

Treatment

In patients with a megakaryocytic thrombocytope-nia and active bleeding, transfusion of platelet concentrates is highly recommended. In patients with MDS, supportive care with platelet concentrates must be evaluated individually [25]. Prophylactic platelet transfusions are indicated in all patients with acute leukemia on chemotherapy, when their platelet count drops below $10 \times 10^9/L$. This threshold should be increased to 20–$30 \times 10^9/L$, when additional risk factors for bleeding are present (such as fever, infections, sepsis) [26].

In ITP, treatment with steroids is indicated for asymptomatic patients with platelet counts below 20–$30 \times 10^9/L$. For patients with active bleeding,

treatment should be given also if the platelet count is higher than $30 \times 10^9/L$ (the recommended initial dosage is 1 mg/kg daily, which should gradually be reduced after 10–14 days) [7]. However, steroid ther-apy must be carefully evaluated in elderly people, due to its important side effects, such as arterial hyper-tension, diabetes, and osteoporosis, and its relatively lower efficacy. In poor responders or in patients who require unacceptably high doses of steroids, alternative treatments may be considered, includ-ing the anti-CD20 monoclonal antibody rituximab or other immunosuppressive agents. Splenectomy should be considered in patients who are resistant to medical treatment and have persistently very low platelet counts, with bleeding manifestations, even though a lower percentage of response, a higher intraoperative mortality, and high risk of bacterial infections have been reported in the elderly, com-pared to younger patients [7,27]. High-dose intrave-nous immunoglobulin therapy, particularly useful in young patients, must be carefully evaluated in the elderly, because thrombotic events during this treat-ment have been reported [28]. In thrombocytopenia associated with autoimmune disease, treatment of the underlying disease is recommended, and usually improves the platelet count.

In drug-induced thrombocytopenias, discontinu-ing the administration of the drug may be sufficient to obtain a normalization in the platelet count. In HIT with thrombosis, heparin therapy must be dis-continued and replaced with other anticoagulants, such as lepirudin or danaparoid sodium [29].

Most cases of thrombocytopenia due to vitamin B_{12} or folate deficiency improve with vitamin treatment.

The current established treatment of TTP is plasma exchange with fresh frozen plasma or cryo-supernatant, which is rich in ADAMTS13 and poor in VWF multimers [30]. In patients with DIC, treat-ment of the underlying cause is very important. Supportive therapy with fresh frozen plasma (10–15 mL/kg) is indicated in patients with high risk of bleeding. A beneficial role for low-molecular-weight heparin (LMWH) anticoagulation is also shown in the management of DIC (e.g., malignancies, sepsis) [21].

Inherited disorders of platelet function

Inherited disorders of platelet function are generally classified based on the functions or responses that are abnormal. However, since platelet functions are intimately related, a clear distinction between disorders of platelet adhesion, aggregation, activation, secretion, and procoagulant activity is in many instances problematic. For this reason, we propose a classification that is based on abnormalities of platelet components that share common characteristics [31]: (1) platelet receptors for adhesive proteins, (2) platelet receptors for soluble agonists, (3) platelet granules, (4) signal-transduction pathways, and (5) procoagulant phospholipids. Inherited disorders of platelet function that are less well characterized will be lumped in a sixth category of miscellaneous disorders (Table 28.4).

Abnormalities of the platelet receptors for adhesive proteins

Abnormalities of the GPIb/V/IX complex

Bernard–Soulier syndrome
Characterized by autosomal recessive, prolonged bleeding time, thrombocytopenia, giant platelets, and decreased platelet survival, Bernard–Soulier syndrome (BSS) is associated with quantitative or qualitative defects of the platelet glycopotein complex GPIb/V/IX [31]. The degree of thrombocytopenia may be overestimated when the platelet count is performed with automatic counters, because giant platelets, which may be as frequent as 70–80% in occasional patients, may reach the size of red blood cells and, as a consequence, are not recognized as platelets by the counters. Typically, BSS platelets do not agglutinate to ristocetin and this defect is not corrected by the addition of normal plasma. The platelet responses to physiologic agonists is normal, with the exception of low concentrations of thrombin. Bleeding events, which may be very severe, can be controlled by platelet transfusion. Most heterozygotes, with few exceptions, do not have a bleeding diathesis.

Table 28.4. Inherited disorders of platelet function.

Abnormalities of the platelet receptors for adhesive proteins
  GPIb/V/IX complex (Bernard–Soulier syndrome, Platelet-type von Willebrand disease, Bolin–Jamieson syndrome)
  GPIIb/IIIa (α_{IIb}/β_3) (Glanzmann thrombasthenia)
  GPIa/IIa (α_2/β_1)
  GPVI
  GPIV

Abnormalities of the platelet receptors for soluble agonists
  Thromboxane A_2 receptor
  α_2-adrenergic receptor
  $P2Y_{12}$ receptor

Abnormalities of the platelet granules
  δ-granules (δ-Storage Pool Deficiency, Hermansky–Pudlak syndrome, Chediak–Hygashi syndrome, thrombocytopenia with absent radii syndrome, Wiskott–Aldrich syndrome)
  α-granules (Gray platelet syndrome, Quebec platelet disorder, Paris–Trousseau–Jacobsen syndrome)
  α- and δ-granules (α, δ-storage pool deficiency)

Abnormalities of the signal-transduction pathways
  Abnormalities of the arachidonate/thromboxane A_2 pathway, $G\alpha q$ deficiency, partial selective PLC-$\beta 2$ isozyme deficiency, defects in pleckstrin phosphorylation, defective Ca^{2+} mobilization, hyperresponsiveness of platelet $Gs\alpha$

Abnormalities of membrane phospholipids
  Scott syndrome
  Stormorken syndrome

Miscellaneous abnormalities of platelet function
  Primary secretion defects
  Other platelet abnormalities (Montreal platelet syndrome, osteogenesis imperfecta, Ehlers–Danlos syndrome, Marfan syndrome, hexokinase deficiency, glucose-6-phosphate dehydrogenase deficiency)

Platelet-type, or pseudo, von Willebrand disease
Von Willebrand disease (VWD) is a disorder of primary hemostasis that is due to complete or partial defects of von Willebrand factor (VWF), an adhesive protein that plays an essential role in platelet adhesion and aggregation under high shear forces [32]. Platelet-type (or pseudo) VWD is not due to defects

of VWF, but to gain of function phenotype of the platelet GPIbα, which has an increased avidity for VWF, leading to the binding of the largest VWF multimers to resting platelets and their clearance from the circulation. Since the high-molecular-weight VWF multimers are the most hemostatically active, their loss is associated with bleeding risk, as in type 2B VWD, which is caused by a gain of functional abnormality of the VWF molecule.

Bolin–Jamieson syndrome

This is a rare, autosomal dominant mild bleeding disorder associated with a larger form of GPIbα in one allele [33], which is probably associated with a large multimer form of the size polymorphism occurring in the mucin-like domain.

Abnormalities of GPIIb/IIIa (αIIb/β3) (Glanzmann thrombasthenia)

Glanzmann thrombasthenia (GT) is an autosomal recessive disease that is caused by lack of expression or qualitative defects of one of the two glycoproteins forming the integrin α_{IIb}/β_3, which in activated platelets binds the adhesive glycoproteins that bridge adjacent platelets, securing platelet aggregation [31]. The diagnostic hallmark of the disease is the lack or severe impairment of platelet aggregation induced by all agonists; severe forms are characterized by lack of fibrinogen in the platelet α-granules. Platelet clot retraction is defective. GT platelets normally bind to the subendothelium, but they fail to spread. The disease is associated with bleeding manifestations that are similar to those of patients with BSS, although of lower severity. The molecular defects that are responsible for GT have been recently reviewed [34].

Abnormalities of GPIa/IIa (α_2/β_1)

Two patients with mild bleeding disorders associated with deficient expression of the platelet receptor for collagen GPIa/IIa (α_2/β_1) and selective impairment of platelet responses to collagen have been described [35,36]. Their platelet defect spontaneously recovered after menopause, suggesting that α_2/β_1 expression is under hormonal control.

Abnormalities of GPVI

A selective defect of collagen-induced platelet aggregation was also described in another mild bleeding disorder, characterized by the deficiency of the platelet GPVI [37], a member of the immunoglobulin superfamily of receptors, which mediates platelet activation by collagen.

Abnormalities of GPIV

GPIV binds collagen, thrombospondin, and probably other proteins. Its physiological role is unclear, because its deficiency, which is common in healthy individuals from Japan and other East Asian populations, is not associated with an abnormal phenotype [31].

Abnormalities of the platelet receptors for soluble agonists

Thromboxane A$_2$ (TxA$_2$) receptor

Two patients with abnormal platelet responses to TxA$_2$ have been described, who display an Arg^{60} to Leu mutation in the first cytoplasmic loop of the TxA$_2$ receptor [38], affecting both isoforms of the receptor. The mutation was found exclusively in the affected members of the two unrelated families, and was inherited as an autosomal dominant trait.

ADP receptors

Platelets possess two P2 receptors for ADP: P2Y$_{12}$ and P2Y$_1$ [39]. Only patients with congenital defects of the platelet P2Y$_{12}$ receptors have been described so far [40–42]. These patients have lifelong histories of excessive bleeding, prolonged bleeding time, and abnormalities of platelet aggregation that are similar to those observed in patients with defects of platelet secretion (reversible aggregation in response to weak agonists and impaired aggregation in response to low concentrations of collagen or thrombin), except that the aggregation response to ADP is severely impaired. Other abnormalities of platelet function found in these patients were: (1) no inhibition by ADP of PGE_1-stimulated platelet adenylyl cyclase; (2) normal shape change and normal (or mildly reduced) mobilization of cytoplasmic ionized calcium induced by ADP; and (3) presence of about 30% of the normal number of platelet binding sites for $[^{33}P]2MeSADP$ or $[^3H]ADP$. These patients display deletions in the open reading frame, which shift the reading frame before introducing a stop codon, causing a premature truncation of the protein.

Another patient with congenital bleeding disorder associated with abnormal $P2Y_{12}$-mediated platelet responses to ADP has more recently been characterized [43]. The platelet phenotype is very similar to that of patients with $P2Y_{12}$ deficiency, except that the number and affinity of $[^{33}P]$-2MeSADP binding sites was normal. Analysis of the patient $P2Y_{12}$ gene revealed, in one allele, a G-to-A transition changing the codon for Arg^{256} in the sixth transmembrane domain to Gln and, in the other, a C-to-T transition changing the codon for Arg^{265} in the third extracellular loop to Trp. Neither mutation interfered with receptor surface expression but both altered function, since ADP inhibited the forskolin-induced increase of cAMP markedly less in CHO cells transfected with either mutant $P2Y_{12}$ than wild-type receptor.

Abnormalities of the platelet granules

Abnormalities of the δ-granules (δ-storage pool deficiency)

The term δ-storage pool deficiency (δ-SPD) defines a congenital abnormality of platelets characterized by deficiency of dense granules in megakaryocytes and platelets. It may present as an isolated platelet function defect or associate with a variety of congenital disorders. Between 10% and 18% of patients with congenital abnormalities of platelet function have SPD [44,45]. The inheritance is autosomal recessive in some families and autosomal dominant in others [46].

δ-SPD is characterized by a bleeding diathesis of variable degree, mildly to moderately prolonged skin bleeding time, abnormal platelet secretion induced by several platelet agonists, and impaired platelet aggregation. Typically, δ-SPD platelets have decreased levels of δ-granule constituents. The bleeding time is usually prolonged, and the extent of its prolongation is inversely related to the amount of ADP or serotonin contained in the granules.

Normal aggregation responses to ADP or epinephrine have been observed in some patients [47], indicating that there is a large variability in platelet aggregation in patients with δ-SPD; this has been well documented in a large study of 106 patients with δ-SPD, which showed that about 25% of the patients had normal aggregation responses, while only 33% had aggregation tracings typical for a platelet secretion defect [45]. Lumiaggregometry, which measures platelet aggregation and secretion simultaneously, may prove a more accurate technique than platelet aggregometry for diagnosing patients with δ-SPD and, more generally, with platelet secretion defects.

The *Hermansky–Pudlak syndrome* (HPS) and the *Chediak–Hygashi syndrome* (CHS) are rare syndromic forms of δ-SPD. HPS is an autosomal recessive disease of subcellular organelles of many tissues, involving abnormalities of melanosomes, platelet δ-granules, and lysosomes [46]. It is characterized by tyrosinase-positive oculocutaneous albinism, a bleeding diathesis due to δ-SPD and ceroid-lypofuscin lysosomal storage disease. HPS can arise from mutations in different genetic loci. CHS is also an autosomal recessive disorder, characterized by variable degrees of oculocutaneous albinism, very large peroxidase-positive cytoplasmic granules in a variety of hematopoietic (neutrophils) and non-hematopoietic cells, easy bruisability due to δ-SPD, and recurrent infections, associated with neutropenia, impaired chemotaxis and bactericidal activity, and abnormal NK function. The syndrome is lethal, leading to death usually in the first decade of life [46].

Abnormalities of the α-granules (gray platelet syndrome)

Gray platelet syndrome (GPS)

The condition owes its name to the gray appearance of the patient's platelets in peripheral blood smears as a consequence of the rarity of platelet granules

[48]. The inheritance pattern seems to be autosomal recessive, although in a single family it seemed to be autosomal dominant. Affected patients have a life-long history of mucocutaneous bleeding, which may vary from mild to moderate in severity, prolonged bleeding time, mild thrombocytopenia, abnormally large platelets, and isolated reduction of the platelet α-granule content. Mild to moderate myelofibrosis has been described in some patients and hypothetically ascribed to the action of cytokines that are released by the hypogranular platelets and megakaryocytes in the bone marrow. The basic defect in GPS is probably defective targeting and packaging of endogenously synthesized proteins in platelet α-granules.

Quebec platelet disorder

The Quebec platelet disorder is an autosomal dominant qualitative platelet abnormality, characterized by severe post-traumatic bleeding complications unresponsive to platelet transfusion, abnormal proteolysis of α-granule proteins, severe deficiency of platelet factor V, deficiency of multimerin (a large protein that binds factor V and its activated form, factor Va), reduced-to-normal platelet counts, and markedly decreased platelet aggregation induced by epinephrine [46].

Jacobsen or Paris–Trousseau syndrome

This is a rare syndrome that is associated with a mild hemorrhagic diathesis and is characterized by congenital thrombocytopenia, normal platelet lifespan, increased number of marrow megakaryocytes, many of which presenting with signs of abnormal maturation, and intramedullary lysis. A fraction of the circulating platelets has giant α-granules, which are unable to release their content upon platelet stimulation with thrombin. A deletion of the distal part of one chromosome 11 [del(11)q23.3>qter] was found in the affected patients [46].

Abnormalities of the α- and δ-granules (α, δ-storage pool deficiency)

α, δ-storage pool deficiency is characterized by deficiencies of both α- and δ-granules. The clinical picture and the platelet aggregation abnormalities are similar to those of patients with GPS or δ-SPD [46].

Abnormalities of the signal-transduction pathways

Congenital abnormalities of the arachidonate/thromboxane A_2 pathway, involving the liberation of arachidonic acid from membrane phospholipids, defects of cyclooxygenase or thromboxane synthetase, are associated with platelet function defects and mild bleeding. Other congenital abnormalities of the platelet signal-transduction pathways that have been described involve G-proteins (Gαq deficiency), the phosphatidylinositol metabolism (partial selective PLC-β2 isozyme deficiency), and defects in pleckstrin phosphorylation [31].

Three patients were recently described with a polymorphism of the gene encoding the extra-large stimulatory G-protein α-subunit (XLSα), associated with hyper-responsiveness of platelet Gsα, enhanced intraplatelet cAMP generation, and a bleeding syndrome [49]. The functional polymorphism in these patients involves the imprinted region of the *XLSα* gene, a phenomenon not described previously for platelet disorders but already known for defects expressing phenotypically in other tissues.

Abnormalities of membrane phospholipids

Scott syndrome

Scott syndrome is a rare bleeding disorder associated with the maintenance of the asymmetry of the lipid bilayer in the membranes of blood cells, including platelets [50], leading to reduced thrombin generation and defective wound healing. The cause of the defect is still unclear.

Stormorken syndrome

Resting platelets from patients with this syndrome display a full procoagulant activity [51]. Therefore, compared with the Scott syndrome, this condition represents the other side of the coin; yet, surprisingly, it is also associated with a bleeding tendency. Platelets respond normally to all agonists, with the exception of collagen.

Miscellaneous abnormalities of platelet function

Primary secretion defects

The term *primary secretion defect* was probably used for the first time by Weiss [52], to indicate all those ill-defined abnormalities of platelet secretion not associated with platelet granule deficiencies. The term was later used to indicate the platelet secretion defects not associated with platelet granule deficiencies and abnormalities of the arachidonate pathway, or, more generally, all the abnormalities of platelet function associated with defects of signal transduction. With the progression in our knowledge of platelet pathophysiology, this heterogeneous group, which lumps together the majority of patients with congenital disorders of platelet function, will become progressively thinner, losing those patients with better-defined biochemical abnormalities responsible for their platelet secretion defect. An example is given by patients with heterozygous $P2Y_{12}$ deficiency, who were included in this group of disorders until their biochemical abnormality was identified [31].

Other platelet abnormalities

Spontaneous platelet aggregation and decreased responses to thrombin are observed in patients with the *Montreal platelet syndrome*, a rare and poorly characterized congenital thrombocytopenia with large platelets [31].

Platelet function abnormalities have been reported in osteogenesis imperfecta, the Ehlers–Danlos syndrome, the Marfan syndrome, hexokinase deficiency, and glucose-6-phosphate dehydrogenase deficiency.

Treatment

Platelet transfusions should be used only in severe bleeding episodes, which are usually seen in patients with BSS, or, less frequently, GT. Recombinant factor VIIa is a good, albeit rather expensive, alternative to platelet transfusions. Anti-fibrinolytic agents, such as aprotinin and tranexamic acid, or the vasopressin analog desmopressin (DDAVP), should be used in all other circumstances, because they are relatively cheap, do not cause platelet refractoriness, and do not bear the risk of transmitting blood-borne viral diseases [53].

REFERENCES

1. Kaufman RM, Airo R, Pollack S, Crosby WH. Circulating megakaryocytes and platelet release in the lung. *Blood* 1965; **26**: 720–8.
2. Nilsson Ehle H, Jagenburg R, Landahl S, Svanborg A, Westin J. Haematological abnormalities and reference intervals in the elderly: A cross-sectional comparative study of three Swedish population samples aged 70, 75 and 81 years. *Acta Med Scand* 1988; **224**: 595–604.
3. Carraro MC, Rossetti L, Gerli GC. Prevalence of retinopathy in patients with anemia or thrombocytopenia. *Eur J Haematol* 2001; **67**: 238–44.
4. Chong BH, Chesterman C. Thrombocytopenias due to bone marrow disorders. In Gresele P, Page C, Fuster V, Vermylen J, eds, *Platelets in Thrombotic and Non-Thrombotic Disorders* (Cambridge: Cambridge University Press, 2002), 528–41.
5. Aul C. Establishing the incidence of MDS. International Conference, Up-dating in Myelodysplastic Syndrome, Pavia, Italy, September 26–27, 2002.
6. Greenberg P, Cox C, LeBeau MM, *et al.* International scoring system for evaluating prognosis in myelodysplastic syndromes. *Blood* 1997; **89**: 2079–88.
7. George JN, Woolf SH, Raskob GE *et al.* Idiopathic thrombocytopenic purpura: a practice guideline developed by explicit methods for the American Society of Hematology. *Blood* 1996; **88**: 3–40
8. Frederiksen H, Schmidt K. The incidence of idiopathic thrombocytopenic purpura in adults increases with age. *Blood* 1999; **94**: 909–13.
9. Jonsson H, Nived O, Sturfelt G, Silman A. Estimating the incidence of systemic lupus erythematosus in a defined population using multiple sources of retrieval. *Br J Rheumatol* 1990; **29**: 185–8.
10. Webert KE, Kelton JG. Immune-mediated thrombocytopenia. In Gresele P, Page C, Fuster V, Vermylen J, eds,

Platelets in Thrombotic and Non-Thrombotic Disorders (Cambridge: Cambridge University Press, 2002), 542–5.

11. Aster RH. Drug-induced thrombocytopenia. In Michelson AD, ed, *Platelets* (Amsterdam: Academic Press, 2002), 593–606.

12. Kaufman DW, Kelly JP, Johannes CB, *et al*. Acute thrombocytopenic purpura in relation to the use of drugs. *Blood* 1993; **82**: 2714–18.

13. Visentin GP, Bacsi S, Aster RH. Molecular immunopathogenesis of heparin-induced thrombocytopenia. In Warkentin TE, Greinacher A, eds, *Heparin-Induced Thrombocytopenia* (New York, NY: Marcel Dekker, 2001), 149–65.

14. Warkentin TE: Clinical picture of heparin-induced thrombocytopenia. In Warkentin TE, Greinacher A, eds, *Heparin-Induced Thrombocytopenia* (New York, NY: Marcel Dekker, 2001), 43–86.

15. Chong BH. Heparin-induced thrombocytopenia. *Blood Rev* 1988; **2**: 108–14.

16. Murphy S. Platelet storage and transfusion. In Gresele P, Page C, Fuster V, Vermylen J, eds, *Platelets in Thrombotic and Non-Thrombotic Disorders* (Cambridge: Cambridge University Press, 2002), 707–23.

17. Furlan M, Robles R, Galbusera M, *et al*. Von Willebrand factor-cleaving protease in thrombotic thrombocytopenic purpura and the hemolytic-uremic syndrome. *N Engl J Med* 1998; **339**: 1578–84.

18. Tsai HM, Lian ECY. Antibodies to von Willebrand factor-cleaving protease in acute thrombotic thrombocytopenic purpura. *N Engl J Med* 1998; **339**: 1585–94.

19. George JN. The role of ADAMTS13 in the pathogenesis of thrombotic thrombocytopenic purpura-hemolytic uremic syndrome. *Clin Adv Hematol Oncol* 2005; **3**: 627–32.

20. George JN. How I treat patients with thrombotic thrombocytopenic purpura-hemolytic uremic syndrome. *Blood* 2000; **96**: 1223–9.

21. Levi M, ten Cate H. Dissiminated intravascular coagulation. *N Engl J Med* 1999; **341**: 587–92.

22. Hoffbrand AV, Pettit JE, Moss PAH. Disseminated intravascular coagulation. In *Essential Haematology*, 4th edn (London: Blackwell, 2001), 268–70.

23. George JN. Thrombocytopenia: pseudothrombocytopenia, hypersplenism, and thrombocytopenia associated with massive transfusion. In Beutler E, Lichtman MA, Coller BS, Kipps TJ, eds, *Williams Hematology* (New York, NY: McGraw-Hill, 1995), 1355–60.

24. Bizzarro N. Pseudothrombocytopenia. In Michelson AD, ed, *Platelets*, 2nd edn (Burlington, MA: Academic Press, 2006), 999–1008.

25. Bernasconi C. Evidence-based approach to treatment of myelodysplastic syndromes. *Haematologica* 2001; **86**: 897–9.

26. Rebulla P, Finazzi G, Marangoni F, *et al*. A multicenter randomized study of the threshold for prophylactic platelet transfusions in adults with acute myeloid leukemia. *N Engl J Med* 1997; **337**: 1870–5.

27. Difino SM, Lachant NA, Kirshner JJ, Gottlieb AJ. Adult idiopathic thrombocytopenic purpura. Clinical findings and response to therapy. *Am J Med* 1980; **69**: 430–42.

28. Woodruff RK, Grigg AP, Firkin FC, Smith IL. Fatal thrombotic events during treatment of autoimmune thrombocytopenia with intravenous immunoglobulin in elderly patients. *Lancet* 1986; **2**: 217–18.

29. Greinacher A, Warkentin TE. Treatment of heparin-induced thrombocytopenia: an overview. In Warkentin TE, Greinacher A, eds, *Heparin-Induced Thrombocytopenia* (New York, NY: Marcel Dekker, 2001), 291–322.

30. Rock G, Shurnak KH, Sutton DM, Buskard NA, Nair RC. Cryosupernatant as replacement fluid for plasma exchange in thrombotic thrombocytopenic purpura. Members of the Canadian Apheresis Group. *Br J Haematol* 1996; **94**: 383–6.

31. Cattaneo M. Inherited platelet-based bleeding disorders. *J Thromb Haemost* 2003; **1**: 1628–36.

32. Ruggeri ZM. Structure of von Willebrand factor and its function in platelet adhesion and thrombus formation. *Best Pract Res Clin Haematol* 2001; **14**: 257–79.

33. Bolin RB, Okumra T, Jaieson GA. New polymorphism of platelet membrane glycoproteins. *Nature* 1977; **269**: 69–70.

34. Nurden AT, Nurden P. Inherited disorders of platelet function. In Michelson AD, ed, *Platelets*, 2nd edn (Burlington, MA: Academic Press, 2006), 1029–50.

35. Nieuwenhuis HK, Sakariassen KS, Houdijk WP, Nievelstein PF, Sixma JJ. Deficiency of platelet membrane glycoprotein Ia associated with a decreased platelet adhesion to subendothelium: a defect in platelet spreading. *Blood* 1986; **68**: 692–5.

36. Kehrel B, Balleisen L, Kokott R, *et al*. Deficiency of intact thrombospondin and membrane glycoprotein Ia in platelets with defective collagen-induced aggregation and spontaneous loss of disorder. *Blood* 1988; **71**: 1074–8.

37. Moroi M, Jung SM, Okuma M, Shinmyozu K. A patient with platelets deficient in glycoprotein VI that lack both collagen-induced aggregation and adhesion. *J Clin Invest* 1989; **84**: 1440–5.

38. Hirata T, Kakizuka A, Ushikubi F, Fuse I, Okuma M, Narumiya S. Arg60 to Leu mutation of the human thromboxane A2 receptor in a dominantly inherited bleeding disorder. *J Clin Invest* 1994; **94**: 1662–7.

39. Cattaneo M, Gachet C. ADP receptors and clinical bleeding disorders. *Arterioscler Thromb Vasc Biol* 1999; **19**: 2281–5

40. Cattaneo M, Lecchi A, Randi AM, McGregor JL, Mannucci PM. Identification of a new congenital defect of platelet function characterized by severe impairment of platelet responses to adenosine diphosphate. *Blood* 1992; **80**: 2787–96.

41. Cattaneo M, Lecchi A, Lombardi R, Gachet C, Zighetti ML. Platelets from a patient heterozygous for the defect of P2CYC receptors for ADP have a secretion defect despite normal thromboxane A2 production and normal granule stores: further evidence that some cases of platelet "primary secretion defect" are heterozygous for a defect of P2CYC receptors. *Arterioscler Thromb Vasc Biol* 2000; **20**: E101–E106.

42. Nurden P, Savi P, Heilmann E, *et al.* An inherited bleeding disorder linked to a defective interaction between ADP and its receptor on platelets. Its influence on glycoprotein IIb-IIIa complex function. *J Clin Invest* 1995; **95**: 1612–22.

43. Cattaneo M, Zighetti ML, Lombardi R, *et al.* Molecular bases of defective signal transduction in the platelet P2Y12 receptor of a patient with congenital bleeding. *Proc Natl Acad Sci USA* 2003; **100**: 1978–83.

44. Nieuwenhuis HK, Akkerman JW, Sixma JJ. Patients with a prolonged bleeding time and normal aggregation tests may have storage pool deficiency: studies on one hundred six patients. *Blood* 1987; **70**: 620–3.

45. Rao AK. Congenital disorders of platelet secretion and signal transduction. In Colman RW, Hirsh J, Marder VJ, Clowes AW, George JN, eds, *Hemostasis and Thrombosis: Basic Principles and Clinical Practice* (Philadelphia, PA: Lippincott Williams & Wilkins, 2001), 893–904.

46. Cattaneo M. Congenital disorders of platelet secretion. In Gresele P, Page C, Fuster V, Vermylen J, eds, *Platelets in Thrombotic and Non-Thrombotic Disorders* (Cambridge: Cambridge University Press, 2002), 655–73.

47. Lages B, Weiss HJ. Biphasic aggregation responses to ADP and epinephrine in some storage pool deficient platelets: relationship to the role of endogenous ADP in platelet aggregation and secretion. *Thromb Haemost* 1980; **43**: 147–53.

48. Raccuglia G. Gray platelet syndrome: a variety of qualitative platelet disorder. *Am J Med* 1971; **51**: 818–28.

49. Freson K, Hoylaerts MF, Jaeken J, *et al.* Genetic variation of the extra-large stimulatory G protein alpha-subunit leads to Gs hyperfunction in platelets and is a risk factor for bleeding. *Thromb Haemost* 2001; **86**: 733–8.

50. Weiss HJ. Scott syndrome: a disorder of platelet coagulant activity. *Semin Hematol* 1994; **31**: 312–19.

51. Solum NO. Procoagulant expression in platelets and defects leading to clinical disorders. *Arterioscler Thromb Vasc Biol* 1999; **19**: 2841–6.

52. Weiss HJ. Congenital disorders of platelet function. *Semin Hematol* 1980; **17**: 228–41.

53. Cattaneo M. Qualitative platelet disorders. In O'Shaughnessy D, Makris M, Lillicrap D, eds, *Practical Hemostasis and Thrombosis* (Oxford: Blackwell, 2005), 83–90.

29

Gene–environment interactions and vascular risk in the elderly

Daniela Mari

Introduction

Prospective studies have demonstrated a positive association between plasma levels of proteins involved in hemostatic mechanisms and the development of atherothrombotic disease in individuals of either sex [1]. The genetic factors that modulate the individual susceptibility to multifactorial diseases such as cardiovascular diseases are common polymorphisms which generally have a modest effect at an individual level, but, because of their high frequency in the population, can be associated with a high attributable risk. Potential synergistic gene–environment interaction can reveal or facilitate the phenotypic expression of such susceptibility genes. Common biallelic polymorphisms of many genes encoding for coagulation and fibrinolysis proteins influence the plasma levels of these proteins [2,3]. Cardiovascular diseases (e.g., myocardial infarction, angina, and stroke) reach epidemic proportions in the elderly and are the primary limits to survival in humans. In the last decades particular attention has been paid to cardiovascular risk factors in the elderly, and genetic epidemiological studies of the diseases of aging are increasing rapidly [4]. Many aspects of aging involve inflammation [5]. Age-related disease such as atherosclerosis are triggered or worsened by systemic chronic inflammation. Some traditional risk factors lose importance as predictors of atherothrombotic diseases, and the role of novel cardiovascular risk factors such as clotting and fibrinolytic proteins emerges.

Polymorphisms in the hemostatic system in the elderly

Fibrinogen

Elevated plasma levels of fibrinogen are consistently associated with arterial thrombotic disorders. Prospective studies of both healthy subjects and patients with atherothrombotic diseases have shown an association between fibrinogen levels and myocardial infarction, stroke and peripheral vascular disease. The Northwick Park Heart Study was the first to report the association between high fibrinogen levels and ischemic heart disease (IHD). Subsequently many studies and meta-analyses have confirmed the initial report [6–11]. Fibrinogen levels are affected by age, physical inactivity, smoking, infection, body weight, alcohol consumption, hypertension, insulin resistance pattern, and seasonal changes in elderly people [12]. Fibrinogen, moreover, is an acute-phase reactant. During acute-phase inflammation the genes that encode fibrinogen are upregulated by interleukin 6 [13].

The GA-455 biallelic polymorphism involving the promoter region of the beta-fibrinogen gene has been evaluated in many clinical studies. The allele containing the polymorphic cutting site for the restriction enzyme HaeIII is identified as G-455, and the allele without the cutting site is identified as A-455. Carriers of the less frequent allele A-455 (approx. 0.20 in the general population) have higher fibrinogen levels (approx. 20–30%) than carriers of the G-455 allele [14]. In a population-based study of 482 healthy middle-aged men, of whom 231 were smokers, the β-fibrinogen GA-455 polymorphism genotype was determined, along with plasma fibrinogen levels. Smokers had the highest plasma fibrinogen levels (2.92 g/L), ex-smokers the next (2.73 g/L), and those who had never smoked had the lowest levels (2.66 g/L, $p < 0.001$). Those with one or two A-455 alleles had significantly higher plasma fibrinogen levels in never-smokers and ex-smokers (8.2% and 9.0%, respectively, $p < 0.05$), and the effect was larger in younger men (45–55 years, 11.6%, $p = 0.002$) than in older men (>65 years, 4.5%, NS), but was not significant in smokers (2.4%, $p > 0.05$). Allele frequencies were calculated and compared across age groups and between smokers and non-smokers. The difference in frequency of the GA-455 allele between smokers and non-smokers varied significantly with age ($p < 0.01$), with the frequency of the A-455 allele being significantly lower in smokers than in non-smokers in subjects aged over 65 years ($p < 0.05$), but not in younger men. [15].

Recently, in a population-based longitudinal study, the Cardiovascular Health Study (CHS), 5888 American adults aged 65 and over have been followed for up to 10 years to assess the roles of traditional and novel cardiovascular risk factors in the development of coronary heart disease [16,17]. Primary endpoints of this study included "years of life" as well as "years of healthy life," defined as the number of persons in good health in the 10 years after the enrollment. Plasma fibrinogen was a predictor of total mortality, confirming the results of other cohort studies of older adults [18,19]. No association with longevity was observed, however, for the GA-455 beta-fibrinogen promoter polymorphism [20]. The explanation of this negative result may lie in the small, insignificant part of the overall variance in fibrinogen levels explained by the GA-455 polymorphism in the promoter region of the fibrinogen gene. This fact was observed also in a twin study consisting of 129 monozygotic twin pairs and 153 dizygotic same-sex twins aged 73 to 94 years who participated in the Longitudinal Study of Aging of Danish Twins [21]. As expected, the effects of genetic factors are smaller in the elderly twins

because of the presence of many inflammatory triggers, such as cardiovascular disease and other age-associated diseases.

It is not completely explained how much of the difference in heritability can be attributed to age as opposed to other population characteristics. The association between the GA-455 polymorphism of the fibrinogen Bβ gene and plasma fibrinogen levels and myocardial infarction, and potential synergistic gene–environment interaction involving this polymorphism, have been explored in a case–control study (Stockholm Heart Epidemiology Program, SHEEP) [22]. A total of 2246 cases (1485 men and 761 women) were enrolled. Of these, 1643 (1105 men and 538 women) survived at least 28 days after myocardial infarction and 1169 survivors (826 men aged 58.2 ± 7.1 years and 343 women aged 61.6 ± 6.8 years) were genotyped for the GA-455 polymorphism. The results were compared with those of 1517 individuals without known heart disease (1028 men aged 58.8 ± 7.1 years and 489 women aged 61.9 ± 6.7 years). Smoking, job stress, overweight, diabetes mellitus, physical inactivity, hypertension, hypercholesterolemia, high low-density lipoprotein cholesterol/high-density lipoprotein cholesterol (LDL/HDL) rate, and hypertriglyceridemia were included as environment–gene interaction factors. Presence of the A allele at the GA-455 polymorphic site was associated with higher plasma fibrinogen levels than the presence of the G allele, but the difference was statistically significant for men only. No association was found between the A-455 allele and increased risk of myocardial infarction. In addition no gene–environment interactions were detected for any of the environmental exposures studied.

Factor VII (FVII)

The coagulation cascade is triggered when circulating FVII reacts with tissue factor which is usually not expressed in the intact vasculature. Factor VII plasma levels progressively increase with age, from a mean of 95 units/dL in subjects aged 20 years to over 110 units/dL in subjects over 50 years [23]. Environmental factors other than age also influence plasma levels of FVII, including body mass index and plasma tryglicerides. The correlation between plasma triglyceride levels and FVII coagulant activity might suggest a combined role of FVII and hypertriglyceridemia in arterial thrombotic disease. Thrombotic disorders have been shown to be more frequent in subjects with higher plasma levels of FVII [24], but the data have not been confirmed in other studies [25]. Discrepant results might have been due to differences in FVII coagulant assay methodologies in the different studies. In the CHS [18], FVII concentrations were associated with risk of angina (RR = 1.44) in men and with death in women (RR, middle quintile compared with first = 0.66). However, in general, FVII was not consistently associated with cardiovascular events in this population [26].

A common polymorphism in the FVII gene that is detected by the presence or absence of the cleavage site for Msp1 is strongly associated with FVII coagulant activity (factor VIIc) [27]. The variable site is located in exon 8 of the gene and is detected using in-vitro gene amplification. The base change that creates the Msp1 polymorphism is a G-to-A substitution, leading to the replacement of arginine (Arg) with glutamine (Gln) in the protein product of the M2 allele. There are conflicting data in the literature regarding the results of clinical studies carried out in young-adult populations on the association between the FVII polymorphism and arterial thrombosis. Reports of a protective effect of the Q allele against myocardial infarction in several Italian studies [28–30] are counterbalanced by numerous reports showing no such findings in other populations [31–34], including the Framingham Heart Study [35]. Recently, the results of a case–control genetic study based on the Jerusalem Longitudinal Study, carried out in the elderly, were published [36]. R353Q FVII polymorphism was examined in approximately 400 subjects. The mean age of the population at the time of DNA sampling was 75 years. There were 150 males and 74 females in the older Ashkenazi group. The younger control group (21.89 years, range 13–33 years) included 121 Ashkenazi males and 320 females. The only significant difference between the young and old population involved a reduced percentage (30.6% versus 19.2%) of the A allele in older Ashkenazi men (chi-square = 4.027, $p = 0.045$, 1 df) and a corresponding marked decrease (9.7–2.1%) in the percentage of AA homozygous (chi-square = 5.790, $p = 0.055$, 2 df). Thus, these data confirm that if there is any effect of FVII genotypes on atherothrombotic disease, it is very small and detectable only in highly selected populations.

Jeffery et al. [37] have suggested a protective contribution of the Q allele of the R353Q polymorphism of FVII, in individuals with chronic stable angina. Patients attending the hospital for routine day-case angiography over a 20-month period were followed up prospectively. Factor VIIa, VIIc and VIIAg levels, genotype for R353Q, lipid status, smoking history, and the degree of vessel disease were determined. Of 519 cases, 400 had no previous myocardial infarction or coronary artery bypass surgery; in 153 of these no coronary artery disease had been demonstrable. The genotype was QQ in 9 (2%) cases; RQ in 78 (20%), and RR in 313 (78%). Compared with RR subjects, heterozygous subjects were 2.7 years older (95% CI 0.3–5.0, $p = 0.027$), but no significant differences were observed regarding gender, cholesterol, extent of vessel disease, or smoking history. When individuals with coronary artery disease were included, the RQ heterozygous were 3.5 years older than the RR homozygous (95% CI 0.6–6.4, $p = 0.016$). The Q allele was associated with lower levels of FVII. There was no significant association between the degree of vessel disease and genotype, but a moderate protective effect of the Q allele in relation to the severity of angina was demonstrated. The protective effect might have been mediated by reduced levels of FVII. Only five individuals presented the QQ genotype and for this reason the influence of homozygosity on severity and age of appearance of angina could not be investigated. The effect size for age at presentation was similar for each gender separately: women 3.9 years ($p = 0.27$), men 3.4 years ($p = 0.03$). For smokers the difference in age at presentation disappeared, being only 1.2 years higher for RQ than for RR smokers (95% CI 1.3–3.7, $p = 0.3$).

The relation of food intake and R353Q transition was explored in 1158 individuals representing the extreme quintiles of the FVII clotting activity (FVII:C) distribution, among subjects enrolled in the Rotterdam study, a population-based cohort study of 7893 persons. The quintiles were combined for linear regression analyses. FVII:C was inversely associated with fiber and protein intake, and positively with saturated fat. The inverse association of FVII with fiber was stronger in subjects with the RR genotype ($\beta = -0.76\%$ pooled plasma [PP/g], 95% CI -1.23 to -0.29), than in those with RQ/QQ genotypes ($\beta = -0.19\%$ PP/g, 95% CI -0.97 to 0.59). The association of FVII:C with saturated fat was positive in those with the RR allele and inverse in subjects with the Q allele [38]. In spite of the limits of the study, it is well known that the RR genotype of the R353Q polymorphism of factor VII is a risk indicator for myocardial infarction through increased FVII levels. Environmental dietary factors, such as high intake of saturated fat and low intake of fiber and protein, may modulate the thrombotic risk of the RR genotype.

Factor XIII (FXIII)

Factor XIII catalyzes cross-linking of fibrin in the last step of coagulation. A common G>T polymorphism leading to a valine (Val) to leucine (Leu) substitution 3 amino acids from the thrombin activation site, described in exon 2 of the FXIII A-subunit gene (FXIII Val34Leu), has been associated with decreased risk of coronary artery and cerebrovascular disease [39]. Because of the complexity of gene–gene and gene–environment interactions between polymorphisms in the fibrinogen-chain gene and FXIII Val34Leu polymorphism, fibrinogen plasma levels are modulated, influencing the permeability of a clot. As intermediaries for environmental effects, fibrinogen concentrations are an important candidate for interacting with fibrinogen and FXIII coding polymorphisms to alter vascular risk [40]. Clinical studies confirm this gene–gene and gene–environment interaction. Elbaz et al. [41] studied the relation between brain infarction (BI) and the

FXIII Val34Leu polymorphism in 456 patients with a median age of 69 years, consecutively recruited after confirmation of BI by imaging, and 456 matched controls. The distribution of genotypes was different in cases (63.2% Val/Val; 30.9% Val/Leu; 5.9% Leu/Leu) compared with controls (49.8% Val/Val; 42.8% Val/Leu; 7.4% Leu/Leu; $p < 0.001$). Carrying the Leu allele was associated with an odds radio (OR) of 0.58 (95% CI 0.44–0.75). In addition, the effect of smoking was modified by the polymorphism ($p = 0.05$), and was weaker among Leu carriers than among non-carriers, suggesting that among Leu carriers the protective effect of the polymorphism outweighed the effect of smoking.

Factor V (FV)

A common missense mutation in coagulation FV (Arg506 Gln), FV Leiden [42], creates phenotypic resistance to the anticoagulant effects of activated protein C and predisposes carriers to venous thrombosis [43].

The Women's Health Initiative Estrogen Plus Progestin trial was a double-blind controlled trial of 16 608 postmenopausal women randomized to receive hormone replacement therapy or placebo. The age at enrollment varied between 50 and 79 years and the median follow-up was 5.6 years [44]. Together with other gene variants related to thrombosis risk (prothrombin 20120A, methylenetetrahydrofolate reductase C677F, FXIII Val34Leu, PAI-1 4G/5G), FV Leiden was measured in the first 147 women who developed thrombosis and in 513 controls. Estrogen plus progestin was associated with a doubled risk of venous thrombosis. Only FV Leiden enhanced the hormone-associated risk of venous thrombosis in postmenopausal women, with a 6.69-fold increased risk compared with women in the placebo group without the mutation.

In young individuals who have experienced at least one episode of arterial thromboembolism the role of FV mutation has been extensively studied, without conclusive results [45]. The prevalence of the FV mutation was determined in a group of elderly patients (64 ± 9 years old) with stroke and compared with its prevalence in several control patient groups (older controls 66 ± 8 years old, young controls 46 ± 14 years old) [46]. The prevalence was the same in older individuals with or without stroke and was lower in elderly individuals than in the younger ones. In conclusion, FV Leiden does not appear to influence the risk of arterial thrombosis in the elderly.

Factor VIII/von Willebrand factor (FVIII/VWF)

It is well known that increased plasma levels of FVIII are associated with an increased risk of venous thrombosis [47]. The plasma FVIII levels are modulated by VWF antigen (VWF:Ag), the carrier molecule of FVIII in plasma [48,49], and ABO blood group [50]. In the CHS, FVIII concentrations showed a positive association with risk of coronary heart disease among men and risk of cerebrovascular disease, i.e., transient ischemic attacks and stroke, among women [51].

VWF has been identified as a risk factor for recurrent myocardial infarction in the general population and is associated with cerebrovascular disease [52–54]. In the Rotterdam study [55] a strong correlation was demonstrated in elderly individuals (mean age 78) between VWF and atrial fibrillation, myocardial infarction, diabetes, and smoking in a large community-based study. Seemingly, VWF concentrations were a marker of endothelial damage [55].

Recently, the results of a 20-year follow-up examination of all surviving men (aged 60–79 years) enrolled in the British Regional Heart Study were published [56]. In this prospective study of cardiovascular diseases, non-diabetic older men with no history of cardiovascular heart disease or stroke showed a significant association between insulin resistance and inflammatory markers (C-reactive protein and white cell count), coagulation factors VII–IX, markers of endothelial dysfunction (VWF and tissue-plasminogen activator), and blood viscosity. These relationships were independent of age, smoking, physical activity, alcohol intake, social class, use of statin and aspirin, and persisted after further adjustment for abdominal obesity. In particular, fasting insulin was

the factor associated most strongly with VWF and FVIII. Only fasting insulin was independently associated with VWF, whereas FVIII, which was highly correlated with VWF ($r = 0.69$), showed independent relationships with blood glucose and fasting insulin.

Plasminogen activator inhibitor 1 (PAI-1)

PAI-1 is a major determinant of fibrinolytic activity. There is substantial experimental and epidemiologic evidence that PAI-1 might contribute to the development of ischemic cardiovascular disease [57]. Elevated PAI-1 plays a role in the metabolic syndrome [58], and strong associations have been described between PAI-1 plasma levels and excess weight, abdominal obesity, diabetes mellitus, and insulin concentration. A common deletion/insertion polymorphism (4G/5G) has been identified in the 5′ promoter region. The guanine insertion/deletion polymorphism is located at position –675, where one allele has a sequence of four guanines (4G) and the other has a fifth guanine inserted (5G) [59]. The 4G allele has been correlated with high levels of gene transcription and elevated PAI-1 plasma levels in comparison with the 5G allele. This PAI-1 polymorphism modulates phenotypes associated with the metabolic syndrome [60].

The Leiden 85-plus study is a population-based study including 1258 subjects aged 85 years or older [61]. Six hundred sixty-six individuals (188 men and 478 women), successfully genotyped for angiotensin-I-converting enzyme and PAI-1 gene variants, were followed up over 10 years. The primary result of this prospective study was that men $\geqslant 85$ years old carrying the PAI-1 4G/5G genotype were at a threefold increased risk of death due to ischemic heart disease within the 10-year follow-up (95% CI 1.2–7.6). Plasma levels of PAI-1 increase with age in a population characterized by a relatively high prevalence of obesity, hypertension, and diabetes mellitus [62]. Stratifying by genotype, significant associations were found between age and PAI-1 antigen in 4G/4G and in 4G/5G groups, helping to identify a subgroup of people with an increasing risk of cardiovascular disease with age.

Recently, Reiner and coworkers examined the association between promoter polymorphisms of several thrombosis and inflammation genes with longevity in the CHS. Genotyping assays were performed at baseline on a subset of 2224 CHS individuals (1874 whites and 350 blacks). The mean age at the study entry was 73 years (84% whites, 54% women). After 10 years of follow-up, PAI-1 4G/4G genotype was associated with increased cardiovascular mortality in women and lower noncardiovascular mortality in men [19].

The Quebec Family Study genotyped 666 subjects for five PAI-1 gene polymorphisms and is the first to show an association with direct measures of fat mass and abdominal fat, thus suggesting that PAI-1 may influence fat mass accretion, particularly in women. Stratified analyses were performed with analysis of covariance in men ($n = 280$) and women ($n = 386$) separately. PAI-1-675 4G/5G polymorphism was strongly associated with body mass index ($p = 0.01$) and fat mass ($p = 0.05$) in women. The PAI-1-675 4G/5G promoter polymorphism and the c.43G. A (p.A15T, rs6092) variant within the exon 1 were associated with abdominal visceral fat but only in postmenopausal women ($p = 0.05$). No association was observed in men [63]. Hormone replacement therapy, in a group of postmenopausal women with coronary artery disease, decreased circulating PAI-1 levels in those with the 4G/5G phenotype [64]. From this study it is not clear whether estrogen is beneficial for these individuals. A study on Italian centenarians suggests that the 4G allele carriers reached longevity despite high circulating PAI-1 levels [65].

Another important gene–environment interaction was identified by Brown *et al.* [66], who demonstrated a significant interactive effect of salt intake and PAI-1 4G/5G genotype on PAI-1 antigen. The activation of the renin–angiotensin–aldosterone system increased the effects of PAI-1 genotype on the risk of thrombotic cardiovascular events, associated with PAI-1 antigen. As renin production decreases with age, it is not surprising that the association between PAI-1 4G/5G genotype and myocardial infarction was stronger in the young [67] than in the older population [68,69].

Thrombin activatable fibrinolysis inhibitor (TAFI)

TAFI is a plasma carboxypeptidase that regulates fibrinolysis by removing the C-terminal lysine and arginine residues from fibrin, thereby decreasing plasminogen on its surface [70].

A single nucleotide polymorphism in the coding region of the TAFI gene, 1040C/T, results in the Thr325Ile substitution [71]. This polymorphism is of particular interest because TAFI-Ile325 has a 60% greater antifibrinolytic activity than TAFI-Thr325. Many other polymorphisms are described in the TAFI gene, nine in promoter region, two in the 3′ untranslated region, and three in the coding region. These polymorphisms are in strong linkage disequilibrium and form four main haplotypes. Circulating levels of TAFI are strongly determined by polymorphic variations in the promoter and the 3′ region of the TAFI gene [72,73].

Because of its role in the fibrinolytic system, the TAFI gene may be involved in the pathogenesis of atherothrombotic diseases. However, epidemiologic data evaluating the relations between plasma TAFI levels and the risk of cardiovascular disease have given conflicting results. In some studies, high TAFI levels were found to be protective against myocardial infarction [74] and to be negatively correlated with development of refractory angina pectoris [75]. In other studies, high TAFI levels were associated with increased risk of acute coronary artery disease [76] or angina pectoris [77–79]. The difference between studies may be due to the methods used for TAFI determination, because some enzyme-linked immunosorbent assays (ELISA) had decreased antibody reactivity towards the TAFI-Ile325 isoform and consequently produced abnormally low result of TAFI.

From 1991 until 1994 the Prospective Epidemiological Study of Myocardial Infarction (PRIME) recruited 9758 men aged 50–59 years with no previous cardiovascular events, living in France and Northern Ireland, and they were followed up for 5 years. A total of 248 cases of cardiovascular disease and 493 matched controls were used for the genetic study. TAFI levels, when measured with a truly reliable method, were strongly influenced by polymorphisms of the TAFI gene but not associated with risk of cardiovascular heart disease [80].

The results of CHS [19] highlighted the role of TAFI-438A/A genotype in predicting mortality from all causes. Older white men (mean age at enrollment was 73) with this genotype had a reduced 10-year mortality rate. Survival was increased by 0.9 years, and they had 1.1 additional years of active life expectancy. No significant effect of TAFI-438G/A on survival was observed in women. It should be noted that the prevalence of the TAFI-438G/A promoter genotype in this population was significantly different from that reported in another study of a healthy middle-aged population of European descent [74]. The influence of TAFI genotype on survival could be age- and sex-specific.

The mortality reduction associated with the TAFI-438A/A genotype involved all causes of mortality, not just that from thromboembolic or cardiovascular disease. Activated TAFI may cleave different substrates and regulate the course of inflammation [81]. This enzyme significantly contributes to the inactivation of C5a, the most potent of complement-derived anaphylatoxins [82]. This TAFI-438A/A genotype may have provided our ancestors with enhanced anti-inflammatory and anti-thrombotic mechanisms, to improve wound healing and facilitate reproduction.

Hyperhomocysteinemia

Homocysteine is a sulfur-containing amino acid, which results from the hydrolysis of S-adenosyl-homocysteine in the methionine metabolic cycle. Several conditions may determine an increase of blood homocysteine, such as an inadequate folate intake with diet, smoking, drugs (i.e., methotrexate, hormones, antiepileptic), renal failure, and inherited gene polymorphism of methylene-tetra-hydro-folate reductase (MTHFR). This common functional polymorphism, C677T, is associated with decreased enzymatic activity and increased homocysteine concentration.

Increased levels of circulating homocysteine may trigger endothelial dysfunction through oxidative damage and induce increased oxidation of low-density lipoprotein, stimulation of smooth muscle cell proliferation, and hypercoagulable state. Hyperhomocysteinemia represents a modifiable cardiovascular risk factor, since vitamin supplementation has been shown to effectively lower plasma homocysteine levels.

The association between moderately high plasma levels of total homocysteine (tHcy) with the risk of cardiovascular disease, coronary artery disease, cerebrovascular disease, peripheral artery disease, and venous thromboembolism has been reported in several case–control, cross-sectional, and prospective studies reviewed by Cattaneo [83]. In the Homocysteine Studies Collaboration meta-analysis [84] a weak association was observed between tHcy and coronary heart disease, and in the prospective studies considered a plasma tHcy reduction of 25% was associated with an 11% lower risk of ischemic heart disease (OR 0.89, 95% CI 0.83–0.96).

A recent meta-analysis presents new evidence that an increased tHcy may be a causal risk factor for stroke [85]. If homocysteine increases the risk of stroke, MTHFR polymorphism should increase the risk of stroke by increasing circulating levels of homocysteine. Among 15 635 people without cardiovascular disease, the weighted mean difference in homocysteine concentration between TT and CC homozygotes was 1.93 μmol/L (95% CI 1.38–2.47). The expected odds ratio for stroke corresponding to this difference, based on previous observational studies, was 1.20 (1.10–1.31). In this genetic meta-analysis ($n = 13\,928$) the odds ratio for stroke was 1.26 (1.14–1.40) for TT versus CC homozygotes, similar to the expected odds ratio ($p = 0.29$).

Many ongoing clinical trials have the aim to demonstrate that decreasing tHcy with folic acid (with or without B vitamins) is associated with a reduction in cardiovascular risk [86]. The influence of age on tHcy plasma levels in patients with different genotypes has been investigated in three North American studies: a study of mothers of children with spina bifida (three age groups, <34 years, 34–40 years,

>40 years), the National Heart, Lung, and Blood Family Heart Study (three age groups, <45 years, 45–59 years, >60 years) and a Mayo Clinic study of patients undergoing coronary angiography (three age groups, <56 years, 56–67 years, >67 years) [87]. Plasma homocysteine levels increased with age in the C/C and C/T genotype groups ($p < 0.0001$ and $p < 0.001$, respectively), but not in the T/T genotype. Genotype was significantly associated with plasma homocysteine levels in the whole population and in the youngest group ($p = 0.002$ and $p = 0.005$, respectively), but not in the two older age groups. The subjects of these studies were highly selected. The family heart study and the Mayo Clinic study involved individuals at high risk for cardiovascular disease, while only mothers of children with spina bifida were involved in the spina bifida study. The prevalence of MTHFR genotypes in this selected population may not reflect the prevalence in the general population.

Higher plasma homocysteine levels have been associated with low vitamin status in the elderly [88], and thus the non-genetic causes of hyperhomocysteinemia may be more important in the aged population. The treatment of hyperhomocysteinemia in older individuals is safe and not expensive [89,90]. The Nutrition Committee of the American Heart Association has recommended 0.4 mg of folic acid, 2 mg of vitamin B_6, and 6 mg of vitamin B_{12} daily.

The centenarians

All studies on coagulation factors in elderly subjects have been performed in individuals under the age of 80. In general aging is associated with increased concentration of clotting factors, which may be a harbinger of increased coagulability, or alternatively may represent a harmless manifestation of the aging process. The study of centenarians, who present a natural model of successful aging, may help to identify the biological basis of longevity. In 1995 Mari et al. [91] for the first time showed the results of an extended study of coagulation and fibrinolysis in 25 Italian centenarians. The results were compared with those obtained in two control groups of healthy adults, 25 aged 18–50 years and 25 aged 51–69 years. Older controls had, in general, slightly higher values of several coagulation and fibrinolysis measurements than younger controls. Centenarians had striking signs of heightened coagulation enzyme activity, as assessed directly by measuring activated FVII in plasma ($p < 0.01$, compared with either control group) or indirectly by measuring the plasma levels of the activation peptides of prothrombin, FIX, FX, and thrombin–antithrombin complexes (all $p < 0.001$). Heightened coagulation enzyme activity was accompanied by signs of fibrin formation (high fibrinopeptide A, $p < 0.001$) and secondary hyperfibrinolysis (high D-dimer and plasmin–antiplasmin complex [PAP], $p < 0.001$). Plasma concentrations of fibrinogen and FVIII were higher than in controls, whereas other coagulation factors were not elevated.

In conclusion, this study showed that the very elderly did not escape the state of hypercoagulability associated with aging, but that this phenomenon is compatible with health and longevity. Hence, high plasma levels of the coagulation activation markers in older populations do not necessarily predict a high risk of arterial or venous thrombosis. Gene polymorphisms associated with the plasma levels of fibrinogen, FVII, and PAI-1, hemostasis proteins that help to predict the risk of atherothrombotic disease, were compared in 124 healthy individuals over 100 years old and 130 young, healthy individuals to identify genetic influences on extreme longevity [65]. The restriction fragment length polymorphism GA-455, located in the promoter of the β-fibrinogen gene, the guanine insertion/deletion polymorphism 4G/5G in the promoter of the PAI-1 gene, and the R353Q substitution polymorphism in exon 8 of the FVII gene have been investigated. Alleles and genotypes associated with elevated plasma levels of fibrinogen and FVII were found with similar frequencies in centenarians and in the comparison group. However, in centenarians there was a significantly higher frequency of the 4G allele and of the homozygous 4G/4G genotype associated with high

PAI-1 levels. Since high PAI-1 is considered a predictor of recurrent myocardial infarction in young men, it is intriguing that the corresponding genetic marker is more frequent in centenarians who have escaped major age-related atherothrombotic disease and reached the extreme limits of human life. Homozygosity for the 4G allele, despite its association with impaired fibrinolysis, is compatible with successful aging. Rizzo *et al.* [92] showed that healthy centenarians have significantly higher plasma PAI-1 levels than non-centenarians, but these levels were not associated with the same degree of insulin resistance found in non-centenarians. Bladbjerg *et al.* [93] showed that polymorphisms of hemostasis genes do not predict longevity because the allele distributions were similar in Danish centenarians and younger individuals. We described the same allele frequency of mutant F/V, an established risk factor for idiopathic and recurrent venous thrombosis, in Italian centenarians and in non-centenarians, without thrombotic events [94]. A slightly lower allele frequency in French centenarians was detected [95], unchanged allele frequency was found with low prevalence of venous thrombosis in Danish centenarians and one female homozygous for the FV mutation gene without history of thrombosis [96].

Regarding endothelial integrity, we have described significantly higher levels of VWF:Ag and VWF:Rco in centenarians than in controls without significant difference between blood group O and non-O. Fifty-one percent of centenarians have a reduction of the relative proportion of high-molecular-weight multimers (HMV); furthermore VWF-cleaving protease was lower than in young controls [97].

The finding that the VWF:CP levels are low when VWF levels are high in centenarians could be a corollary of the previously described paradox of successful aging [90], adding another marker of increased risk of atherothrombosis to the scenario. The laboratory evidence of heightened coagulation enzyme activity does not necessarily indicate an increased thrombotic risk. Among centenarians, striking biochemical signs of hypercoagulability have been documented, as assessed by measurements of plasma-activated FVII, F1+2, the activation peptides of FIX and FX, TAT, FpA, and DD. The accelerated generation of activated FX, resulting in increased conversion of prothrombin into thrombin and eventually in fibrin formation, may be due to enhanced FVII–tissue factor interaction at the site of endothelial damage, or may be a consequence of impaired availability of glycosaminoglycans that modulate antithrombin III activity in vivo on the vascular surface. In addition, centenarians display high immune-reactivity against human beta-2-glycoprotein I, but low binding to the bovine molecule in the anticardiolipin assay. In spite of the presence of antibodies comparable to those found in patients with the antiphospholipid syndrome, no vascular events were reported, suggesting the presence of unknown protective factors and/or the lack of triggering factors [98]. Centenarians possess also high-risk alleles for many polymorphisms related to the cardiovascular diseases, even in homozygous form [65, 92–95].

Thus, the state of hypercoagulability and the possession of several high-risk alleles and well-known atherothrombotic risk markers [97] appear to be compatible with longevity and/or health. In the oldest old, the risk factors may play a different role than in young-adult subjects: for example, high total cholesterol concentrations are associated with longevity owing to lower mortality from cancer and infection [99].

Conclusions

Atherosclerotic disease has reached epidemic proportions only within the last century. In fact, given that genetic polymorphisms have surely been present between populations for thousands of years, it is only the quite recent development of adverse genetic and environmental interactions that can explain the incidence and prevalence of this disorder. Gene–environment interactions are important because genes produce their effects in an indirect way (through proteins) and, therefore, the ultimate outcome of gene action may be different in different circumstances. In addition, perhaps thousands of gene variations escaped the force of natural selection and thus play roles in the genesis of different patterns of aging in humans. The study of environmental factors is important especially when behavioral or rehabilitative interventions may compensate for the functional decline of aging.

The recent studies of cardiovascular risk factors, assessed late in life, have highlighted some novel, promising candidates among markers of hemostatic activation and hemostatic proteins [19,26]. Specifically, the modulation of fibrinolysis may influence aging and age-related diseases. For example, PAI-1 links two pathophysiological situations, obesity and diabetes, both of which are conditions at risk for cardiovascular diseases. On the other hand, numerous studies indicate that the increase in cardiovascular risk cannot be ascribed solely to the role of PAI-1 in either obesity or insulin resistance, but many environmental factors could interfere with PAI-1 plasma levels and 4G/5G genotype, including salt intake, physical activity, and triglyceride levels [66,69,100]. Oral antidiabetic drugs, such as metformin, reduce plasma PAI-1 levels [101]. The use of a small-molecule PAI-1 antagonist to reduce plasma PAI-1 activity and tissue remodeling would appear to be a promising strategy [102].

Recently, for the first time, it has been demonstrated that a hemostasis-associated gene can contribute to human longevity, in the shape of a common promoter variant of the TAFI gene [19]. This fact suggests that the modulation of fibrinolysis may result in longevity, perhaps because reduced plasma levels of TAFI are associated with reduced inflammatory activity. To a large extent genetics influences the levels of clotting factors that predict increased risk of cardiovascular disease even in elderly individuals. The combination of genotype and environmental factors determines individual disease susceptibility. Future studies, including of the oldest old, will help to clarify the importance of traditional and newer risk factors and lead to better estimates of individual cardiovascular risk.

REFERENCES

1. Meade TW. Haemostatic function, arterial disease and the prevention of arterial thrombosis. *Baillieres Clin Haematol* 1994; **7**: 733–55.
2. Green F, Humphries S. Genetic determinants of arterial thrombosis. *Baillieres Clin Haematol* 1994; **7**: 675–92.
3. Voetsch B, Loscalzo J. Genetic determinants of arterial thrombosis. *Arterioscler Thromb Vasc Biol* 2004; **24**: 216–29.
4. Cauley JA, Dorman JS, Ganguli M. Genetic and aging epidemiology: the merging of two disciplines. *Neurol Clin* 1996; **14**: 467–75.
5. Franceschi C, Bonafe M, Valensin S, *et al*. Inflamm-aging: an evolutionary perspective on immunosenescence. *Ann NY Acad Sci* 2000; **908**: 244–54.
6. Meade TW, Mellows S, Brozovic M, *et al*. Haemostatic function and ischaemic heart disease: principal results of the Northwick Park Heart Study. *Lancet* 1986; **2**: 533–7.
7. MacCallum PK, Meade TW. Haemostatic function, arterial disease and the prevention of arterial thrombosis. *Baillieres Best Pract Res Clin Haematol* 1999; **12**: 577–9.
8. Wilhelmsen L, Svardsudd K, Korsan-Bengsten K, Larsson B, Welin L, Tibblin G. Fibrinogen as a risk factor for stroke and myocardial infarction. *N Engl J Med* 1984; **31**: 501–5.
9. Balleisen L, Bailey J, Epping PH, Schulte H, van De Loo J. Epidemiological study on factor VII, factor VIII and fibrinogen in industrial population: baseline data on the relation to age, gender, body-weight, smoking, alcohol, pill-using and menopause. *Thromb Haemost* 1985; **54**: 475–9.
10. Maresca G, Di Blasio A, Marchioli R, Di Minno G. Measuring plasma fibrinogen to predict stroke and myocardial infarction: an update. *Arterioscleros Thromb Vasc Biol* 1999; **19**: 1368–77.
11. Heinrich J, Balleisen L, Schulte H, Assmann G, van de Loo J. Fibrinogen and factor VII in the prediction of coronary risk: results from the PROCAM study in healthy men. *Arterioscler Thromb* 1994; **14**: 54–9.
12. Crawford VLS, McNerlan SE, Stout RS. Seasonal changes in platelets, fibrinogen, and factor VII in elderly people. *Age Ageing* 2003; **32**: 661–5.
13. Duan HO, Simpson-Haidaris PJ. Functional analysis of interleukin 6 response elements (IL-6REs) on the human gamma-fibrinogen promoter: binding of hepatic stat3

correlates negatively with transactivation potential of type II IL-6REs. *J Biol Chem* 2003; **17**: 41270–81.

14. Thomas A, Green F, Kelleher C, *et al.* Variation in the promotor region of the β fibrinogen gene is associated with plasma fibrinogen levels in smokers and non-smokers. *Thromb Haemost* 1991; **65**: 487–90.

15. Thomas AE, Green FR, Humphries SE. Association of genetic variation at the beta-fibrinogen gene locus and plasma fibrinogen levels: interaction between allele frequency of the G/A-455 polymorphism, age and smoking. *Clin Genet* 1996; **50**: 184–90.

16. Diehr P, Patrick DL, Bild DE, Burke GL, Williamson JD. Predicting future years of healthy life for older adults. *J Clin Epidemiol* 1998; **51**: 343–53.

17. Diehr P, Newman AB, Jackson SA, Kuller L, Powe N. Weight modification trials in older adults: what should the outcome measure be? *Curr Control Trials Cardiovasc Med* 2002; **3**: 1–8.

18. Tracy RP, Arnold AM, Ettinger W, Fried L, Meilahn E, Savage P. The relationship of fibrinogen and factors VII and VIII to incident cardiovascular disease and death in the elderly: results from the Cardiovascular Health Study. *Arterioscler Thromb Vasc Biol* 1999; **19**: 1776–83.

19. Reiner AP, Diehr P, Browner WS, *et al.* Common promoter polymorphisms of inflammation and thrombosis genes and longevity in older adults: the Cardiovascular Health Study. *Atherosclerosis* 2005; **181**: 175–83.

20. Yano K, Grove JS, Chen R, Rodriguez BL, Curb JD, Tracy RP. Plasma fibrinogen as a predictor of total and cause-specific mortality in elderly Japanese-American men. *Arterioscler Thromb Vasc Biol* 2001; **2**: 1065–70.

21. de Maat MP, Bladbjerg EM, Hjelmborg JB, Bathum L, Jespersen J, Christensen K. Genetic influence on inflammation variables in the elderly. *Arterioscler Thromb Vasc Biol* 2004; **24**: 2168–73.

22. Leander K, Wyman B, Hallqvist J, Falk G, De Faire U. The G-455A polymorphism of the fibrinogen beta-gene relates to plasma fibrinogen in male cases, but does not interact with environmental factors in causing myocardial infarction in either men or women. *J Intern Med* 2002; **252**: 332–41.

23. Balleisen L, Bailey J, Epping PH, Schulte H, van De Loo J. Epidemiological study on factor VII, factor VIII and fibrinogen in industrial population: baseline data on the relation to age, gender, body-weight, smoking, alcohol, pill-using and menopause. *Thromb Haemost* 1985; **54**: 475–9.

24. Meade TW, Chakrabarti R, Haines AP, North Y, Thompson SG, Brozovic M. Haemostatic function and cardiovascular death: early results of a prospective study. *Lancet* 1980; **1**: 1050–5.

25. Folsom AR, Wu KK, Rosamond WD, Sharrett AR, Chambless LE. Prospective study of hemostatic factors and incidence of coronary heart disease: the Atherosclerosis Risk in Communities (ARIC) study. *Circulation* 1997; **96**: 1102–8.

26. Tracy RP, Arnold AM, Ettinger W, Fried L, Meilahn E, Savage P. The relationship of fibrinogen and factors VII and VIII to incident cardiovascular disease and death in the elderly: results from the Cardiovascular Health Study. *Arterioscler Thromb Vasc Biol* 1999; **19**: 1776–8.

27. Humphries SE, Green FR, Temple A, *et al.* Genetic factors determining thrombosis and fibrinolysis. *Ann Epidemiol* 1992; **2**: 371–85.

28. Iacoviello L, Di Castelnuovo A, De Knijff P, *et al.* Polymorphisms in the coagulation factor VII gene and the risk of myocardial infarction. *N Engl J Med* 1998; **338**: 79–85.

29. Di Castelnuovo A, D'Orazio A, Amore C, Falanga A, Donati MB, Iacoviello L. The decanucleotide insertion/deletion polymorphism in the promoter region of the coagulation factor VII gene and the risk of familial myocardial infarction. *Thromb Res* 2000; **98**: 9–17.

30. Girelli D, Russo C, Ferraresi P, *et al.* Polymorphisms in the factor VII gene and the risk of myocardial infarction in patients with coronary artery disease. *N Engl J Med* 2000; **343**: 774–80.

31. Doggen CJ, Manger Cats V, Bertina RM, Reitsma PH, Vandenbroucke JP, Rosendaal FR. A genetic propensity to high factor VII is not associated with the risk of myocardial infarction in men. *Thromb Haemost* 1998; **80**: 281–5.

32. Lane A, Green F, Scarabin PY, *et al.* Factor VII Arg/Gln353 polymorphism determines factor VII coagulant activity in patients with myocardial infarction (MI) and control subjects in Belfast and in France but is not a strong indicator of MI risk in the ECTIM study. *Atherosclerosis* 1996; **119**: 119–27.

33. Lievers KJ, Mennen LI, Rattink AP, *et al.* The -323Ins10 polymorphism for factor VII is not associated with coronary atherosclerosis in symptomatic men. The REGRESS Study Group. *Thromb Res* 2000; **97**: 275–80.

34. Wang XL, Wang J, McCredie RM, Wilcken DE. Polymorphisms of factor V, factor VII, and fibrinogen genes: relevance to severity of coronary artery disease. *Arterioscler Thromb Vasc Biol* 1997; **17**: 246–51.

35. Feng D, Tofler GH, Larson MG, *et al.* Factor VII gene polymorphism, factor VII levels, and prevalent

cardiovascular disease: the Framingham Heart Study. *Arterioscler Thromb Vasc Biol* 2000; **20**: 593–600.

36. Stessman J, Maaravi Y, Hammerman-Rozenberg R, *et al*. Candidate genes associated with ageing and life expectancy in the Jerusalem longitudinal study. *Mech Ageing Dev* 2005; **126**: 333–9.

37. Jeffery S, Poloniecki J, Leatham E, *et al*. A protective contribution of the Q allele of the R353Q polymorphism of the factor VII gene in individuals with chronic stable angina? *Int J Cardiol* 2005; **100**: 395–9.

38. Mennen LI, De Maat MPM, Schouten EG, *et al*. Dietary effects on coagulation factor VII vary across genotypes of the R/Q353 polymorphism in elderly people. *J Nutr* 1998; **128**: 870–4.

39. Ariens RA, Lai TS, Weisel JW, Greenberg CS, Grant PJ. A role of factor XIII in fibrin clot formation and effects of genetic polymorphisms. *Blood* 2002; **100**: 743–75.

40. Lim B, Ariens R, Carter A, Weisel J, Grant P. Genetic regulation of fibrin structure and function: complex gene–environment interactions may modulate vascular risk. *Lancet* 2003; **361**: 1424–31.

41. Elbaz A, Poirier O, Canaple S, Chedru F, Cambien F, Amarenco P. The association between the Val34Leu polymorphism in the factor XIII gene and brain infarction. *Blood* 2000; **95**: 586–91.

42. Bertina RM, Koeleman BP, Koster T, *et al*. Mutation in blood coagulation factor V associated with resistance to activated protein C. *Nature* 1994; **369**: 64–7.

43. Ridker PM, Hennekens CH, Lindpaintner K, Stampfer MJ, Eisenberg PR, Miletich JP. Mutation in the gene coding for coagulation factor V and the risk of myocardial infarction, stroke, and venous thrombosis in apparently healthy men. *N Engl J Med* 1995; **332**: 912–17.

44. Cushman M, Kuller LH, Prentice R, *et al*. Estrogen plus progestin and risk of venous thrombosis. *JAMA* 2004; **292**: 1573–80.

45. Reiner AP, Siscovick DS, Rosendaal FR. Hemostatic risk factors and arterial thrombotic disease. *Thromb Haemost* 2001; **85**: 584–95.

46. Press RD, Liu XY, Beamer N, Coull BM. Ischemic stroke in the elderly: role of the common factor V mutation causing resistance to activated protein C. *Stroke* 1996; **27**: 44–8.

47. Kamphuisen PW, Eikenboom JCJ, Bertina, RM. Elevated factor VIII levels and the risk of thrombosis. *Arterioscler Thromb Vasc Biol* 2001; **21**: 731–8.

48. Weiss HJ, Hoyer IW. Von Willebrand factor: dissociation from antihemophilic factor procoagulant activity. *Science* 1973; **182**: 1149–51.

49. Wise RJ, Dorner AJ, Krane M, Pittman DD, Kaufman RJ. The role of von Willebrand factor multimers and propeptide cleavage in binding and stabilization of factor VIII. *J Biol Chem* 1991; **266**: 21948–55.

50. Orstavik KH, Magnus P, Reisner H, Berg K, Graham JB, Nance W. Factor VIII and factor IX in a twin population: evidence for a major effect of ABO locus on factor VIII level. *Am J Hum Genet* 1985; **37**: 89–101.

51. Tracy RP, Arnold AM, Ettinger W, Fried L, Meilahn E, Savage P. The relationship of fibrinogen and factors VII and VIII to incident cardiovascular disease and death in the elderly: results from the cardiovascular health study. *Arterioscler Thromb Vasc Biol* 1999; **19**: 1776–83.

52. Lip GY, Blann AD. Von Willebrand factor and its relevance to cardiovascular disorders. *Br Heart J* 1995; **74**: 580–3.

53. Catto AJ, Carter AM, Barrett JH, Bamford J, Rice PJ, Grant PJ. Von Willebrand factor and factor VIII:C in acute cerebrovascular disease: relationship to stroke subtype and mortality. *Thromb Haemost* 1997; **77**: 1104–8.

54. Jansson JH, Nilsson TK, Johnson O. Von Willebrand factor in plasma: a novel risk factor for recurrent myocardial infarction and death. *Br Heart J* 1991; **66**: 351–5.

55. Conway DS, Heeringa J, Van Der Kuip DA, *et al*. Atrial fibrillation and the prothrombotic state in the elderly: the Rotterdam study. *Stroke* 2003; **34**: 413–17.

56. Wannamethee SG, Lowe GD, Shaper AG, Rumley A, Lennon L, Whincup PH. The metabolic syndrome and insulin resistance: relationship to haemostatic and inflammatory markers in older non-diabetic men. *Atherosclerosis* 2005; **181**: 101–8.

57. Kohler HP, Grant PJ. Plasminogen-activator inhibitor type 1 and coronary artery disease. *N Engl J Med* 2000; **342**: 1792–801.

58. Juhan-Vague I, Alessi MC, Vague P. Increased plasma plasminogen activator inhibitor 1 levels: a possible link between insulin resistance and atherothrombosis. *Diabetologia* 1991; **34**: 457–62.

59. Dawson S, Wiman B, Hamsten A, Green F, Humphries S, Henney AM. The two allele sequences of a common polymorphism in the promoter of the plasminogen activator inhibitor-1 (PAI-1) gene responds differently to IL-1 in Hep G2 cells. *J Biol Chem* 1993; **268**: 10739–45.

60. Juhan-Vague I, Morange PE, Frere C, *et al*. The plasminogen activator inhibitor-1-675 4G/5G genotype influences the risk of myocardial infarction associated with elevated plasma proinsulin and insulin

concentrations in men from Europe: the HIFMECH study. *J Thromb Haemost* 2003; **1**: 2322–9.

61. Heijmans BT, Westendorp RG, Knook DL, Kluft C, Slagboom PE. Angiotensin I-converting enzyme and plasminogen activator inhibitor-1 gene variants: risk of mortality and fatal cardiovascular disease in an elderly population-based cohort. *J Am Coll Cardiol* 1999; **34**: 1176–83.

62. Bonfigli AR, Sirolla C, Cenerelli S, *et al*. Plasminogen activator inhibitor-1 plasma level increases with age in subjects with the 4G allele at position -675 in the promoter region. *Thromb Haemost* 2004; **92**: 1164–5.

63. Bouchard L, Mauriege P, Vohl MC, Bouchard C, Perusse L. Plasminogen-activator inhibitor-1 polymorphisms are associated with obesity and fat distribution in the Quebec family study: evidence of interactions with menopause. *Menopause* 2005; **12**: 136–43.

64. Grancha S, Estelles A, Tormo G, *et al*. Plasminogen activator inhibitor-1 (PAI-1) promoter 4G/5G genotype and increased PAI-1 circulating levels in postmenopausal women with coronary artery disease. *Thromb Haemost* 1999; **81**: 516–21.

65. Mannucci PM, Mari D, Merati G, *et al*. Gene polymorphisms predicting high plasma levels of coagulation and fibrinolysis proteins: a study in centenarians. *Arterioscler Thromb Vasc Biol* 1997; **17**: 755–9.

66. Brown NJ, Murphey LJ, Srikuma N, Koschachuhanan N, Williams GH, Vaughan DE. Interactive effect of PAI-1 4G/5G genotype and salt intake on PAI-1 antigen. *Arterioscler Thromb Vasc Biol* 2001; **21**: 1071–7.

67. Iacoviello L, Burzotta F, Di Castelnuovo A, Zito F, Marchioli R, Donati MB. The 4G/5G polymorphism of PAI-1 promoter gene and the risk of myocardial infarction: a meta-analysis. *Thromb Haemost* 1998; **80**: 1029–30.

68. Roest M, van der Schouw YT, Banga JD, *et al*. Plasminogen activator inhibitor 4G polymorphism is associated with decreased risk of cerebrovascular mortality in older women. *Circulation* 2000; **101**: 67–70.

69. Vaisanen SB, Humphries SE, Luong LA, Penttila I, Bouchard C, Rauramaa R. Regular exercise, plasminogen activator inhibitor-1 (PAI-1) activity and the 4G/5G promoter polymorphism in the PAI-1 gene. *Thromb Haemost* 1999; **82**: 1117–20.

70. Bouma BN, Meijers JC. New insights into factors affecting clot stability: a role for thrombin activatable fibrinolysis inhibitor (TAFI; plasma procarboxypeptidase B, plasma procarboxypeptidase U, procarboxypeptidase R). *Semin Hematol* 2004; **41**: 13–19.

71. Brouwers GJ, Vos HL, Leebeek FW, *et al*. A novel, possibly functional, single nucleotide polymorphism in the coding region of the thrombin-activatable fibrinolysis inhibitor (TAFI) gene is also associated with TAFI levels. *Blood* 2001; **98**: 1992–3.

72. Henry M, Aubert H, Morange PE, *et al*. Identification of polymorphisms in the promoter and the 3′ region of the TAFI gene: evidence that plasma TAFI antigen levels are strongly genetically controlled. *Blood* 2001; **97**: 2053–8.

73. Crainich P, Tang Z, Macy EM. A polymorphism at position -438 in the promoter region of thrombin-activatable fibrinolysis inhibitor (TAFI) is strongly associated with plasma antigen levels in healthy older men and women. *Circulation* 2000; **102**: 866.

74. Juhan-Vague I, Morange PE, Aubert H, *et al*. Plasma thrombin-activatable fibrinolysis inhibitor antigen concentration and genotype in relation to myocardial infarction in the north and south of Europe. *Arterioscler Thromb Vasc Biol* 2002; **22**: 867–73.

75. Brouwers GJ, Leebeek FW, Tanck MW, Wouter Jukema J, Kluft C, de Maat MP. Association between thrombin-activatable fibrinolysis inhibitor (TAFI) and clinical outcome in patients with unstable angina pectoris. *Thromb Haemost* 2003; **90**: 92–100.

76. Santamaria A, Martinez-Rubio A, Borrell M, Mateo J, Ortin R, Fontcuberta J. Risk of acute coronary artery disease associated with functional thrombin activatable fibrinolysis inhibitor plasma level. *Haematologica* 2004; **89**: 880–1.

77. Silveira A, Schatteman K, Goossens F, *et al*. Plasma procarboxypeptidase U in men with symptomatic coronary artery disease. *Thromb Haemost* 2000; **84**: 364–8.

78. Morange PE, Juhan-Vague I, Scarabin PY, *et al*. Association between TAFI antigen and Ala147Thr polymorphism of the TAFI gene and the angina pectoris incidence: the PRIME study (Prospective Epidemiological Study of MI). *Thromb Haemost* 2003; **89**: 554–60.

79. Schroeder V, Chatterjee T, Mehta H, *et al*. Thrombin activatable fibrinolysis inhibitor (TAFI) levels in patients with coronary artery disease investigated by angiography. *Thromb Haemost* 2002; **88**: 1020–5.

80. Morange PE, Tregouet DA, Frere C, *et al*. TAFI gene haplotypes, TAFI plasma levels and future risk of coronary heart disease: the PRIME study. *J Thromb Haemost* 2005; **3**: 1503–10.

81. Bajzar L, Jain N, Wang P, Walker JB. Thrombin activatable fibrinolysis inhibitor: not just an inhibitor of fibrinolysis. *Crit Care Med* 2004; **32**: S320–S324.

82. Campbell WD, Lazoura E, Okada N, Okada H. Inactivation of C3a and C5a octapeptides by carboxypeptidase R and carboxypeptidase N. *Microbiol Immunol* 2002; **46**: 131–4.

83. Cattaneo M. Hyperhomocysteinemia and thrombosis. *Lipids* 2001; **36**: S13–S26.

84. Homocysteine Studies Collaboration. Homocysteine and risk of ischemic heart disease and stroke: a meta-analysis. *JAMA* 2002; **288**: 2015–22.

85. Casas JP, Bautista LE, Smeeth L, Sharma P, Hingorani AD. Homocysteine and stroke: evidence on a causal link from Mendelian randomisation. *Lancet* 2005; **365**: 224–32.

86. Yap S, Boers GH, Wilcken B, *et al.* Vascular outcome in patients with homocystinuria due to cystathionine beta-synthase deficiency treated chronically: a multicenter observational study. *Arterioscler Thromb Vasc Biol* 2001; **21**: 2080–5.

87. Spotila LD, Jacques PF, Berger PB, Ballman KV, Ellison RC, Rozen R. Age dependence of the influence of methylenetetrahydrofolate reductase genotype on plasma homocysteine level. *Am J Epidemiol* 2003; **158**: 871–7.

88. Selhub J, Jacques PF, Wilson PW, Rush D, Rosenberg IH. Vitamin status and intake as primary determinants of homocysteinemia in an elderly population. *JAMA* 1993; **270**: 2693–8.

89. Malinow MR, Bostom AG, Krauss RM. Homocyst(e)ine, diet, and cardiovascular diseases: a statement for healthcare professionals from the Nutrition Committee, American Heart Association. *Circulation* 1999; **99**: 178–82.

90. Cattaneo M. Homocysteine and cardiovascular diseases. *Circulation* 1999; **100**: e151.

91. Mari D, Mannucci PM, Coppola R, Bottasso B, Bauer KA, Rosenberg RD. Hypercoagulability in centenarians: the paradox of successful aging. *Blood* 1995; **85**: 3144–9.

92. Rizzo MR, Ragno E, Barbieri M, *et al.* Elevated plasma activator inhibitor 1 is not related to insulin resistance and to gene polymorphism in healthy centenarians. *Atherosclerosis* 2002; **160**: 385–90.

93. Bladbjerg EM, Andersen-Ranberg K, de Maat MPM, *et al.* Longevity is independent of common variations in genes associated with cardiovascular risk. *Thromb Haemost* 1999; **82**: 1110–15.

94. Mari D, Duca F, Mannucci PM, Franceschi C. Mutant factor V (Arg506Gln) in healthy centenarians. *Lancet* 1996; **347**: 1044.

95. Faure-Delanef L, Quéré I, Zouali H, Cohen D. Human longevity and R506Q factor V gene mutation. *Thromb Haemost* 1997; **78**: 1160.

96. Kristensen SR, Andersen-Ranberg K, Bathum L, Jeune B. Factor V Leiden and venous thrombosis in Danish centenarians. *Thromb Haemost* 1998; **80**: 860–1.

97. Coppola R, Mari D, Lattuada A, Franceschi C. Von Willebrand factor in Italian centenarians. *Haematologica* 2003; **88**: 39–43.

98. Meroni PL, Mari D, Monti D, *et al.* Anti-beta 2 glycoprotein I antibodies in centenarians. *Exp Gerontol* 2004; **39**: 1459–65.

99. Weverling-Rijnsburger AW, Blauw GJ, Lagaay AM, Knook DL, Meinders AE, Westendorp RG. Total cholesterol and risk of mortality in the oldest old. *Lancet* 1997; **350**: 1119–23.

100. De Taeye B, Smith LH, Vaughan DE. Plasminogen activator inhibitor-1: a common denominator in obesity, diabetes and cardiovascular disease. *Curr Opin Pharmacol* 2005; **5**: 149–54.

101. Grant PJ, Stickland MH, Booth NA, Prentice CR. Metformin causes a reduction in basal and post-venous occlusion plasminogen activator inhibitor-1 in type 2 diabetic patients. *Diabet Med* 1991; **8**: 361–5.

102. Weisberg AD, Albornoz F, Griffin JP, *et al.* Pharmacological inhibition and genetic deficiency of plasminogen activator inhibitor-1 attenuates angiotensin II/salt-induced aortic remodeling. *Arterioscler Thromb Vasc Biol* 2004; **25**: 365–71.

30

Antithrombotic therapy: guidelines for the elderly

Chiara Cerletti, Holger Schünemann, Giovanni de Gaetano

Introduction

The purpose of this chapter is to summarize anti-thrombotic therapy guidelines that specifically address the elderly. Guidelines for elderly patients differ from those for younger populations because advanced age often represents an exclusion criterion in epidemiologic and clinical studies. Guidelines that focus on the elderly are also required because of differences in baseline risks for both target outcomes that need to be prevented and adverse outcomes that develop as a consequence of an intervention. The latter point is of importance because management decisions always involve a tradeoff between benefits and downsides (harms, burden, and cost of an action).

Methods

In this chapter we focus on existing clinical practice guidelines. We searched the Seventh ACCP Conference on Antithrombotic and Thrombolytic Therapy: Evidence-based Guidelines (AT7) for guidelines related to elderly patients. AT7 is one of the leading international resources for the treatment and prevention of thromboembolic disorders, compiled by over 80 panel members who produced a series of 22 chapters published in a supplement of the journal *Chest* [1]. The guidelines are based on comprehensive evaluations of the literature and include graded evidence-based recommendations that consider the quality of evidence and the strength of a recommendation. Grade 1 recommendations are strong, and indicate that the benefits do, or, for recommendations to not take an action, do not, outweigh the harms, burdens, and costs. Grade 2 recommendations suggest that individual patients' values may lead to different choices (for a full understanding of the grading, see [2]). We searched electronically all chapters of this supplement (except for the methodologic chapters on grading, development, or implementation of recommendations, and the chapters for disorders in pregnancy and childhood). We used the following text-words: elderly, old(er), age. All relevant citations were reviewed to establish whether they were related to recommendations for the elderly.

We found mention of the text-words relating to old age in eight chapters: one dealt with the pharmacology and management of vitamin K antagonists [3], one with hemorrhagic complications of anticoagulant treatment [4], and the other six were related to antithrombotic therapy in the following clinical conditions:

atrial fibrillation [5]
valvular heart disease [6]
ischemic stroke [7]
coronary artery disease [8]
acute myocardial infarction [9]
peripheral arterial occlusive disease [10]

No specific recommendations for the elderly were included among those proposed by the Seventh ACCP Conference, with a few of exceptions. We report below, chapter by chapter, a selection of paragraphs related to elderly patients.

Blood Disorders in the Elderly, ed. Lodovico Balducci, William Ershler, Giovanni de Gaetano.
Published by Cambridge University Press. © Cambridge University Press 2008.

The pharmacology and management of the vitamin K antagonists

Initiation and maintenance dosing

Following the administration of warfarin, an initial effect on the prothrombin time (PT) usually occurs within the first two or three days, depending on the dose administered, and an antithrombotic effect occurs within the next several days [11,12]. Heparin should be administered concurrently when a rapid anticoagulant effect is required, and its administration should be overlapped with warfarin until the INR has been in the therapeutic range for at least two days. A loading dose (>20 mg) of warfarin is not recommended. A number of randomized studies have supported the use of a lower initiation dose. Thus, there is room for flexibility in selecting a starting dose of warfarin. Some clinicians prefer to use a larger starting dose (e.g., 7.5–10 mg), while a starting dose of <5 mg might be appropriate in the elderly. When the INR has been in the therapeutic range (for most indications an INR target range of 2.0–3.0) on two measurements approximately 24 hours apart, heparin therapy is discontinued. If treatment is not urgent (e.g., chronic stable atrial fibrillation), warfarin administration, without concurrent heparin administration, can be commenced out-of-hospital with an anticipated maintenance dose of 4–5 mg per day.

Initiation of anticoagulation in the elderly

The dose required to maintain a therapeutic range for patients over 60 years of age decreases with increasing age [13–15], possibly because of a reduction in the clearance of warfarin with age [16,17]. Therefore in the elderly the initial dose of warfarin should not be more than 5 mg [18], and in some cases (i.e., in patients with a high risk of bleeding, and in those who are undernourished or have congestive heart failure or liver disease) it should be less. Other factors that may influence the response to anticoagulation in the elderly include the potential for a greater number of other medical conditions and/or concurrent drug use [13]. Consequently, it is advisable to monitor older patients more frequently in order to maximize their time in the therapeutic range (TTR) [19].

A specific recommendation for the elderly is made as follows. In the elderly, and in patients who are debilitated, malnourished, have congestive heart failure, or have liver disease, the use of a starting dose of ≤5 mg is suggested (Grade 2C).

Adverse events and their management

The relationship between older age and anticoagulant-associated bleeding is controversial. Several reports [14,20–33] have indicated that older individuals are not at increased risk for bleeding, while others [34–43] have described such an association. The discrepancy may be partly explained by the wide range in the mean age of the patients enrolled in the various studies, the relative lack of representation in most studies of patients over 80 years of age, and the selection and survivorship biases in non-inception cohort studies. When investigators attempt to separate the effect of age from comorbid conditions associated with age, some have concluded that age in and of itself is not a major independent risk factor [13,20,24,44] while others have found it to be an independent risk factor [36,45], even after controlling for the intensity of the anticoagulant effect. It has also been suggested [19] that older patients who have high-quality anticoagulation management, such as that provided by an anticoagulation clinic (ACC), have the same risk of bleeding as their younger counterparts. Last, the location of major bleeding may be a factor, and there is reasonable evidence [20,36] to suggest that there is a real increase in intracranial hemorrhage in the elderly. Based on these findings, individuals who are otherwise good candidates for anticoagulation therapy should not have it withheld because of their age. However, elderly patients should be monitored more frequently in order to maximize their time in the therapeutic range and to reduce the number of adverse events.

Hemorrhagic complications of anticoagulant treatment

Patient characteristics

The risk of major bleeding during warfarin therapy can be related to specific comorbid conditions or patient characteristics. An increasing body of evidence supports age as an independent risk factor for major bleeding [34,37–40,42,44–56]. For example, Pengo *et al.* [56] evaluated the relationship of age and other risk factors to the incidence of major bleeding. Major bleeding occurred more frequently in patients over 75 years of age (5.1% per year) than in younger patients (1% per year). Multivariate analysis indicated that age >75 years was the only variable independently related to primary bleeding (i.e., bleeding unrelated to organic lesion). Also, risk for intracranial hemorrhage may be increased among older patients, especially those ≥75 years old, when the INR is above therapeutic levels [36,40,57,58]. The mechanism by which aging causes anticoagulant-related bleeding is not known.

Atrial fibrillation

The efficacy of warfarin in preventing stroke in patients with nonvalvular atrial fibrillation (AF) has been consistently demonstrated in a number of randomized controlled trials (RCTs) and in meta-analyses of randomized trials. Overall, the rates of warfarin-related bleeding in these studies have been low.

Treating 1000 patients with AF for 1 year with oral anticoagulants rather than aspirin would prevent 23 additional ischemic strokes while causing nine additional major bleeds [59].

Because 50% or more of patients with AF are over 75 years old, the risk–benefit of oral anticoagulant therapy in this clinical subgroup is of particular interest. One study (SPAF II) [60] raised concern that the risk for warfarin-related bleeding, especially intracranial hemorrhage, may be increased substantially in patients ≥75 years old. The rate of major bleeding while receiving warfarin was 2.3% per year, compared with 1.1% per year for patients receiving aspirin, 325 mg/day. However, the rate of major warfarin-related bleeding was 4.2% per year in patients ≥75

years old, compared with 1.7% per year in younger patients; the corresponding rates for intracranial bleeding were 1.8% and 0.6% per year, respectively. The reason why these rates are substantially higher than those observed in the other clinical trials of warfarin in patients with AF is likely related to the intensity of anticoagulant therapy: virtually all intracranial hemorrhages in SPAF II, as in the other clinical trials, were associated with an INR >3.0 [60]. In contrast, in the SPAF III trial (targeted INR, 2.0–3.0), the mean age was 71 years and the rate of intracranial hemorrhage was 0.5% per year [35].

The relative risk–benefit of warfarin therapy at a targeted INR of 1.5–2.1 compared with warfarin therapy at a targeted INR of 2.2–3.5 has been evaluated in a randomized trial in patients with atrial fibrillation [61]. Major bleeding occurred in 6 of 55 patients in the conventional-intensity group (rate, 6.6%/year), compared with none of the 60 patients (0%/year) in the low-intensity group ($p = 0.01$). The six patients with major bleeding were all elderly (mean 74 years) and older than the other 109 patients without major bleeding (mean 66 years; $p < 0.01$). The INR before bleeding was below 3.0 in four patients, and was 3.1 and 3.6 in the remaining two patients, respectively.

A systematic review [62] compared the rates of stroke, intracranial bleeding, and major bleeding from studies of patients treated in actual clinical practice with the pooled data from RCTs. Patients in clinical practice were older and had more comorbid conditions than the patients in clinical trials. Nevertheless, the rates of ischemic stroke were similar between clinical practice and the clinical trials (1.8 and 1.4 per 100 patient-years, respectively), as were the corresponding rates of intracranial bleeding (0.1 and 0.3) and major bleeding (1.1 and 1.3) [62]. There was a higher rate of minor bleeding in clinical practice (12.0 per 100 patient-years) than in clinical trials (7.9 per 100 patient-years; $p = 0.002$).

Relationship between the risk of bleeding and patient risk factors

There is good evidence that comorbid conditions, particularly recent surgery or trauma, are very important risk factors for heparin-induced bleeding [50,63,64]. Some studies [65,66] have reported that older patients had a higher risk of heparin-induced bleeding. In an analysis of a randomized trial [67], age >70 years was associated with a clinically important increased risk of major bleeding.

Antithrombotic therapy in atrial fibrillation

Risk of ICH during anticoagulation

Intracerebral hemorrhage (ICH) is the only hemorrhagic complication that regularly produces deficits as great or greater than the ischemic strokes antithrombotic therapy is designed to prevent. Overall, the rates of ICH were reassuringly low in the initial AF randomized trials comparing anticoagulation with control or placebo. However, a substantially higher rate of ICH was observed in the SPAF II study [60], with seven ICHs observed among 385 patients >75 years old for an annualized rate of 1.8%, compared with 0.8% in patients receiving aspirin. In contrast, in the primary prevention trials, the rate of ICH was only 0.3% per year among those older than 75 years [68]. In the secondary prevention EAFT study [69], the average age at entry was 71 years and no ICHs were diagnosed, although a CT scan was not done in all patients with symptoms of stroke [46,69]. In the high-risk arm of SPAF III [35], (mean age 71 years, mean INR 2.4), the rate of ICH was 0.5% per year, compared to 0.9% per year in the aspirin plus low-dose warfarin arm. The AFASAK 2 study [70] reported two ICHs in the INR 2.0–3.0 arm, for an annual rate of 0.6%, compared to 0–0.3% in the three other treatment arms during a shorter period of follow-up.

The reasons for the high ICH rate in the SPAF II trial [40] in patients over the age of 75, as compared with the other studies, are not entirely clear, but the patients were older than in any other AF trial, and the target anticoagulation intensity was high (INR 2.0–4.5).

Efficacy of oral anticoagulant therapy versus aspirin

The SPAF II trial [60] included two separate trials, one for individuals aged 75 years or older, and one for those under 75. In the younger group (mean age, 65 years), adjusted-dose warfarin decreased the rate of stroke by 33%, compared with a 27% reduction in the older patients (mean age, 80 years); neither difference was statistically significant. The SPAF II study [60] included the experience of patients who had participated in group 1 of SPAF I [71], in which aspirin-treated patients had an extremely low event rate; moreover, many of the strokes in the warfarin arm of SPAF II occurred in individuals who had stopped warfarin.

Antithrombotic therapy for AF in clinical practice

Despite the extensive data from randomized trials demonstrating the efficacy of adjusted-dose warfarin for prevention of thromboembolism, concerns persist about how generalizable these findings are when applied to "real-world" clinical practice settings [62,72–78]. The trials enrolled only a small proportion of screened patients (e.g., <10% in SPAF [71]), relatively few very elderly patients (only 10% >80 years old [57]), and they used especially careful and frequent monitoring of anticoagulation intensity.

Comparison and validation of stroke risk stratification schemes

The AFI- and SPAF-based risk stratification schemes are largely consistent with each other. Prior stroke or TIA, older age, hypertension, and diabetes emerge from both analyses as risk factors for stroke in patients with AF.

Additional validation efforts have also been conducted comparing AFI, SPAF, and the previous Sixth ACCP Consensus Conference [79] risk schemes. Among 259 elderly (≥65 years old) participants with nonvalvular AF in the Cardiovascular Health Study [83], annual rates of stroke using modified

AFI/ACCP-6 criteria were 2.7% (95% CI 1.7–4.1%) for high-risk subjects (prior stroke or TIA, hypertension, diabetes, congestive heart failure, or coronary heart disease) and 2.4% (95% CI 0.9–5.1%) for moderate-risk subjects (age ≥65 years and no high-risk features) not receiving anticoagulation. Using the SPAF III criteria, annual stroke rates were relatively similar, ranging from 3.7% (95% CI 2.1–5.8%) for high risk (prior stroke or TIA, women >75 years old, systolic BP >160 mm Hg, or impaired left-ventricular systolic function), 2.0% (95% CI 0.7–4.7%) for moderate risk (history of hypertension and no high-risk features), and 1.7% (95% CI 0.6–3.8%) for low risk (no moderate or high-risk features). Among 1073 patients without prior stroke or TIA who participated in the SPAF III trial aspirin plus low-dose warfarin arm or the SPAF III aspirin cohort study, the AFI, ACCP, and SPAF I-II criteria were evaluated [81]. The stroke rates for each risk stratum differed across the different risk schemes: while stroke risks were low in the low-risk categories for all schemes, there was significant variation in the moderate- to high-risk categories as well as in the proportion of subjects in each category.

Patient preferences and decision analyses

Anticoagulation poses a significant hemorrhagic risk in all age groups. Oral vitamin K anticoagulants (VKAs) also impose other lifestyle constraints on patients such as dietary modifications and frequent monitoring of anticoagulation intensity. As a result, patient education and involvement in the anticoagulation decision is important. Many patients with AF have a great fear of ischemic stroke and choose warfarin even for a relatively small decrease in the absolute risk of stroke [82], while others at relatively low risk for stroke want to avoid the burdens and risks of VKAs and opt for aspirin [82–84]. The safe use of anticoagulants depends on patient cooperation and a monitoring system that can achieve INR targets on a regular basis. Findings of the randomized trials suggest that anticoagulation at an INR of 2.0–3.0 can be adequately safe even for elderly patients, and the Italian Study on Complications of

Oral Anticoagulant Therapy [34,85] and ATRIA [86] experiences demonstrate that low hemorrhage rates can be achieved in clinical practice outside of trials, particularly if well-organized anticoagulation clinics are involved [57,70,85,86].

Recommendations

In patients with persistent (also known as "sustained," and including patients categorized as "permanent" in certain classification schemes [87]) or paroxysmal (intermittent) AF at high risk of stroke (i.e., having any of the following features: prior ischemic stroke, TIA, or systemic embolism, age >75 years, moderately or severely impaired left ventricular systolic function and/or congestive heart failure, history of hypertension, or diabetes mellitus), anticoagulation with an oral VKA, such as warfarin (target INR 2.5, range 2.0–3.0) is recommended (Grade 1A).

AF following cardiac surgery

When AF persists for more than 48 hours in the postoperative period following CABG surgery, anticoagulation with heparin or an oral VKA is appropriate [88], but the potential for bleeding in surgical patients poses a particular challenge. The choice of drug (heparin and/or oral anticoagulant) must be based on the individual clinical situation. Optimal protection against ischemic stroke for high-risk patients with AF involves anticoagulation with an oral VKA, such as warfarin (INR 2.0–3.0). This is associated with a considerable risk of bleeding among the elderly during the early postoperative period, but no adequate study has specifically addressed the relative efficacy and toxicity in this clinical situation.

Cardioversion of AF of known duration of under 48 hours

For AF of short (<48 hours) duration, a common practice is to cardiovert without transesophageal echocardiography (TEE) or prolonged precardioversion anticoagulation. This practice was called into question when a study reported a 13% prevalence of atrial thrombi on TEE among patients with AF of <72 h duration [89]. Subsequently, data were reported from a study of 357 patients who had a symptomatic duration of AF for under 48 hours [90]: 250 patients converted spontaneously and 107 patients underwent pharmacologic or electrical cardioversion, all without screening TEE or a month of warfarin prior to cardioversion. Clinical thromboembolism occurred in three subjects (<1%), all of whom were elderly women without a history of prior AF and with normal left-ventricular systolic function. Though a low stroke risk was seen in these studies, it may be prudent to initiate heparin anticoagulation and to perform TEE (or delay cardioversion for one month) for high-risk patients. Even without use of TEE, anticoagulation with heparin (e.g., IV heparin with target partial thromboplastin time [PTT] of 60 s [range 50–70 s] or LMWH at full DVT treatment doses) immediately prior to cardioversion may be appropriate. Many of these patients will require anticoagulation after cardioversion should AF recur, and the use of heparin will decrease the risk of thrombus formation during the pericardioversion period. There are no randomized trials comparing these approaches in patients with AF of under 48 hours in duration.

Rate versus rhythm control in AF: implications for use of anticoagulants

Three randomized trials [91–93] have compared rhythm-control and rate-control approaches; each gave similar results, showing equivalent outcomes in both arms, with the predominance of thromboembolic events among patients not receiving warfarin at a dose sufficient to maintain the INR in the target range. The largest trial, AFFIRM [91], included 4060 patients with recurrent AF. Study subjects were over 65 years old or had other risk factors for stroke or death and no contraindications to anticoagulation therapy. All patients were initially anticoagulated, but warfarin could be withdrawn from those in the rhythm-control arm who maintained normal sinus

rhythm (NSR). At five years, 35% of rate-control patients were in NSR compared to 63% of those in the rhythm-control group. Over 85% of patients in the rate-control arm were treated with warfarin as compared to 70% in the rhythm-control arm. After a mean follow-up of 3.5 years, all-cause mortality (the primary endpoint) was not reduced by rhythm control (rhythm-control group 26.7% vs. rate-control group 25.9%, $p = 0.08$), and there was a trend toward a higher risk of ischemic stroke (7.1% with rhythm control vs. 5.5% for rate control, $p = 0.79$). Importantly, 72% of strokes occurred in patients receiving no warfarin or with INR below 2.0. There was no significant difference in functional status or quality of life in the two groups.

Antithrombotic therapy in valvular heart disease: native and prosthetic

Patients with mitral valve disease in sinus rhythm

Despite the powerful thromboembolic potential of AF, the rheumatic mitral valve disease patient in sinus rhythm still has a substantial risk of systemic embolism and is, therefore, a possible candidate for long-term oral anticoagulant (OAC) therapy. This is particularly true if the patient has had prior AF or is being treated with antiarrhythmic medications to maintain sinus rhythm [91–93]. It is not yet clear whether periodic echocardiography to detect atrial thrombus is indicated in older patients with mitral stenosis who remain in sinus rhythm. Other than age, there are no reliable clinical markers in such cases, so the decision to treat is problematic. Because the risk of AF is high in the rheumatic mitral disease patient with a very large atrium, some authorities suggest that patients in normal sinus rhythm with a left atrial diameter >55 mm should receive anticoagulant therapy [94].

Mitral annular calcification

The clinical syndrome of mitral annular calcification (MAC) includes a strong female preponderance and may be associated with mitral stenosis and regurgitation, calcific aortic stenosis, conduction disturbances, arrhythmias, embolic phenomena, and endocarditis.

Many factors contributing to the risk of thromboembolism in MAC include AF, the hemodynamic consequences of the mitral valve lesion itself (stenosis and regurgitation), fragmentation of calcific annular tissue, and diffuse vascular atherosclerosis. In light of these observations, a good argument can be made for prophylactic anticoagulant therapy in patients with AF or a history of an embolic event. However, since most of these patients are elderly (mean age, 73–75 years) [95,96], the risks of anticoagulation with VKAs will be increased. Therefore, if the mitral lesion is mild or if an embolic event is clearly identified as calcific rather than thrombotic, the risks from anticoagulation may outweigh the benefit of OAC therapy in patients without AF. Certainly the clinician should be discouraged from initiating anticoagulant therapy merely on the basis of radiographic evidence of MAC. Antiplatelet drugs might represent an uncertain compromise for those with advanced lesions, although to our knowledge no studies indicate that this therapy is effective in preventing thromboembolism in MAC. For patients with repeated embolic events despite OAC therapy, or in whom multiple calcific emboli are recognized, valve replacement should be considered.

Elderly patients, patients with AF or myocardial infarction, or other risk factors

Higher rates of thromboembolic complications with valves in the mitral position may be attributed to a higher incidence of AF, left atrial enlargement, and perhaps endocardial damage from rheumatic mitral valve disease [97]. A low left-ventricular ejection fraction, old age, and history of prior thromboembolism also are associated with thromboembolic complications [98].

Cannegieter and associates [99] showed that the risk of thromboembolism and of bleeding was highest among patients over 70 years of age. However,

among elderly patients ($\geq$70 years), a retrospective case series [100] suggested that a low level of VKAs was satisfactory with St. Jude Medical valves in the aortic position. Many of these patients were treated before the INR was in use, but in recent years an INR of 1.8–2.5 was satisfactory.

Antithrombotic and thrombolytic therapy for ischemic stroke

The benefits of tPA were consistent regardless of patient age, stroke subtype, stroke severity, or prior use of aspirin. While patients with severe neurologic deficits at baseline were less likely to have a good outcome, regardless of treatment, a subgroup analysis of patients over 75 years old with an initial NIH Stroke Scale (NIHSS) of >20 demonstrated a reduction in death or severe disability with tPA compared with placebo [101]. This benefit occurred despite the increased risk of ICH in patients with severe strokes (adjusted odds ratio [OR] 4.3, 95% CI 1.6–11.9).

Phase IV studies

Two formal prospective phase IV studies have examined outcomes with use of tPA in National Institute of Neurological Disorders and Stroke (NINDS)-derived protocols restricted to a three-hour treatment window in clinical practice.

The Standard Treatment with Alteplase to Reverse Stroke study [102] was conducted in 75 medical centers in the USA (24 academic and 33 community). A total of 389 patients were treated in a median time of 2 hours and 44 minutes from stroke onset to treatment. The median NIHSS at baseline was 13; the mean age was 69 years. At 30 days, 35% of patients had very favorable outcomes (modified Rankin scale [RS] 0–1), 43% were functionally independent (modified RS 0–2), and 13% had died. The rate of symptomatic ICH was 3.3%; seven of the 13 patients with symptomatic ICH died. Predictors of favorable outcome included baseline NIHSS score <10, absence of major abnormalities on baseline CT, age $\geq$85 years, and lower mean arterial pressures at baseline.

The Canadian Activase for Stroke Effectiveness Study [103] was conducted in 60 centers in Canada (25 academic and 35 community). A total of 1132 patients were treated, with median time to treatment of 150 minutes. The median NIHSS at baseline was 14, and the mean age was 70 years. At 90 days, 36% of patients had very favorable outcomes. The overall mortality rate was 21%. The rate of symptomatic ICH was 4.6%. Multivariate analysis showed that only elevated glucose (OR 1.6, 95% CI 1.2–2.3) and onset-to-treatment time (OR 1.2, 95% CI 1.0–1.5) were predictors of symptomatic ICH.

The results of these two phase IV studies demonstrate comparable safety and clinical outcomes to the NINDS trial, with a trend to lower rates of symptomatic ICH.

Published reports from routine clinical practice

Published reports of the use of tPA in routine clinical experience have generally been favorable [104–114], with reported rates of symptomatic ICH usually below 7%. The largest multi-center survey of the use of tPA in clinical practice reported a 6% symptomatic ICH rate in 1205 patients analyzed both retrospectively and prospectively [114]. Logistic regression models identified age, stroke severity, elevated glucose, low platelets, and early major CT changes as predictors of symptomatic ICH. Strict adherence to protocols and experience are important to ensure appropriate use and adequate safety. Increased rates of symptomatic ICH associated with protocol violations have been reported by several groups [107,111,112,114].

Stroke prevention: the Antithrombotic Trialists' meta-analysis

The Antithrombotic Trialists [115] also analyzed the differences in the response of patients over 65 and under 65 years of age, and by sex. While some variation is seen, all groups – young and old, men and women – benefit to a similar proportionate degree from antiplatelet therapy. The same is true for patients with hypertension compared to those without hypertension, and diabetes compared to no diabetes.

Antithrombotic therapy for coronary artery disease

The GUSTO trial

The Global Use of Strategies to Open Occluded Coronary Arteries (GUSTO) IIb trial [116] was one of the first large-scale attempts to study the spectrum of patients presenting with acute chest pain, stratifying the randomization on the basis of their initial ECG findings (ST-segment elevation or not). GUSTO IIb results showed that patients without ST-segment elevation represent a different population from those with ST-segment elevation. They were older, more likely to be female, and had more comorbidity than the group with ST-segment elevation. For descriptive purposes, these patients were being categorized not on the basis of their admitting diagnosis, but rather on the diagnosis that became clear 12–24 hours later, namely unstable angina (UA) or myocardial infarction (MI), typically non-Q-wave infarction.

Fondaparinux

Fondaparinux elimination is prolonged in patients with renal impairment [117]. Total clearance is reduced by 25% in patients with mild renal impairment (CrCl 50–80 mL/min), approximately 40% lower among patients with moderate renal impairment (CrCl 30–50 mL/min) and 55% lower in the setting of severe renal impairment (CrCl <30 mL/min). Fondaparinux elimination is also reduced (by 25%) in patients >75 years old (compared with patients <65 years old). There are insufficient data to recommend fondaparinux in patients presenting with non-ST-segment elevation (NSTE) acute coronary syndrome (ACS). Large randomized trials are under way evaluating the safety and efficacy of fondaparinux among patients presenting with both ST-segment elevation and NSTE ACS.

Streptokinase and aspirin: ISIS-2 trial

The early reduction in mortality with aspirin persisted when the patients were observed for a mean of 15 months [118]. Aspirin reduced the risk of non-fatal reinfarction by 49% and non-fatal stroke by 46%. The increased rate of early non-fatal reinfarction noted when streptokinase therapy was used alone is consistent with marked platelet activation after fibrinolytic therapy, and was completely resolved when aspirin was added (3.8% vs. 1.3%). Aspirin added to the benefit of streptokinase therapy in all groups examined. In particular, among patients over 70 years old, the combination markedly reduced the mortality rate from 23.8% to 15.8% ($p < 0.001$) without increasing the risk of hemorrhage or stroke. Because of poor prognosis in older patients who have experienced actue MIs, the absolute number of lives saved with aspirin and thrombolytic therapy increases dramatically with age (2.5 per 100 treated patients <60 years of age and 7–8 per 100 treated patients ≥60 years of age).

Primary prevention

Aspirin therapy reduced ischemic cardiac events in four of the five trials, the effect being most marked for non-fatal MI. Although there were trends to increased total stroke and hemorrhagic stroke with aspirin in the US Physicians Trial and the UK Doctors Trial [119], there were trends toward a lower number of total strokes with aspirin in the TPT and virtually no difference in the fourth trial (HOT) [120]. A main distinguishing characteristic between the first two trials and the other three was the considerably lower dose of aspirin, 75 mg/day in the TPT and HOT trials and 100 mg in the Primary Prevention Project [121]. There is a consistent failure in all five trials to show a reduction in all-cause mortality by aspirin, although this is not surprising, as none of the single trials was sufficiently large to demonstrate or exclude an effect on all-cause mortality. In the US Physicians Trial, the risk of MI among men aged 40–49 years was only 0.1% per year (one MI per year per 1000 men), whereas among men aged 60–69 years the rate of MI was 0.82% per year (8.2 MIs per year per 1000 men). Among the older men, the absolute risk reduction with aspirin was approximately 4.4 infarcts per year per 1000 men treated. Similarly, the absolute benefits were greater

among men with diabetes mellitus, with systolic or diastolic hypertension, who smoked cigarettes, and who had a lack of exercise. It is possible that aspirin increases the number of fatal events of coronary heart disease in older men, although this observation requires confirmation or refutation in other trials.

The UK and US Physicians trials recruited doctors not ineligible on account of previous cardiovascular events or receiving aspirin for other reasons, but otherwise specified no risk factors for selection into the trial (although these were recorded at entry for comparison between the active and placebo-treated groups and, in the case of the US trial, for subgroup analyses according to various risk factors). UK and US physicians may have been at somewhat higher risk than participants in the other trials on account of the inclusion of large proportions of older men. The higher risk of cardiovascular and coronary events in the TPT was due to the inclusion of a larger number of risk factors for defining eligibility than for the other trials.

Thrombolysis and adjunctive therapy in acute myocardial infarction

Streptokinase

The Fibrinolytic Therapy Trialists' Collaborative Group combined trials investigating streptokinase for treatment of acute MI in a meta-analysis [122]. The authors observed an overall benefit among patients with ST-segment elevation or bundle-branch block irrespective of age, sex, blood pressure, heart rate, prior MI, or diabetic status.

GUSTO I trial

Despite the aggressive regimens of fibrinolysis, aspirin, and heparin, ICH was uncommon in GUSTO I [123]. For each of the streptokinase arms, 0.5% of patients suffered an ICH, compared with 0.7% of patients treated with accelerated alteplase and 0.9% of patients treated with combination fibrinolytic therapy. To put the results in full perspective, the GUSTO I investigators developed the concept of "net clinical benefit," that is, the avoidance of either death or non-fatal disabling stroke. When comparing the net clinical benefit among the four regimens, accelerated alteplase still provided a clear benefit compared with the other three regimens. The benefit of accelerated alteplase was seen in nearly every subgroup analyzed, including patients with anterior or inferior MI and in the young and the elderly. The absolute benefit was greater in higher-risk patients, for example, those with anterior MI.

ASSENT 2 trial

In ASSENT 2 [124], the rates of ICH were nearly identical for tenecteplase and alteplase (0.93% and 0.94%, respectively), as were the overall rates of stroke (1.78% and 1.66%). The group at the highest risk for ICH was elderly female patients weighing ≤ 67 kg, which has been noted in two previous multivariate analyses [125,126]. It is encouraging that the rate of ICH in this high-risk group was only 1.1% after treatment with tenecteplase, compared with 3.0% for those treated with alteplase (multivariable adjusted OR 0.30, 95% CI 0.09–0.98, $p < 0.05$). In all other patients, the ICH rates were similar between the two groups.

ASSENT 3 PLUS trial

The ASSENT 3 PLUS trial [127] evaluated the feasibility, efficacy, and safety of prehospital treatment with either tenecteplase plus enoxaparin or tenecteplase plus UFH. The primary efficacy and efficacy-plus-safety endpoints were identical to those utilized in the main ASSENT 3 trial. Consistent with ASSENT 3, there was a trend toward a lower rate of the composite of 30-day mortality, in-hospital reinfarction, or in-hospital refractory ischemia in the enoxaparin group (14.2% vs. 17.4%, $p = 0.08$). However, the lower rates of reinfarction (3.6% vs. 5.9%, $p = 0.028$) and refractory ischemia (4.4% vs. 6.5%, $p = 0.067$) were offset by a significantly higher rate of ICH (2.2% vs. 0.97%, $p = 0.048$) and a tendency toward more major bleeding (4% vs. 2.8%, $p = 0.17$). The risk for ICH and major bleeding was mainly confined to patients over 75 years old; it

remains uncertain whether this is due in part to the prehospital administration of fibrinolysis and the initial non-weight-adjusted bolus of enoxaparin therapy given to the generally older and higher-risk population included in the trial, who presumably had reduced renal function (the dose of enoxaparin was not adjusted for in the analysis).

Rates of the primary efficacy endpoint in the groups receiving enoxaparin, combination abciximab, and standard therapy were 11.4%, 11.1%, and 15.4%, respectively ($p = 0.0001$). Rates of all stroke (1.49% vs. 1.52%) as well as ICH (0.94% vs. 0.93%) were similar for combination therapy as compared to standard treatment. Total, major, and minor bleeding were all significantly higher with combination treatment, and once again there was no benefit and a tendency toward harm seen in the elderly. Rates of the primary efficacy endpoint in the groups receiving enoxaparin, combination abciximab, and standard therapy were 11.4%, 11.1%, and 15.4%, respectively ($p = 0.0001$). Rates of all stroke (1.49% vs. 1.52%) as well as ICH (0.94% vs. 0.93%) were similar for combination therapy as compared to standard treatment. Total, major, and minor bleeding were all significantly higher with combination treatment, and once again there was no benefit and a tendency toward harm seen in the elderly.

Primary angioplasty versus thrombolysis

There is an absolute benefit of 1–3.4 lives saved per 100 patients treated with fibrinolytic therapy in the patients aged over 75 years [122,128]. The elderly are, however, at increased risk of ICH, and the proven clinical benefit has not been observed in retrospective review of large observational databases [129,130]. When primary angioplasty is readily available, preferential reperfusion with angioplasty is recommended [131,132].

Antithrombotic therapy during percutaneous coronary intervention

Bivalirudin may be particularly useful for patients at high risk for bleeding, such as the elderly or those with renal insufficiency. It also may be better than heparin for patients who do not get adjunctive treatment with a GPIIb-IIIa inhibitor [133].

Antithrombotic therapy in peripheral arterial occlusive disease (PAOD)

Chronic limb ischemia

Atherosclerotic PAOD is symptomatic with intermittent claudication in 2–3% of men and 1–2% of women over 60 years of age [134–136]. However, the prevalence of asymptomatic PAOD, generally proven by a reduced ankle/brachial systolic pressure index, is three to four times as great [137,138]. After 5–10 years, 70–80% of patients remain unchanged or improved, 20–30% have progression of symptoms and require intervention, and 10% require amputation [139,140]. Progression of disease is greatest in patients with multilevel arterial involvement, low ankle-to-brachial pressure indices, chronic renal insufficiency, diabetes mellitus and, possibly, heavy smoking [139].

The prevalence of PAOD increases with age and is a significant cause of hospital admission and an important predicator of cardiovascular and stroke mortality, which is increased twofold to threefold [134,135,140,141].

Summary and discussion

In this chapter we have reviewed the available evidence relating to antithrombotic therapy specifically for the elderly, based on one of the most widely known guidelines on this topic, the AT7.

Elderly patients will generally require lower dosing of oral anticoagulation with VKAs antagonists and should receive lower starting doses. The age-specific increase in adverse effects with OAC is somewhat controversial and may be overcome by closer monitoring of anticoagulation in the elderly. In addition, age in itself may not be a risk factor for increased bleeding risk from OAC after adjustment for comorbidities. In patients with AF the elderly will have the greatest net benefit from OAC, as expressed by a Grade 1A recommendation for patients older than 75 years. However, as in almost any therapeutic decision, the administration of OAC requires careful consideration of patients' values and preferences.

Increase benefit in the elderly is also seen in patients being treated with tPA for acute ischemic stroke who qualify for treatment (i.e., early presentation), despite increased ICH risk.

Similarly, antiplatelet therapy is equally efficacious for secondary stroke prevention in the elderly compared to younger patients. In acute coronary syndrome, difficulties are posed by the higher prevalence of atypical presentation in the elderly, which often does not allow straightforward diagnosis of acute MI with ST-segment elevation and thrombolysis, but if administered to older patients greater net benefits are seen in many trials. This is also seen in trials of antiplatelet therapy in the elderly for secondary prevention in patients with coronary artery disease. Since PAOD is more prevalent in the elderly, and complication rates are higher in the elderly, greater net benefit is also expected from antiplatelet therapy in this condition.

While age is frequently reported as a prognostic as well as an effect-modifying factor, age-specific recommendations are rarely made (except in rare cases such as for patients with AF). This is most important for the evaluation of the benefits and downsides of therapy. Both the relative risk reductions for prevented endpoints and the relative risk increase for adverse outcomes will often be similar or the same in the elderly. It is the baseline risk or event rate that may increase in the elderly (e.g., the baseline risk for a stroke in patients with AF increases in the elderly, and the risk for ICH may increase in elderly patients receiving thrombolysis). However, if this increase is either linear or proportional for both wanted and unwanted outcomes, then the clinical net benefit will be higher for many interventions in the elderly. Thus, extrapolation of results from trials may be justified, and may support the administration of therapies that have been examined in younger patients. This is seen for aspirin therapy in acute MI, for secondary prevention of cardiovascular disease, and for stroke prevention in AF, if oral anticoagulation is managed carefully in the elderly.

Our review of the AT7 demonstrates that there is a need to increase age-specific recommendations based on an assessment of baseline risk in the elderly. This could be achieved by producing age-specific measures of net clinical benefit, such as in the case of aspirin therapy for the prevention of secondary outcomes in patients post MI. Meta-analysis – following the rules of when to trust a subgroup analysis [142] – should provide subgroup analyses for age strata when possible, because for many interventions net benefits increase with age. An alternative to subgroup analysis and extrapolation is the conduct of trials that focus on elderly patients.

Making recommendations in the elderly is hindered by another problem, the higher prevalence of comorbidities. This problem can complicate clinicians' efforts to follow clinical practice guidelines because of the possibility of conflicting recommendations, drug interaction, polypharmacy, and cost. Clinicians need to be aware of this concern. As described above, clinical research should focus on the elderly and be less restrictive in inclusion criteria (i.e., conduct pragmatic or management trials rather than explanatory trials in the elderly) and trials should include patients with comorbidities.

In summary, clinical practice guidelines require careful evaluation of interventions in the elderly, but this is not always done. What is clear, however, is that for many interventions the elderly may experience greater net benefit than younger patients and that – in the absence of contraindications – guidelines should not be ignored because of age.

ACKNOWLEDGEMENTS

This work was partially supported by the Italian Ministry of University and Research (MIUR, Programma Triennale di Ricerca, decreto 1588).

REFERENCES

1. The Seventh ACCP Consensus Conference on Antithrombotic and Thrombolytic Therapy. *Chest* 2004; **126** (3 Suppl): 163S–696S.
2. Guyatt G, Schunemann HJ, Cook D, Jaeschke R, Pauker S. Applying the grades of recommendation for antithrombotic and thrombolytic therapy: the Seventh ACCP Conference on Antithrombotic and Thrombolytic Therapy. *Chest* 2004; **126** (3 Suppl.): 179S–187S.
3. Ansell J, Hirsh J, Poller L, Bussey H, Jacobson A, Hylek E. The pharmacology and management of the vitamin K antagonists: the Seventh ACCP Conference on Antithrombotic and Thrombolytic Therapy. *Chest* 2004; **126** (3 Suppl.): 204S–233S.
4. Levine MN, Raskob G, Beyth RJ, Kearon C, Schulman S. Hemorrhagic complications of anticoagulant treatment: the Seventh ACCP Conference on Antithrombotic and Thrombolytic Therapy. *Chest* 2004; **126** (3 Suppl.): 287S–310S.
5. Singer DE, Albers GW, Dalen JE, Go AS, Halperin JL, Manning WJ. Antithrombotic therapy in atrial fibrillation: the Seventh ACCP Conference on Antithrombotic and Thrombolytic Therapy. *Chest* 2004; **126** (3 Suppl.): 429S–456S.
6. Salem DN, Stein PD, Al-Ahmad A, *et al.* Antithrombotic therapy in valvular heart disease–native and prosthetic: the Seventh ACCP Conference on Antithrombotic and Thrombolytic Therapy. *Chest* 2004; **126** (3 Suppl.): 457S–482S.
7. Albers GW, Amarenco P, Easton JD, Sacco RL, Teal P. Antithrombotic and thrombolytic therapy for ischemic stroke: the Seventh ACCP Conference on Antithrombotic and Thrombolytic Therapy. *Chest* 2004; **126** (3 Suppl.): 483S–512S.
8. Harrington RA, Becker RC, Ezekowitz M, *et al.* Antithrombotic therapy for coronary artery disease: the Seventh ACCP Conference on Antithrombotic and Thrombolytic Therapy. *Chest* 2004; **126** (3 Suppl.): 513S–548S.
9. Menon V, Harrington RA, Hochman JS, *et al.* Thrombolysis and adjunctive therapy in acute myocardial infarction: the Seventh ACCP Conference on Antithrombotic and Thrombolytic Therapy. *Chest* 2004; **126** (3 Suppl.): 549S–575S.
10. Clagett GP, Sobel M, Jackson MR, Lip GY, Tangelder M, Verhaeghe R. Antithrombotic therapy in peripheral arterial occlusive disease: the Seventh ACCP

Conference on Antithrombotic and Thrombolytic Therapy. *Chest* 2004; **126** (3 Suppl): 609S–626S.

11. Harrison L, Johnston M, Massicotte MP, *et al.* Comparison of 5 mg and 10 mg loading doses in initiation of warfarin therapy. *Ann Intern Med* 1997; **126**: 133–6.

12. O'Reilly RA, Aggeler PM. Studies on coumarin anticoagulant drugs: initiation of warfarin therapy with a loading dose. *Circulation* 1968; **38**: 169–77.

13. Gurwitz JH, Avorn J, Ross-Degnan D, *et al.* Aging and the anticoagulant response to warfarin therapy. *Ann Intern Med* 1992; **116**: 901–4.

14. Redwood M, Taylor C, Bain BJ, *et al.* The association of age with dosage requirement for warfarin. *Age Ageing* 1991; **20**: 217–20.

15. James AH, Britt RP, Raskino CL, *et al.* Factors affecting the maintenance dose of warfarin. *J Clin Pathol* 1992; **45**: 704–6.

16. Mungall D, White R. Aging and warfarin therapy. *Ann Intern Med* 1992; **117**: 878–9.

17. Bowles SK. Stereoselective dispostion of warfarin in young and elderly subjects. *Clin Pharmacol Ther* 1994; **55**: 172.

18. O'Connell MB, Kowal PR, Allivato CJ, *et al.* Evaluation of warfarin initiation regimens in elderly inpatients. *Pharmacotherapy* 2000; **20**: 923–30.

19. McCormick D, Gurwitz JH, Goldberg J, *et al.* Long-term anticoagulation therapy for atrial fibrillation in elderly patients: efficacy, risk, and current patterns of use. *J Thromb Thrombolysis* 1999; **7**: 157–63.

20. Fihn SD, McDonell M, Martin D, *et al.* Risk factors for complications of chronic anticoagulation: a multicenter study. Warfarin Optimized Outpatient Follow-up Study Group. *Ann Intern Med* 1993; **118**: 511–20.

21. Forfar JC. Prediction of hemorrhage during long-term oral coumarin anticoagulation by excessive prothrombin ratio. *Am Heart J* 1982; **103**: 445–6.

22. Charney R, Leddomado E, Rose DN, *et al.* Anticoagulation clinics and the monitoring of anticoagulant therapy. *Int J Cardiol* 1988; **18**: 197–206.

23. Errichetti AM, Holden A, Ansell J. Management of oral anticoagulant therapy: experience with an anticoagulation clinic. *Arch Intern Med* 1984; **144**: 1966–8.

24. Petty GW, Lennihan L, Mohr JP, *et al.* Complications of long-term anticoagulation. *Ann Neurol* 1988; **23**: 570–4.

25. Bussey HI, Rospond RM, Quandt CM, *et al.* The safety and effectiveness of long-term warfarin therapy in an anticoagulation clinic. *Pharmacotherapy* 1989; **9**: 214–19.

26. Sixty Plus Reinfarction Study Research Group. Risks of long-term oral anticoagulant therapy in elderly patients after myocardial infarction: second report of the Sixty Plus Reinfarction Study Research Group. *Lancet* 1982; **1**: 62–8.

27. McInnes GT, Helenglass G. The performance of clinics for outpatient control of anticoagulation. *J R Coll Physicians Lond* 1987; **21**: 42–5.

28. Wickramasinghe LSP, Basu SK, Bansal SK. Long-term oral anticoagulant therapy in elderly patients. *Age Ageing* 1988; **17**: 388–96.

29. Joglekar M, Mohanaruban K, Bayer AJ, *et al.* Can old people on oral anticoagulants be safely managed as outpatients? *Postgrad Med J* 1988; **64**: 775–7.

30. Issacs C, Paltiel O, Blake G, *et al.* Age-associated risks of prophylactic anticoagulation in the setting of hip fracture. *Am J Med* 1994; **96**: 487–91.

31. Davis FB, Estruch MT, Samson-Cervera EB, *et al.* Management of anticoagulation in outpatients: experience with an anticoagulation service in a municipal hospital setting. *Arch Intern Med* 1977; **137**: 197–202.

32. Graves DJ, Wenger NK, Clark WS. Lack of excessive bleeding risk in elderly patients receiving long-term oral anticoagulation. *Cardiol Elderly* 1995; **3**: 273–80.

33. Copland M, Walker ID, Tait RC. Oral anticoagulation and hemorrhagic complications in an elderly population with atrial fibrillation. *Arch Intern Med* 2001; **161**: 2125–8.

34. Palareti G, Leali N, Coccheri S, *et al.* Bleeding complications of oral anticoagulant treatment: an inception-cohort, prospective collaborative study (ISCOAT): Italian Study on Complications of Oral Anticoagulant Therapy. *Lancet* 1996; **348**: 423–8.

35. Stroke Prevention in Atrial Fibrillation III Investigators. Adjusted-dose warfarin versus low-intensity, fixed dose warfarin plus aspirin for high risk patients with atrial fibrillation: Stroke Prevention in Atrial Fibrillation III randomized clinical trial. *Lancet* 1996; **348**: 633–8.

36. Hylek EM, Singer DE. Risk factors for intracranial hemorrhage in outpatients taking warfarin. *Ann Intern Med* 1994; **120**: 897–902.

37. Landefeld CS, Goldman L. Major bleeding in outpatients treated with warfarin: incidence and prediction by factors known at the start of outpatient therapy. *Am J Med* 1989; **87**: 144–52.

38. van der Meer FJM, Rosendaal FR, Vandenbroucke JP, *et al.* Bleeding complications in oral anticoagulant therapy: an analysis of risk factors. *Arch Intern Med* 1993; **153**: 1557–62.

39. Launbjerg J, Egeblad H, Heaf J, *et al.* Bleeding complications to oral anticoagulant therapy: multivariate analysis of 1010 treatment years in 551 outpatients. *J Intern Med* 1991; **229**: 351–5.

40. Stroke Prevention in Atrial Fibrillation Investigators. Bleeding during antithrombotic therapy in patients with atrial fibrillation. *Arch Intern Med* 1996; **156**: 409–16.

41. Fihn SD, Callahan CM, Martin DC, *et al.* The risk for and severity of bleeding complication in elderly patients treated with warfarin. *Ann Intern Med* 1996; **124**: 970–9.

42. Steffensen FH, Kristensen K, Ejlersen E, *et al.* Major haemorrhagic complications during oral anticoagulant therapy in a Danish population-based cohort. *J Intern Med* 1997; **242**: 497–503.

43. Palareti, Hirsh J, Legnani C, *et al.* Oral anticoagulation treatment in the elderly: a nested, prospective, case–control study. *Arch Intern Med* 2000; **160**: 470–8.

44. Petitti DB, Strom BL, Melmon KL. Duration of warfarin anticoagulation therapy and the probabilities of recurrent thromboembolism and hemorrhage. *Am J Med* 1986; **81**: 255–9.

45. Landefeld CS, Rosenblatt MW, Goldman L. Bleeding in outpatients treated with warfarin: relation to the prothrombin time and important remediable lesions. *Am J Med* 1989; **87**: 153–9.

46. European Atrial Fibrillation Trial (EAFT) Study Group. Optimal oral anticoagulant therapy in patients with nonrheumatic atrial fibrillation and recent cerebral ischemia. *N Engl J Med* 1995; **333**: 5–10.

47. Peyman MA. The significance of hemorrhage during treatment of patients with coumarin anticoagulants. *Acta Med Scand* 1958; **162**: 1–62.

48. Roos J, van Joost HE. The cause of bleeding during anticoagulant treatment. *Acta Med Scand* 1965; **178**: 129–31.

49. Pollard JW, Hamilton MJ, Christensen NA, *et al.* Problems associated with long-term anticoagulant therapy. *Circulation* 1962; **25**: 386–92.

50. Coon WW, Willis PW. Hemorrhagic complications of anticoagulant therapy. *Arch Intern Med* 1974; **133**: 386–92.

51. Kuijer PM, Hutten BA, Prins MH, *et al.* Prediction of the risk of bleeding during anticoagulant treatment for venous thromboembolism. *Arch Intern Med* 1999; **159**: 457–60.

52. Hutten BA, Lensing AW, Kraaijenhagen RA, *et al.* Safety of treatment with oral anticoagulants in the elderly: a systematic review. *Drugs Aging* 1999; **14**: 303–12.

53. Chenhsu R, Chiang SC, Chou MH, Lin MF. Long-term treatment with warfarin in Chinese population. *Ann Pharmacother* 2000; **334**: 1395–401.

54. Yasaka M, Minematsu K, Yamaguchi T. Optimal intensity of international normalized ratio in warfarin therapy for secondary prevention of stroke in patients with non-valvular atrial fibrillation. *Intern Med* 2001; **40**: 1183–8.

55. Pengo V, Legnani C, Noventa F, *et al.* on behalf of the ISCOAT Study Group. Oral anticoagulant therapy in patients with nonrheumatic atrial fibrillation and risk of bleeding: a multicenter inception cohort study. *Thromb Haemost* 2001; **85**: 418–22.

56. Kearon C, Ginsberg JS, Kovacs MJ, *et al.* Comparison of low-intensity warfarin therapy with conventional-intensity warfarin therapy for long-term prevention of recurrent venous thromboembolism. *N Engl J Med* 2003; **349**: 631–9.

57. Atrial Fibrillation Investigators. Risk factors for stroke and efficacy of antithrombotic therapy in atrial fibrillation: analysis of pooled data from five randomized controlled trials. *Arch Intern Med* 1994; **154**: 1449–57.

58. Albers GW. Atrial fibrillation and stroke: three new studies, three remaining questions. *Arch Intern Med* 1994; **154**: 1443–8.

59. van Walraven C, Hart RG, Singer DE, *et al.* Oral anticoagulants versus aspirin in nonvalvular atrial fibrillation: an individual patient meta-analysis. *JAMA* 2002; **288**: 2441–8.

60. Warfarin versus aspirin for prevention of thromboembolism in atrial fibrillation: Stroke Prevention in Atrial Fibrillation II study. *Lancet* 1994; **343**: 687–91.

61. Yamaguchi T. Optimal intensity of warfarin therapy for secondary prevention of stroke in patients with nonvalvular atrial fibrillation: a multicenter, prospective, randomized trial. Japanese Nonvalvular Atrial Fibrillation–Embolism Secondary Prevention Cooperative Study Group. *Stroke* 2000; **31**: 817–21.

62. Evans A, Kalra L. Are the results of randomized controlled trials on anticoagulation in patients with atrial fibrillation generalizable to clinical practice. *Arch Intern Med* 2001; **161**: 1443–7.

63. Wilson JR, Lampman J. Heparin therapy: a randomized prospective study. *Am Heart J* 1979; **97**: 155–8.

64. Hull RD, Raskob G, Rosenbloom D, *et al.* Heparin for 5 days as compared with 10 days in the initial treatment of proximal venous thrombosis. *N Engl J Med* 1990; **322**: 1260–4.

65. Jick H, Slone D, Borda IT, *et al*. Efficacy and toxicity of heparin in relation to age and sex. *N Engl J Med* 1968; **279**: 284–6.

66. Basu D, Gallus AS, Hirsh J, *et al*. A prospective study of the value of monitoring heparin treatment with the activated partial thromboplastin time. *N Engl J Med* 1972; **287**: 324–7.

67. Campbell NR, Hull R, Brant R, *et al*. Aging and heparin-related bleeding. *Arch Intern Med* 1996; **156**: 857–60.

68. Connolly SJ. Stroke Prevention in Atrial Fibrillation II study. *Lancet* 1994; **343**: 1509.

69. European Atrial Fibrillation Trial Study Group. Secondary prevention in non-rheumatic atrial fibrillation after transient ischaemic attack or minor stroke. *Lancet* 1993; **342**: 1255–62.

70. Gullov AL, Koefoed BG, Petersen P. Bleeding during warfarin and aspirin therapy in patients with atrial fibrillation: The AFASAK 2 Study. *Arch Intern Med* 1999; **159**: 1322–8.

71. Stroke Prevention in Atrial Fibrillation Investigators. Stroke Prevention in Atrial Fibrillation study: final results. *Circulation* 1991; **84**: 527–39.

72. Evans A, Perez I, Yu G, *et al*. Should stroke subtype influence anticoagulation decisions to prevent recurrence in stroke patients with atrial fibrillation? *Stroke* 2001; **32**: 2828–32.

73. Kalra L, Yu G, Perez I, *et al*. Prospective cohort study to determine if trial efficacy of anticoagulation for stroke prevention in atrial fibrillation translates into clinical effectiveness. *BMJ* 2000; **320**: 1236–9.

74. Gage BF, Boechler M, Doggette AL, *et al*. Adverse outcomes and predictors of underuse of antithrombotic therapy in Medicare beneficiaries with chronic atrial fibrillation. *Stroke* 2000; **31**: 822–7.

75. Caro JJ, Flegel KM, Orejuela ME, *et al*. Anticoagulant prophylaxis against stroke in atrial fibrillation: effectiveness in actual practice. *Can Med Assoc J* 1999; **161**: 493–7.

76. Aronow WS, Ahn C, Kronzon I, *et al*. Incidence of new thromboembolic stroke in persons 62 years and older with chronic atrial fibrillation treated with warfarin versus aspirin. *J Am Geriatr Soc* 1999; **47**: 366–8.

77. Goldenberg GM, Silverstone FA, Rangu S, *et al*. Outcomes of long-term anticoagulation in frail elderly patients with atrial fibrillation. *Clin Drug Invest* 1999; **17**: 483–8.

78. Gottlieb LK, Salem-Schatz SR. Anticoagulation in atrial fibrillation: does efficacy in clinical trials translate into effectiveness in practice? *Arch Intern Med* 1994; **154**: 1945–53.

79. Albers GW, Dalen JE, Laupacis A, *et al*. Antithrombotic therapy in atrial fibrillation. *Chest* 2001; **119**: 194S–206S.

80. Feinberg WM, Kronmal RA, Newman AB, *et al*. Stroke risk in an elderly population with atrial fibrillation. *J Gen Intern Med* 1999; **14**: 56–9.

81. Pearce LA, Hart RG, Halperin JL. Assessment of three schemes for stratifying stroke risk in patients with nonvalvular atrial fibrillation. *Am J Med* 2000; **109**: 45–51.

82. Man-Son-Hing M, Laupacis A, O'Connor AM, *et al*. Warfarin for atrial fibrillation: the patient's perspective. *Arch Intern Med* 1996; **156**: 1841–8.

83. Man-Son-Hing M, Laupacis A, O'Connor AM, *et al*. A patient decision aid regarding antithrombotic therapy for stroke prevention in atrial fibrillation: a randomized controlled trial. *JAMA* 1999; **282**: 737–43.

84. Gage BF, Cardinalli AB, Owens DK. The effect of stroke and stroke prophylaxis with aspirin or warfarin on quality of life. *Arch Intern Med* 1996; **156**: 1829–36.

85. Palareti G, Manotti C, D'Angelo A, *et al*. Thrombotic events during anticoagulant treatment: results of the inception-cohort, prospective, collaborative ISCOAT study: ISCOAT study group (Italian Study on Complications of Oral Anticoagulant Therapy). *Thromb Haemost* 1997; **78**: 1438–43.

86. Go AS, Hylek EH, Chang Y, *et al*. Anticoagulation for stroke prevention in atrial fibrillation: how well do randomized trials translate into clinical practice? *JAMA* 2003; **290**: 2685–92.

87. Fuster V, Ryden LE, Asinger RW, *et al*. ACC/AHA/ESC guidelines for the management of patients with atrial fibrillation: executive summary. A report of the American College of Cardiology/American Heart Association Task Force on Practice Guidelines and the European Society of Cardiology Committee for Practice Guidelines and Policy Conferences (Committee to Develop Guidelines for the Management of Patients With Atrial Fibrillation) developed in collaboration with the North American Society of Pacing and Electrophysiology. *Circulation* 2001; **104**: 2118–50.

88. Taylor GJ, Malik SA, Colliver JA, *et al*. Usefulness of atrial fibrillation as a predictor of stroke after isolated coronary artery bypass grafting. *Am J Cardiol* 1987; **60**: 905–7.

89. Mitchell MA, Hughes GS, Ellenbogen KA, *et al*. Cardioversion-related stroke rates in atrial fibrillation and atrial flutter. *Circulation* 1997; **96** (Suppl. I): I-453.

90. Weigner MJ, Caulfield TA, Danias PG, *et al.* Risk for clinical thromboembolism associated with conversion to sinus rhythm in patients with atrial fibrillation lasting less than 48 hours. *Ann Intern Med* 1997; **126**: 615–20.

91. Wyse DG, Waldo AL, DiMarco JP, *et al.* A comparison of rate control and rhythm control in patients with atrial fibrillation. *N Engl J Med* 2002; **347**: 1825–33.

92. Van Gelder IC, Hagens VE, Bosker HA, *et al.* A comparison of rate control and rhythm control in patients with recurrent persistent atrial fibrillation. *N Engl J Med* 2002; **347**: 1834–40.

93. Hohnloser SH, Kuck KH, Lilienthal J. Rhythm or rate control in atrial fibrillation: Pharmacological Intervention in Atrial Fibrillation (PIAF); a randomised trial. *Lancet* 2000; **356**: 1789–94.

94. Pumphrey CW, Fuster V, Chesebro JH. Systemic thromboembolism in valvular heart disease and prosthetic heart valves. *Mod Concepts Cardiovasc Dis* 1982; **51**: 131–6.

95. Nishimura RA, McGoon MD, Shub C, *et al.* Echocardiographically documented mitral-valve prolapse: long-term follow-up of 237 patients. *N Engl J Med* 1985; **313**: 1305–9.

96. Fulkerson PK, Beaver BM, Auseon JC, *et al.* Calcification of the mitral annulus: etiology, clinical associations, complications and therapy. *Am J Med* 1979; **66**: 967–77.

97. Horstkotte D, Schulte H, Bircks W, *et al.* Unexpected findings concerning thromboembolic complications and anticoagulation after complete 10 year follow up of patients with St. Jude Medical prostheses. *J Heart Valve Dis* 1993; **2**: 291–301.

98. Horstkotte D, Scharf RE, Schultheiss HP. Intracardiac thrombosis: patient-related and device-related factors. *J Heart Valve Dis* 1995; **4**: 114–20.

99. Cannegieter SC, Rosendaal FR, Wintzen AR, *et al.* Optimal oral anticoagulant therapy in patients with mechanical heart valves. *N Engl J Med* 1995; **333**: 11–17.

100. Arom KV, Emery RW, Nicoloff DM, *et al.* Anticoagulant related complications in elderly patients with St. Jude mechanical valve prostheses. *J Heart Valve Dis* 1996; **5**: 505–10.

101. A randomized trial of anticoagulants versus aspirin after cerebral ischemia of presumed arterial origin. The Stroke Prevention in Reversible Ischemia Trial (SPIRIT) Study Group. *Ann Neurol* 1997; **42**: 857–65.

102. Albers GW, Bates VE, Clark WM, *et al.* Intravenous tissue-type plasminogen activator for treatment of acute stroke: the Standard Treatment with Alteplase to Reverse Stroke (STARS) study. *JAMA* 2000; **283**: 1145–50.

103. Hill MD, Buchan AM. Methodology for the Canadian Activase for Stroke Effectiveness Study (CASES). CASES Investigators. *Can J Neurol Sci* 2001; **28**: 232–8.

104. Grond M, Stenzel C, Schmulling S, *et al.* Early intravenous thrombolysis for acute ischemic stroke in a community-based approach. *Stroke* 1998; **29**: 1544–9.

105. Chiu DKD, Villar-Cordova C. Intravenous tissue plasminogen activator for acute ischemic stroke. *Stroke* 1998; **29**: 18–22.

106. Trouillas P, Nighoghossian N, Derex L, *et al.* Thrombolysis with intravenous rtPA in a series of 100 cases of acute carotid territory stroke: determination of etiological, topographic, and radiological outcome factors. *Stroke* 1998; **29**: 2529–40.

107. Tanne D, Bates VE, Verro P, *et al.* Initial clinical experience with IV tissue plasminogen activator for acute ischemic stroke: a multicenter survey. The t-PA Stroke Survey Group. *Neurology* 1999; **53**: 424–7.

108. Akins PT, Delemos C, Wentworth D, *et al.* Can emergency department physicians safely and effectively initiate thrombolysis for acute ischemic stroke? *Neurology* 2000; **55**: 1801–5.

109. Katzan I, Furlan AF, Lloyd LE, *et al.* Use of tissue-type plasminogen activator for acute ischemic stroke: the Cleveland area experience. *JAMA* 2000; **283**: 1151–8.

110. Wang DZ, Rose JA, Honings DS. Treating acute stroke patients with intravenous tPA: the OSF Stroke Network experience. *Stroke* 2000; **31**: 77–81.

111. Lopez-Yunez A, Bruno A, Williams L, *et al.* Protocol violations in community-based rtPA stroke treatment are associated with symptomatic intracerebral hemorrhage. *Stroke* 2001; **32**: 12–16.

112. Bravata DM, Kim N, Concato J, *et al.* Thrombolysis for acute stroke in routine clinical practice. *Arch Intern Med* 2002; **162**: 1994–2001.

113. Merino JG, Silver B, Wong E, *et al.* Extending tissue plasminogen activator use to community and rural stroke patients. *Stroke* 2002; **33**: 141–6.

114. Tanne D, Kasner SE, Demchuk AM, *et al.* Markers of increased risk of intracerebral hemorrhage after intravenous recombinant tissue plasminogen activator therapy for acute ischemic stroke in clinical practice: the Multicenter rt-PA Stroke Survey. *Circulation* 2002; **105**: 1679–85.

115. Antithrombotic Trialists' Collaboration. Collaborative meta-analysis of randomised trials of antiplatelet therapy for prevention of death, myocardial infarction, and stroke in high risk patients. *BMJ* 2002; **324**: 71–86.

116. The Global Use of Strategies to Open Occluded Coronary Arteries (GUSTO) IIb investigators. A comparison of recombinant hirudin with heparin for the treatment of acute coronary syndromes. *N Engl J Med* 1996; **335**: 775–82.

117. Vullemenot A, Schiele F, Meneveau N, *et al*. Efficacy of a synthetic pentasaccharide, a pure factor Xa inhibitor, as an antithrombotic agent- a pilot study in the setting of coronary angioplasty. *Thromb Haemost* 1999; **81**: 214–20.

118. ISIS-2 (Second International Study of Infarct Survival) Collaborative Group. Randomized trial of intravenous streptokinase, oral aspirin, both, or neither among 17, 187 cases of suspected acute myocardial infarction: ISIS-2. *Lancet* 1988; **2**: 349–60.

119. Hennekens CH, Peto R, Hutchison GB, *et al*. An overview of the British and American aspirin studies. *N Engl J Med* 1988; **318**: 923–4.

120. Hansson L, Zanchetti A, Carruthers SG, *et al*. Effects of intensive blood-pressure lowering and low-dose aspirin in the patients with hypertension: principal results of the Hypertension Optimal Treatment (HOT) randomized trial. *Lancet* 1998; **351**: 1755–62.

121. de Gaetano G. Low-dose aspirin and vitamin E in people at cardiovascular risk: a randomized trial in general practice; Collaborative Group of the Primary Prevention Project. *Lancet* 2001; **357**: 89–95.

122. Indications for fibrinolytic therapy in suspected acute myocardial infarction: collaborative overview of early mortality and major morbidity results from all randomised trials of more than 1000 patients. Fibrinolytic Therapy Trialists' (FTT) Collaborative Group. *Lancet* 1994; **343**: 311–22.

123. An international randomized trial comparing four thrombolytic strategies for acute myocardial infarction. The GUSTO investigators. *N Engl J Med* 1993; **329**: 673–82.

124. Single-bolus tenecteplase compared with front-loaded alteplase in acute myocardial infarction: the ASSENT-2 double-blind randomised trial. Assessment of the Safety and Efficacy of a New Thrombolytic Investigators. *Lancet* 1999; **354**: 716–22.

125. Gurwitz JH, Gore JM, Goldberg RJ, *et al*. Risk for intracranial hemorrhage after tissue plasminogen activator treatment for acute myocardial infarction. Participants in the National Registry of Myocardial Infarction 2. *Ann Intern Med* 1998; **129**: 597–604.

126. Simoons ML, Maggioni AP, Knatterud G, *et al*. Individual risk assessment for intracranial haemorrhage during thrombolytic therapy. *Lancet* 1993; **342**: 1523–8.

127. Wallentin L, Goldstein P, Armstrong PW, *et al*. Efficacy and safety of tenecteplase in combination with the low-molecular-weight heparin enoxaparin or unfractionated heparin in the prehospital setting: the Assessment of the Safety and Efficacy of a New Thrombolytic Regimen (ASSENT)-3 PLUS randomized trial in acute myocardial infarction. *Circulation* 2003; **108**: 135–42.

128. White HD. Thrombolytic therapy in the elderly. *Lancet* 2000; **356**: 2028–30.

129. Berger AK, Radford MJ, Wang Y, *et al*. Thrombolytic therapy in older patients. *J Am Coll Cardiol* 2000; **36**: 366–74.

130. Thiemann DR, Coresh J, Schulman SP, *et al*. Lack of benefit for intravenous thrombolysis in patients with myocardial infarction who are older than 75 years. *Circulation* 2000; **101**: 2239–46.

131. Holmes DR Jr, White HD, Pieper KS, *et al*. Effect of age on outcome with primary angioplasty versus thrombolysis. *J Am Coll Cardiol* 1999; **33**: 412–19.

132. OONeill WW, de Boer MJ, Gibbons RJ, *et al*. Lessons from the pooled outcome of the PAMI, ZWOLLE and Mayo Clinic randomized trials of primary angioplasty versus thrombolytic therapy of acute myocardial infarction. *J Invasive Cardiol* 1998; **10** (Suppl. A): 4A–10A.

133. Antman E. Should bivalirudin replace heparin during percutaneous coronary interventions? *JAMA* 2003; **289**: 903–5.

134. Reunanen A, Takkunen H, Aromaa A. Prevalence of intermittent claudication and its effect on mortality. *Acta Med Scand* 1982; **211**: 249–56.

135. Jelnes R, Gaardsting O, Hougaard Jensen K, *et al*. Fate in intermittent claudication: outcome and risk factors. *BMJ* 1986; **293**: 1137–40.

136. Skau T, Jonsson B. Prevalence of symptomatic leg ischaemia in a Swedish community: an epidemiological study. *Eur J Vasc Surg* 1993; **7**: 432–7.

137. Criqui MH, Fronek A, Barrett-Connor E, *et al*. The prevalence of peripheral arterial disease in a defined population. *Circulation* 1985; **71**: 510–15.

138. Newman AB, Siscovick DS, Manolio TA, *et al*. Ankle-arm index as a marker of atherosclerosis in the cardiovascular health study. *Circulation* 1993; **88**: 837–45.

139. Cox GS, Hertzer NR, Young JR, *et al*. Nonoperative treatment of superficial femoral artery disease: long-term follow-up. *J Vasc Surg* 1993; **17**: 172–82.

140. Howell MA, Colgan MP, Seeger RW, *et al*. Relationship of severity of lower limb peripheral vascular disease to mortality and morbidity: a six-year follow-up study. *J Vasc Surg* 1989; **9**: 691–7.

141. Ogren M, Hedblad B, Isacsson SO, *et al*. Non-invasively detected carotid stenosis and ischaemic heart disease in men with leg arteriosclerosis. *Lancet* 1993; **342**: 1138–41.

142. Oxman A Guyatt G. A consumer's guide to subgroup analyses. *Ann Intern Med* 1992; **116**: 78–84.

Index